Skin and the Heart

Carmen Salavastru
Dedee F. Murrell • James Otton
Editors

Skin and the Heart

Springer

Editors
Carmen Salavastru
Paediatric Dermatology Department
Colentina Clinical Hospital, "Carol Davila",
University of Medicine and Pharmacy
Bucharest
Romania

Dedee F. Murrell
Professor of Dermatology
University of New South Wales
Sydney, NSW
Australia

James Otton
Department of Cardiology
Liverpool Hospital
University of New South Wales
Sydney, NSW
Australia

ISBN 978-3-030-54778-3 ISBN 978-3-030-54779-0 (eBook)
https://doi.org/10.1007/978-3-030-54779-0

This Springer imprint is published by the registered company Springer Nature Switzerland AG
The registered company address is: Gewerbestrasse 11, 6330 Cham, Switzerland

Preface

The concept for this book, which covers the links between skin diseases and cardiac diseases, was first derived at the EADV Congress in Copenhagen in 2015 during a meeting between Drs Salavastru and Murrell.

Having learned that, while training as a dermatologist, Dr Salavastru had completed her PhD in medical science in a cardiology-related topic, Dr Murrell, who herself had considered cardiology as a career after training with some of the leading cardiologists in the UK and USA, thought that the many under-recognised links between cardiovascular disease and skin disease would be fascinating topics to bring together under one cover.

Dr James Otton, an academic cardiologist in Sydney with a PhD and an interest in dermatology thanks to his cardiac imaging work and his dermatologist wife, Dr Linda Martin, was the icing on the cake in terms of finding a cardiovascular co-editor.

Having worked with Springer before on the specialised topic of *Blistering Diseases*, published in 2015, the editors know that this publisher values books that cover in-depth and diverse topics, and we are grateful for their enduring assistance with this effort.

The book covers the embryology of the skin and heart and their relationship. Genetic diseases with overlapping manifestations in the skin and heart then follow, including epidermolysis bullosa, cardiocutaneous disorders, connective tissue diseases (including Marfan, Ehlers–Danlos, cutis laxa and pseudoxanthoma elasticum), tuberous sclerosis, incontinentia pigmenti and neurofibromatosis.

Then follows inflammatory skin diseases, including lupus, vasculitis and Behcet and Kawasaki disease.

Infectious diseases are particularly topical, with the COVID-19 pandemic and the link between its involvement of blood vessels, the skin and the heart. Lyme disease, syphilis and childhood infectious viral diseases complete this topic.

Endocrine diseases—diabetes, xanthomas and Fabry disease—all produce protean manifestations in the skin and cardiac system.

Lastly, we have included drug reactions which damage the heart and skin as well as miscellaneous conditions linking the two.

Clearly, with a such a large range of pertinent subject material, not all possible topics could be covered. Hopefully with the popularity of this first edition, we will be able to expand these topics in a future edition.

Bucharest, Romania Carmen Salavastru
Sydney, NSW, Australia Dedee F. Murrell
Sydney, NSW, Australia James Otton

Contents

Contributors

Erkan Alpsoy Department of Dermatology and Venereology, Akdeniz University School of Medicine, Antalya, Turkey

Cătălina Andrei "Carol Davila" University of Medicine and Pharmacy, Cardiology, SCU "Bagdasar-Arseni", Bucharest, Romania

Anamaria Balić Department of Dermatology and Venereology, University Hospital Centre Zagreb, School of Medicine University of Zagreb, Zagreb, Croatia

Can Baykal Dermatology and Venereology, Istanbul, Faculty of Medicine, Istanbul, Istanbul, Turkey

Christina Bergqvist Assistance Publique-Hôpital Paris (AP-HP), Hôpital Henri-Mondor, Department of Dermatology, Créteil, France

Université Paris-Est Creteil (UPEC), Faculty of medicine, Créteil, France

A. Bilgic Department of Dermatology and Venereology, Akdeniz University, School of Medicine, Antalya, Turkey

Mihai Ceaușu "Carol Davila" University of Medicine and Pharmacy, Department of Pathology, INML "Mina Minovici", Bucharest, Romania

Elena Chiticariu Service of Dermatology and Venerology, CHUV, FBM-UNIL, Lausanne, Switzerland

Eliza Cinteza Cardiology Department "Marie Curie" Emergency Children's Hospital, Pediatrics Department "Carol Davila" University of Medicine and Pharmacy, Bucharest, Romania

Stefana Cretu Dermatology Department, Carol Davila University of Medicine and Pharmacy, Bucharest, Romania

Gonzalo del Monte-Nieto Australian Regenerative Medicine Institute, Monash University, Clayton, VIC, Australia

E. Ellenbogen Department of Dermatology, Tel Aviv Sourasky Medical Center, Tel Aviv, Tel Aviv, Israel

Sackler Faculty of Medicine, Tel Aviv University, Tel Aviv, Israel

J. W. Frew Clinical Investigation, Laboratory for Investigative Dermatology, The Rockefeller University, New York, NY, USA

P. Geenty Cardiology Department, Westmead Hospital, Westmead, NSW, Australia

Mohamad Goldust University of Rome G. Marconi, Rome, Italy

Department of Dermatology, University Hospital Basel, Basel, Switzerland

Vasu D. Gooty University of Tennessee Heath Science Center, LeBonheur Children's Hospital, Memphis, TN, USA

Muhammed Burak Günay Dermatology and Venereology, Istanbul Faculty of Medicine, Istanbul, Turkey

Atula Gupta Department of Dermatology, Skin-Aid Clinic, Gurugram, Haryana, India

Richard Paul Harvey Developmental and Stem Cell Biology Division, Victor Chang Cardiac Research Institute, Darlinghurst, NSW, Australia

St. Vincent's Clinical School and School of Biotechnology and Biomolecular Science, UNSW Sydney, Kensington, Australia

Jana Hercogová Department of Dermatovenereology, 2nd Medical Faculty, Charles University Prague and Na Bulovce Hospital, Prague, Czech Republic

Department of Dermatovenereology, Institute for Clinical and Experimental Medicine, Prague, Czech Republic

Department of Dermatovenereology, Prague, Czech Republic

Angela Hernández-Martín Department of Dermatology, Hospital Infantil Niño Jesús, Madrid, Spain

Daniel Hohl Service of Dermatology and Venerology, CHUV, FBM-UNIL, Lausanne, Switzerland

Tarique Hussain Department of Pediatrics, UT Southwestern Medical Center, Congenital Cardiac MR Service, Office: Children's Medical Center, Dallas, TX, USA

Michel Janier STD Clinic, Hôpital Saint-Louis AP-HP and Hôpital Saint-Joseph, Paris, France

Richmond Jeremy University of Sydney, Sydney, Australia

Royal Prince Alfred Hospital Sydney, Sydney, Australia

Marfan and Aortic Disease Clinic, Royal Prince Alfred Hospital, Camperdown, Australia

Sergiusz Jóźwiak Department of Child Neurology, Medical University of Warsaw, Warszawa, Poland

Jana Kazandjieva Department of Dermatology, Medical University, Sofia, Bulgaria

Birgül Özkesici Kurt Clinic of Dermatology and Venereology, Adiyaman University Training and Research Hospital, Adiyaman, Turkey

Olivier Lairez Excellence Centre for Mastocytosis (CEREMAST), Toulouse, France

Department of Cardiology, Toulouse University Hospital, Paul Sabatier University, Toulouse, France

J. W. J. Lasschuit Department of Endocrinology, St Vincent's Hospital Sydney, Darlinghurst, NSW, Australia

Clinical Diabetes, Appetite and Metabolism, Garvan Institute of Medical Research, Darlinghurst, NSW, Australia

Faculty of Medicine, University of New South Wales, Sydney, NSW, Australia

Cristina Bulai Livideanu Excellence Centre for Mastocytosis (CEREMAST), Toulouse, France

Department of Dermatology, Toulouse University Hospital, Paul Sabatier University, Toulouse, France

Sonya Marina Department of Dermatology, Medical University, Varna, Bulgaria

Branka Marinović Department of Dermatology and Venereology, University Hospital Centre Zagreb, School of Medicine University of Zagreb, Zagreb, Croatia

Zrinka Bukvić Mokos Department of Dermatology and Venereology, University Hospital Centre Zagreb, School of Medicine University of Zagreb, Zagreb, Croatia

Dedee F. Murrell Faculty of Medicine, Department of Dermatology, St George Hospital, University of New South Wales, Sydney, NSW, Australia

James Otton Department of Cardiology, Liverpool Hospital, University of New South Wales, Sydney, NSW, Australia

Marijan Pašalić Department of Cardiovascular Diseases, University Hospital Centre Zagreb, School of Medicine University of Zagreb, Zagreb, Croatia

Carle Paul Excellence Centre for Mastocytosis (CEREMAST), Toulouse, France

Department of Dermatology, Toulouse University Hospital, Paul Sabatier University, Toulouse, France

Patrick Pender Department of Cardiology, Liverpool Hospital, Sydney, NSW, Australia

Justin Phan Department of Cardiology, St Vincent's Hospital, Darlinghurst, NSW, Australia

University of New South Wales, Kensington, NSW, Australia

Monica Popescu "Carol Davila" University of Medicine and Pharmacy, Bucharest, Romania

Dermato-oncology Research Unit, "Colentina" Clinical Hospital, Bucharest, Romania

Shruti Rateesh Department of Cardiology, Liverpool Hospital, Sydney, NSW, Australia

Carmen Salavastru Paediatric Dermatology Department, Colentina Clinical Hospital, "Carol Davila" University of Medicine and Pharmacy, Bucharest, Romania

Robert A. Schwartz Dermatology, Pediatric, Medicine, and Pathology, Rutgers New Jersey Medical School, Newark, NJ, USA

Kristina Semkova St John's Institute of Dermatology, St Thomas' Hospital, London, UK

Adelina Sendrea "Carol Davila" University of Medicine and Pharmacy, Bucharest, Romania

Dermato-Oncology Research Unit, "Colentina" Clinical Hospital, Bucharest, Romania

Kavita Sharma Department of Pediatrics, UT Southwestern Medical Center, Office: Children's Medical Center, Dallas, TX, USA

Monika Słowińska Department of Child Neurology, Medical University of Warsaw, Warszawa, Poland

J. R. Snaith Department of Diabetes and Endocrinology, St Vincent's Hospital Sydney, Darlinghurst, NSW, Australia

Efthymia Soura 1st University Department of Dermatology – Venereology, Andreas Syggros Hospital, National and Kapodistrian Medical School of Athens, Athens, Greece

Rajesh Subbiah Department of Cardiology, St Vincent's Hospital, Darlinghurst, NSW, Australia

University of New South Wales, Kensington, NSW, Australia

Victor Chang Cardiac Research Institute, Darlinghurst, NSW, Australia

Alina Suru Paediatric Dermatology Department, "Carol Davila" University of Medicine and Pharmacy, Bucharest, Romania

Amalia Tamariz-Martel Department of Cardiology, Hospital Infantil Niño Jesús, Madrid, Spain

M. Tchan Genetic Medicine Department, Westmead Hospital, Westmead, NSW, Australia

L. Thomas Cardiology Department, Westmead Hospital, Westmead, NSW, Australia

George-Sorin Ţiplica "Carol Davila" University of Medicine and Pharmacy, Dermatology II, Colentina Clinical Hospital, Bucharest, Romania

Pierre Wolkenstein Assistance Publique-Hôpital Paris (AP-HP) Hôpital Henri-Mondor, Department of Dermatology, Créteil, France

Université Paris-Est Creteil (UPEC), Faculty of medicine, Créteil, France

INSERM, Centre d'Investigation Clinique 006, Assistance Publique-Hôpital Paris (AP-HP), Hôpital Henri-Mondor, Referral Center of Neurofibromatosis, Créteil, France

INSERM U955 Neurofibromatosis and Lymphoma oncogenesis, Créteil, France

Part I

Embryology

Embryology of the Skin

1

Eran Ellenbogen

Introduction

Attempts to uncover the causal relation of morphogenetic structures, their functions and the underlying molecular machinery that created such processes is frequently ellucidated by observing the effects of mutation of the gene studied in simpler organisms. This approach began with John S. Dexter in 1914, when he noticed the appearance of a notch in the wings of the fruit fly "Drosophila melanogaster". This lead almost a century later to the formation of a general theory anchored by a large experimental body of work identifying the *Notch* signaling pathway as a conserved evolutionary pathway, a signaling mechanism crucial for proper embryonic development in living organisms. The case of the morphogenesis of embryonic skin is a remarkable story that could not be unveiled solely by genetic study, devoid of its physiological and molecular causal chains.

We survey the development of the embryonic skin and its regenerative power, while we examine the discovery of a binary trigger and molecular mechanism which underlie the regulation of epidermal development. Understanding of molecular signal transduction operating as a regulator of cascading specific commands to form an organ such as the skin during natal and postnatal development culminated only a little over a decade ago. We review the central role of the Notch signaling switch in the morphogenesis of skin. Through the study of *Drosophila melanogaster,* we follow and identify the successful use of diverse tools which lead to the hypothesis that skin and its epigenetic expression in response to the environment is mediated by a signaling path caused by the action of a binary switch. The Notch signaling path as well as its cascading proteins are regulated by a biological process shared universally across the entire gamut of biological species.

E. Ellenbogen (✉)
Department of Dermatology, Tel Aviv Sourasky Medical Center, Tel Aviv, Israel

Sackler Faculty of Medicine, Tel Aviv University, Tel Aviv, Israel
e-mail: ellenbogen.md@gmail.com

C. Salavastru et al. (eds.), *Skin and the Heart*,
https://doi.org/10.1007/978-3-030-54779-0_1

Mammalian skin is the most regenerative organ, and as such is constantly in need to be rebuilt and repaired. The primary function of the skin is to preserve internal hydrostatic pressure and prevent fluid loss from the body, with the outermost layer, the epidermis, protecting the body from mechanical trauma and microbial insult. This protective layer is separated from the basement membrane. This organ structure is responsible for the formation of dermal appendages, including hair follicles, mammary glands, and sebaceous glands. There must exist a means during development whereby stem cells are able to selectively differentiate into the necessary specialized cells.

Human skin can typically be divided into three distinct layers, the outermost epidermis, the dermis, and the basal hypodermis [1]. Epidermal thickness is 0.1 mm in average, and is a squamous stratified epithelium consisting primarily of keratinocytes and surficial structures such as follicles and sweat glands. Dermal thickness typically ranges from 1.0–2.0 mm and is separated from the epidermis by an epidermal basement complex which supports function such as: nails, blood, lymph vessels and nerve endings. Lastly, Hypodermal thickness ranges from 1.0–2.0 mm and is made up of adipose tissue which directly fuses to muscles and bones beneath the skin.

Epidermal & Epidermal Cells Development

Epidermal development is a process consisting of different phases; epidermal specification, commitment, stratification, terminal differentiation, and appendageal growth. Each and every step of epidermal development is closely linked to development of dermis and mesenchyme.

The specification of embryonic skin development begins right after the process of gastrulation, which is an early stage of embryonic development occurring after fertilization. In gastrulation, there is invagination of the epiblast along the primitive streak and proliferation and downward migration of epiblast cells. Gastrulation results in formation of three germ layers: the ectoderm, mesoderm, and endoderm (Fig. 1.1).

The human epithelium originates from embryonic ectoderm. Once it acquires a destiny via Wnt signaling as an epidermal cell expressing keratin (I.e. Keratinocytes), formation of ectodermal cells layer covering the growing embryo is established. The newly formed embryonic basal keratinocytes express keratin 5/14 which is considered the hallmark for the event referred to as epidermal commitment. At a fetal age of 4–6 weeks; Primordial keratinocytes generate a transient protective layer from the amniotic fluid, the periderm, a single cell layer overlying the developing epidermis and referred to as the "stratum germinativum", this layer is shed once epidermis starts stratification at approximately 8 weeks and eventually replaced by the cornified cell layer.

At a fetal age of 8–11 weeks; an intermediate layer will be formed between the periderm and basal layer which consists of proliferating cells, thus able to accommodate the accelerated growth phase of the evolving embryo. This layer will eventually mature into the spinous skin layer expressing keratin 1/10.

Intermediate layer and spinous cells express K1, their expression is induced by Notch signaling. This pathway controls spinous cells to continue differentiate, mature, and eventually migrate towards the skin surface to form the granular and cornified layers. The literature on the embryonic skin development indicates that the responsible actor for the process is a differentiating binary switch associated with Notch signaling mechanism which remains crucial in the postnatal epidermis for inhibiting basal cell proliferation and initiating terminal differentiation.

The process of terminal differentiation where the intermediate layer differentiates into spinous and granular layer may be observed early as the 15th week at the hair canal, and at around 22–24 at the inter-follicular epidermis. Subsequently, by week 24–26 the cornified layer starts to form while the periderm layer is detached and sloughed to form among other the waxy newborn coat referred to as the Vernix caseosa. [2, 3].

Neural crest cells are almost the sole contributor to the development of melanocyte formation. These specialized cells may travel either ventrally with a neurogenic fate forming glial cells and peripheral sensory neurons, or to a dorsolateral route leading to a melanogenic fate with cells finally residing in the epidermis [4]. Langerhans cells are developed from myeloid embryonic precursors from fetal liver and yolk sac, Langerhans Cells appear within the fetal skin already as soon as the first trimester [5]. Merkel cells may appear in the skin at around 8 weeks of gestation at the lower parts of the epidermis, their origin has remained debatable and different authors postulate that their origin is either from neural crest cells while others support the claim of epithelial lineage origin based upon the expression of epithelial keratins (CK 8, 18, 20), another hypothesis suggests a consolidation combining a neural crest and epidermal lineage [6].

Development of the Dermis and Subcutis

The origin of the dermis, unlike epidermis, is variable. Facial and cranial dermis is derived from neural crest ectoderm, excluding occipital and otic areas which originates from mesoderm. In the back, the dorsal trunk originates from segmental units of the paraxial mesoderm referred to as somites, while limbs and ventral trunk are derived from mesoderm plate. At 8 weeks embryonic dermal cells are able to produce collagen, mainly types 1, 3, and 4 although not sufficient to assemble as complex fibers, acquiring a cellular and amorphous figure with very little organized fibers. By third month, collagen production accumulates into fibers starting to reside in the reticular dermis. The dermis is becoming vascularized by capillaries layered to larger blood vessels. After the eighth week the growing foetus is already able to feel mother movements as fondling mainly d/t growth of skin sensory nerve fibers intervening through dermis and epidermis. The lymphatic system derived from venous endothelial cells and follows the same developments pattern of blood vessels. Adipocytes begin to acquire fat, and by the third trimester fat lobules and septae are established [7, 8].

Dermal-Epidermal Junction

The junction between the dermis and epidermis (DEJ) controls the connections between basal keratinocytes and dermis, the interaction between the epidermis and dermis is also the foundation for the emergence of epidermal appendages. Animal studies have shown that an enzymatic separation between ectoderm to mesenchyme will eventually lead to ectoderm tissue alone, thus the human dermis will regulate or control the fate of the epidermal tissue. Furthermore, the dermal mesenchyme is the tissue determining the tissue origin and not the epidermis, thus dermal tissue can be combined experimentally with different epithelium from other origin in order to have the fate of the mesenchyme original tissue.

The embryonic DEJ is composed of the different elements and proteins known for the full term foetus as type 4 collagen, laminin, heparan sulfate and proteoglycans, by the 12th week, DEJ maturation is almost completed and the majority of membrane proteins as well as vital structures, are by now in place; hemidesomosomes, anchoring filaments, fibrils, etc. As foetal development advances, the flat DEJ gains morphology of a mature DEJ characterized by interdigitate dermal papillae and processes of rete ridges [7].

Development of Skin Appendages

Hair follicle development is first observed between 11–12 weeks, embryonic epidermis forms local condensations called placodes, dermal cells than thicken to form the dermal papilla. Placodes proliferate and deepen into the dermis forming a hair germ, the follicle base outgrows around the dermal papilla forming a peg with the appearance of, a future hair follicle. The developing follicle has two noticeable lumps, an upper portion that marks the formation of sebaceous gland and a lower one where stem cells accumulate. The second trimester of pregnancy follows a maturation process forming seven layers of cells, and at week 21 a hair canal is established followed immediately by hair shaft growth.

A strong connection is required between the different signalling pathways for proper development of hair shafts. Reciprocation is established between Notch, Wnt, Hedghog and bone morphogenetic protein (BMP). Hair cycle pattern through adult life, consisting of the well-known three phases; anagen, catagen and telogen are repeating continuously, while during the perinatal period telogen is initiated, leading to lanugo hair shedding in utero [9].

At approximately 12 week of gestation, dorsal digital epidermal condensations indicate the initiation of nail development. Signaling of both BMP and Wnt pathways are required for proper nail orientation. The proximal matrix is formed by cells proliferating in the nail field, which eventually attributes to the formation of nail plate. At first the entire nail plate is covered by epidermis, but later on goes through degeneration, leaving a thin band at the proximal nail. The brim between dorsal and ventral skin is marked by the hyponichium located at the very end part of the nail as a thick epidermis. The hand nails are fully grown at week 32 while the toe nails grow at a slower pace until week 36.

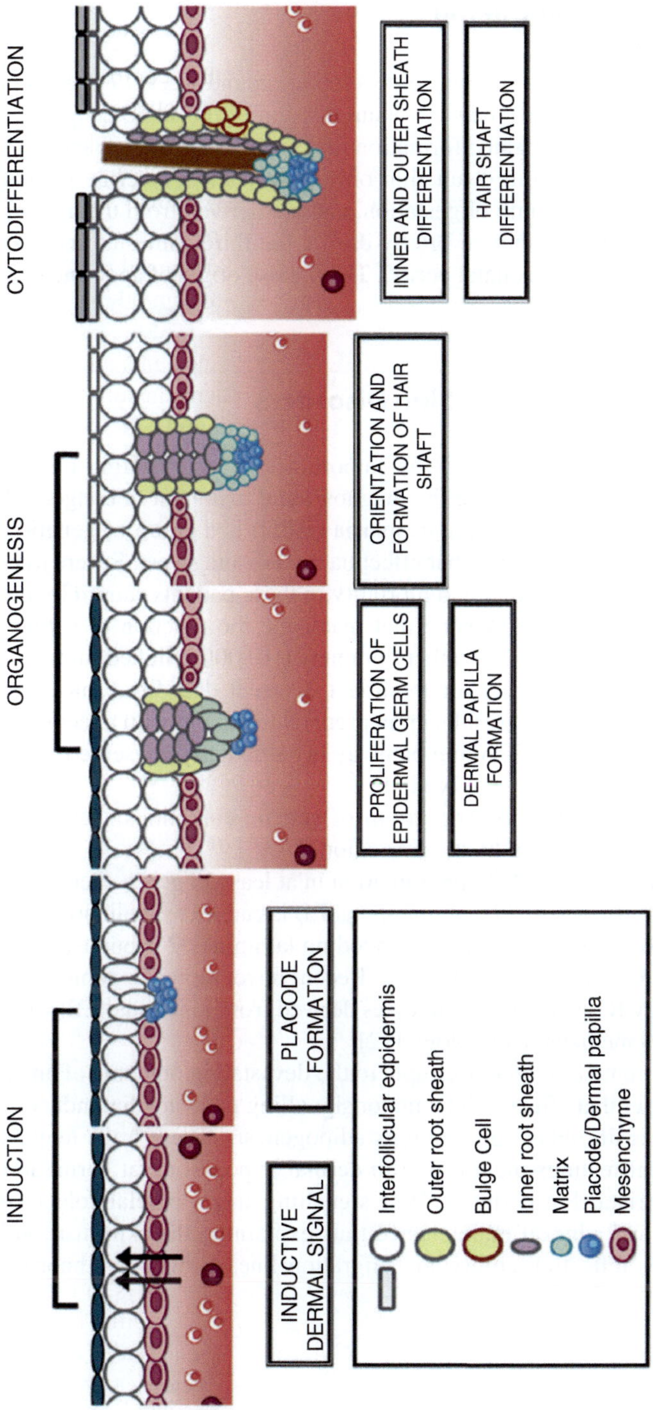

Fig. 1.1 Hair follicle formation (Forni et al., 2012)

Sweat Gland Development

Eccrine sweat glands are starting to develop at around week 17 and upon stimulation of mesenchymal BMP causing a suppression of the sonic hedgehog signaling pathway, allowing sweat gland formation first on palms and soles and later on at the rest of the body, but acquire function only post-nataly. Apocrine glands begin to form only at the fifth month of gestation, and are derived from the upper portion of the hair follicle. They function briefly during the third trimester and become dormant for the rest of the neonatal period. The precise origin of apocrine glands is still poorly known [10].

Treatment of Congenital Skin Disorders

From a clinician point of view, the importance of understating embryonic skin development is fundamental for the diagnosis and treatment of congenital skin disorders. Hypohidrotic ectodermal dysplasia (HED) is a group of genetic disorders, sharing some striking features that effect hair, teeth and sweat. Severe hyperthermia is a major cause of morbidity and mortality in these patients caused by the inability to sweat. Mutations in EDA gene that inactivate the function of ectodysplasin A (EDA) are responsible for the rather common 1:10,000 x-linked mutation in males and thus a convenient target for treatment. Current data from mice studies have demonstrated encouraging results upon prenatal treatment with a recombinant EDA protein, and since EDA signalling pathway is particularly conserved, animal model may be applicable to human as well [11].

Epidermolysis bullosa (EB) a group of genetic conditions sharing the clinical features of fragile skin and blister formation.

EB may be caused by different mutation in at least 20 genes encoding DEJ components. The most severe type of junctional EB is caused by a mutation in one of the genes (LAMB3, LAMC2, LAMA3) encoding laminin 332 subunits, a crucial component of the lamina lucida of the DEJ. Recent novel reports exhibit the in situ correction of LAMB3 gene in keratinocytes derived from junctional EB patient using a CRISPR/Cas9 mediated technology [12].

Goltz syndrome is another example to the devastating outcome of an uncommon genetic disorder that effects Wnt a major signalling pathway that induces osteogenesis, stimulates fibroblasts and inhibits adipogenesis. These traits may explain the disease clinical features manifesting in dermal hypoplasia, fat herniation and dermatopathia striata. Furthermore, Wnt signalling has a crucial role in epidermal regeneration and adnexal maintenance thus explaining the skin distribution along blaschko lines reflecting embryonic migration lines as well as abnormal adnexal structures [13].

References

1. Forni FF, Trombetta-Lima M, Mari CS. Stem cells in embrionic skin developmen. Biol Res. 2012:215–22.
2. Liu S, Zhang H, Duan E. Epidermal development in mammals: key regulators, signals from beneath, and stem cells. Int J Mol Sci. 2013;14(6):10869–95.
3. Veltri A, Lang C, Lien WH. Concise review: wnt signaling pathways in skin development and epidermal stem cells. Stem cells (Dayton, Ohio). 2018;36(1):22–35.
4. Vandamme N, Berx G. From neural crest cells to melanocytes: cellular plasticity during development and beyond. Cell Mol Life Sci. 2019;76(10):1919–34.
5. Hashimoto-Hill S, Friesen L, Park S, Im S, Kaplan MH, Kim CH. RARalpha supports the development of Langerhans cells and langerin-expressing conventional dendritic cells. Nat Commun. 2018;9(1):3896.
6. Abraham J, Mathew S. Merkel cells: a collective review of current concepts. Int J Appl Basic Med Res. 2019;9(1):9–13.
7. Fine JD, Smith LT, Holbrook KA, Katz SI. The appearance of four basement membrane zone antigens in developing human fetal skin. J Invest Dermatol. 1984;83(1):66–9.
8. Couly GF, Coltey PM, Le Douarin NM. The developmental fate of the cephalic mesoderm in quail-chick chimeras. Development. 1992;114(1):1–15.
9. Rishikaysh P, Dev K, Diaz D, Qureshi WM, Filip S, Mokry J. Signaling involved in hair follicle morphogenesis and development. Int J Mol Sci. 2014;15(1):1647–70.
10. Lu C, Fuchs E. Sweat gland progenitors in development, homeostasis, and wound repair. Cold Spring Harbor perspectives in medicine. 2014;4(2).
11. Margolis CA, Schneider P, Huttner K, Kirby N, Houser TP, Wildman L, et al. Prenatal treatment of X-linked Hypohidrotic ectodermal dysplasia using recombinant Ectodysplasin in a canine model. J Pharmacol Exp Ther. 2019;370(3):806–13.
12. Benati D, Miselli F, Cocchiarella F, Patrizi C, Carretero M, Baldassarri S, et al. CRISPR/Cas9-mediated in situ correction of LAMB3 Gene in keratinocytes derived from a Junctional Epidermolysis Bullosa patient. Molecular Therapy: the journal of the American Society of Gene Therapy. 2018;26(11):2592–603.
13. Bostwick B, Van den Veyver IB, Sutton VR. Focal dermal hypoplasia. In: Adam MP, Ardinger HH, Pagon RA, Wallace SE, Bean LJH, Stephens K, et al., editors. GeneReviews((R)). Seattle (WA): University of Washington, Seattle. University of Washington, Seattle. GeneReviews is a registered trademark of the University of Washington, Seattle. All rights reserved.; 1993.

Embryology of the Heart

2

Gonzalo del Monte-Nieto and Richard Paul Harvey

The Primitive Heart

Cardiogenic Field Formation The heart is the first functional organ formed in the developing embryo. The cardiac progenitors arise just after gastrulation from the mesodermal layer and more precisely from the splanchnic lateral mesoderm. In response to signals from the embryonic endoderm, the cardiac progenitors migrate rostrally forming a crescent in the cephalo-medial region of the embryo (Fig. 2.1a) [1]. In the cardiac crescent, two different populations of cardiac progenitor cells have been described, the so-called first and second heart fields (FHF and SHF) [2], that will mainly contribute to the endocardium and myocardial layers of the heart (Fig. 2.1a). There has been considerable controversy over the interpretation of these proposed heart fields, in particular whether they are truly distinct fields or a unified field that ingresses the heart and differentiates into cardiac tissue in 2 different temporal waves [3]. Recent studies using lineage tracing and single cell transcriptomics analysis of cardiac progenitor cells (Mesp1^{+}) appear to show that FHF and SHF progenitors are distinct cardiomyocyte populations specified during gastrulation [4]. Nevertheless, at the cardiac crescent stage, FHF and SHF cardiac progenitors differentially express genes such as *Mlc2a* and *Islet1* respectively [5]. As development proceeds, cardiac progenitors migrate forming two endocardial bilateral tubes surrounded by a myocardial epithelium in the middle region of the human

G. del Monte-Nieto (✉)
Australian Regenerative Medicine Institute. Monash University, Clayton, VIC, Australia
e-mail: gonzalo.delmontenieto@monash.edu

R. P. Harvey
Developmental and Stem Cell Biology Division, Victor Chang Cardiac Research Institute, Darlinghurst, NSW, Australia

St. Vincent's Clinical School and School of Biotechnology and Biomolecular Science, UNSW Sydney, Kensington, Australia
e-mail: r.harvey@victorchang.edu.au

C. Salavastru et al. (eds.), *Skin and the Heart*,
https://doi.org/10.1007/978-3-030-54779-0_2

embryo. These two endocardial tubes then fuse forming a single straight tube called the primitive heart tube (Fig. 2.1b). This primitive heart is likely formed exclusively from FHF cardiac progenitors organized in two cellular layers, the endocardium and the myocardium, separated by a thick extracellular matrix layer called the cardiac jelly (Fig. 2.1b). Once the primitive cardiac tube is formed, cells located in the SHF proliferate and ingress into the heart from both inflow and outflow poles, contributing to formation of the right ventricle and the outflow tract (OFT) for those cells entering the arterial pole, and to the atrium and associated large vessel and atrioventricular conduction tissue in the case of the cells entering the venous pole [6–8]. The only chamber formed exclusively from FHF progenitors is the left ventricle [5]. During this early phase, cardiomyocytes forming the heart tube, called primary myocardium, are characterized by their automaticity or pacemaker activity, and their slow conduction capabilities, critical for the peristaltic contraction from venous to arterial pole in the early heart [1].

Cardiac Looping As the heart develops, progressive cell ingression of SHF progenitors from both poles of the embryonic heart promotes the elongation and loop-

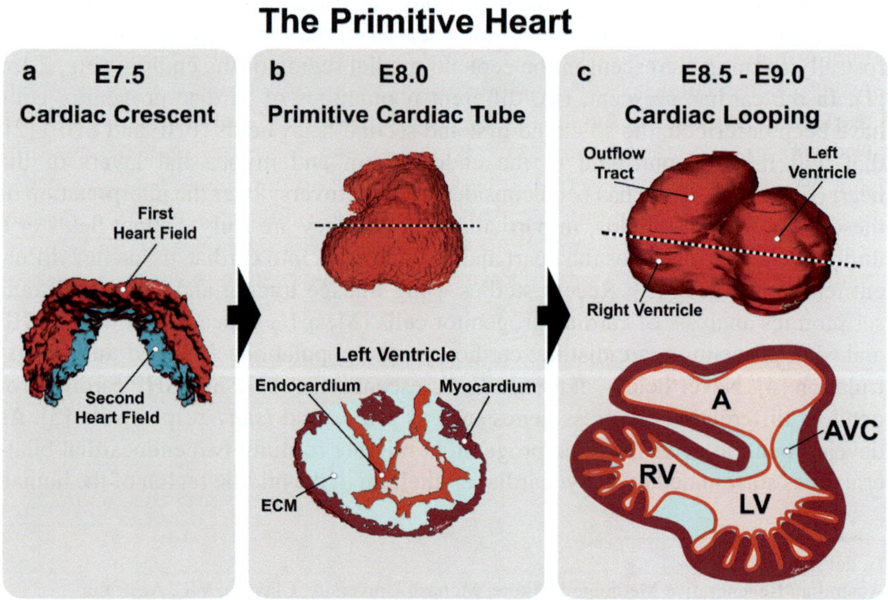

Fig. 2.1 The Primitive Heart. (**a**) Diagram based on 3D reconstructions of the cardiac crescent showing the First (red) and Second (blue) Heart Fields of the mouse. (**b**) Top: 3D reconstruction of the primitive heart tube at E8.0. Bottom: section of the 3D reconstruction showing the tissue and ECM distribution of the primitive cardiac tube at E8.0. (**c**) Top: 3D reconstruction of a looped embryonic heart at E9.0. Compare 3D reconstructions in B and C to see the transition from a straight to a looped heart. Bottom: diagram depicting a heart section with the tissue and ECM distribution at E9.0. In section: red: myocardium; orange: endocardium; blue: ECM. A: atrium; AVC: atrioventricular canal; LV: left ventricle; RV: right ventricle.

ing of the cardiac tube (Fig. 2.1c) [1]. The consistent rightwards looping of the heart tube is governed by a molecular left/right signalling pathway originating within and around a key organising centre of the early gastrulating embryo called the node, initiating a cascade of events leading to left/right asymmetries in multiple organs including heart [9]. Left-right asymmetries in the ingression of SHF progenitors were recently demonstrated to play a critical role in the cardiac looping process [10]. During heart looping, the straight cardiac tube assumes a rightward spiral, promoting the relocation of its ventral and dorsal walls to become the outer and inner curvatures of the looped heart, respectively (Fig. 2.1c). This asymmetric morphogenesis during cardiac looping is the first evidence of left-right asymmetries taking place during heart development and is controlled by differential expression of transcription factor and signalling factor genes such as *Pitx2* or *Bone morphogenetic protein* (*Bmp*) *4*, respectively, as early as the cardiac crescent stage.

Cardiac Chambers

Cardiac Chamber Specification As described in the previous section, the primitive heart is mainly formed by migration of cardiac progenitors that form the cardiac tube and subsequent migration of SHF progenitors into the heart. The early myocardium is mainly quiescent with proliferation centres located outside of the heart tube in the caudo-medial pericardial wall, which are the source of progenitors for the heart [11]. However, as the heart loops, cardiomyocytes located specifically at the outer curvature begin to proliferate (Figs. 2.1c and 2.2a) [12]. At the same time, gene regulatory networks controlling myocardial differentiation are activated in these cardiomyocytes in order to induce the specification of specialised chamber myocardium [13–15]. The current model for how cardiac chambers form, called the “ballooning model” [13], replaced a previous textbook notion in which all the heart

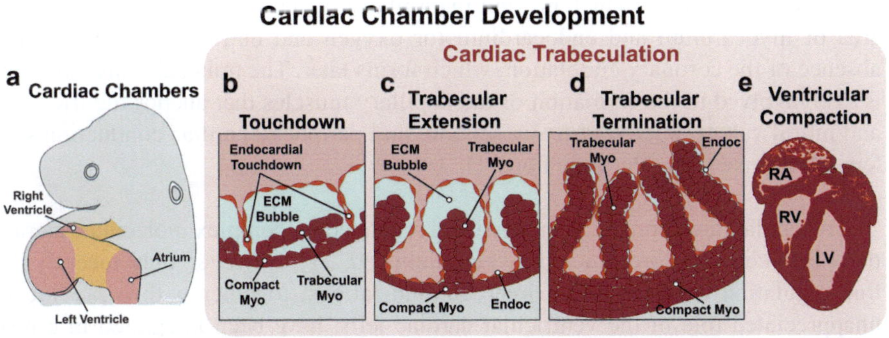

Fig. 2.2 Cardiac Chamber Development. (**a**) Cartoon of a mouse embryo showing the cardiac chambers at E9.5. (**b–e**) Trabeculation process. (**b**) Touchdown, (c) Extension, (**d**) Termination and (**e**) Compaction phases of the trabeculation process. See the dynamics of endocardium, myocardium and ECM during the process. Endocardium: orange; chamber myocardium: red; ECM: blue. Myo: myocardium; Endoc: endocardium; RA: right atrium; LV: left ventricle; RV: right ventricle

regions were thought to be preconfigured in a segmental pattern along the primitive heart tube. The ballooning model proposes that the cardiomyocyte domains located at the outer curvature of the forming heart wall will form the chamber myocardium by activating proliferation and chamber differentiation programs and "ballooning out" from the primitive tubular heart (Fig. 2.2a). During this process, the automaticity and low conductivity of the primary cardiomyocytes is lost as the expression of genes involved in high conductivity and cardiomyocyte conduction coupling allow the synchronous contraction of the entire chamber. In addition, chamber cardiomyocytes are characterized by the presence of a more elaborated contractile machinery including sarcomeres and sarcoplasmic reticulum, compared to the primary myocardium. The chamber myocardium will form the atrial and ventricular chambers of the heart (Figs. 2.1c and 2.2a). However, while this process occurs at the outer curvature, at the inner curvature the chamber-specific genetic program is repressed by the T-box family transcription factor genes *Tbx2* and *Tbx3* [16, 17]. This non-chamber tissue will give rise to the cardiac valves, atrial and ventricular septa, and some cardiac conduction system components, that will be covered in the following sections.

Ventricular trabeculation Soon after chambers are specified, cardiomyocytes comprising the chamber myocardium will acquire different fates during the process of trabeculation (Fig. 2.2b-e). Trabeculae are the muscular ridges that project towards the lumen of the forming heart chambers. Their formation is the first morphological evidence of ventricular specification [18]. Trabeculation occurs first and in a more extensive way in the ventricular chambers, whereas it is more limited in the atrial chambers where trabeculae form the pectinate muscles. During trabeculation, the initially smooth epithelial layer of myocardium of the ventricular wall is transformed into a convoluted sponge-like myocardium. Trabeculae are critical for force generation in the early heart, for directing blood efficiently in the absence of mature cardiac valves (which prevent regurgitation), and for increasing the surface area of myocardium and endocardium for oxygen and nutrient exchange in the absence of the coronary circulation, which forms later. The trabecular myocardium is also involved in the formation of the papillary muscles that anchor the tricuspid and mitral valves, inter-ventricular septum, and peripheral cardiac conduction system giving rise to the Purkinje fibres [1, 19].

Trabecular development is induced and regulated by complex molecular interactions between endocardium and myocardium [20, 21]. However, only recently the fine regulation of these tissue intercommunications, together with a previously unappreciated role of the ventricular cardiac jelly, have been integrated in a new model for trabeculation in the mouse [22]. The model predicts that trabeculation begins as early as the heart tube assembly stage (E8.0), not at E9.5 as previously described. During the early phases of trabeculation, fine regulation of cardiac jelly synthesis and degradation by the Nrg1 and Notch pathways, respectively, promotes the formation of endocardial sprouts in a process similar to sprouting angiogenesis in developing vascular beds. Endocardial sprouts tunnel through the cardiac jelly forming the so-called endocardial touchdowns, that end up contacting the outer compact myocardial layer (Fig. 2.2b). In 3D, this process leads to the segmentation of the ventricular chamber in distinct dome-like structures that are rich in cardiac jelly and encapsulate the protruding trabecular myocardium, which likely occurs via extrusion of cardiomyocytes from the outer layer (Fig. 2.2b) [23]. Once the trabecular units are defined in this way, cardiac jelly degradation continues from the trabecular base to apex, and this is also finely controlled by Notch-Nrg1 pathway interaction (Fig. 2.2c). This progressive cardiac jelly degradation continues until E14.5, when total degradation of the cardiac jelly promotes trabecular growth arrest in the so-called termination phase [22], which is associated with a spike in expression of the metalloprotease ADAMTS1 (Fig. 2.2d) [24]. Once trabeculation finishes around E14.5 in mice, the chamber wall undergoes a process called compaction, in which the trabecular myocardium is simplified (Fig. 2.2e). During this process, myocardium of the outer ventricular wall (compact myocardium) undergoes proliferation and actively expands into the trabecular zone, effectively incorporating the trabecular myocardium into the ventricular wall and leading to ventricular wall thickening (Fig. 2.2e) [25].

In humans, severe defects in early trabeculation are most likely embryonic lethal, as they are in mouse, whereas defects in later trabecular development and the compaction process lead to congenital heart disease and adult cardiomyopathies including hypoplastic left heart or non-compaction cardiomyopathy [26]. Mutations in the Notch pathway components has been related to these disease conditions [27–30], confirming that the Notch pathway as a critical regulator of trabeculation.

Cardiac Valves and Septation

Cardiac Valves The cardiac valves are one of the earliest cardiac structures formed during heart development although their growth and maturation extends until after birth. In vertebrates, there are two different types of valves associated with the atrioventricular canal (AVC) and outflow tract (OFT), respectively, each functioning to ensure unidirectional blood flow in the heart (Fig. 2.3a). The valvulogenic regions are specified early in heart tube formation along with the cardiac chambers, and are controlled by the Bmp2 pathway and downstream transcription factors Tbx2 and Tbx3 [31, 32]. These regions are also characterized by the presence of thick swelling of cardiac jelly formed from extracellular matrix (ECM) components secreted mainly by the myocardium [33], and constrained by the endocardial cell layer, together forming the so-called endocardial cushions (Fig. 2.3b) [34].

In mice, the endocardium lining the AVC canal at E9.0 and the OFT canal one day later undergoes an endothelial-to-mesenchymal transition (EndMT) in response to molecular cues originating from the underlining myocardium (Fig. 2.3c) [35, 36]. EndMT is finely regulated by a signalling network integrating Transforming Growth Factor (Tgf)β, Bmp and the Notch signalling pathways [37]. During valve EndMT, BMPs first promote endocardial cushion formation to create a pro-EndMT environment [31, 38, 39]. After that, Notch promotes EndMT initiation, and together with

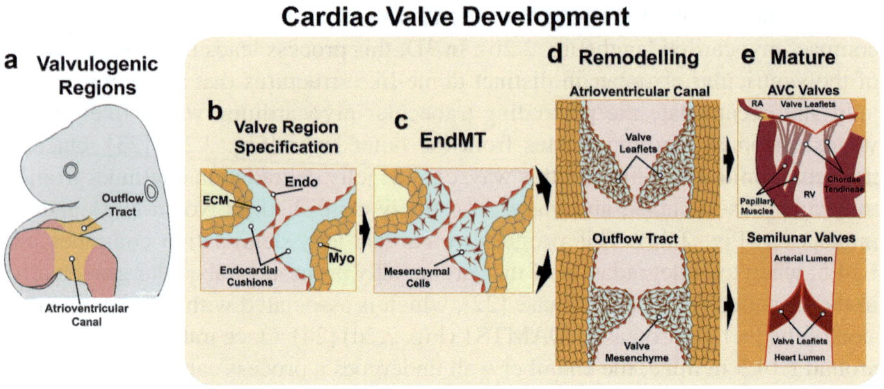

Fig. 2.3 Cardiac Valve Development. (**a**) Cartoon of an embryo showing the valvulogenic regions of the mouse heart at E9.5. (**b–e**) Valvulogenic process. (**b**) Valve Region Specification, (**c**) EndMT, (**d**) Remodlling and (**e**) Maturation phases of the valvulogenic process. See the dynamics of endocardium, myocardium, mesenchymal cells and ECM during the process. Endocardium: orange; valve myocardium: yellow; mesenchymal cells: brown; ECM: blue. Myo: myocardium; Endo: endocardium; RA: right atrium; RV: right ventricle

the Bmp and Tgfβ pathways induces the endocardial transition towards a mesenchymal and invasive cell phenotype [40, 41]. The endocardial cells undergoing EndMT become hypertrophic, lose apico-basal cell polarity, extend filopodia towards the cardiac jelly, and invade the endocardial cushions [36]. Once the endocardial cells ingress into the cardiac jelly, the endocardial layer proliferates to ensure its integrity. During the EndMT process, endocardial cells undergo a molecular switch involving reduction in endothelial gene expression and upregulation of mesenchymal gene expression, endowing them with a highly migratory and invasive potential that allows them to colonize the endocardial cushions [42]. The signalling pathways involved activate specific gene regulatory networks formed by transcriptional activators and repressors including Snail, Slug, Zeb1, Zeb2 and Twist1. Although all of these factors have been described to repress the transcription of the gene encoding the vascular endothelial (VE)-cadherin cell adhesion protein among others, they also perform other overlapping roles during EndMT. The transcription factors Snail and Slug are described to play key roles during EndMT induction, whereas Zeb1/2 and Twist1 are involved in the maintenance of the invasive phenotype [43]. These transcription factors form a self-supporting network, cross-regulating each other's expression as well as their own, reinforcing the metastable regulatory state underlying EndMT [44–47].

Linage tracing analyses have demonstrated the contribution of endocardial EndMT-derived cells to the valvular mesenchyme [48]. However, they have also shown that the AVC valve mesenchyme receives cellular contributions from epicardial derived cells (EPDCs) [49]. In contrast, the OFT valve mesenchyme is formed mainly by neural crest cells derivatives [50], even though the final contribution of these cells to the mature valve leaflets is minimal [51]. The epicardium and neural crest are extra-cardiac cell populations, themselves originating by an EMT process. They will be described in detail in the following sections. The valve cushion mesenchyme also contribute to the formation of the inter-atrial and inter-ventricular septa [52].

Therefore, the valvular primordia constitute the basic component from which the aortic and pulmonary semilunar valves, and the tricuspid and mitral valves, will mature. Until birth, valvular primordia undergo maturation and remodelling, giving rise to the functional valve leaflets seen in adults ((Fig. 2.3d, e). Defects in the formation of the valve primordia or their maturation can lead to a number of congenital heart diseases affecting not only the cardiac valves themselves, but also the formation of the cardiac chambers or septa. These include atrial septal defects (ASD), ventricular septal defects (VSD), transposition of the great arteries (TGA), tetralogy of Fallot, valvular atresia, valvular stenosis, Ebstein's anomaly and hypoplastic left heart (HLH) syndrome, among others [53]. Aberrant expression of most of the regulatory factors described above have been described to cause valve defects. Furthermore, mouse mutants for the *Neurofibromatosis Type 1* (*Nf1*) gene show structural OFT defects and enlarged AVC cushions due to excessive EndMT [54, 55], and in humans, *Nf1* mutations are associated to defects in many other organ systems including the skin. Interestingly, these defects can be recapitulated by the forced activation of the Ras pathway [56].

Atrial Septation During formation of the venous pole of the heart, morphogenetic processes leading to the incorporation of the major inflow veins into the atrial chambers are critical for the process of atrial septation. The primary atrial septum has its origins in myocardial progenitors located at the venous pole of the heart which grow from the dorsal atrial wall towards the AVC cushion to form a muscular crescent (Fig. 2.4a, green). During growth, the leading edge of the septum becomes covered with a thick cardiac jelly cellularized with mesenchymal cells, resembling endocardial cushions (Fig. 2.4a) [57]. This primary atrial septum forms on the right side of the pulmonary vein inlet and continues growing until it contacts and fuses with the cushion tissue of the AVC (Fig. 2.4b). The closure of the intercommunication between atrial chambers (primary atrial foramen) by the forming atrial septum leads to complete separation between the left and right atria. However, soon after, perforations in the primary septum form by apoptosis, re-establishing a communication between the two atria called the secondary foramen (Fig. 2.4b). As development proceeds, a secondary muscular septum forms from an infolding of the interatrial myocardial wall on the right side of the primary septum, but this never closes completely, retaining an oval-shaped opening termed the foramen ovale ((Fig. 2.4c). The secondary atrial foramen (in the primary atrial septum) and foramen ovale (in the secondary septum) are off-set, and in combination act as a type of flap valve allowing the one-way transit of blood from the right to the left atria during development ((Fig. 2.4c) [58]. This configuration of the inter-atrial septum is critical during foetal life allowing blood to bypass the lungs, which are not yet expanded; however, at birth, when the lungs expand, the right atrial pressure rises, and the flap valve is permanently closed by fusion of the primary and secondary septa. Failure of fusion leads to the condition known as patent foramen ovale

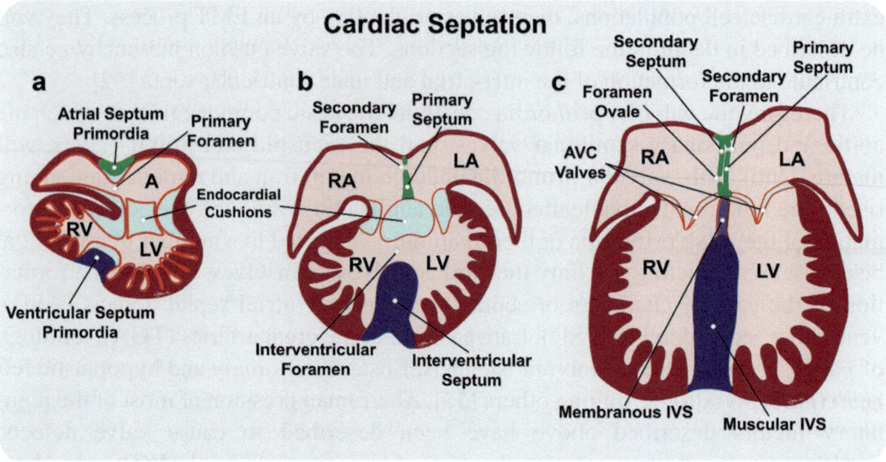

Fig. 2.4 Cardiac Septation. (**a–c**) Diagram showing a mouse heart section at (**a**) E10.5, (**b**) E12.5 and (**c**) E14.5 where the atrial (green) and ventricular (purple) septum development is depicted. The diagrams also show the disposition of the AVC endocardial cushions and their evolution during the AVC septation process. Endocardium: orange; myocardium: red; ECM: blue; atrial septum: green; Ventricular septum: purple. A: atrium; RA: right atrium; LA: left atrium; RV: right ventricle; LV: left ventricle; AVC: atrioventricular canal; IVS: inter-ventricular septum

(PFO). Defects in the formation of any of the components of the atrial septum leads to atrial septal defects (ASD).

Ventricular Septation The separation of the left and right ventricles begins at the outer curvature with an infolding of the chamber wall, which is likely a continuation of the bulbo-ventricular groove created during heart looping and chamber expansion (Fig. 2.4a, purple). In the early heart, a ring of cardiomyocytes called the "primary ring" can be recognised with molecular markers lying between the primitive left ventricle and the outflow region [1, 59]. Recent detailed 3D mapping and lineage tracing have defined this ring as containing precursors of elements of the cardiac conduction system of the heart, including the atrioventricular node, atrioventricular bundle, and left and right bundle branches [1]. The cardiac conduction system will be described in Sect. 5 (Fig. 2.6).

As the heart develops, the primary ring intersects with a ring of cardiomyocytes surrounding the AVC, which also contributes to the central conduction system of the heart. As anterior SHF cells are added to create the right ventricle and definitive OFT, the primary ring becomes positioned more caudally at the inter-ventricular junction encompassing the outer curvature, which corresponds to the position of the future inter-ventricular septum. By E11.5, the primary and AV canal rings become distorted due to expansion of the AV canal and addition of the definitive right ventricle and outflow tract. A distinct inter-ventricular septum forms as myocardial cells protrude inwards at the outer curvature, with cells of primary ring origin being retained at the crest of the growing septum (Fig. 2.4b). In mouse, the primary ring expresses the transcription factor *Tbx3* [60], detected as early as E8.0, suggesting a very early specification of the zone within the heart tube that will give rise to parts of the cardiac conduction system and inter-ventricular septum.

During ventricular septum formation, the inward growth of the muscular septum has been considered by morphologists to involve aggregation and subsequent condensation or compaction of part of the trabecular meshwork [61]. However, molecular markers of compact and trabecular cardiomyocytes reveal that the septum is heterogeneous in cellular composition, showing a compact myocardium identity in the septal core and trabecular myocardium signature evident only at its flanks. Patterns of cell clones in lineage tracing analysis suggest an apical/basal gradient in proliferative growth of the septum as it protrudes inwards [62]. As in the formation of the inter-atrial septum, the leading edge of the forming ventricular septal displays a cellularized cushion-like ECM, most likely secreted by primary ring cardiomyocytes. Upon closure of the ventricular foramen, this cushion component fuses with the AVC cushions to become part of the larger membranous atrioventricular septal complex (Fig. 2.4c). T-box transcription factors play important roles in ventricular septation with genetic deletion of *Tbx5* leading to complete loss of the septum [63]. Under-development or misalignment of the membranous septum is a common cause of ventricular septal defects (VSD) in humans.

Cardiac Cushion Septation Like the primary atrial and ventricular chambers, both the AVC and the OFT regions also undergo a type of septation processes. The AVC, originally connecting the common atrium and the primitive left ventricle, becomes divided into right and left canals by a mesenchymal septum derived from part of the AVC cushion as it expands to bridge both ventricles and atrial chambers ((Fig. 2.4a–c). The AVC septum will divide the original AVC cushions into the different cushion components that give rise to the valve leaflets of the mitral and tricuspid valves [64]. Septation of the OFT region will be described in the next section (Fig. 2.5). Once all the different cardiac regions and septa are completely developed, the fully functional and mature four chambered heart incorporates fully separated systemic and pulmonary pumps.

Cardiac Neural Crest Cells and OFT Septation

Cardiac Neural Crest Cells Neural crest cells originate in the ectodermal layer at the edges of the dorsal neural tube (Fig. 2.5a). Once released, they migrate throughout the body and take their place in multiple developmental processes, often involving cell types originated from the 3 germ layers. Neural crest cells are classified based on their origins as trunk and cranial neural crest cells, with the latter type giving rise to mesenchymal cells that ingress into the heart and populate exclusively the endocardial cushions of the OFT region [50]. The cardiac neural crest cells con-

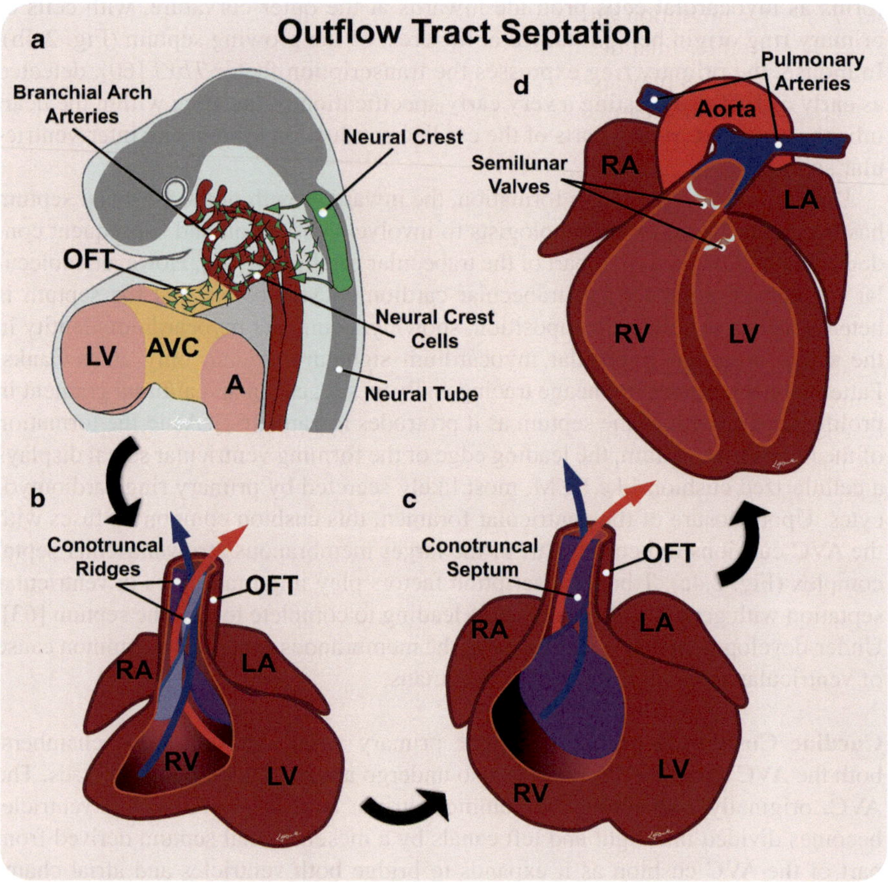

Fig. 2.5 Outflow Tract Septation. (**a**) Diagram depicting an E9.5 mouse embryo during the process of cardiac neural crest (green) migration to the branchial arch arteries and outflow tract. (**b–d**) conotruncal septation process. Neural crest cells in the outflow tract regions contribute first to the conotruncal ridges that will fuse and spiral, forming the conotruncal septum (**c**). This process is critical for the separation of the aortic and pulmonary tracts and to connect each tract to its corresponding ventricle (**d**). red arrow: aortic tract; blue arrow: pulmonary tract. A: atrium; LV: left ventricle; AVC: atrioventricular canal; OFT: outflow tract; RA: right atrium; LA: left atrium; RV: right ventricle

trol the development and septation of the OFT by forming the aorticopulmonary septum that divides the arterial pole into the systemic and the pulmonary outlets (Fig. 2.5a–d). However, the cardiac neural crest cells also contribute to the development and patterning of the smooth muscle component of the thoracic arteries, the parasympathetic innervation of the heart and the connective tissue of the glands in the neck [50, 65].

During cardiac neural crest cell development, induction factors from the different germ layers are required, first for neural crest formation and specification in the ectoderm, then for their detachment from the ectodermal layer via an EMT process, and finally for migration throughout the body following local signalling cues that direct them to their final destinations. Among these signalling cues, Bmp and Wnt signalling pathways play significant roles.

Once specified, the cardiac neural crest cells migrate first to the aortic arch arteries where they proliferate (Fig. 2.5a). A subset of these cells continues to the heart and ingress via the arterial pole to colonize the thick cardiac jelly forming the endocardial cushions of the OFT. This migration pattern was identified first by cell tracking in quail-chick chimaeras [50] and then confirmed by genetic linage tracing in the mouse [66].

OFT Septation As cardiac neural crest cells ingress into the OFT, the cells follow the shape of the cushions and condense forming the aorticopulmonary septation complex (Fig. 2.5b) [67]. The cells form an inverted U-shaped condensation of mesenchymal tissue with the sharp ends located inside of each of the OFT cushions and the main body located in between the fourth and the sixth pairs of aortic arch arteries, the precursors of the aorta and the ductus arteriosus, respectively.

As the OFT develops, the entire cono-truncal region spirals, as does the aorticopulmonary septation complex, likely as a result of left/right asymmetry cues (Fig. 2.5b, c). During this process, the OFT cushions become "myocardialized" as a front of OFT myocardium protrudes inwards. This promotes the fusion of the two ends of the U-shaped complex at the middle region of the OFT, subdividing the OFT cushions into the aortic and pulmonary valve forming regions (Fig. 2.5c, d) [67]. Therefore, the cellular composition of the mesenchyme of the forming OFT valves differs from that of the AVC valves, as it is formed by cells derived from the pharynx, neural crest, and endocardium lining via EndMT. However, the neural crest component is transient, with the mature valve leaflets mainly formed by the endocardial-derived component [51]. The aortic and pulmonary valves, also known as semilunar valves, have 3 leaflets that will mature during development until they acquire their final functional shape after birth.

Defective formation or migration of cardiac neural crest cells has been associated with abnormal patterning of the great arteries, defects in the pharyngeal glands and, most importantly, defects in OFT septation including persistent truncus arteriosus (PTA), double-outlet right ventricle (DORV) and ventricular septal defects (VSD) [68]. Defects are also associated with DiGeorge syndrome in humans [69, 70].

Cardiac Conduction System

As discussed, the process of heart development involves a series of morphogenetic events that will shape the organ into its mature form. During the process, its contractile cells, the cardiomyocytes, specialize into different functional components in order to adapt to the increasing demand of the heart during development and postnatally. During early development, the primitive and early looping heart tubes contract in a peristaltic fashion, where caudal cardiomyocytes have dominant pacemaker activity. At this stage, peristalsis and slow conductivity are sufficient to pump blood from the venous to arterial pole, and to satisfy the oxygen and nutrient requirement

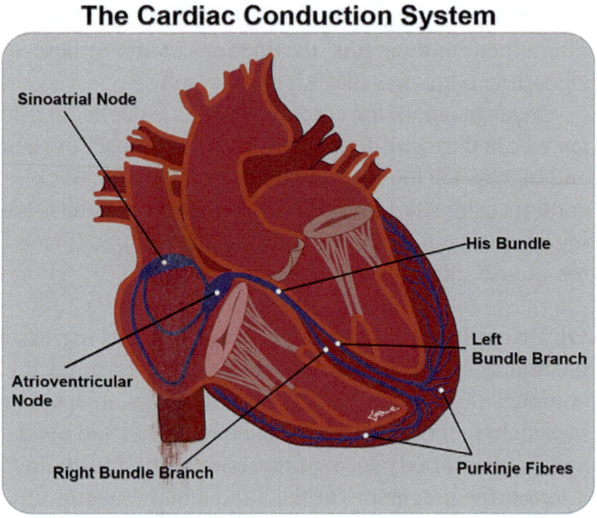

Fig. 2.6 Cardiac Conduction System. Diagram depicting the cardiac conduction system (purple) in the adult heart

of the early embryo. However, as the embryo grows and the heart develops into a four-chamber organ, this contraction pattern is no longer efficient, and the heart undergoes cardiomyocyte specializations to develop the complex sequential and coordinated contraction pattern that we can observe in an electrocardiogram. This involves simultaneous contraction of entire chambers, and cardiomyocytes specialized as pacemakers and conducting tissue conduits that transmit and coordinate the contraction pattern across different regions of the heart [1].

The cardiac conduction system can be divided into slow and fast conducting elements. The slow-conducting elements include the sinoatrial node and the atrioventricular node, whereas the atrioventricular bundle, the left and right bundle branches and the Purkinje fibre network, also known as the ventricular conduction system, are the fast conducting elements (Fig. 2.6).

The sinoatrial node, located at the intersection between the vena cava and the right atrium, constitutes the pacemaker of the heart (Fig. 2.6). It is formed by cardiomyocytes maintaining the automaticity present in the primitive myocardium, and is innervated and controlled by the autonomic nervous system [71]. The impulse generated in the sinoatrial node spreads through the atrial myocardium in a diffuse pattern, promoting its contraction. The impulse then travels to the atrioventricular node, located at the junction between the atria and the ventricles at the base of the atrial septum (Fig. 2.6). The atrioventricular node imposes a delay on the impulse, allowing the full contraction of the atria to occur before the ventricles contract. In order to prevent transmission of the impulse directly from the atria to the ventricles, specialize connective tissue forming the annulus fibrosus and the central fibrous body insulates the two chamber types and prevents synchronized contraction. Therefore, the electrical impulse can only be transmitted to the ventricles through the connection between the atrioventricular node and the fast-conducting atrioventricular bundle (His bundle), located at the tip of the ventricular septum (Fig. 2.6). Once passed this point, the impulse travels through the fast conducting components of the conduction system including the His bundle and left and right bundle branches, and spreads throughout the entire ventricular wall via the Purkinje fibre network (Fig. 2.6) [1].

From the developmental biology perspective, the slow components of the cardiac conduction system derive from the specialization of the primary myocardium. During the regional specialisation of the heart leading to chamber induction, the chamber myocardium acquires fast conductivity and loses automaticity mainly by the activation of genes encoding subunits of the high conductance gap junctions Cx40 and Cx43 (Gja5 and Gja1), and the cardiac sodium channel Scn5a (Nav1.5). In contrast, the non-chamber myocardium retains slow conduction and automaticity, features of the primitive myocardium [72]. As mentioned above, in non-chamber myocardium, the chamber-specific genetic program is repressed by the T-box family genes *Tbx2* and *Tbx3* [16, 17]. The pacemaker activity of the sinoatrial node can be recognized at the venous pole as early as E9.0 in the mouse. Similarly, the primary non-chamber myocardium forming the AVC has been described as the precursor for the atrioventricular node and the atrioventricular bundle [73]. In contrast, the bundle branches and the Purkinje fibre network derive from the differentiation of a subendocardial population of fast conducting ventricular cardiomyocytes located in the interventricular septum and trabecular myocardium respectively [74]. Defective cardiac conduction system development has been associated with disease conditions including atrioventricular conduction disease, and Wolff-Parkinson-White, Long QTL and Brugada syndromes [75–78].

Epicardium and Coronary Vasculature

The Epicardium In vertebrate hearts, the epicardium originates from a cluster of about 200 cells called the proepicardium (PE), positioned in the anterior region of the *septum transversum* [79] and originally derived from progenitors located in the lateral plate mesoderm (Fig. 2.7a). The PE is formed mainly by two different cell types, one with epithelial features covering a core enriched in ECM secreted by core mesenchymal cells (Fig. 2.7a) [80]. The mechanisms regulating PE induction are still unknown, but both endodermal signals from the hepatic primordia [81] and inductive signals from the sino-atrial myocardium [82] have been suggested as PE inductive signals. Among them, a complex balance between Bmp and Fibroblast Growth Factor (Fgf) signalling pathways has been described to regulate differentiation processes in the *septum transversum* region that will give rise to the myocardium of the *sinus venosus* and the PE [83, 84]. Other molecules expressed in the PE from the beginning of its development are the T-box transcription factor family gene *Tbx18* [84], Wilms tumour protein gene *Wt1* [85], encoding a transcription factor described as a cell adhesion regulator during epicardium development [86] and as a repressor of the epithelial phenotype of the epicardium [87], and *Raldh2*, a gene implicated in retinoic acid (RA) synthesis and PE survival [88]. Furthermore, the Notch pathway controls proepicardial and epicardial differentiation [89].

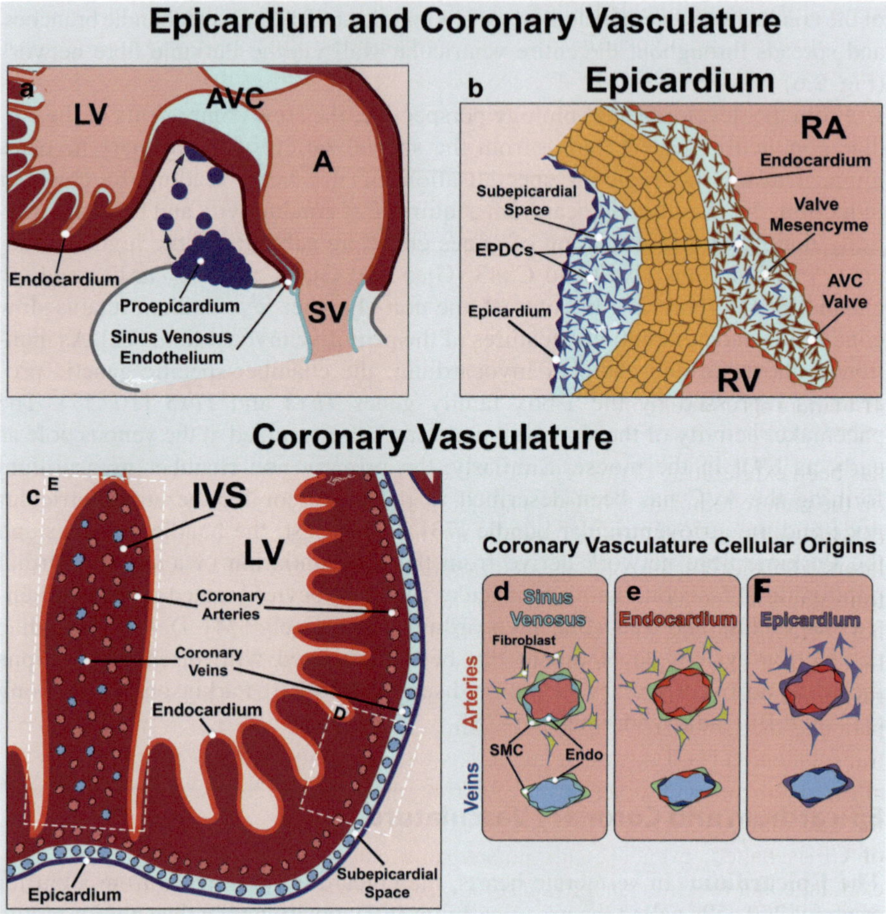

Fig. 2.7 Epicardium and Coronary Vasculature. (**A**) Diagram showing the different sources of cell progenitors for the coronary vasculature in the mouse: endocardium (orange), sinus venosus endothelium (light blue) and proepicardium (purple). The image also shows the process of proepicardial cell cluster release to the pericardial cavity and proepicardial cell attachment to the myocardial wall to form the epicardium. (**B**) Diagram showing the process of formation of the epicardial derived cells (EPDCs; light purple) from the epicardium and their contribution to the AVC mesenchyme. (**C**) Diagram depicting a late foetal left ventricle and septum with the distribution of coronary arteries and veins in the ventricular compact wall and the inter-ventricular septum. The dashed squares delimiting the inter-ventricular septum and ventricular wall, refer to the different contributions of different cell types to the coronary vasculature in panels E and D respectively. (**D–F**) Diagrams depicting a coronary artery and a coronary vein containing the different cell types forming them following a colour code (red: arterial endothelium, blue: vein endothelium; green: smooth muscle cells; yellow: fibroblasts) that is replace by the defining colour from the tissue of origin: sinus venosus (**D**, light blue); endocardium (**E**, orange) and epicardium (**F**; purple). Endocardium: orange; myocardium: red; ECM: blue; proepicardium/epicardium: purple; sinus venosus endothelium: light blue; mesenchymal cells: brown; EPDCs: light purple; coronary arteries: red; coronary veins: blue; smooth muscle cells: green; fibroblasts: yellow. A: atrium; LV: left ventricle; AVC: atrioventricular canal; SV: sinus venosus; RA: right atrium; RV: right ventricle; EPDCs: epicardial derived cells; IVS: inter-ventricular septum; Endo: endothelium; SMCs: smooth muscle cells

At E9.0, in mammals [90], the PE sheds cell clusters to the pericardial cavity that attach to the myocardial wall [91]. Once these PE cells contact the myocardium, they spread and grow as a monolayer to cover the whole outer-most wall of the heart, forming the epicardium (Fig. 2.7a, b) [92]. Once formed, the epicardium releases paracrine factors implicated in proliferation and differentiation of the compact myocardium [93, 94]. All of the mouse mutants with defective epicardial formation show a reduction in myocardial proliferation and a thin compact myocardium, demonstrating that induction of compact myocardium proliferation is dependent on the epicardium [94–98].

At the same time as the epicardium is covering the heart surface, both the epicardium and the myocardium secrete an extracellular matrix between them called the subepicardium (Fig. 2.7b). The composition of the subepicardium is critical for epicardial adhesion and stabilization, with fibronectin as a key molecule for adhesion and migration of epicardial cells [99]. The generation of the subepicardial space precedes the epicardial EMT forming the EPDCs that cellularize the subepicardium and subsequently the myocardial wall (Fig. 2.7b). EPDCs are the progenitor cells for the smooth muscle and fibroblastic components of the coronary vessels, being also able to contribute to the AVC mesenchyme (Fig. 2.7b, f) [100, 101].

The Coronary Vasculature The heart, as for any other major vessel, has its own *vasa vasorum*. The coronary vasculature is a complex network of arteries, veins and capillaries that takes blood from the aortic region at the base of the aortic valve, and irrigates the entire heart. The heart also has a lymphatic vasculature [102]. The developmental process giving rise to coronary vessel formation and the tissue origins for the different cell types forming these vessels have been under intense debate over the last decade.

The epicardium and the EPDCs were considered for many years as the main tissue origin of the endothelium, smooth muscle and fibroblast components of the coronary arteries [103, 104]. However, recent studies have demonstrated that whereas the smooth muscle and fibroblastic components of the coronary arteries are indeed derived from EPDCs, the endothelium has multiple origins (Fig. 2.7f) [105, 106]. Indeed, three different sources have been proposed [107]. The majority of the venous and arterial endothelium appears to originate by endothelial sprouting from the endothelium forming the *sinus venosus* region (Fig. 2.7a, c, d). These sprouting vessels form a coronary venous plexus in the subepicardium which then ingresses into the myocardial wall to form the coronary arterial endothelium (Fig. 2.7a). The primordial coronary arteries inside the myocardium then recruit the smooth muscle and fibroblastic components in order to form the mature coronary arteries [105]. The other identified source of arterial endothelium is the endocardium [106], that ingress the myocardium from the luminal side and contributes to the arterial endothelium of the coronary arteries in the interventricular septum (Fig. 2.7a, c, e). Finally, a minor proportion of the coronary endothelium originates from EPDCs (Fig. 2.7f) [107]. Coronary vessel development has been described as a combined process of vasculogenesis, where a primitive plexus unconnected to the systemic flow is initially formed, and then by angiogenesis, whereby the now perfused arterial coronary plexus will reach its definitive shape [99]. Typical signalling pathways involved in vessel development including Notch and VEGF [89, 108]. Congenital coronary artery malformations include fistulae, anomalous coronary artery origin, and defects in the patterning of the hierarchical coronary plexus [109].

References

1. Moorman AF, Christoffels VM. Cardiac chamber formation: development, genes, and evolution. Physiol Rev. 2003;83:1223–67.
2. Meilhac SM, Esner M, et al. The clonal origin of myocardial cells in different regions of the embryonic mouse heart. Dev Cell. 2004;6:685–98.
3. Moorman AF, Christoffels VM, et al. The heart-forming fields: one or multiple? Philos Trans R Soc Lond Ser B Biol Sci. 2007;362:1257–65.
4. Lescroart F, Chabab S, et al. Early lineage restriction in temporally distinct populations of Mesp1 progenitors during mammalian heart development. Nat Cell Biol. 2014;16:829–40.
5. Cai CL, Liang X, et al. Isl1 identifies a cardiac progenitor population that proliferates prior to differentiation and contributes a majority of cells to the heart. Dev Cell. 2003;5:877–89.
6. De La Cruz MV, Sanchez Gomez C, et al. Experimental study of the development of the Truncus and the Conus in the Chick embryo. J Anat. 1977;123:661–86.
7. De La Cruz MV, Sanchez-Gomez C, et al. The primitive cardiac regions in the straight tube heart (stage 9) and their anatomical expression in the mature heart: an experimental study in the Chick embryo. J Anat. 1989;165:121–31.
8. Van Den Berg G, Moorman AF. Concepts of cardiac development in retrospect. Pediatr Cardiol. 2009;30:580–7.
9. Hamada, H. & Tam, P. P. 2014. Mechanisms of left-right asymmetry and patterning: driver, mediator and responder. *F1000prime Rep,* 6, 110.
10. Le Garrec JF, Dominguez JN, et al. A predictive model of asymmetric morphogenesis from 3d reconstructions of mouse heart looping dynamics. elife. 2017;6
11. Van Den Berg G, Abu-Issa R, et al. A caudal proliferating growth center contributes to both poles of the forming heart tube. Circ Res. 2009;104:179–88.
12. Soufan AT, Van Den Berg G, et al. Regionalized sequence of myocardial cell growth and proliferation characterizes early chamber formation. Circ Res. 2006;99:545–52.
13. Christoffels VM, Habets PE, et al. Chamber formation and morphogenesis in the developing mammalian heart. Dev Biol. 2000;223:266–78.
14. Moorman AF, Schumacher CA, et al. Presence of functional sarcoplasmic reticulum in the developing heart and its confinement to chamber myocardium. Dev Biol. 2000;223:279–90.
15. Thomas T, Yamagishi H, et al. The Bhlh factors, Dhand and Ehand, specify pulmonary and systemic cardiac ventricles independent of left-right sidedness. Dev Biol. 1998;196:228–36.
16. Christoffels VM, Hoogaars WM, et al. T-box transcription factor Tbx2 represses differentiation and formation of the cardiac chambers. Dev Dyn. 2004;229:763–70.
17. Hoogaars WM, Tessari A, et al. The transcriptional repressor Tbx3 delineates the developing central conduction system of the heart. Cardiovasc Res. 2004;62:489–99.
18. Ben-Shachar G, Arcilla RA, et al. Ventricular Trabeculations in the Chick embryo heart and their contribution to ventricular and muscular Septal development. Circ Res. 1985;57:759–66.
19. Sedmera D, Pexieder T, et al. Developmental patterning of the myocardium. Anat Rec. 2000;258:319–37.
20. Negro A, Brar BK, et al. Essential roles of Her2/Erbb2 in cardiac development and function. Recent Prog Horm Res. 2004;59:1–12.
21. Grego-Bessa J, Luna-Zurita L, et al. Notch signaling is essential for ventricular chamber development. Dev Cell. 2007;12:415–29.

22. Del Monte-Nieto G, Ramialison M, et al. Control of cardiac jelly dynamics by Notch1 and Nrg1 defines the building plan for Trabeculation. Nature. 2018;557:439–45.
23. Cherian AV, Fukuda R, et al. N-cadherin Relocalization during cardiac Trabeculation. Proc Natl Acad Sci U S A. 2016;113:7569–74.
24. Stankunas K, Hang CT, et al. Endocardial Brg1 represses Adamts1 to maintain the microenvironment for myocardial morphogenesis. Dev Cell. 2008;14:298–311.
25. Tian X, Li Y, et al. Identification of a hybrid myocardial zone in the mammalian heart after birth. Nat Commun. 2017;8:87.
26. Jenni R, Oechslin E, et al. Echocardiographic and Pathoanatomical characteristics of isolated left ventricular non-compaction: a step towards classification as a distinct cardiomyopathy. Heart. 2001;86:666–71.
27. Bourke LM, Del Monte-Nieto G, et al. Loss of rearranged L-Myc fusion (Rlf) results in defects in heart development in the mouse. Differentiation. 2016;94:8–20.
28. D'amato, G., Luxan, G., et al. 2016. Sequential notch activation regulates ventricular chamber development. *Nat Cell Biol,* 18**,** 7-20.
29. Kobayashi J, Yoshida M, et al. Directed differentiation of patient-specific induced pluripotent stem cells identifies the transcriptional repression and epigenetic modification of Nkx2-5, Hand1, and Notch1 in Hypoplastic left heart syndrome. PLoS One. 2014;9:E102796.
30. Luxan G, Casanova JC, et al. Mutations in the notch pathway regulator Mib1 cause left ventricular noncompaction cardiomyopathy. Nat Med. 2013;19:193–201.
31. Ma L, Lu MF, et al. Bmp2 is essential for cardiac cushion epithelial-Mesenchymal transition and myocardial patterning. Development. 2005;132:5601–11.
32. Yamada M, Revelli JP, et al. Expression of Chick Tbx-2, Tbx-3, and Tbx-5 genes during early heart development: evidence for Bmp2 induction of Tbx2. Dev Biol. 2000;228:95–105.
33. Krug EL, Runyan RB, et al. Protein extracts from early embryonic hearts initiate cardiac endothelial Cytodifferentiation. Dev Biol. 1985;112:414–26.
34. Eisenberg LM, Markwald RR. Molecular regulation of Atrioventricular Valvuloseptal morphogenesis. Circ Res. 1995;77:1–6.
35. Markwald RR, Fitzharris TP, et al. Structural development of Endocardial cushions. Am J Anat. 1977;148:85–119.
36. Markwald RR, Fitzharris TP, et al. Structural analysis of Endocardial Cytodifferentiation. Dev Biol. 1975;42:160–80.
37. Garside VC, Chang AC, et al. Co-Ordinating notch, bmp, and Tgf-Beta signaling during heart valve development. Cell Mol Life Sci. 2013;70:2899–917.
38. Sugi Y, Yamamura H, et al. Bone morphogenetic Protein-2 can mediate myocardial regulation of Atrioventricular cushion Mesenchymal cell formation in mice. Dev Biol. 2004;269: 505–18.
39. Rivera-Feliciano J, Tabin CJ. Bmp2 instructs cardiac progenitors to form the heart-valve-inducing field. Dev Biol. 2006;295:580–8.
40. Timmerman LA, Grego-Bessa J, et al. Notch promotes epithelial-Mesenchymal transition during cardiac development and oncogenic transformation. Genes Dev. 2004;18: 99–115.
41. Luna-Zurita L, Prados B, et al. Integration of a notch-dependent Mesenchymal gene program and Bmp2-driven cell invasiveness regulates murine cardiac valve formation. J Clin Invest. 2010;120:3493–507.
42. Hay ED. The Mesenchymal cell, its role in the embryo, and the remarkable signaling mechanisms that create it. Dev Dyn. 2005;233:706–20.
43. Peinado H, Olmeda D, et al. Snail, Zeb and Bhlh factors in tumour progression: an Alliance against the epithelial phenotype? Nat Rev Cancer. 2007;7:415–28.
44. Lander R, Nasr T, et al. Interactions between twist and other Core epithelial-Mesenchymal transition factors are controlled by Gsk3-mediated phosphorylation. Nat Commun. 2013;4:1542.
45. Peiro S, Escriva M, et al. Snail1 transcriptional repressor binds to its own promoter and controls its expression. Nucleic Acids Res. 2006;34:2077–84.

46. Takkunen M, Grenman R, et al. Snail-dependent and -independent epithelial-Mesenchymal transition in Oral squamous carcinoma cells. J Histochem Cytochem. 2006;54:1263–75.
47. Wels C, Joshi S, et al. Transcriptional activation of Zeb1 by slug leads to cooperative regulation of the epithelial-Mesenchymal transition-like phenotype in melanoma. J Invest Dermatol. 2011;131:1877–85.
48. Kisanuki YY, Hammer RE, et al. Tie2-Cre transgenic mice: a new model for endothelial cell-lineage analysis in vivo. Dev Biol. 2001;230:230–42.
49. Gittenberger-De Groot AC, Vrancken Peeters MP, et al. Epicardium-derived cells contribute a novel population to the Myocardial Wall and the Atrioventricular cushions. Circ Res. 1998;82:1043–52.
50. Kirby ML, Gale TF, et al. Neural crest cells contribute to Normal Aorticopulmonary Septation. Science. 1983;220:1059–61.
51. Plein A, Fantin A, et al. Neural crest cells in cardiovascular development. Curr Top Dev Biol. 2015;111:183–200.
52. Runyan RB, Markwald RR. Invasion of mesenchyme into three-dimensional collagen gels: a regional and temporal analysis of interaction in embryonic heart tissue. Dev Biol. 1983;95:108–14.
53. Ransom J, Srivastava D. The genetics of cardiac birth defects. Semin Cell Dev Biol. 2007;18:132–9.
54. Brannan CI, Perkins AS, et al. Targeted disruption of the Neurofibromatosis Type-1 gene leads to developmental abnormalities in heart and various neural crest-derived tissues. Genes Dev. 1994;8:1019–29.
55. Jacks T, Shih TS, et al. Tumour predisposition in mice heterozygous for a targeted mutation in Nf1. Nat Genet. 1994;7:353–61.
56. Lakkis MM, Epstein JA. Neurofibromin modulation of Ras activity is required for Normal Endocardial-Mesenchymal transformation in the developing heart. Development. 1998;125:4359–67.
57. Jensen B, Wang T, et al. Evolution and development of the atrial septum. Anat Rec (Hoboken). 2019;302:32–48.
58. Anderson RH, Brown NA, et al. Development and structure of the atrial septum. Heart. 2002;88:104–10.
59. Poelmann RE, Gittenberger-De Groot AC, et al. Evolution and development of ventricular Septation in the Amniote heart. PLoS One. 2014;9:E106569.
60. Mohan RA, Mommersteeg MTM, et al. Embryonic Tbx3(+) Cardiomyocytes form the mature cardiac conduction system by progressive fate restriction. Development. 2018;145
61. Anderson RH, Spicer DE, et al. The development of Septation in the four-chambered heart. Anat Rec (Hoboken). 2014;297:1414–29.
62. Franco D, Meilhac SM, et al. Left and right ventricular contributions to the formation of the Interventricular septum in the mouse heart. Dev Biol. 2006;294:366–75.
63. Koshiba-Takeuchi K, Mori AD, et al. Reptilian heart development and the molecular basis of cardiac chamber evolution. Nature. 2009;461:95–8.
64. Lamers WH, Moorman AF. Cardiac Septation: a late contribution of the embryonic primary myocardium to heart morphogenesis. Circ Res. 2002;91:93–103.
65. Jiang X, Rowitch DH, et al. Fate of the mammalian cardiac neural crest. Development. 2000;127:1607–16.
66. Lo CW, Cohen MF, et al. Cx43 gap junction gene expression and gap Junctional communication in mouse neural crest cells. Dev Genet. 1997;20:119–32.
67. Waldo K, Miyagawa-Tomita S, et al. Cardiac neural crest cells provide new insight into Septation of the cardiac outflow tract: aortic sac to ventricular Septal closure. Dev Biol. 1998;196:129–44.
68. Nishibatake M, Kirby ML, et al. Pathogenesis of persistent Truncus Arteriosus and Dextroposed aorta in the Chick embryo after neural crest ablation. Circulation. 1987;75:255–64.

69. Bockman DE, Kirby ML. Dependence of thymus development on derivatives of the neural crest. Science. 1984;223:498–500.
70. Van Mierop LH, Kutsche LM. Cardiovascular anomalies in Digeorge syndrome and importance of neural crest as a possible Pathogenetic factor. Am J Cardiol. 1986;58:133–7.
71. Gordan R, Gwathmey JK, et al. Autonomic and endocrine control of cardiovascular function. World J Cardiol. 2015;7:204–14.
72. De Jong F, Opthof T, et al. Persisting zones of slow impulse conduction in developing chicken hearts. Circ Res. 1992;71:240–50.
73. Aanhaanen WT, Brons JF, et al. The Tbx2+ primary myocardium of the Atrioventricular Canal forms the Atrioventricular node and the base of the left ventricle. Circ Res. 2009;104:1267–74.
74. Van Weerd JH, Christoffels VM. The formation and function of the cardiac conduction system. Development. 2016;143:197–210.
75. Benson DW. Genetics of Atrioventricular conduction disease in humans. Anat Rec A Discov Mol Cell Evol Biol. 2004;280:934–9.
76. Brugada P, Brugada R, et al. The Brugada syndrome. Arch Mal Coeur Vaiss. 2005;98:115–22.
77. Clancy CE, Kass RS. Inherited and acquired vulnerability to ventricular arrhythmias: cardiac Na+ and K+ channels. Physiol Rev. 2005;85:33–47.
78. Gollob MH, Green MS, et al. Identification of a gene responsible for familial Wolff-Parkinson-white syndrome. N Engl J Med. 2001;344:1823–31.
79. Manner J, Perez-Pomares JM, et al. The origin, formation and developmental significance of the Epicardium: a review. Cells Tissues Organs. 2001;169:89–103.
80. Nahirney PC, Mikawa T, et al. Evidence for an extracellular matrix bridge guiding Proepicardial cell migration to the myocardium of Chick embryos. Dev Dyn. 2003;227:511–23.
81. Ishii Y, Iwanaga M, et al. Protein-protein interactions between rat hepatic cytochromes P450 (P450s) and Udp-Glucuronosyltransferases (Ugts): evidence for the functionally active Ugt in P450-Ugt complex. Drug Metab Pharmacokinet. 2007;22:367–76.
82. Wessels A, Perez-Pomares JM. The Epicardium and Epicardially derived cells (Epdcs) as cardiac stem cells. Anat Rec A Discov Mol Cell Evol Biol. 2004;276:43–57.
83. Kruithof BP, Van Wijk B, et al. Bmp and Fgf regulate the differentiation of multipotential pericardial mesoderm into the myocardial or Epicardial lineage. Dev Biol. 2006;295:507–22.
84. Schlueter J, Manner J, et al. Bmp is an important regulator of Proepicardial identity in the Chick embryo. Dev Biol. 2006;295:546–58.
85. Moore AW, Schedl A, et al. Yac transgenic analysis reveals Wilms' tumour 1 gene activity in the proliferating Coelomic epithelium, developing diaphragm and limb. Mech Dev. 1998;79:169–84.
86. Kirschner KM, Wagner N, et al. The Wilms tumor suppressor Wt1 promotes cell adhesion through transcriptional activation of the Alpha4integrin gene. J Biol Chem. 2006;281:31930–9.
87. Martinez-Estrada OM, Lettice LA, et al. Wt1 is required for cardiovascular progenitor cell formation through transcriptional control of snail and E-cadherin. Nat Genet. 2009;42:89–93.
88. Jenkins SJ, Hutson DR, et al. Analysis of the Proepicardium-Epicardium transition during the malformation of the Rxralpha−/− Epicardium. Dev Dyn. 2005;233:1091–101.
89. Del Monte G, Casanova JC, et al. Differential notch signaling in the Epicardium is required for cardiac inflow development and coronary vessel morphogenesis. Circ Res. 2011;108:824–36.
90. Komiyama M, Ito K, et al. Origin and development of the Epicardium in the mouse embryo. Anat Embryol (Berl). 1987;176:183–9.
91. Viragh S, Challice CE. The origin of the Epicardium and the embryonic myocardial circulation in the mouse. Anat Rec. 1981;201:157–68.
92. Hiruma T, Hirakow R. Epicardial formation in embryonic Chick heart: computer-aided reconstruction, scanning, and transmission electron microscopic studies. Am J Anat. 1989;184:129–38.
93. Lavine KJ, Yu K, et al. Endocardial and Epicardial derived Fgf signals regulate myocardial proliferation and differentiation in vivo. Dev Cell. 2005;8:85–95.

94. Pennisi DJ, Ballard VL, et al. Epicardium is required for the full rate of Myocyte proliferation and levels of expression of Myocyte Mitogenic factors Fgf2 and its receptor, Fgfr-1, but not for Transmural myocardial patterning in the embryonic Chick heart. Dev Dyn. 2003;228:161–72.
95. Kastner P, Grondona JM, et al. Genetic analysis of Rxr alpha developmental function: convergence of Rxr and Rar signaling pathways in heart and eye morphogenesis. Cell. 1994;78:987–1003.
96. Kreidberg JA, Sariola H, et al. Wt-1 is required for early kidney development. Cell. 1993;74:679–91.
97. Kwee L, Baldwin HS, et al. Defective development of the embryonic and Extraembryonic circulatory systems in vascular cell adhesion molecule (Vcam-1) deficient mice. Development. 1995;121:489–503.
98. Manner J. Experimental study on the formation of the Epicardium in Chick embryos. Anat Embryol (Berl). 1993;187:281–9.
99. Kalman F, Viragh S, et al. Cell surface Glycoconjugates and the extracellular matrix of the developing mouse embryo Epicardium. Anat Embryol (Berl). 1995;191:451–64.
100. Dettman RW, Denetclaw W Jr, et al. Common Epicardial origin of coronary vascular smooth muscle, perivascular fibroblasts, and Intermyocardial fibroblasts in the avian heart. Dev Biol. 1998;193:169–81.
101. Perez-Pomares JM, Macias D, et al. The origin of the Subepicardial mesenchyme in the avian embryo: an Immunohistochemical and quail-Chick chimera study. Dev Biol. 1998;200:57–68.
102. Norman S, Riley PR. Anatomy and development of the cardiac lymphatic vasculature: its role in injury and disease. Clin Anat. 2016;29:305–15.
103. Mikawa T, Gourdie RG. Pericardial mesoderm generates a population of coronary smooth muscle cells migrating into the heart along with ingrowth of the Epicardial organ. Dev Biol. 1996;174:221–32.
104. Perez-Pomares JM, Phelps A, et al. Experimental studies on the spatiotemporal expression of Wt1 and Raldh2 in the embryonic avian heart: a model for the regulation of myocardial and Valvuloseptal development by Epicardially derived cells (Epdcs). Dev Biol. 2002;247:307–26.
105. Red-Horse K, Ueno H, et al. Coronary arteries form by developmental reprogramming of venous cells. Nature. 2010;464:549–53.
106. Wu B, Zhang Z, et al. Endocardial cells form the coronary arteries by angiogenesis through myocardial-Endocardial Vegf signaling. Cell. 2012;151:1083–96.
107. Tian X, Pu WT, et al. Cellular origin and developmental program of coronary angiogenesis. Circ Res. 2015;116:515–30.
108. Wang Y, Wu B, et al. Uncontrolled Angiogenic precursor expansion causes coronary artery anomalies in mice lacking Pofut1. Nat Commun. 2017;8:578.
109. Dodge-Khatami A, Mavroudis C, et al. Congenital heart surgery nomenclature and database project: anomalies of the coronary arteries. Ann Thorac Surg. 2000;69:S270–97.

Part II

Genetic Diseases

Cardiac Involvement in Epidermolysis Bullosa

3

A. Bilgic and Dedee F. Murrell

Introduction

Epidermolysis bullosa (EB) is a vast group of chronic debilitating skin disorders characterized by skin fragility, widespread painful blistering, erosions, scar formation and systemic organ abnormalities and involvement. It is a spectrum of genetic disorders in which adhesion of the skin and other epithelia to the underlying connective tissue is compromised. The severity of the condition ranges from mild to lethal, with an estimated prevalence of 56.8 per million individuals worldwide [1]. The most recent classification proposes four subtypes: Epidermolysis bullosa simplex (EBS), Junctional epidermolysis bullosa (JEB), Dystrophic epidermolysis bullosa (DEB), and Kindler syndrome. EBS covers several subtypes in which mechanical fragility and blistering is limited to the epidermis. On the other hand, JEB includes EB subtypes where blisters develop within the lamina lucida of the skin basement membrane zone (BMZ) and DEB encompasses the subtypes with blistering occurring within the upper papillary dermis below the lamina densa of the skin BMZ. Another form is Kindler syndrome, a specific entity characterized by photosensitivity and other specific clinical phenotypic features and blistering occurring in multiple levels within and/ or beneath the BMZ [2].

Several defective proteins and gene mutations have been identified in the pathogenesis of EB types causing various degrees of skin fragility. Those defective proteins are also expressed in internal organs and have structural functions. Thus, some

A. Bilgic
Department of Dermatology and Venereology, Akdeniz University, School of Medicine, Antalya, Turkey

D. F. Murrell (✉)
Department of Dermatology, St George Hospital, Sydney, Australia

Faculty of Medicine, University of New South Wales, Sydney, Australia
e-mail: d.murrell@unsw.edu.au

C. Salavastru et al. (eds.), *Skin and the Heart*,
https://doi.org/10.1007/978-3-030-54779-0_3

types of EB have complications in internal organs such as kidneys, heart, etc. [3]. Furthermore, secondary complications (anemia, etc.) due to EB might contribute to cardiac problems or contribute to the existing cardiac involvement.

Prevalence/ Population Affected

Cardiac involvement and problems due to EB are seen rarely in the literature as EB itself is a rare disease. However, both EB and cardiac involvement of EB debilitating diseases, creating life-long problems for patients and for the health system and may be fatal. The most common cardiac problem/involvement seen in EB is cardiomyopathy (CM) most notably dilated cardiomyopathy (DCM) [4]. The exact prevalence of cardiomyopathy and/or cardiac involvement in EB is not established in large prospective studies yet. However, Fine et al. reported that the highest cumulative risk of cardiomyopathy was demonstrated in patients with recessive DEB-generalized severe (RDEB-gen sev) (4.5%, ≥20 years of age), with lesser risks in JEB, generalized intermediate(JEB-gen intermed) and recessive DEB-generalized intermediate (RDEB-gen intermed) (1.1% and 0.4%, respectively). When congestive heart failure is also included, the cumulative lifetime risk in RDEB-gen sev increased to 5.5% [5].

EB forms proven to have association with cardiac involvement (DCM and/or other cardiac problems) are; RDEB, JEB, EBS- Muscular Dystrophy (EBS-MD), Lethal acantholytic epidermolysis bullosa (LAEB), EBS due to KLHL24 mutations and cardiocutaneous syndromes such as Skin Fragility–Woolly Hair Syndrome [2]. Previous and current nomenclature of these specific EB forms are described in Table 3.1 in order to prevent any confusion.

Table 3.1 List of EB subtypes associated with cardiac involvement/ previous nomenclature and target proteins

Type of EB	Subtypes	Previous nomenclature	Subclass	Targeted protein
EBS, Suprabasal				
	Acantholytic EBS (EBS-acanth)	–	–	Desmoplakin, plakoglobin
	Skin fragility syndromes	–	-Desmoplakin deficiency (EBS-desmoplakin; Skin fragility-woolly hair syndrome)	Desmoplakin
			-Plakoglobin deficiency (EBS-plakoglobin; Skin fragility-plakoglobin deficiency)	Plakoglobin

Table 3.1 (continued)

Type of EB	Subtypes	Previous nomenclature	Subclass	Targeted protein
			-Plakophilin deficiency (EBS-plakophilin; skin Fragility-ectodermal dysplasia syndrome)	Plakophilin 1
EBS, basal				
	EBS with muscular dystrophy (EBS-MD)		–	Plectin
JEB				
	JEB, generalized Severe (JEB-gen sev)	JEB, Herlitz	–	Laminin-332
	JEB, generalized Intermediate (JEB-gen intermed)	JEB, non-Herlitz	–	Laminin-332
DEB				
	RDEB, generalized severe (RDEB, gen sev)	RDEB, Hallopeau-Siemens	–	Collagen VII: Absent or markedly Reduced
	RDEB, generalized intermediate (RDEB, gen intermed)	RDEB, non-Hallopeau-Siemens	–	Collagen VII: Reduced

EB epidermolysis bullosa, *EBS* epidermolysis bullosa simplex, *JEB* junctional epidermolysis bullosa, *DEB* dystrophic epidermolysis bullosa, *RDEB* recessive dystrophic epidermolysis bullosa

Pathophysiology of Disease

Desmosomes are intercellular junctions found especially in tissues which are under mechanical stress such as epithelia, myocardium, bladder and gastrointestinal mucosa. Their primary function is cell adhesion. They have three major component protein groups: the desmosomal cadherins which consist of desmogleins (DSG1–4) and desmocollins (DSC1–3), the plakin family member desmoplakin (DSP), and the arm (armadillo) proteins plakoglobin (PG) and plakophilins (PKP1–3) [27]. Mutations in these proteins might result in either only inherited skin and /or hair abnormalities (such as mutations of the genes encoding PKP1, DSP, PG, DSG1, DSG4, DSC2, DSC3 and corneodesmosin) or both skin /hair abnormalities with heart muscle pathology (like mutations in the genes encoding DSP, PG or DSC2) [27, 28]. Several EB types and subtypes are seen as a consequence of these mutations.

DSP is the most abundantly expressed component of the desmosome [29]. DSP-I is the main isoform in the heart and DSP-II is mainly expressed in the skin [30]. Over the past decades, DSP mutations have been implicated in several clinical syndromes featuring skin, hair and/or cardiac abnormalities [7] such as striate palmoplantar keratoderma, arrhythmogenic right ventricular cardiomyopathy, Carvajal syndrome, Naxos-like syndrome and skin fragility–woolly hair syndrome [31, 32].

The most severe form of phenotypes due to DSP mutations is lethal acantholytic epidermolysis bullosa (LAEB) which was firstly described by Jonkman et al. [23]. Vahlquist et al. presented a case with clinical features of LAEB with sparse, thin hair, widespread skin erosions, and focal hyperkeratosis on her soles and around the thickened nails (pachyonychia). Later, she further developed shortening of cardiac ejection fraction, low-voltage electrocardiogram with T-wave changes over the left ventricle, a pathologically dilated left ventricle and severely impaired systolic function in spite of being asymptomatic [6]. In a report of Asimaki et al., a case of compound heterozygosity for two novel nonsense DSP mutations presented with a unique phenotype of palmoplantar hyperkeratosis, complete alopecia and early onset CM, leading to hemiparesis and sudden cardiac death in childhood [7].

Plectin is a large adhesive protein and an essential part of hemidesmosomes in the skin, interacting with keratin intermediate filaments and b4 integrin. However, it is expressed in several tissues and cell types such as the sarcolemma of the muscle. Mutations in the PLEC gene cause EBS basal subtypes in 8% of cases [33] and cause several forms of EB [34]. Specifically, mutations in PLEC are responsible for at least three disease subtypes: [35] EBS-Ogna (EBS-Og) [36], a recessive form of EB associated with pyloric atresia and severe loss of skin, EBS with pyloric atresia (EBS-PA) [37], and a recessive form of EBS -MD [38].

Plakoglobin is an intracellular armadillo protein and desmosomal component. The encoding gene is JUP [39]. The first human JUP mutation associated with cardiomyopathy, PPK and woolly hair (Naxos disease) was reported in 2000 [40]. A new severe phenotype caused by a homozygous nonsense JUP mutation, leading to complete loss of PG, was recently reported [8]. The clinical features, which led to neonatal lethality, comprised generalized epidermolysis, total alopecia and onycholysis; no cardiac abnormality was noted (although post-mortem examination was not performed). The phenotype closely resembled LAEB but the molecular pathology was in JUP gene rather than DSP. The authors labelled the disorder 'lethal congenital epidermolysis bullosa' (LCEB) [8].

Desmocollins (DSC) are components of desmosomes. They have three different forms, DSC1, DSC2 and DSC3. DSC1 and DSC3 are expressed in the suprabasal layers of the epidermis but not in the heart [41]. The first case regarding DSC2 mutation with a skin phenotype with mild palmoplantar keratoderma and woolly hair and arrhythmogenic right ventricular cardiomyopathy (with significant left ventricular involvement and a history of cardiac arrest) was reported in 2009 [42]. Moreover, heterozygotic DSC2 mutations results in cardiomyopathy without skin and hair abnormalities [43].

Dermatological and Cardiological Manifestations

Specific EB Forms Associated with Cardiac Involvement

There are several case reports describing the association of different EB subtypes and cardiac pathologies. These reports are summarized in Table 3.2.

Table 3.2 Literature about cardiac involvement/ cardiomyopathy in EB

Literature	Study type/ group	EB type	Possible aetiological factors cited
Vahlquist et al. [6]	Case report (n = 1)	(LAEB)	DSP mutations
Asimaki et al. [7]	Case report (n = 1)	(LAEB)	DSP mutations
Pigors et al. [8]	Case report (n = 1)	(LCEB)	JUP mutation
Brook et al. [9]	Case report (n = 1)	RDEB	Long term transfusion therapy with secondary iron overload
Melville et al. [10]	Case series (n = 25)	RDEB	Selenium deficiency
Sidwell et al. [11]	Case series (n = 6)	RDEB	Carnitine deficiency
Morelli et al. [12]	Case report (n = 1)	RDEB	Viral myocarditis
Taibjee et al. [13]	Case report (n = 1)	RDEB	Cardiotoxic drugs (amitriptyline)
Ergül et al. [14]	Case report (n = 1)	RDEB	Selenium deficiency
Oh et al. [15]	Case report (n = 1)	RDEB	No obvious reason or any evidence
Ryan et al. [16]	Retrospective chart review (n = 45)	RDEB	Having severe forms of RDEB (generalized or intermediate)
Batalla et al. [17]	Descriptive, cross-sectional chart-review (n = 57)	EBS (n = 19), JEB (4 Herlitz and 6 non-Herlitz), DEB (14 dominant and 13 recessive), 1 Kindler syndrome.	Anemia, iron overload (secondary hemosiderosis), chronic kidney failure, carnitine, selenium, zinc and other nutritional deficiency, hypoalbuminemia and hypoaminoacidemia.
Ryan et al. [18]	Case report (n = 1)	RDEB	No obvious reason-left ventricular noncompaction (LVNC), a novel cardiomyopathy type
Fine et al.[5]	Retrospective review (n = 15)	JEB non-Herlitz subtypes (JEB-O); RDEB, Hallopeau–Siemens (RDEB-HS); RDEB, non-Hallopeau–Siemens (RDEB-nHS)	Chronic renal failure as an important risk factor
Lara-Corrales et al. [19]	A multi-centered, retrospective study (n = 15)	RDEB subtypes and JEB, non-Herlitz subtype	Abnormal hemoglobin levels, low serum iron, low albumin, low selenium and total carnitine levels, potential cardiotoxic drug use (either amitriptyline, cisapride or both)
Çelik et al. [20]	Case report (n = 1)	EBS-MD	Cardiotoxic drug (amitriptyline, cisapride) use and/or plectin mutation
Villa et al. [21]	Case report (n = 1)	EBS-MD	No obvious reason-left ventricular noncompaction (LVNC) cardiomyopathy

(continued)

Table 3.2 (continued)

Literature	Study type/ group	EB type	Possible aetiological factors cited
Gostyńska et al. [22]	Case report (n = 2)	EBS-MD	A new PLEC isoform due to alternative splicing of exon 8
Jonkman et al. [23]	Case report (n = 1)	LAEB	DSP mutations
Yenamandra et al. [24]	Case report (n = 1)	EBS	Mutations in the KLHL24 gene
Hedberg-Olfers et al. [25]	Case report (n = 1)	EBS	Mutations in the KLHL24 gene
Schwieger-Briel et al. [26]	Case report (n = 20)	EBS	Mutations in the KLHL24 gene

EBS Epidermolysis bullosa simplex, *JEB* Junctional epidermolysis bullosa, *DEB* Dystrophic epidermolysis bullosa, *LAEB* Lethal acantholytic epidermolysis bullosa, *LCEB* Lethal congenital epidermolysis bullosa, *EBS-MD* EBS- Muscular Dystrophy, *RDEB-HS* recessive DEB-Hallopeau-Siemens, *JEB-nH* JEB, non-Herlitz, *DSG* desmogleins, *DSC* desmocollins, *DSP* desmoplakin, *PG* plakoglobin, *PKP* plakophilins

Recessive Dystrophic EB (RDEB), Generalized Severe

RDEB is characterized by the absence or reduction of collagen VII levels in stratified squamous epithelia. RDEB-gen sev form is one of the most severe forms of EB which was previously named RDEB, Hallopeau-Siemens. It is a result of two mutation in the COL7A1 gene [2]. Its dermatological findings consist of generalized blisters and skin fragility at birth and onwards, oral mucosa fragility, healing with milia and atrophic scarring, dystrophic or absent nails, scalp alopecia and granulation tissue in chronic wounds. Extracutaneous involvement of RDEB encompasses anemia, growth retardation, delayed puberty, osteoporosis, dental caries, gastrointestinal problems, ocular problems, pseudosyndactyly, glomerulonephritis, renal amyloidosis, CM and increased risk of skin cancers [2].

Brook et al. was first to describe a 17-year-old patient with RDEB as having congestive heart failure (CHF) and CM [9]. In their report, chronic anemia, long-term transfusion therapy and secondary hemosiderosis were suggested as possible contributors for CHF and CM. Later Melville et al. described two unrelated patients with RDEB developing fatal dilated CM. Then, they investigated a cohort of patients in terms of cardiac problems and possible factors. As reduced serum selenium level was found in 14 of 25 other children with DEB, the authors suggested that micronutrient deficiency, most probably selenium deficiency was the most probable cause for the cardiomyopathy. Eighteen patients out of 25 showed no evidence of cardiomyopathy in echocardiographic screening [10]. Sidwell et al. reported an analysis of patients with RDEB who were screened regularly for 7 years. During the study period, six of 61 children developed DCM. Patients were monitored for different nutrient levels and assessed for cardiac function. Free and total carnitine concentrations were found significantly lower in the RDEB with DCM than others [11]. However, baseline selenium levels and overall mean carnitine and selenium concentrations did not have significant difference [11]. Morelli et al. described a patient with RDEB suffered from a heart failure due to viral myocarditis. Their case recovered spontaneously and fully being different from the others [12]. Another case report of a 6-year-old girl this time with RDEB, who had regular laboratory and cardiological follow-up, was presented by Taibjee et al. This patient had been introduced to amitriptyline and cisapride, the two potentially cardiotoxic drugs used for chronic pain and chronic gastroesophageal reflux, respectively. After using amitriptyline and cisapride treatment, the patient started to have deterioration in her cardiac function presented by clinically (breathlessness, acute dyspnea and tachycardia) and also echocardiologically (left ventricular function at only 20%, massive cardiomegaly) reduced cardiac function and died to a suspected tachycardic arrhythmia [13]. Ergül et al. presented a 16-year-old boy with the diagnosis of RDEB having respiratory distress and heart failure symptoms. Clinical and laboratory investigations yielded low plasma selenium level and DCM in echocardiography. Partial improvement in cardiac functions was achieved with selenium replacement and anti-congestive treatment [14]. In some cases, such as a 25-month-old Korean girl, with RDEB-gen sev reported by Oh et al., no obvious reason or any evidence was shown to be the reason for CM [15]. However, it seems that the mutations in COL7A1 do not cause DCM in DEB patients directly, because the cardiac tissue does not express type VII collagen [11]. One of our cohort of RDEB-gen sev patients developed DCM presenting with breathlessness when in her late 20s; she had been given regular iron infusions as a child but when transitioned to the adult EB service, she was investigated for thalassemia trait, which was positive from her maternal Asian side and iron infusions were ceased in favor of blood transfusions. She was known to have had a low selenium level chronically and had not been taking the supplements. Upon resuming selenium supplementation, her cardiac function improved after some months, but she still requires management with an ACE inhibitor due to renal impairment.

Another of our RDEB-gen sev patients who had severe blistering of his upper back and failure to thrive, developed breathlessness from cardiomyopathy at age 9 and passed away despite medical therapy (Fig. 3.1).

Ryan et al. published a retrospective chart review regarding patients with RDEB examined between 1987 and 2014. They compared the results of laboratory data and echocardiographic findings of patients with EB and results of age-appropriate controls. A total number of 154 echocardiograms in 45 patients with RDEB were examined. The most common findings in the available patient data were left ventricular dilation (18% of patients), increased left ventricular mass (LFM) (26%), shortening of ejection fraction (11%), depressed right ventricular systolic function (11%) and dilated aortic root (18%). Patients with abnormal echocardiographic findings included 38 patients with RDEB-gen sev type, only one patient with RDEB,

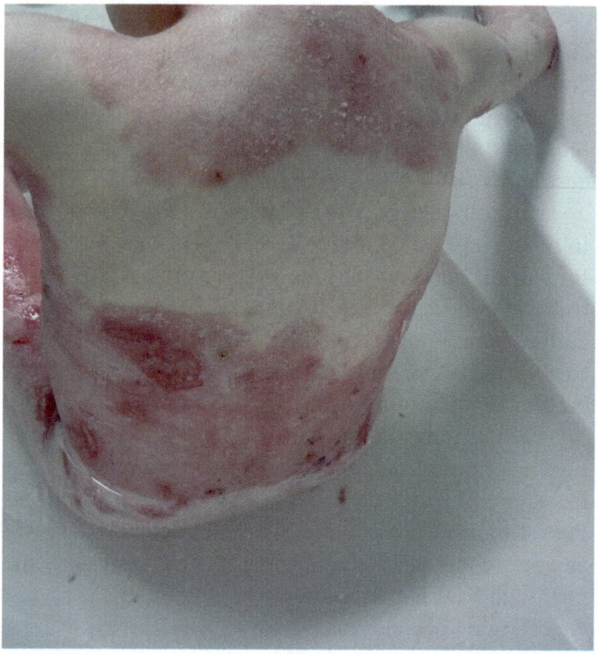

Fig. 3.1 A RDEB-gen sev patient with EB skin involvement who also had growth retardation and cardiomyopathy

localized (RDEB-loc) (an elevated LVM) and another patient with RDEB-gen intermed type (depressed right ventricular systolic function) [16].

Batalla et al. recently published a descriptive, cross-sectional chart-review study to determine the prevalence of DC in patients with EB seen in a pediatric referral hospital in Barcelona, Spain, between 1986 and 2015. The type and main subtypes of EB and the presence or absence of DC in these patients were investigated. In this chart-review, 57 patients were included. Nineteen had EBS, 10 had JEB (4 JEB-gen sev and 6 JEB-gen intermed), 27 had DEB (14 dominant and 13 recessive), and 1 had Kindler syndrome. In 19 patients, cardiological and echocardiographic assessment were performed. Only two patients with recessive DEB were diagnosed with DC. CM associated factors were identified as anemia, iron overload (secondary hemosiderosis), chronic kidney failure, carnitine, selenium, zinc and other nutritional deficiency, hypoalbuminemia and hypoaminoacidemia. Other factors found in the literature are cardiotoxic drugs (amitriptyline, cisapride) and viral infections [17].

Ryan et al. presented the first case with EB and left ventricular noncompaction (LVNC), a novel cardiomyopathy type. In routine echocardiogram, 5-year-old boy with RDEB showed spongiform myocardium, with 4 segments of the left ventricle affected showing deep trabeculations without any sign of classic DCM [18]. Although this patient had no sign for DCM, it is noteworthy that LVNC might evolve into a DCM phenotype. Thus, patients with LVNC are at risk of DCM in their lifetime.

There are 7 subtypes of LVNC, including isolated that accounts for 25% of cases, isolated with arrhythmias, dilated, hypertrophic, hypertrophic and dilated, restrictive, and LVNC with congenital heart disease. The most commonly used diagnostic criteria focus on the ratio of the thickness of noncompacted to compacted left ventricular wall at the midpapillary level as measured by echocardiography or magnetic resonance imaging. Overall, outcomes in patients with LVNC are poor because of early death from heart failure or sudden death related to arrhythmias or stroke [18, 44].

Junctional Epidermolysis Bullosa (JEB)

JEB is the EB form caused by reduced dermal-epidermal adhesion due to deficiencies of one of the proteins described in the literature such as laminin-332, type XVII collagen, integrin $\alpha6\beta4$ or integrin $\alpha3$. Dermatological manifestations of JEB are somewhat similar to RDEB [2].

Fine et al. analyzed all data in the US National Epidermolysis Bullosa Registry between 1986 and 2002 regarding the frequencies of CHF and CM documented with patient self-reporting, medical histories and medical records [5]. Twenty-one patients were identified as having CHF or CM; however, 15 of them were included in the analysis after careful review of the available data. CHF and CM were reported in only three EB subtypes JEB-gen intermed; RDEB-gen sev; RDEB-gen intermed among all of the participants in the registry. The most common EB subtype affected was RDEB-gen sev, with about 7% reporting at least one of these complications. In their analysis, Fine et al. showed that CHF is significant especially among patients with RDEB-gen sev and chronic renal failure is an important risk factor for CHF in these specific EB subtypes. CHF or CM were the cause of death in 30% of patients with RDEB-gen sev [5].

A multi-centered, retrospective study was established by Lara-Corrales et al. in order to determine the existence of DC among patients with EB seen between 1990 and 2006 [19]. They identified 15 EB patients with DC, most notably among the subtypes of RDEB (87%) and JEB-gen intermed (13%). At the time of diagnosis of DC, the majority of patients had few or no symptoms. Dyspnea / tachypnea (46.7%) and change in effort tolerance (40.0%) were reported as the most common symptoms and tachycardia was the most common sign of DC (85.7%). Available laboratory data showed abnormal hemoglobin levels, low serum iron, low albumin, low selenium and low total carnitine levels in patients. Potential cardiotoxic drug use (either amitriptyline, cisapride or both) was reported in 5 patients whom one of died. Initial echocardiogram results of 13 patients out of 15 showed mild reduction in qualitative systolic function in 6 / 15 patients, moderate reduction in 4 / 15 patients and severe reduction in 2 / 15 patients. The mean follow-up period was 6.3 ± 4.8 years and seven (46.7%) out of the 15 patients diagnosed with DC died during the follow-up period [19]. One of our cohort of JEB-gen sev patients due to LAMC2 mutations died in his early 20s due to cardiomyopathy which presented quite suddenly. He had significant involvement of his upper back and buttock areas and had been relatively immobile due to involvement of his feet for years. (Fig. 3.2).

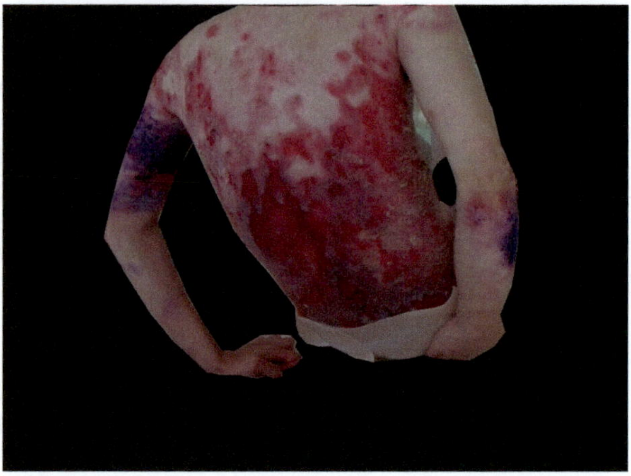

Fig. 3.2 Extensive involvement of the back in the patient with JEB due to LAMC2 splice mutations who developed cardiac failure in early 20s

Epidermolysis Bullosa Simplex- Muscular Dystrophy (EBS-MD)

This EBS variant is characterized by skin fragility, late-onset muscular dystrophy, visual, oropharyngeal, gastrointestinal, and genitourinary system symptoms [2, 20].

Celik et al. described a distinct variant of EB called EBS-MD with cardiac involvement for the first time. Clinical and laboratory examination showed atrial fibrillation, pericardial effusion, and hypokinetic left ventricular cardiac walls. After eliminating other factors, authors suggested the cardiotoxic drug (amitriptyline, cisapride) use as the probable reason for CM in their case. However, they also underlined that cardiac involvement in EBS-MD could be due to plectin mutation as expression of plectin is seen in cardiac muscles [20].

An 18-year-old patient with EBS-MD was reported as having left ventricular noncompaction. This was the first report this phenomenon described [21]. In left ventricular non-compaction (LVNC) cardiomyopathy, characteristic morphologic appearance composed of a dual layered myocardium: a thin, epicardial layer and a thick, endocardial layer with "spongy" trabeculations is characteristic findings [45]. Some of the possible results of LVNC cardiomyopathy are heart failure, arrhythmia, sudden death and thromboembolism [46, 47]. Altogether, authors underlined the importance of cardiac evaluation and imaging for early diagnosis and treatment of this complication [21].

Gostyńska et al. described the presence of a new PLEC isoform due to alternative splicing of exon 8, which results in a moderate EBS-MD phenotype, found in skin, myocardium, and striated muscle of healthy human controls. In their report, family had history of cardiac death in two members and cardiomyopathy. Thus, this new mutation could be another factor for CM in specific EB forms [22].

Lethal Acantholytic Epidermolysis Bullosa (LAEB)

Bolling et al. described the second report of lethal acantholytic epidermolysis bullosa (LAEB). Different from the first case reported by Jonkman et al. in 2005, cardiomyopathy was observed in addition to other classical findings (extensive non-bullous epidermal dislodgment, universal alopecia, dystrophic or absent nails and rapid postnatal demise) of this EB form [23]. The findings of poor contractility and dilated myocardium in LAEB cases supports the association of LAEB with cardiomyopathy. As all previous reports about DSP mutations affecting the DP C-terminus were associated with cardiomyopathy, cardiac abnormality is thought to be a possible extracutaneous involvement site in LAEB. In LAEB cardiac problems are present at birth, maybe due to the severity of the mutations [48].

EBS- KLHL24 Mutations

Mutations in KRT5 (keratin 5) and KRT14 (keratin 14) were the most commonly reported ones for autosomal dominant localized forms of EBS [49]. However, several phenotypes and genotypes of EBS were also reported due to different mutations such as mutations in PLEC (plectin), ITGA6 (a6 integrin subunit), ITGB4 (b4 integrin subunit), PKP1, DSP, JUP, TGM5 (transglutaminase 5), EXPH5 (exophilin-5), and DST (dystonin, 230-kDa bullous pemphigoid antigen) [2]. In spite of these findings, there is a large group of EBS patients where specific mutations have not been established. In 2016, a new gene and mutation for dominant EBS has been described by Lin et al. in the methionine start codon of KLHL24 (Kelch-like family member 24) [50]. More than 25 patients have been reported since then. The phenotypic features include skin defects and blistering at birth, typically healing with atrophic stellate scarring, skin fragility, and macular hyperpigmentation or hypopigmentation in childhood, and additional nail defects, oral ulceration and hair loss. Yenamandra et al. recently presented a Dutch family with EBS due to mutations in the KLHL24 gene. The difference of this case was the accompanying cardiomyopathy [24]. Previously, two patients with a homozygous KLHL24 nonsense mutation and with associated hypertrophic cardiomyopathy were presented and the association were validated by Hedberg-Olfers et al. [25]. Thus, they suggested the mutations in the KLHL24 gene could result in not only purely skin involvement of EB, but also a syndromic type with organ involvement such as the heart.

Furthermore, in a recent report, 18 patients with EBS-KLHL24 from nine families were presented (10 of them have been previously reported by He et al.) by Schwieger-Briel et al. [26, 51]. In addition to 8 new patients in this cohort, two additional individuals (patients 19 and 20) belonging to family 9, had skin fragility and history of death due to dilated cardiomyopathy. Overall, 17 (85%) patients showed evidence of cardiac involvement either with elevated cardiac biomarkers or with documented DCM (40%), and two of them died due to the cardiac pathology in their cohort with EBS-KLHL24 mutations. This report supported the previously described association of EBS with KLHL24 mutations and cardiomyopathy [26].

Specific Cardiac Involvement of EB (Dilated Cardiomyopathy)

Although CM have three different forms (dilated, hypertrophic, and restrictive), DCM is the most common form seen in patients with EB. It is a rare disease in pediatric populations with an incidence of 0.6–0.7 / 10,000 children [52]. The WHO defines DCM as the progressive dilatation and impaired contractility of the left or both ventricles [53]. An association has been suggested between EB and DCM as described above. However, the exact etiology of DCM is not clear. Some drugs, viral infections, anemia, iron loading, micronutrient deficiencies such as selenium and carnitine have been implicated in its ethology [11].

Chronic anemia is very common in severe EB and it is recognized as a cause for DCM. The anemia seen in EB is multifactorial. Chronic blood loss secondary to wounds and bleeding, poor gastrointestinal absorption, chronic inflammation results in chronic iron-deficient state. Folic acid or vitamin B12 deficiencies are not considered as contributing factors to the anemia seen in EB. Response to treatment is also poor in these patients and could cause secondary hemosiderosis due to iron overload by repeated transfusions. Both chronic/ recurrent anemia and secondary hemosiderosis could be the leading factors for cardiomyopathy. Thus, each patient should be evaluated individually for anemia therapy and followed for their hematologic status and cardiac functions closely [4, 9].

Carnitine is a compound with an essential role in the transport of long chain fatty acids into the mitochondria where they then undergo fatty acid oxidation: a major source of energy for the heart [11]. Carnitine and selenium deficiency have been suggested as a factor for DCM, although there have been different reports regarding these associations [10, 54, 55].

Amitriptyline, increasingly used for chronic pain in this condition, may cause CM. Tricyclic antidepressants like amitriptyline are well known causes of arrhythmia, especially in overdose. Furthermore, even at recommended doses, it is also associated with cardiomyopathy, cardiomegaly, and ventricular failure, in some cases reversed by stopping the drug [13]. Cisapride is another cardiotoxic drug which might cause QT prolongation and serious ventricular arrhythmias. Caution has been advised in patients with pre-existing cardiac disease and with interacting drugs including amitriptyline [13].

Viral myocarditis is another possible mechanism result in CM for EB patients. These patients can manifest flu-like symptoms before the onset of cardiomyopathy. However, although it is thought as a possible reason, not many cases have been reported [12].

Diagnosis/Investigations

In terms of assessing any cardiac involvement and problems in patients with EB, annual blood tests with complete blood count, metabolic tests, albumin levels, total and free carnitine levels, selenium and zinc levels, thyroid hormone measurement, and cardiac assessment (cardiological examination, electrocardiogram and echocardiogram which should include prospective measurement of ventricular and atrial muscle dimensions, not just valves and ejection fractions; normal dimensions in adults do not apply to most EB patients) should be evaluated regularly. In addition, serology for viral infections should be performed and treated if any sign occurs [17].

Treatment/ Follow-Up

With regard to the literature, the first challenge for physicians/ dermatologists is identifying the exact diagnosis by clinicopathological confirmation and/or searching out for any sign associated with cardiocutaneous syndromes. Careful clinical evaluation and close long-term follow-up is essential for all EB patients but especially for the ones associated with cardiac involvement. However, the treatment is extremely limited.

The management of EB-associated cardiomyopathy includes the correction of possible nutritional deficiencies, treatment of anemia, avoidance of potentially cardiotoxic drugs, and the use of medications, including angiotensin-converting enzyme inhibitors, diuretics, and digoxin, although these drugs may be insufficient to stabilize or reverse cardiac impairment in some patients [4].

Prevention

- Treatment of wounds on the skin and mucosal surfaces might be helpful to reduce blood loss and associated anemia.
- It is especially important to avoid iron overload while treating the existing anemia.
- Thalassemia trait should be considered in patients with at risky genetic backgrounds as if present, iron supplementation should be avoided to prevent cardiac and liver damage from iron overload; if anemia develops, transfusions are better than iron infusions for such patients.
- The use of cardiotoxic drugs should be limited during the follow-up period of EB patients unless they are essential.
- Maintain normal Selenium, Magnesium, Zinc and Carnitine levels
- Any sign of viral infection should be evaluated under caution.
- Regular cardiac examination and laboratory investigations (cardiac markers, electrocardiogram and echocardiogram) should be done even in asymptomatic JEB and RDEB patients every 12 months and if they become symptomatic, more regularly.
- Medications for cardiac involvement in each individual EB patient should be given as soon as the diagnosis of cardiac involvement is established.

References

1. Gowran RJ, Kennan A, Marshall S, Mulcahy I, Ní Mhaille S, Beasley S, Devlin M. Adopting a sustainable Community of Practice Model when developing a service to support patients with Epidermolysis Bullosa (EB): a stakeholder-centered approach. Patient. 2015;8(1):51–63.
2. Fine JD, Bruckner-Tuderman L, Eady RA, Bauer EA, Bauer JW, Has C, Heagerty A, Hintner H, Hovnanian A, Jonkman MF, Leigh I, Marinkovich MP, Martinez AE, McGrath JA, Mellerio JE, Moss C, Murrell DF, Shimizu H, Uitto J, Woodley D, Zambruno G. Inherited epidermolysis bullosa: updated recommendations on diagnosis and classification. J Am Acad Dermatol. 2014;70(6):1103–26.

3. Murat-Susˇic´ S, Husar K, Skerlev M, Marinovic´ B, Babic´ I. Inherited epidermolysis bullosa—the spectrum of complications. Acta Dermatovenerol Croat ADC 2011; 19(4): 255–263.
4. Fine JD, Mellerio JE. Extracutaneous manifestations and complications of inherited epidermolysis bullosa: part II. Other organs J Am Acad Dermatol. 2009;61(3):387–402.
5. Fine JD, Hall M, Weiner M, Li KP, Suchindran C. The risk of cardiomyopathy in inherited epidermolysis bullosa. Br J Dermatol. 2008;159:677–82.
6. Vahlquist A, Virtanen M, Hellström-Pigg M, Dragomir A, Ryberg K, Wilson NJ, Östman--Smith I, Lu L, McGrath JA, Smith FJ. A Scandinavian case of skin fragility, alopecia and cardiomyopathy caused by DSP mutations. Clin Exp Dermatol. 2014;39(1):30–4.
7. Asimaki A, Syrris P, Ward D, Guereta LG, Saffitz JE, McKenna WJ. Unique epidermolytic bullous dermatosis with associated lethal cardiomyopathy related to novel desmoplakin mutations. J Cutan Pathol. 2009;36(5):553–9.
8. Pigors M, Kiritsi D, Krumpelmann S, et al. Lack of plakoglobin leads to lethal congenital epidermolysis bullosa: a novel clinico-genetic entity. Hum Mol Genet. 2011;20:1811–9.
9. Brook MM, Weinhouse E, Jarenwattananon M, Nudel DB. Dilated cardiomyopathy complicating a case of epidermolysis bullosa dystrophica. Pediatr Dermatol. 1989;6(1):21–3.
10. Melville C, Atherton D, Burch M, Cohn A, Sullivan I. Fatal cardiomyopathy in dystrophic epidermolysis bullosa. Br J Dermatol. 1996;135(4):603–6.
11. Sidwell RU, Yates R, Atherton D. Dilated cardiomyopathy in dystrophic epidermolysis bullosa. Arch Dis Child. 2000;83(1):59–63. Review
12. Morelli S, Dianzani C, Sgreccia A, Porciello R, Bottoni U, Calvieri S. Reversible acute global left ventricular dysfunction in a patient with autosomal recessive dystrophic epidermolysis bullosa. Int J Cardiol. 2001;79(2–3):321–3.
13. Taibjee SM, Ramani P, Brown R, Moss C. Lethal cardiomyopathy in epidermolysis bullosa associated with amitriptyline. Arch Dis Child. 2005;90(8):871–2.
14. Ergül Y, Nişli K, Avcı B, Omeroğlu RE. Dilated cardiomyopathy associated with dystrophic epidermolysis bullosa: role of micronutrient deficiency? Turk Kardiyol Dern Ars. 2011;39(4):328–31.
15. Oh SW, Lee JS, Kim MY, Choi JY, Kim SC. Recessive dystrophic epidermolysis bullosa associated with dilated cardiomyopathy. Br J Dermatol. 2007;157(3):610–2.
16. Ryan TD, Lucky AW, King EC, Huang G, Towbin JA, Jefferies JL. Ventricular dysfunction and aortic dilation in patients with recessive dystrophic epidermolysis bullosa. Br J Dermatol. 2016;174(3):671–3.
17. Batalla A, Vicente A, Bartrons J, Prada F, Fortuny C, González-Enseñat MA. Cardiomyopathy in patients with hereditary bullous Epidermolysis. Actas Dermosifiliogr. 2017;108(6):544–9.
18. Ryan TD, Ware SM, Lucky AW, Towbin JA, Jefferies JL, Hinton RB. Left ventricular noncompaction cardiomyopathy and aortopathy in a patient with recessive dystrophic epidermolysis bullosa. Circ Heart Fail. 2012;5(5):81–2.
19. Lara-Corrales I, Mellerio JE, Martinez AE, et al. Dilated cardiomyopathy in epidermolysis bullosa: a retrospective, multicenter study. Pediatr Dermatol. 2010;27:238–43.
20. Celik C, Uysal H, Heper AO, Karaoglan B. Epidermolysis bullosa simplex associated with muscular dystrophy and cardiac involvement. J Clin Neuromuscul Dis. 2005;6(4):157–61.
21. Villa CR, Ryan TD, Collins JJ, Taylor MD, Lucky AW, Jefferies JL. Left ventricular noncompaction cardiomyopathy associated with epidermolysis bullosa simplex with muscular dystrophy and PLEC1 mutation. Neuromuscul Disord. 2015 Feb;25(2):165–8.
22. Gostyńska KB, Lemmink H, Bremer J, Pas HH, Nijenhuis M, van den Akker PC, Sinke RJ, Jonkman MF, Pasmooij AMG. A PLEC isoform identified in skin, muscle, and heart. J Invest Dermatol. 2017;137(2):518–22.
23. Jonkman MF, Pasmooij AM, Pasmans SG, et al. Loss of desmoplakin tail causes lethal acantholytic epidermolysis bullosa. Am J Hum Genet. 2005;77:653–60.
24. Yenamandra VK, van den Akker PC, Lemmink HH, Jan SZ, Diercks GFH, Vermeer M, van den Berg MP, van der Meer P, Pasmooij AMG, Sinke RJ, Jonkman MF, Bolling MC. Cardiomyopathy in patients with epidermolysis bullosa simplex with mutations in KLHL24. Br J Dermatol. 2018;179(5):1181–3.

25. Hedberg-Oldfors C, Danielsson O, Hubbert L, Nennesmo I, Abramsson A, Banote R, et al. Hypertrophic cardiomyopathy and abnormal glycogen storage in heart and skeletal muscle associated with inactivation of KLHL24. Neuromuscul Disord. 2016;26:S88–S212.
26. Schwieger-Briel A, Fuentes I, Castiglia D, Barbato A, Greutmann M, Leppert J, Duchatelet S, Hovnanian A, Burattini S, Yubero MJ, Ibañez-Arenas R, Rebolledo-Jaramillo B, Gräni C, Ott H, Theiler M, Weibel L, Paller AS, Zambruno G, Fischer J, Palisson F, Has C. Epidermolysis Bullosa simplex with KLHL24 mutations is associated with dilated cardiomyopathy. J Invest Dermatol. 2019;139(1):244–9.
27. Holthofer B, Windoffer R, Troyanovsky S, et al. Structure and function of desmosomes. Int Rev Cytol. 2007;264:65–163.
28. Petrof G, Mellerio JE, McGrath JA. Desmosomal genodermatoses. Br J Dermatol. 2012;166(1):36–45.
29. Mueller H, Franke WW. Biochemical and immunological characterization of desmoplakins I and II, the major polypeptides of the desmosomal plaque. J Mol Biol. 1983;163:647–71.
30. Uzumcu A, Norgett EE, Dindar A, et al. Loss of desmoplakin isoform I causes early onset cardiomyopathy and heart failure in a Naxos-like syndrome. J Med Genet. 2006;43:e5.
31. Lai-Cheong JE, Arita K, McGrath JA. Genetic diseases of junctions. J Invest Dermatol. 2007;127:2713–25.
32. Bouameur JE, Favre B, Borradori L. Plakins, a versatile family of cytolinkers: roles in skin integrity and in human diseases. J Invest Dermatol. 2014;134(4):885–94.
33. Bolling MC, Jongbloed JDH, Boven LG, Diercks GFH, Smith FJD, Irwin McLean WH, Jonkman MF. Plectin mutations underlie epidermolysis bullosa simplex in 8% of patients. J Invest Dermatol. 2014;134(1):273–6.
34. Pfendner E, Rouan F, Uitto J. Progress in epidermolysis bullosa: the phenotypic spectrum of plectin mutations. Exp Dermatol. 2005;14(4):241–9. Review
35. McMillan JR, Akiyama M, Rouan F, Mellerio JE, Lane EB, Leigh IM, Owaribe K, Wiche G, Fujii N, Uitto J, Eady RA, Shimizu H. Plectin defects in epidermolysis bullosa simplex with muscular dystrophy. Muscle Nerve. 2007;35(1):24–35.
36. Koss-Harnes D, Hoyheim B, Anton-Lamprecht I, Gjesti A, Jorgensen RS, Jahnsen FL, et al. A site-specific plectin mutation causes dominant epidermolysis bullosa simplex ogna: two identical de novo mutations. J Invest Dermatol. 2002;118:87–93.
37. Pfendner E, Uitto J. Plectin gene mutations can cause epidermolysis bullosa with pyloric atresia. J Invest Dermatol. 2005;124:111–5.
38. Shimizu H, Takizawa Y, Pulkkinen L, Murata S, Kawai M, Hachisuka H, et al. Epidermolysis bullosa simplex associated with muscular dystrophy: phenotype-genotype correlations and review of the literature. J Am Acad Dermatol. 1999;41:950–6.
39. Delva E, Tucker DK, Kowalczyk AP. The desmosome. Cold Spring Harb Perspect Biol. 2009;1:a002543.
40. McKoy G, Protonotarios N, Crosby A, et al. Identification of a deletion in plakoglobin in arrhythmogenic right ventricular cardiomyopathy with palmoplantar keratoderma and woolly hair (Naxos disease). Lancet. 2000;355:2119–24.
41. Nuber UA, Schafer S, Schmidt A, et al. The widespread human desmocollin Dsc2 and tissue-specific patterns of synthesis of various desmocollin subtypes. Eur J Cell Biol. 1995;66:69–74.
42. Simpson MA, Mansour S, Ahnood D, et al. Homozygous mutation of desmocollin-2 in arrhythmogenic right ventricular cardiomyopathy with mild palmoplantar keratoderma and woolly hair. Cardiology. 2009;113:28–34.
43. Syrris P, Ward D, Evans A, et al. Arrhythmogenic right ventricular dysplasia /cardiomyopathy associated with mutations in the desmosomal gene desmocollin-2. Am J Hum Genet. 2006;79:978–84.
44. Towbin JA. Left ventricular noncompaction: a new form of heart failure. Heart Fail Clin. 2010;6(4):453–69.
45. Maron BJ, Towbin JA, Thiene G, et al. Contemporary definitions and classification of the cardiomyopathies an American Heart Association scientific statement from the council on clinical cardiology, heart failure and transplantation committee; quality of care and outcomes research

and functional genomics and translational biology interdisciplinary working groups; and council on epidemiology and prevention. Circulation. 2006;113:1807–16.
46. Oechslin EN, Jost CHA, Rojas JR, Kaufmann PA, Jenni R. Long-term follow-up of 34 adults with isolated left ventricular noncompaction: a distinct cardiomyopathy with poor prognosis. J Am Coll Cardiol. 2000;36:493–500.
47. Murphy RT, Thaman R, Blanes JG, et al. Natural history and familial characteristics of isolated left ventricular non-compaction. Eur Heart J. 2005;26:187–92.
48. Bolling MC, Veenstra MJ, Jonkman MF, Diercks GF, Curry CJ, Fisher J, Pas HH, Bruckner AL. Lethal acantholytic epidermolysis bullosa due to a novel homozygous deletion in DSP: expanding the phenotype and implications for desmoplakin function in skin and heart. Br J Dermatol. 2010;162(6):1388–94.
49. Knöbel M, O'Toole EA, Smith FJ. Keratins and skin disease. Cell Tissue Res. 2015;360:583–9.
50. Lin Z, Li S, Feng C, Yang S, Wang H, Ma D, et al. Stabilizing mutations of KLHL24 ubiquitin ligase cause loss of keratin 14 and human skin fragility. Nat Genet. 2016;48:1508–16.
51. He Y, Maier K, Leppert J, Hausser I. Schwieger- Briel a, Weibel L, et al. Monoallelic mutations in the translation initiation codon of KLHL24 cause skin fragility. Am J Hum Genet. 2016;99:1395e404.
52. Lipshultz SE, Sleeper LA, Towbin JA, et al. The incidence of pediatric cardiomyopathy in two regions of the United States. N Engl JMed. 2003;348:1647–55.
53. Richardson P, McKenna W, Bristow M, et al. Report of the 1995WorldHealthOrganization / international society and federation ofCardiology task force on the definition and classification of cardiomyopathies. Circulation. 1996;93:841–2.
54. Li GS, Wang F, Kang D, Li C. Keshan disease: an endemic cardiomyopathy in China. Hum Pathol. 1985;16:602–9.
55. Li Y, Nan BS. Correlation of selenium, glutathione peroxidase activity and lipoperoxidation rates in dilated cardiomyopathy. Chin Med J. 1989;102:670–1.

Cutaneous Manifestations of Aortic Disease

4

Richmond Jeremy

The Spectrum of Aortic Disease

The principal pathological disorders of the aorta are congenital malformation in infants and children and aortitis, aneurysm and dissection in adults. It is now recognised that a broad spectrum of congenital, genetic and inflammatory disorders can affect the aorta. Aortic aneurysms can present in patients of all ages, including the second and third decades. All too often, progressive aortic disease and aneurysm formation can be clinically silent until a major complication supervenes. Careful physical examination can, however, yield valuable information about the presence of aortic disease, with important signs present in the skin and the eyes.

Congenital Aortic Disease

Congenital disorders of the aorta include the coarctation spectrum and arch interruption syndromes, bilateral aortic arch and the aortic transposition and truncus arteriosus complexes. Cutaneous manifestations are limited. Aplasia cutis congenita has been described in patients with aortic coarctation [1]. The PHACE syndrome is a constellation of developmental abnormalities, including posterior fossa brain malformations, hemangiomas of the face, coarctation of the aorta and optic nerve and retinal features [2]. Affected individuals can also have intracranial vascular lesions akin to Moya Moya disease. The facial haemangiomas appear in infancy and can progress to large size. The cause of the syndrome is unknown.

R. Jeremy (✉)
University of Sydney, Sydney, Australia

Royal Prince Alfred Hospital Sydney, Sydney, Australia

Marfan and Aortic Disease Clinic, Royal Prince Alfred Hospital, Camperdown, Australia
e-mail: Richmond.jeremy@sydney.edu.au

C. Salavastru et al. (eds.), *Skin and the Heart*,
https://doi.org/10.1007/978-3-030-54779-0_4

Turner syndrome (45X) is associated with aortic coarctation and/or bicuspid aortic valve in 10–15% of individuals and aortic dissection can occur at relatively small aortic diameters [3]. Webbing of the neck and excessive skin on the back of the neck are common features. Lymphangiectasia and lymphedema may be observed in childhood or adult life. Important cutaneous features include hypoplastic nails, multiple pigmented naevi, whilst some have increased hirsutism and are prone to keloid scarring.

Inflammatory Aortitis

Inflammatory disease of the aorta and large arteries (aortitis) can be grouped into infectious and non-infectious forms.

Infectious Aortitis

The paradigm of infective aortitis is syphilis, now rarely seen in developed societies. The chancre of primary syphilis and the reddish-pink maculopapular rash of secondary syphilis are well recognised, as are condyloma latum on the mucous membranes, uveitis and interstitial keratitis. Syphilitic aortitis results from inflammation of the vasa vasorum in the ascending aorta and arch, resulting in obliterative endarteritis and ischemic damage to the aortic media and adventitia, with subsequent aneurysm formation [4]. By this stage, however, cutaneous and ophthalmic signs are absent.

Other causes of infectious aortitis include systemic bacteremia, notable *Salmonella spp* and *Staphylococcus aureus* [5]. As with syphilis, the primary pathology involves inflammation of the vasa vasorum. Infectious aortitis can present as a fever of unknown origin, with clinical clues including the cutaneous signs of endocarditis (splinter haemorrhages and Osler's nodes). In the modern era, infection of endovascular stents is an important source of bacterial aortitis.

Non-Infectious Aortitis

A variety of systemic inflammatory syndromes are associated with acute and chronic aortitis, which is often diagnosed at a relatively late stage. These include aortitis associated with the sero-negative spondyloarthropathies, inflammatory bowel disease and chronic granulomatous vasculitis.

The diagnosis of aortitis can be difficult. Non-specific systemic features include malaise and fatigue, weight loss, low grade fever, nocturnal sweats and generalised myalgia. A normochromic, normocytic anaemia may be present and is some cases increased eosinophil count. Systemic inflammatory markers (C reactive protein and erythrocyte sedimentation rate) are often elevated, but are not reliable markers of disease activity. Physical signs may be few, but can include peripheral pulse deficit, systolic bruits over large arteries, a systolic aortic ejection murmur and/or early diastolic murmur of aortic regurgitation. The second heart sound may be prominent in presence of aortic root dilatation. In many of these conditions, informative cutaneous signs may be evident.

Key imaging investigations include echocardiography (aortic valve function and aortic diameter), contrast CT angiography (aortic wall thickening, aortic diameter, conduit artery anatomy) and 18-FDG positron emission tomography (PET) scanning (extent and severity of aortic and vascular inflammation). (Fig. 4.1). Both CT and PET imaging have important roles in monitoring disease activity and response to treatment. For many of these conditions, long term treatment is required and the aortitis can slowly subside over a period of several years.

Reactive Arthritis

Reactive arthritis (also known as Reiter's syndrome), characterised by conjunctivitis, urethritis and arthritis is a post-infectious syndrome, consequent upon urogenital or gastrointestinal infection. A wide variety of bacteria have been implicated including *Salmonella spp., Yersinia spp. and Campylobacter spp.* as well as *Chlamydia spp.* Reactive Arthritis is associated with dilatation of the aortic root and ascending aorta and with aortic valve regurgitation, which may be either acute or chronic [6]. Histopathology has shown active inflammatory infiltrate in the aortic media and adventitia. The cutaneous features of Reactive Arthritis are varied, including circinate balanitis in up to half of affected males and less commonly ulcerative vulvitis in females; nail changes of onycholysis and periungual pustules; oral ulcers and glossitis and keratoderma blennorrhagicum progressing to hyperkeratotic plaques [7].

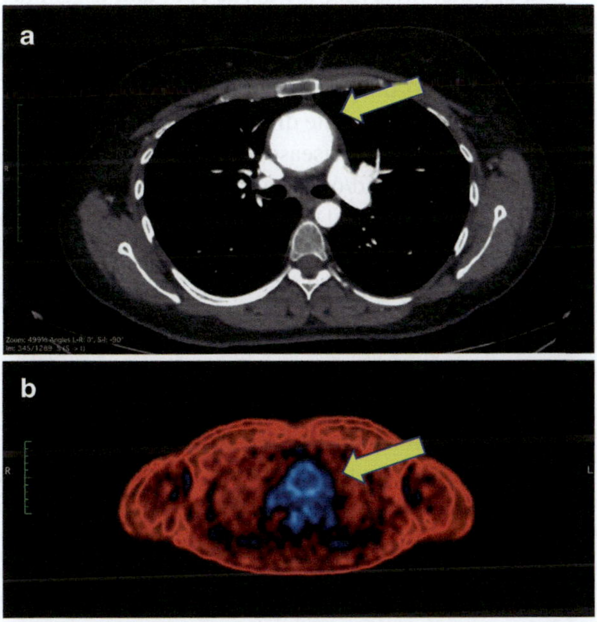

Fig. 4.1 Aortitis in a young female with Behcet's syndrome. Panel A: CT aortogram showing that the ascending aorta is aneurysmal with thickened wall. Note the evidence of intimal irregularity. Panel B: PET scan in same patient showing increased [18] FDG uptake (false colour blue) in ascending aorta

Behcet's Syndrome

Behcet's syndrome is a systemic inflammatory disease of unknown etiology, which may have a genetic predisposition. Usually recognised for the classical clinical features of oral and genital ulceration and ocular inflammation, Behcet's disease is accompanied by a systemic vasculitis in up to half of affected individuals. The ophthalmic manifestations include anterior and posterior uveitis and cutaneous lesions include a pustular folliculitis and erythema nodosum, which may become ulcerative. In the mouth, numerous painful apthous ulcers are observed. In the cardiovascular system, venous inflammation is more common, however systemic arteritis and aortitis do occur [8, 9]. Aneurysms of the thoracic aorta may be large and aortic valve regurgitation may be present. Pulmonary arterial aneurysms and pulmonary haemorrhage may also occur. Treatment is according to disease severity, including local and systemic glucocorticoids, addition of steroid-sparing immunosuppressive agents (eg azathioprine), cyclosporine and TNF-α inhibitors (eg infliximab). Surgery on the aorta or aortic valve is to be avoided in the presence of active inflammation.

Ankylosing Spondylitis

Ankylosing Spondylitis (AS) is a seronegative arthropathy, primarily affecting the lumbo-sacral spine, although other joints can be affected. Between 0.1% and 1% of the population are affected, with men affected more than women. The key cutaneous feature for patients with AS is psoriasis, involving skin and nails, [10]. Other systemic involvement includes lung and bowel. The systemic features of AS are consistent with an apparent disease spectrum across all the sero-negative arthropathies.

An aortitis, involving the aortic root and ascending aorta, may develop later in the course of disease and both aortic regurgitation and atrioventricular heart block can occur [11]. The aortic valve leaflets become thickened and fibrotic. In some patients a periaortitis can extend into the petroperitoneal and retropleural spaces leading to fibrosis. Despite dilatation of the aortic root, aortic rupture and dissection are uncommon in AS. Disease activity can be monitored by structural imaging with echocardiography and/or CT aortography and inflammation by PET scanning.

Management is based upon maintaining flexibility and mobility, with use of non-steroidal anti-inflammatory agents and/or TNF-α inhibitors. There is however no cure. Psoriasis is managed according to usual practice.

Inflammatory Bowel Disease

Inflammatory bowel disease (IBD), notably ulcerative colitis, has been associated with aortitis affecting the aortic root and ascending aorta and also with a more widespread arteritis of the Takayasu spectrum [12]. A variety of aortic complications have been reported in patients with IBD, including aortitis and valvulitis, aortic regurgitation (which may be rapidly progressive) and aortic mural thrombi and systemic embolism [13]. Overall cardiac complications in IBD appear to be uncommon, but it is possible that many instances are subclinical and not detected. Detection of aortic and valvular disease usually requires echocardiography.

Cutaneous manifestations of IBD have been classified as (I) specific lesions with same histopathology as bowel lesions; (II) reactive lesions with immunological triggers; (III) cutaneous disorders associated with IBD and (IV) secondary or complicating cutaneous features [14]. Among group I lesions are stomatitis and apthous ulcers and perianal fissures, whilst features of group II include erythema nodosum, pyoderma gangrenosum and Sweet syndrome. Lesions in group III include psoriasis, secondary amyloidosis and vitiligo. Deficiency of iron, zinc and other essential nutrients can lead to group IV type lesions. Importantly, the cutaneous features of IBD can antedate the gastrointestinal and cardiac manifestations.

Management can be complex, including non-steroidal and steroidal anti-inflammatory agents, steroid-sparing immunosuppressives and anti-TNF-α agents, although many of the drugs used can cause secondary cutaneous manifestations.

IgG4-Related Aortitis

IgG4-related disease (IgG4-RD) is an auto-immune inflammatory disease, characterised by destructive tissue infiltration of lymphocytes and IgG4-secreting plasma cells. Both aortitis and periaortitis occur, affecting approximately 5% and 15% of patients respectively [15]. Aortic aneurysm, dissection and rupture occur. All body tissues can be affected, including the eyes (dacryoadenitis and orbital inflammation) and the skin (angiolymphoid hyperplasia), manifest as pink to brown papules on the head and neck. Approximately half of patients have elevated serum IgG4 levels. Definitive diagnosis requires tissue biopsy and treatment includes systemic glucocorticoids and Rituximab.

Takayasu Arteritis

Takayasu arteritis is a chronic granulomatous inflammation of the aorta and large conduit arteries. A particular feature is massive intimal and medial hyperplasia, resulting in vascular occlusion and the cardinal clinical feature of loss of peripheral pulses. The disease is insidious in onset and may not present until significant vascular damage has occurred. The cause is unknown, although multiple predisposing gene variants have been described. On occasion, cutaneous signs may offer diagnostic information, including tender erythematous nodules on the legs, which may become ulcerated and rarely pyoderma gangrenosum. Biopsy reveals a granulomatous vasculitis [16]. Treatment is with high-dose glucocorticoids and usually a steroid sparing agent such as methotrexate.

Psoriasis and Psoriatic Arthritis

Psoriatic arthritis is one of the sero-negative spondyloarthropathies and predominantly affects the interphalangeal and metacarpophalangeal joints, with sacroiliitis in up to 40% of patients. Individuals with psoriatic arthritis are at increased risk of aortitis and large vessel vasculitis [17]. There is suspicion that psoriasis may contribute to progression of abdominal aortic aneurysm [18]. The presence of typical scaly cutaneous plaques, as well as onycholysis, hyperkeratosis, pitting and ridging of the nails should establish clinical diagnosis.

Genetic Aortopathies

During the last two decades a wide range of genetic aortopathies have been described, with inheritance in an autosomal dominant manner, albeit with variable penetrance, which may be less in females. Thus, examination of first-degree relatives is critically important for detection of other family members at risk.

Some of these conditions exhibit multi-system features (the syndromal aortopathies), whilst others have few if any other features (non-syndromal aortopathies). For many of the genetic aortopathies, physical signs in examination of the skin and integument may be first clue to the presence of underlying aortic disease. The extent of involvement of the vasculature varies between the different phenotypes, ranging from aortic root dilatation to generalised aortic and conduit artery ectasia, multiple aneurysms of elastic arteries, intracranial aneurysms and arterial tortuosity. Full imaging of the vasculature from cranial to lower limb circulations is warranted for affected individuals.

The gene mutations underlying many forms of syndromal aortopathy have been described, such as *FBN1* mutations in Marfan syndrome and *TGFBR1* and *TGFBR2* mutations in Loeys-Dietz syndrome. These mutations can be broadly grouped into those affecting the extracellular matrix, the TGFβ signalling system or the contractile apparatus in the vascular smooth muscle cell. Interestingly, mutations affecting key structural proteins within the aortic wall are rarely associated with aortic aneurysm. Mutations in *COL3A1* underly vascular Ehlers-Danlos syndrome, which is characterised by sudden rupture of conduit and muscular arteries, but rarely by aortic aneurysm formation [19]. Similarly, mutations in *FBLN5* (cutis laxa) and *ABCC6* (pseudoxanthoma elasticum) are not commonly associated with increased risk of aortic or aneurysm, although aortic stiffness is abnormal in pseudoxanthoma elasticum [20].

A variety of gene mutations have been associated with non-syndromal aortic disease, including *ACTA2, MYH11, SMAD4* genes, however at time of writing only 25% of patients with non-syndromal thoracic aortic aneurysm have identifiable gene mutations [19]. Bicuspid aortic valves and associated dilatation or aneurysm of the ascending aorta are common in the general community, however the genetics are largely unknown, with only isolated associations with mutations in *NOTCH1* and *GATA4* genes, among others.

Marfan Syndrome

Marfan syndrome (MFS) is consequent upon mutations in the *FBN1* gene, which encodes the extracellular matrix protein fibrillin-1, responsible for mechanotransduction and regulation of TGFβ signalling in vascular smooth muscle cells [21]. The population prevalence of MFS has been variously calculated at 1.5 to 17.2 per 100,000 population [22]. The diagnosis of MFS is based upon clinical features, as summarised in the revised Ghent criteria [23]. Key features are described in the cardiovascular, ophthalmologic, musculoskeletal, skin and integument systems (Fig. 4.2).

The best recognised cutaneous feature is the presence of striae atrophicae or striae distensae. These are observed over the lower back, shoulders, breasts, hips and thighs (Fig. 4.2). Care must be taken to distinguish isolated lumbar striae consequent upon rapid growth and abdominal striae secondary to pregnancy or overweight. Typically, striae appear in adolescence and are initially of a violaceous hue, fading to pale cream or white colour late in life [24, 25]. Over 90% of Marfan patients have striae, but diagnostic specificity is low compared to case-controls, particularly for striae on buttocks and hips. Striae in other locations had higher specificity (mean 84%, CI = 74–93) with sensitivity of 66% (CI = 54–77) [25].

Other cutaneous features described in Marfan syndrome include increased skin translucency, skin hyperextensibility and papyraceous scars [24]. Abnormal scars (hyperpigmented and hypopigmented) have been reported to have a diagnostic sensitivity of 46% (CI = 34–58) and specificity of 79% (CI = 67–87) [25]. Further musculoskeletal features include pectus deformity (excavatum and carinatum), scoliosis, arachnodactyly (wrist and thumb signs), hyperextensibility, pes planum and abnormal great toe length. Inspection of the face and cranium may reveal malar hypoplasia, dental crowding and a high narrow palate.

Management includes life-long surveillance and use of beta-adrenergic blockers and/or angiotensin receptor blockers for vascular protection. Prophylactic aortic repair is recommended according to aortic size and rate of dilatation.

Loeys-Dietz Syndrome

Originally described as consequent upon mutations in the genes encoding TGFβ receptor subunits (*TGFBR1* and *TGFBR2*) [26], the phenotype now includes patients with mutations in *TGFB2* and *TGFB3* and the downstream SMAD signalling elements (*SMAD3* and *SMAD4*) [27]. The incidence of Loeys-Dietz syndrome (LDS) is less than that of MFS. Like MFS, the phenotype affects multiple body systems, although ectopia lentis is not a feature. The arterial disease appears more aggressive than MFS, with multiple aneurysms occurring throughout the aorta and large elastic arteries. Arterial tortuosity is a common feature and intracranial aneurysms may occur [28].

The musculoskeletal features include scoliosis and arachnodactyly. Characteristic facial features include hypertelorism and downward lateral palpebral fissures. Some

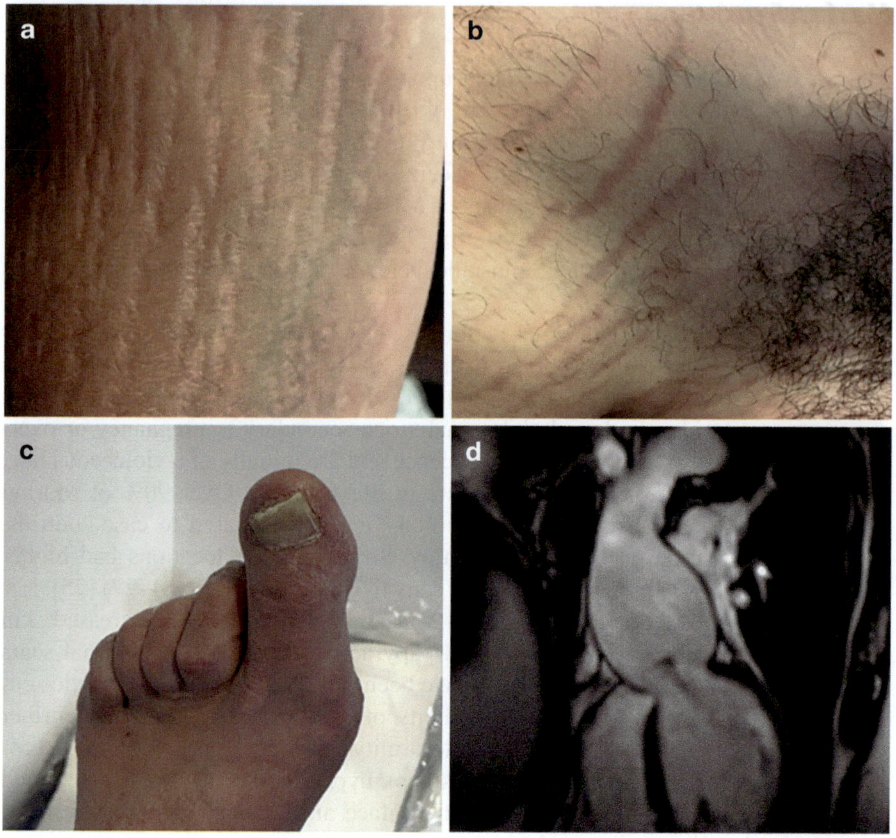

Fig. 4.2 Clinical features of Marfan Syndrome. Panel A and B: Striae atrophicae (old in Panel A and recent in Panel B). Panel C: Abnormal great toe. Panel D: Contrast MR aortogram showing typical dilatation of sinuses of Valsalva, extending into lower ascending aorta. A central jet of aortic regurgitation is also present

individuals have craniosynostosis and the uvula may be bifid or unduly elongated. (Fig. 4.3) Cutaneous findings in LDS include velvety, thin, translucent skin with easy bruising and visible veins. Scars may be atrophic and wound healing may be delayed. In some individuals lacking craniofacial features, these cutaneous features may be a prominent distinguishing feature of LDS from MFS or non-syndromal thoracic aortic aneurysm and dissection [29]. Striae and/or facial milia may also be present [30].

Patients with LDS require life-long surveillance of their entire vasculature and medical management as for MFS. Surgical repair of the aorta is recommended if there is any more than mild dilatation of the aorta. Careful consideration of pregnancy and vascular safety is warranted.

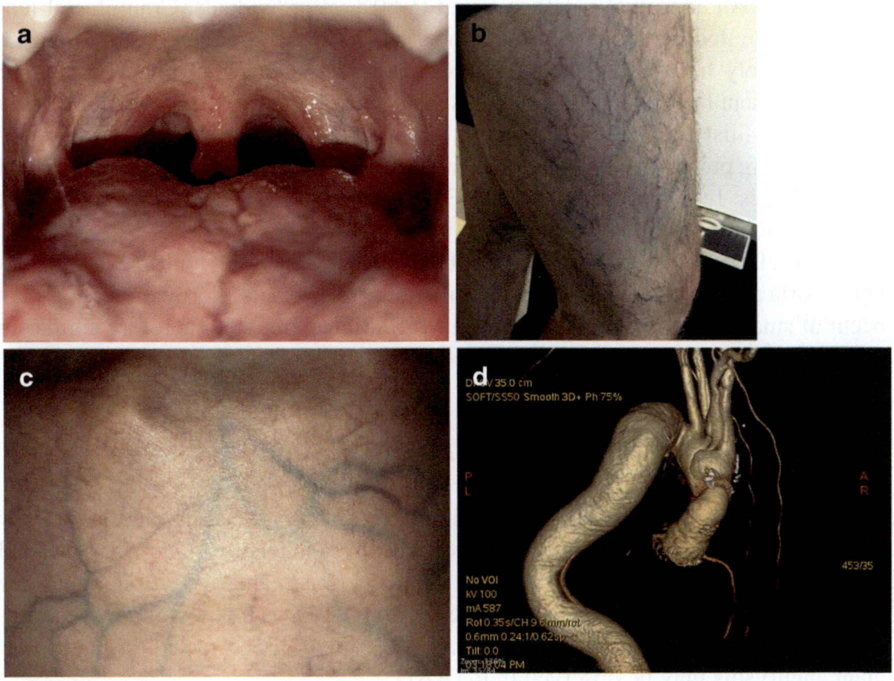

Fig. 4.3 Clinical features of Loeys-Dietz Syndrome. Panel A: Bifid uvula and note also the prominent vascular markings on palate. Panel B:Extensive venous neovascularization on leg. Panel C: Livido reticularis over torso. Panel D: CT aortogram showing dissected and tortuous thoracic aorta. The brachocephalic trunk is aneurysmal

Aneurysm-Osteoarthritis Syndrome

The Aneurysm-Osteoarthritis syndrome (AOS) is consequent upon mutations in the *SMAD3* gene, which encodes the intracellular signalling protein SMAD3, part of the TGFβ signalling pathway. The syndrome is characterized by aneurysms and dissections in the thoracic aorta and other large and medium elastic arteries. A signal feature is early onset of non-inflammatory arthritis. Various musculoskeletal and cutaneous features have been observed [31].

Like MFS, the phenotype can be variable. Striae atrophicae are described in approximately 50% of affected individuals, whilst soft, velvety skin is described in approximately 60% [32]. The skin may be translucent, with prominent thread-like veins across the torso and also on the lower limbs. Easy bruising, atrophic scars and fragile skin may be observed.

The musculoskeletal features can be similar to those of Marfan syndrome, including dolichostenomelia, arachnodactyly, pectus deformity and scoliosis and pes planum. An abnormal palate is found in 50% of individuals. Craniofacial features include hypertelorism, a long face, malar flattening and high forehead. Approximately half of patients have an abnormal uvula, which may be bifid or broad. This can help distinguish patients from those with MFS, in whom the uvula is normal, whilst ectopia lentis does not occur in AOS. Ostoearthritis is a key feature, affecting predominantly the spine and intervertebral discs, the wrists and hands and the knees. In contrast to MFS and Ehlers-Danlos syndrome, joint laxity is not commonly observed.

As with LDS, the arterial disease can be extensive, involving multiple aneurysms in the aorta and great vessels and also intracranial aneurysms. Aortic dissection may occur at smaller aortic diameters than in MFS. Management is therefore similar to that for patients with LDS.

Non-syndromal Thoracic Aortic Aneurysm and Dissection

An increasing number of cases of familial aortic aneurysm and dissection are now recognised, in whom there are minimal external physical features. These are grouped as the non-syndromal heritable thoracic aortic aneurysm and dissection phenotype (h-TAAD). The actual population prevalence of h-TAAD is unknown, however clinical experience indicates that it is more prevalent than MFS. Arterial tortuosity and giant aneurysms may be observed in h-TAAD,

Detection of h-TAAD is difficult and diagnosis is usually incidental discovery of aortic dilatation or after a clinical event eg dissection in a proband. A family history of aortic disease, sudden death or intracranial haemorrhage may be obtained [33]. There may be no external physical signs, or subtle vascular abnormalities may be observed, including prominent veins or early onset venous starring (Fig. 4.4).

A number of gene mutations have been associated with h-TAAD, the most prevalent of which appear to be *ACTA2*, the gene encoding vascular smooth muscle actin [34]. The ACTA2 mutations are associated with systemic smooth muscle dysfunction, including hypotonic bladder, hypoperistalsis of gut, pulmonary hypertension and pupillary dilatation. Intracranial aneurysms also occur and these patients tend to suffer aortic dissection with only mild underlying aortic dilatation.

Overall the prognosis of patients with h-TAAD is comparable to that for MFS and management is similar, however *ACTA2* mutations are considered to convey a worse prognosis, and for those patients a management approach similar to that for LDS is recommended.

Vascular Ehlers-Danlos Syndrome

Vascular Ehlers-Danlos Syndrome (vEDS) is a heritable vasculopathy consequent upon mutations in the *COL3A1* gene. It is characterized by spontaneous arterial dissection and rupture and by rupture of hollow organs eg bowel and uterus. Arterial rupture can occur in the absence of prior aneurysm formation and affects both elastic arteries and large muscular arteries.

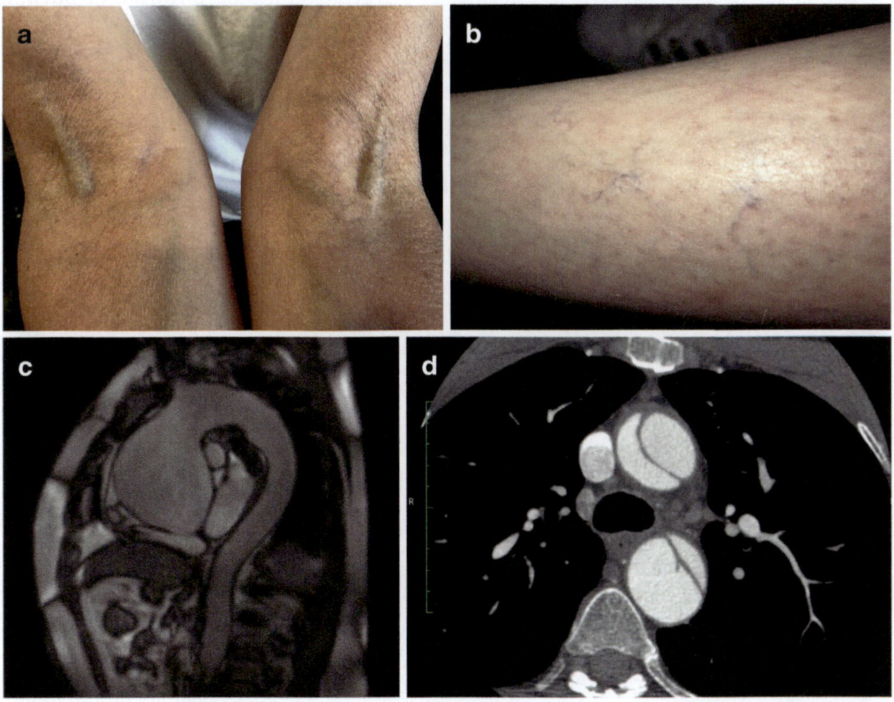

Fig. 4.4 Clinical features of non-syndromal thoracic aortic aneurysm. Panel A: Enlarged cubital fossa veins and valgus deformity. Panel B:Spider veins on lower leg in early life. Panel C: MR aortogram showing giant aneurysm of ascending aorta. Panel D:CT aortogram showing aortic arch dissection and dilatation of ascending and descending aorta

Diagnosis of vEDS can be difficult and presently the multisystem Villefranche criteria underpin clinical diagnosis [35]. Major physical signs include thin, translucent skin, extensive bruising and characteristic facies (prominent eyes, small chin, sunken cheeks, thin nose and lips, reduced ear lobes). Other physical signs may include early onset varicose veins and gingival recession and acrogeria, particularly in the hands and feet (Fig. 4.5).

There is no clearly effective management for v-EDS. The beta-blocker celiprolol may be of use, however clinical data is limited. There is no defined role for prophylactic surgery and therefore management remains reactive to events, coupled with regular surveillance and patient education.

Hereditary Haemorrhagic Telangiectasia

Hereditary haemorrhagic telangiectasia (HHT) is a heritable (autosomal dominant) condition characterised by systemic arteriovenous malformations in skin, brain and gastrointestinal tract. Mutations in *ENG*, *ACVRL1* and *SMAD4* genes are associated with HHT. The telangiectases are seen on both the skin and mucous membranes and can be extensive. Approximately 25% of individuals with HHT have associated

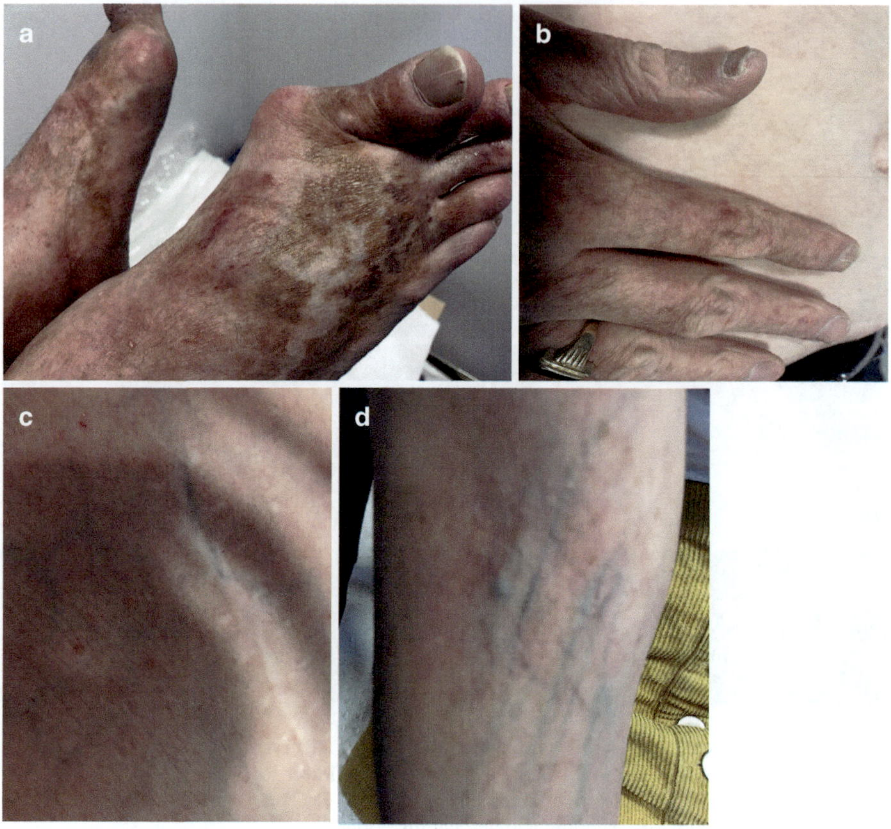

Fig. 4.5 Clinical features of vascular Ehlers Danlos syndrome. Panel A: Easy bruising. Panel B:Acrogeria in hands. Panel C: Paper thin scars. Panel D:Skin translucency

dilatation of the aortic root or ascending aorta, particularly those with *SMAD4* mutations [36].

Management is reactive to complications such as gastrointestinal bleeding, when laser ablation of bleeding telangiectases can be helpful.

Cutis Laxa

Cutis Laxa (CL) describes a phenotype of loose, redundant skin, with reduced elasticity, particularly on the neck, groin and face [37]. Affected individuals may appear prematurely aged. Classification of CL is complex, as the phenotype actually includes several distinct disorders, with differing inheritance, including both autosomal dominant and recessive forms and also X-linked inheritance. Mutations in several genes, including *ELN, FBLN4, FBLN5, ATP6VOA2, ATP7A and PYCR1,* have been associated with CL. The differential diagnosis includes an acquired form of CL, Ehlers-Danlos syndrome and pseudoxanthoma elasticum.

Autosomal dominant CL, consequent upon mutations in the elastin gene, *ELN*, has been associated with aneurysm and dissection of the thoracic aorta [38]. Autosomal recessive CL, consequent upon mutations in *FBLN4/EFEMP2* or *FBLN5* has a more aggressive phenotype than does the autosomal dominant form. Mutations in *FBLN4/EFEMP2* are associated with arterial tortuosity and thoracic aortic aneurysms, but mutations in *FBLN5* are associated with supravalvar aortic stenosis instead. Other autosomal recessive forms of CL, consequent upon *ATP6VOA2, ATP7 and PYCR1* mutations are not associated with aortic disease [37].

A related disorder is arterial tortuosity syndrome (ATS), consequent upon mutations in *SLC2A10*, which encodes the GLUT10 protein, a member of the glucose transporter family. The ATS is characterized by elongation and tortuosity of elastic conduit arteries and by complication of aortic aneurysm and dissection and individuals have variable skin laxity [39]. The phenotype of ATS overlaps that of Loeys-Dietz syndrome, including arachnodactyly, joint laxity, hypertelorism and bifid uvula.

The differential diagnosis of individuals with lax or prematurely wrinkled skin is extensive, including Geoderma osteodysplasticum, Cantu syndrome, Costello syndrome and Hutchinson-Gilford syndrome, none of which are associated with cardiovascular abnormalities. Another differential is Williams syndrome, which is associated with supra-valvar aortic stenosis, but not with aortic aneurysm.

There is no proven medical intervention, although beta-blockers may be used empirically for vascular protection.

Pseudoxanthoma Elasticum

Pseudoxanthoma elasticum (PXE) is a multisystem disorder consequent upon mutations in the *ABCC6* gene, which encodes the protein ATP binding cassette subfamily C member 6, although the physiological role of this protein remains uncertain. The condition is usually first detected because of cutaneous manifestations, including yellow papules, peau d'orange and reduced dermal elasticity in skinfolds. Ophthalmoscopy can reveal angioid streaks and subretinal neovascularization, and in the later stages choroidal atrophy. The pattern of inheritance is autosomal recessive with estimated prevalence of 1 in 50,000. Heterozygotes may have ocular and vascular signs however.

Patients with PXE typically have increased aortic and arterial stiffness, diastolic ventricular stiffness and abnormal vascular calcification [20]. Aortic aneurysm and dissection are rare in PXE. Atherosclerotic disease affecting the carotid and limb arteries is more common in PXE homozygotes.

There is no specific known treatment for PXE, but affected individuals should be treated with aggressive anti-atherosclerotic prevention measures, including statins for lipid control and angiotensin-receptor blockers for limitation of vascular scar formation.

Conclusions

A wide variety of inherited and acquired disorders of the aorta and large arteries are now known, which can carry adverse prognostic implications for affected individuals. All too often, the disease is only discovered when an event such as aortic dissection occurs. Careful physical examination of the skin, integument and peripheral vasculature can yield important diagnostic clues, allowing timely diagnosis and implementation of appropriate management plans. The practitioner should always be alert to the possibility of heritable disease and be prepared to instigate screening of at-risk family members.

References

1. Lataifeh IM, Khriesat WM, Baqain EB, Al Qarqaz FA, Abuekteish F. Aplasia cutis congenita associated with coarctation of the aorta: case report and review of the literature. Int J Dermatol. 2009;48:1222–4.
2. National Organization for Rare Disorders: PHACE syndrome. https://rarediseases.org/rare-diseases/phace-syndrome/
3. Mazzanti L. Cacciari E and the Italian study Group for Turner Syndrome. Congenital heart disease in patients with turner syndrome. J Pediatr. 1998;133:688–92.
4. Heggtveit HA. Syphilitic aortitis. A clinicopathologic study of 100 cases, 1950 to 1960. Circulation. 1964;29:346–55.
5. Foote EA, Postier RG, Greenfield RA, Bronze MS. Infectious aortitis. Curr Treat Options Cardiovasc Med. 2005;7:89–97.
6. Paulus HE, Pearson CM, Pitts W. Aortic insufficiency in five patients with Reiter's syndrome. Am J Med. 1972;53:464–72.
7. Wu IB, Schwartz RA. Reiter's syndrome: the classic triad and more. J Am Acad Dermatol. 2008;5:113–21.
8. Sakane T, Takeno M, Suzuki N, Inaba G. Behcets disease. N Engl J Med. 1999;341:1284–91.
9. Marzban M, Mandegar MH, Karimi A, Abbasi K, Movahedi N, Navabi MA, Abbasi SH, Moshtagi N. Cardiac and great vessel involvement in "Behcet's disease". J Card Surg. 2008;23:765–8.
10. Avalos-Diaz E, Dominguez-Cherit J, Herrera-Esparza R. Cutaneous manifestations of spondyloarthritis. Int J Clin Rheumatol. 2012;7:55–61.
11. Palazzi C, Salvarini C, D'Angelo S, Olivieri I. Aortitis and periaortitis in ankylosing spondylitis. Joint Bone Spine. 2011;78:451–5.
12. Sakhuja V, Gupta KL, Bhasin DK, Malik N, Chugh KS. Takayasu's arteritis associated with idiopathic ulcerative colitis. Gut. 1990;31:831–3.
13. Novacek G, Haumer M, Schima W, Muller C, Miehsler W, Polterauer P, Vogelsang H. Acute mural thrombi in patients with inflammatory bowel disease. Inflamm Bowel Dis. 2004;10:430–5.
14. Huang BL, Chandra S, Shih DQ. Skin manifestations of inflammatory bowel disease. Front Physiol. 2012;3:1–13.
15. Perugino CA, Wallace DS, Meyersohn N, Oliveira G, Stone JR, Stone JH. Large vessel involvement by IgG4-related disease. *Medicine* 2016; 95:28(e3344).
16. Frances C, Boisnic S, Bletry O, Dallot A, Thomas D, Kieffer E, Godeau P. Cutaneous manifestations of Takayasu arteritis. A retrospective study of 80 cases. Dermatologica. 1990;181:266–72.
17. Rose S, Dave J, Milo C, Naik HB, Siegel EL, Mehta NN. Psoriatic arthritis and sacroiliitis are associated with increased vascular inflammation by 18-fluorodeoxyglucose positron emission

tomography: baseline report from the psoriasis atherosclerosis and Cardiometabolic disease initiative. Arthritis Res Ther. 2014;16:R161.
18. No DJ, Armin M, Duan L, Egeberg A, Ahlehoff O, Wu JJ. Risk of aortic aneurysm in patients with psoriasis: a retrospective cohort study. J Eur Acad Dermatol and Venereol. 2018;32:e41–85.
19. Lindsay ME, Dietz HC. The genetics of aortic aneurysm. Cold Spring Harb Perspect Med. 2014;4:a015909.
20. Campens L, Vanakker OM, Trachet B, Segers P, Leroy BP, De Zaeytijd J, Voet D, De Paepe A, De Backer T, De Backer J. Characterization of cardiovascular involvement in pseudoxanthoma elasticum families. Arterioscler Thromb Vasc Biol. 2013;33:2646–52.
21. Jeremy RW, Robertson E, Lu Y, Hambly BD. Perturbations of mechanotransduction and aneurysm formation in heritable aortopathies. Int J Cardiol. 2013;169:7–16.
22. von Koloditsch Y, De Backer J, Schuler H, Bannas P, Behzadi C, Bernhardt AM, Hillebrand M, Fuisting B, Sheikhzadeh S, Rybczynski M, Kolbel T, Puschel K, Blankenberg S, Robinson PN. Perspectives on the revised Ghent criteria for the diagnosis of Marfan syndrome. Application of Clinical Genetics. 2015;8:137–55.
23. Loeys BL, Dietz HC, Braverman AC, Callewaert BL, De Backer J, Devereux RB, Hilhorst-Hoftsee Y, Jondeau G, Faivre L, Milewicz DM, Pyeritz RE, Sponseller PD, Wordsworth P, De Paepe AM. The revised Ghent nosology for the Marfan syndrome. J Med Genet. 2010;47:476–85.
24. Grahame R, Pyeritz RE. The Marfan syndrome: joint and skin manifestations are prevalent and correlated. Br J Rheumatol. 1995;34:126–31.
25. Ledoux M, Beauchet A, Fermanian C, Boileau C, Jondeau G, Saiag P. A case-control study of cutaneous signs in adult patients with Marfan disease: diagnostic value of striae. J Am Acad Dermatol. 2011;64:290–5.
26. Loeys BL, Schwarze U, Holm T, Callewaert BL, Thomas GH, Pannu H, De Backer JF, Oswald GL, Symoens S, Manouvrier S, Roberts AE, Faravelli F, Greco MA, Pyeritz RE, Milewicz DM, Coucke PJ, Cameron DE, Braverman AC, Byers PH, De Paepe AM, Dietz HC. Aneurysm syndromes caused by mutations in the TGF-β receptor. N Engl J Med. 2006;355:788–98.
27. Bertoli-Avella AM, Gillis E, Morisaki H, Verhagen JMA, de Graaf BM, van de Beek G, Gallo E, Kruithof BPT, Venselaar H, Myers LA, Laga S, Doyle AJ, Oswald G, van Cappellen GWA, Yamanaka I, van der Helm RM, Beverloo B, de Klein A, Pardo L, Lammens M, Evers C, Devriendt K, Dumoulein M, Timmermans J, Bruggenwirth HT, Verheijen F, Rodrigus I, Baynam G, Kempers M, Saenen J, van Craenenbroeck EM, Minatoya K, Matsukawa R, Tsukube T, Kubo N, Hofstra R, Goumans MJ, Bekkers JA, Roos-Heselink JW, van de Laar IMBH, Dietz HC, Van Laer L, Morisaki T, Wessels MW, Loeys BL. Mutations in a TGF-β ligand, *TGFB3*, cause syndromic aortic aneurysms and dissections. J Am Coll Cardiol. 2015;65:1324–36.
28. Jondeau G, Ropers J, Regalado E, Braverman A, Evangelista A, Teixedo G, De Backer J, Muino-Mosqueara L, Naudion S, Zordan C, Morisaki T, Morisaki H, Von Koloditsch Y, Dupuis-Gerod S, Morris SA, Jeremy R, Odent S, Ades LC, Bakashi M, Holman K, LeMaire S, Milleron O, Langeois M, Spentchian M, Aubart M, Boileau C, Pyeritz R, Milewicz DM. Montalcino aortic Consortium. International registry of patients carrying TGFBR1 or TGFBR2 mutations: results of the MAC (Montalcino aortic Consortium). Circ Cardiovasc Genet. 2016;9:548–58.
29. MacCarrick G, Black JH, Bowdin S, El-Hamamsy I, Frischmeyer-Guerrerio PA, Guerrerio AL, Sponseller PD, Loeys B, Dietz HC. Loeys-Dietz syndrome: a primer for diagnosis and management. Genet Med. 2014;16:576–87.
30. Lloyd BM, Braverman AC, Anadkat MJ. Multiple facial milia in patients with Loeys-Dietz syndrome. Arch Dermatol. 2011;147:223–6.
31. van de Laar IMBH, Oldenburg RA, Pals G, Roos-Hesselink JW, de Graaf BM, JMA V, Hoedemaekers YM, Willemsen R, Severijnen L-A, Venselaar H, Vriend G, Pattynama PM, Collee M, Majoor-Krakauer D, Poldermans D, IME F-M, Micha D, Timmermans J, Hilhorst-Hoftsee Y, Bierma-Zeinstra SM, Willems PJ, Kros JM, EHG O, Oostra BA, Wessels MW,

Bertoli-Avella AM. Mutations in *SMAD3* cause a syndromic form of aortic aneurysms and dissections with early-onset osteoarthritis. Nat Genet. 2011;43:121–6.

32. van de Laar IMBH, van der Linde D, Oei EHG, Bos PK, Bessems JH, Bierma-Zeinstra SM, van Meer BL, Pals G, Oldenburg RA, Bekkers JA, Moelker A, de Graaf BM, Matyas G, Frohn-Mulder IME, Timmermans J, Hilhorst-Hoftsee Y, Cobben JM, Bruggenwirth HT, van Laer L, Loeys B, de Backer J, Coucke PJ, Dietz HC, Willems PJ, Oostra BA, De Paepe A, Roos-Hesselink JW, Bertoli-Avella AM, Wessels MW. Phenotypic spectrum of the SMAD3-related aneurysms-osteoarthritis syndrome. J Med Genet. 2012;49:47–57.
33. Robertson EN, van der Linde D, Sherrah AG, Vallely MP, Wilson M, Bannon PG, Jeremy RW. Familial non-syndromal thoracic aortic aneurysms and dissections – incidence and family screening outcomes. Int J Cardiol. 2016;25:740–2.
34. Regelado ES, Guo D, Prakash S, Bensend TA, Flynn K, Estrera A, Safi H, Liang D, Hyland J, Child A, Arno G, Boileau C, Jondeau G, Braverman A, Moran R, Morisaki T, Morisaki H, Consortium MA, Pyeritz R, Coselli J, LeMaire S, Milewicz D. Aortic disease presentation and outcome associated with *ACTA2* mutations. Circ Cardiovasc Genet. 2015;8:457–64.
35. Henneton P, Albuisson J, Adham S, Legrand A, Mazzella JM, Jeunemaitre X, Frank M. Accuracy of clinical diagnostic criteria for patients with vascular Ehlers-Danlos syndrome in a tertiary referral Centre. Circ Genom Precis Med. 2019;12:113–20.
36. Vorselaars VMM, Diederick A, Prabhudesai V, Velthuis S, Vos J-A, Snijder RJ, Westermann CJJ, Mulder BJ, Ploos van Amstel JK, Mager JJ, Faughnan ME, Post MC. *SMAD4* gene mutation increases the risk of aortic dilatation in patients with hereditary haemorrhagic telangiectasia. Int J Cardiol. 2017;245:114–8.
37. Berk DR, Bentley DD, Bayliss SJ, Lind A, Urban Z. Cutis laxa: A review. *J Am Acad Dermatol* 2012; 66: 842.e1–17.
38. Szabo Z, Crepeau MW, Mitchell AL, Stephan MJ, Puntel RA, Yin Loke K, Kirk RC, Urban Z. Aortic aneurysmal disease and cutis laxa caused by defect in the elastin gene. J Med Genet. 2006;43:255–8.
39. Coucke PJ, Willaert A, Wessels MW, Callewaert B, Zoppi N, De Backer J, Fox JE, Mancini GMS, Kambouris M, Gardella R, Facchetti F, Willems PJ, Forsyth R, Dietz HC, Barlati S, Colomi M, Loeys B, De Paepe A. Mutations in the facilitative glucose transporter GLUT10 alter angiogenesis and cause arterial tortuosity syndrome. Nat Genet. 2006;38:452–7.

Tuberous Sclerosis Complex: Skin and Heart: Pivotal Common and Early Signs

5

Monika Słowińska, Robert A. Schwartz, and Sergiusz Jóźwiak

Introduction and Pathophysiology

Tuberous sclerosis complex (TSC, Bourneville syndrome) is a genetic neurocutaneous (phakomatosis) disease. It results from a mutation in one of two genes: *TSC1* located on chromosome 9q34 and encoding hamartin or *TSC2* located on chromosome 11p13.3 and encoding tuberin [1, 2]. Hamartin and tuberin form a heterodimer suppressing the mechanistic target of rapamycin (mTOR) pathway, which is responsible for regulating essential cell functions i.e. cell growth and proliferation. Due to a genetic mutation in the *TSC1* or *TSC2* gene, the mTOR pathway is overactivated, resulting in developing multiple tumors (hamartomas) in different organs including skin, heart, brain, kidney, liver, and lungs [1, 2]. Therefore, although TSC is classified as a phakomatosis, it is multi-systemic. However, the clinical presentation and severity of symptoms vary between individuals even among family members.

TSC is a chronic and progressive disease; most of its signs develop with age. The clinical course of TSC includes [1, 2]:

- Epilepsy (70–90%, first seizures usually appear very early, within the first 2 years of life)
- Cognitive impairment (50–60%)
- Autism spectrum disorder and behavioral problems

M. Słowińska · S. Jóźwiak
Department of Child Neurology, Medical University of Warsaw, Warszawa, Poland

R. A. Schwartz (✉)
Dermatology, Pediatric, Medicine, and Pathology, Rutgers New Jersey Medical School, Newark, NJ, USA

C. Salavastru et al. (eds.), *Skin and the Heart*,
https://doi.org/10.1007/978-3-030-54779-0_5

- Brain tumors and abnormalities (cortical dysplasia, subependymal nodules, subependymal giant cell astrocytoma) associated with the risk of epilepsy and hydrocephalus
- Skin manifestations (see Sect. 5. 3)
- Cardiologic manifestations (see Sect. 5. 4)
- Nephrologic manifestations: kidney tumors (angiomyolipomas, renal cancer) and cysts that may result in hemorrhaging and renal failure
- Ophthalmological manifestations: retinal tumors and achromic patches
- Liver tumors (angiomyolipoma)
- Lung lymphangioleiomyomatosis (LAM)

TSC is inherited in an autosomal dominant pattern; however, inherited familial cases are responsible for only 30% of them. In 70% of patients, TSC is caused by *de novo* mutations [1, 2].

Prevalence

It is estimated that TSC affects about 1:6000 to 1:10000 people worldwide [1, 2]. However, due to its variable clinical course including often mild symptomatology and the presence of mosaic forms, the prevalence of TSC may be higher.

Dermatological manifestation

Dermatological manifestations develop in almost all TSC patients and, like other symptoms, they may increase with advancing age.

Hypomelanotic macules (HMs) and "confetti" skin lesions

Hypomelanotic macules are also known as ash-leaf spots or Fitzpatrick patches, and are the earliest detectable and the most common dermatological manifestation of TSC. They may be observed since infancy and are one of the most important signs facilitating early diagnosis of TSC [3]. They are visualized in 90–98% of patients [1]. The presence of at least 3 HMs of a diameter of at least 5 mm is considered a major diagnostic criterion for TSC (Table 5.1) [4].

(a) Clinical [5–8]

HMs are hypopigmented, usually elongated oval or lance-oval shaped spots on the skin asymmetrically distributed mostly on the trunk and buttocks (Figs. 5.1 and 5.2). Polygonal 'thumbprint' shaped HMs may be also observed. The number of HMs may increase with age. They do not cause severe clinical consequences except possible esthetical discomfort.

Table 5.1 Diagnostic criteria for tuberous sclerosis complex [4]

Genetic criteria
Detection of a pathogenic mutation of *TSC1 or TSC2*
Major criteria
Hypomelanotic macules (Fitzpatrick patches) (≥3, at least 5-mm diameter)
Angiofibromas (≥3) or fibrous cephalic plaque
Ungual fibromas (≥2)
Shagreen patch
Multiple retinal hamartomas
Cortical dysplasias (cortical tubers and white matter migration lines)
Subependymal nodules (SEN)
Subependymal giant cell astrocytoma (SEGA)
Cardiac rhabdomyoma
Lymphangioleiomyomatosis (LAM)[a]
Angiomyolipomas (≥2)[a]
Minor criteria
"Confetti" skin lesions
Dental enamel pits (>3)
Intraoral fibromas (≥2)
Retinal achromic patch
Multiple renal cysts
Nonrenal hamartomas
Definite diagnosis: a) detection of a pathogenic mutation (genetic criterion) is sufficient for the diagnosis even in the absence of the clinical features. OR b) 2 major features OR c) 1 major and 2 minor features
Possible diagnosis: either 1 major feature or at least 2 minor.

[a]The presence of LAM and angiomyolipomas without other features does not meet criteria for a definite diagnosis

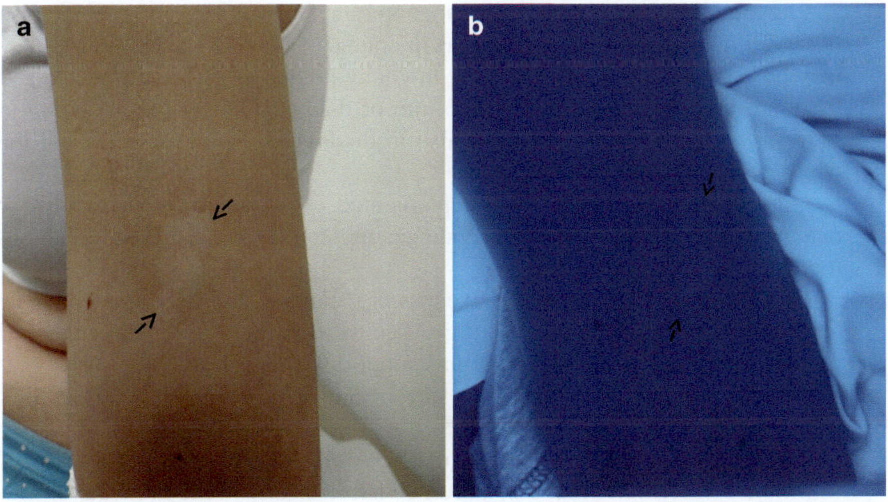

Fig. 5.1 (**a**). Hypomelanotic macule on the arm. (**b**). The same hypomelanotic macule seen in Wood's lamp. Arrows indicate the lesion

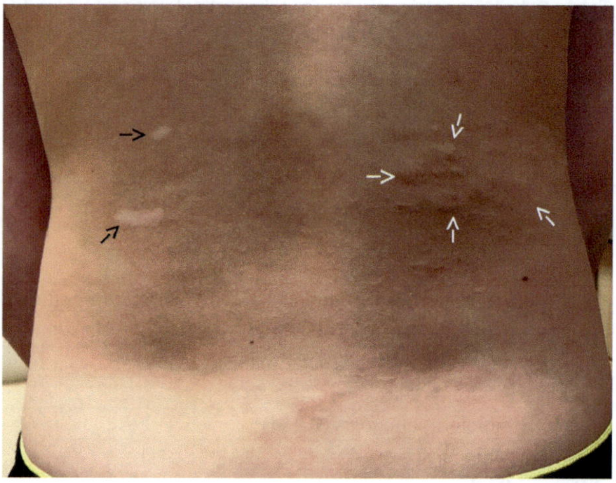

Fig. 5.2 Depigmented spots (black arrows) and shagreen patches (white arrows) in lumbosacral region of a patient with TSC

In some patients smaller so-called *"confetti" lesions* may be also observed. They are a later finding than Fitzpatrick patches and much smaller in size and more numerous, a minor criteria for TSC diagnosis evident as multiple, disseminated hypopigmented tiny macules with a diameter of 1–2 mm, localized mostly on the distal extensive surface of the limbs

(b) Histological [9, 10]

Histochemical and electron microscopic examination revealed that, unlike vitiligo, the number of melanocytes is normal in TSC-associated Fitzpatrick patches. They result from impaired melanogenesis (reduction of the amount of melanin), observed as a reduced and varying number of melanosomes in melanocytes. However, the maturation of melanosomes is normal.

(c) Differential

Fitzpatrick patches are not a pathognomonic sign of TSC and may be also observed in healthy people as well as in course of other diseases. Hence, they may be easily overlooked, especially in young infants. If TSC is suspected and there are less than 3 of them with 5 mm of diameter, careful examination in *Wood's light* should be performed also to distinguish between hypo- and the depigmentation of vitiligo.

Other diseases with localized depigmented or hypopigmented macules or patches in their clinical course include genetic, metabolic, and post-inflammatory etiology i.e.:

- *Vitiligo*—an acquired, progressive loss of melanocytes. There are two types: generalized and segmental vitiligo. Typical distribution, leukotrichia, and associated autoimmune disease may support this diagnosis [6]
- *Halo nevi*—a melanocytic nevus surrounded by a depigmented circle. It is often associated with vitiligo [6].
- *Nevus depigmentosus*—is an irregular but well-defined lesion of several centimeters in diameter that may become visible mostly in the first year of life. They result from cutaneous mosaicism. Some authors distinguish three sub-

types of the nevi depigmentosi: isolated (localized), segmental, and systematized (usually following the Blaschko lines) forms [11].

- *Hypomelanosis of Ito (HOI)*—is also caused by cutaneous mosaicism. Some authors include HOI as a systematized type of the nevus depigmentosus associated with seizures, developmental delay, and eyes and bones abnormalities. The hypopigmentation usually occurs within the first year of life and may be seen as patches, streaks or spiral-shaped areas [11].
- *Post-inflammatory hypopigmentation* (i.e. pityriasis alba, pityriasis versicolor alba, pityriasis lichenoides chronic, lichen striatus, viral infections, insects bites, burns) [6]
- *Piebaldism*—a rare, autosomal dominant disorder characterized by congenital, extensive, symmetric depigmentation. Hair, eyebrows, and eyelashes may be also affected. Lesions are usually significantly more extensive in comparison to these in TSC [6].
- *Waardenburg syndrome*—a rare autosomal dominant disorder associated with deafness and defects of the structures formed from neural crest involving melanocytes [6].

Questions about the age of onset (congenital or acquired Fitzpatrick patches), diffuse or localized involvement, family history, progressive vs stable course, distribution pattern (including distribution following Blaschko lines), shape, associated symptoms or disorders, and the examination with a *Wood's lamp* may be helpful in a differential diagnosis.

Facial angiofibroma (AF)

Facial angiofibromas (AF, previously unproperly called adenoma sebaceum) are one of the most prominent skin lesions in TSC. They usually appear between the second and fifth years of life and are observed in about 70–75% of patients [5, 10]. At least 3 facial AFs are included as a major diagnostic criterion for TSC (Table 5.1) [4]. The name *adenoma sebaceum* is historic; they are not sebaceous adenomas.

(a) Clinical [5, 12]

AFs appear as raised, pink or red-brown papulonodules usually located symmetrically on the face, mostly on the nose and adjacent part of the cheeks nasolabially, and on the chin. Initially they are small, only a few millimeters. However, if untreated, they enlarge with age, especially during the puberty.

Due to the localization and appearance, AF may cause esthetical discomfort and, therefore, psychosocial problems, including anxiety and reduced self-esteem. Extensive AF may cause bleeding or obstructed nasal breathing.

(b) Histological [13]

Histologically AF is a hamartoma of connective tissue and vessels. In microscopic examination, they consist of collagenous stroma with increased spindled to stellate fibroblasts and dilated blood vessels.

(c) Differential [11]

Differential diagnosis should include:

- *Acne vulgaris* - AF, especially in adolescents, may be easily mistaken with *acne vulgaris*.
- *Other benign appendageal tumors* such as trichoepitheliomas
- *Verruca plana* - flat, grayish-yellow, possibly hyperpigmented, and slightly elevated papules of a few millimeters in diameter, due to a human papillomavirus infection.
- *Syringomas* - multiple small, skin-colored to yellow, rounded or flat-topped papules located on the eyelids and cheeks.
- *Basal cell nevus syndrome (Gorlin syndrome)*—a rare genetic syndrome associated with early development of basal cell carcinoma, palmar or plantar pits, skeletal anomalies, facial dysmorphism, and eye anomalies [14–17].
- *Birt-Hogg*-Dube *syndrome*—a rare genetic disorder characterized by the development of multiple benign tumors of the face, neck, and chest, pulmonary cysts and the predisposition for neoplasms, especially renal carcinoma [15].

Fibrous cephalic plaques

Fibrous cephalic plaques are considered as a larger variant of angiofibromas. They can occur at any age and are present in about 20% of TSC patients [16].

(a) Clinical [5, 16]

They appear as raised, firm, flesh-colored or yellow-brown plaques of different shapes that may slowly grow from few millimeters up to several centimeters. They are usually located on the forehead or scalp.

(b) Histological [5, 16]

Fibrous cephalic plaques are histologically classified as angiofibromas, although they tend to have a less pronounced vascular component.

(c) Differentiation

Similar to the differentiation of facial angiofibroma (see Sect. 5. 3. 2), although some fibrous cephalic plaques may resemble scars.

Shagreen patches

Shagreen patches are a type of connective tissue nevus [5, 16, 17]. They are present in about 50% of patients with TSC. Usually, they appear in the first decade of life.

(a) Clinical [5, 16, 17]

They are raised, pink to yellow-brown or skin-colored plaques and orange peel-like in touch located mostly on the back and lumbosacral region but rarely may appear also on the chest or abdomen (Fig. 5.2). In the beginning, they may be small, about few millimeters, but may grow with time to large, irregular lesions. Lesions that are smaller than 1 cm are termed collagenomas. The long axis of shagreen patches tends to fall along Langer lines.

(b) Histological [17]

Microscopic examination reveals increased in number but thickened, disorganized collagen bundles in the reticular dermis and decreased elastin fibers.

(c) Differential

In most patients with TSC, a biopsy may not be required if other characteristic signs of TSC are present. However, in some with suspected TSC, biopsy of the lesion may be helpful in a differential diagnosis that should include:

- *Collagenomas* associated with different diseases (e.g. *Familial cutaneous collagenoma, multiple endocrine neoplasia type 1 (MEN1), Birt-Hogg-Dubé syndrome*).
- *Buschke Ollendorff Syndrome*—a genetic condition characterized by osteopoikilosis and connective tissue nevi. However, in comparison to TSC, skin lesions are usually more yellow, located on the abdomen, chest, limbs and occur in greater number [15, 17].
- *Elastomas of other etiologies*
- *Scars*

Non-traumatic periungual fibromas (Koenen tumors)

Periungual or subungual fibromas, also called *Koenen tumors*, are tumors observed in about 15–80% of patients with TSC [2]. They develop usually in older patients (early adolescence and adulthood) and more often in women than men [1, 2, 5, 16].

(a) Clinical [5, 16]

Koenen tumors are red to skin-colored, firm tumors appearing near the proximal nail fold, more often of the toenails than fingernails (Fig. 5.3). They usually measure 1–5 mm; larger lesions may be easily injured, causing bleeding, pain, and discomfort. They can cause a groove and deformations of the nails.

(b) Histological [18]

Periungual fibromas are compound of stellate-shaped fibroblasts, vertically oriented collagen, and blood vessels. The proportion of vascular and fibrotic components differs between lesions. Elastic fibers are decreased.

(c) Differential

Non-traumatic periungual fibromas are highly associated with TSC, but have to be differentiated from i.e.:

- *Traumatic periungual fibromas*
- *Viral warts*
- *Superficial Acral (Digital) Fibromyxoma*
- *Keloid*

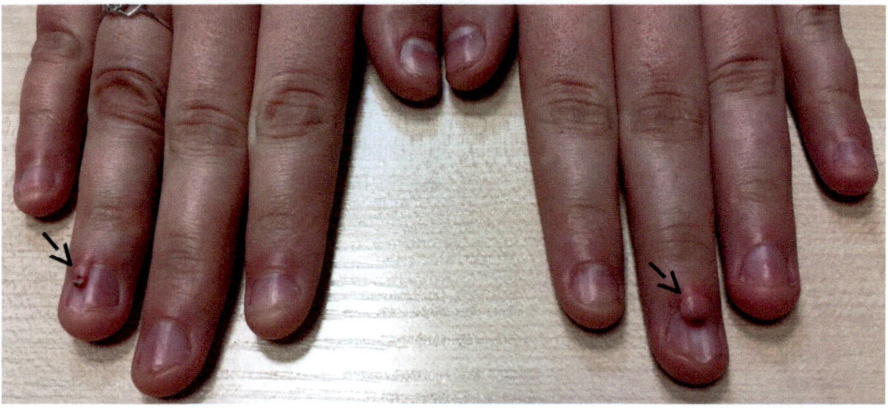

Fig. 5.3 Periungual fibromas

Cardiologic manifestations

(a) Clinical

Cardiac manifestations of TSC include single or multiple cardiac tumors, which are the earliest detectable sign of TSC and may be documented prenatally [3, 19]. Histologically these tumors are benign rhabdomyomas. They usually are located in the ventricles, rarely in the atria (Fig. 5.4) [20].

They are included in the major diagnostic criteria of TSC (Table 5.1) [4]. Multiple cardiac tumors are highly associated with TSC (in about 95%) and may be considered as a clinical biomarker of TSC [19]. However, the presence of a single tumor does not exclude the disease, as about 23–73% of patients with single rhabdomyomas have TSC [19, 21, 22], recalling that cardiac rhabdomyomas are the most frequent pediatric cardiac tumors and may be the earliest detectable sign of TSC.

Unlike the other TSC signs, cardiac tumors usually tend to spontaneously decrease or regress over time. Therefore, their incidence is reduced over time from about 90% in infants to 20% in adults [2]. However, sometimes they may regrow during the adolescence [20].

(b) Investigations

Cardiac tumors, the earliest detectable TSC sign, may be revealed prenatally in fetal echocardiography from 20–22 weeks gestational age onward [3]. They should be monitored during the pregnancy due to their tendency to increase in the third trimester and become a rare cause of cardiac arrhythmia, hydrops fetalis or effusive pericarditis [19].

Although in most cases these tumors do not cause any clinical symptoms, they are the most frequent cause of death in TSC children below 10 years old [23]. Hence, they should be monitored after birth by regular echocardiographic examination with heart function and rhythm assessed, as in some cases these tumors may result in heart failure and cardiac arrhythmias.

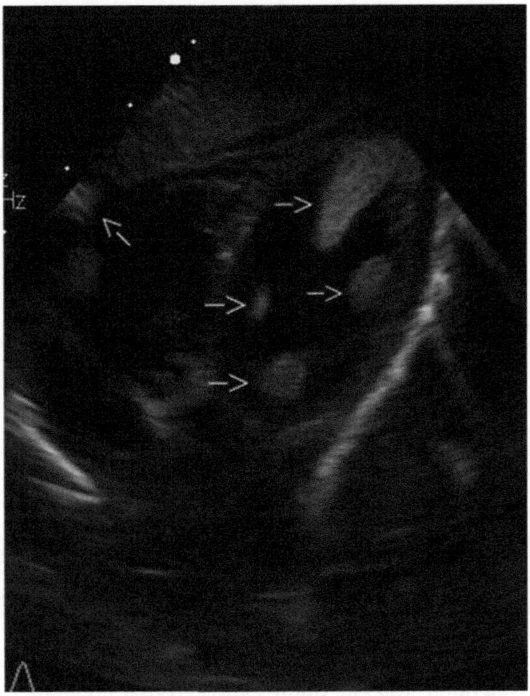

Fig. 5.4 Multiple cardiac rhabdomyomas

Rhabdomyomas are the most common congenital cardiac tumors (40–60%) [24]. However, they should be differentiated with other, especially congenital, heart tumors like teratoma, fibroma, and hemangioma. Myxoma is rare in neonates but more frequent in adults. Echocardiography or heart magnetic resonance imaging (MRI) and the presence of other signs of TSC may facilitate diagnosis. Tumor biopsy with histological assessment is rarely conducted with rhabdomyomas, although histology remains the gold standard for confirmation of this diagnosis [24].

Diagnosis

A diagnosis of TSC is based on diagnostic criteria presented in Table 5.1 [4]. In most cases, a diagnosis is established based on the clinical manifestations. For TSC diagnosis the presence of two major or one major with two minor signs is required. However, one of the difficulties in establishing a TSC diagnosis is a variable clinical presentation and the possibility of the occurrence of signs with advancing age, even if they are not observed at the moment of examination. However, since 2012, a detection of a pathogenic mutation in *TSC1* or *TSC2* is sufficient for the diagnosis even if clinical signs are not prominent. Genetic test detects the mutation in about 90% of patients [3].

Dermatological manifestations may be diagnosed by careful skin examination with aid of a *Wood's lamp*. The presence of other, non-skin manifestations of TSC, history of seizures, and cognitive impairment may facilitate diagnosis.

Cardiac tumors may be detected by pre- or postnatal echocardiography. Children with TSC also require assessment of heart rhythm by electrocardiogram (ECG) or Holter-ECG.

As cardiac tumors are the earliest detectable TSC sign, all children with prenatally detected heart tumors should undergo fetal MRI that in about 2/3 of patients may reveal characteristic brain lesions and confirm a diagnosis. Children with diagnosed or suspected TSC should be referred to a center specialized in the management of TSC, so that a diagnostic workup can be implemented including brain MRI, careful skin examination, echocardiography, abdominal ultrasonography or MRI and ophthalmological evaluation [3].

Treatment

There is no cure for TSC. Patients with TSC require multidisciplinary health care including evaluation by a neurologist, nephrologist, cardiologist, dermatologist, and psychologist [3]. As epilepsy occurs in the vast majority of patients, antiepileptic treatment is necessary in most cases. Rehabilitation and cognitive support are also beneficial. Recent studies showed that epileptic changes on electroencephalography (EEG) precede clinical seizures in TSC patients and early, preventative antiepileptic treatment initiated when ictal discharges are detected on EEG, but before clinical seizures, may improve a neurological and cognitive outcome [25]. Therefore, due to the high risk of developing epilepsy, in all children below 2 years of age, regular electroencephalographic studies (EEG) should be performed every 4 weeks within the first 6 months of life and every 6 weeks thereafter [3]. An early, preventative, antiepileptic treatment with vigabatrin should be considered within first 24 months of life if epileptic discharges occur on EEG record, even without clinical seizures [25, 26].

TSC results from overactivation of the mTOR pathway. Hence the mTOR inhibitors (sirolimus, everolimus) are employed in the therapy. However, as they are immunosuppressive drugs and may cause some side effects, their use is currently recommended to treat growing brain (subependymal giant cell astrocytoma) and kidneys (angiomyolipoma) tumors, lymphangioleiomyomatosis, and some dermatological lesions [27]. However, their antiepileptic properties were also reported [28].

Sometimes surgical treatment is also necessary to treat e.g. subependymal giant cell astrocytoma causing obstructive hydrocephalus, hemorrhagic angiomyolipomas, drug-resistant epilepsy or some dermatological lesions.

Treatment of dermatological manifestations

Most of the dermatological manifestations do not cause clinical symptoms. However, they may result in an esthetical discomfort and associated psychological and sociological problems. Periungual fibromas can be easily injured, causing bleeding and pain. Therefore, sometimes treatment is required, especially of facial angiofibromas and larger periungual fibromas. Regular dermatological assessment is recommended; however, the interval between visits depends on the manifestations in an individual patient.

According to the current recommendation of surveillance and management of TSC, including dermatological aspects, some treatment methods are recommended [29–31]:

1. *Sun protection*—as hypomelanotic macules are prone to sunburn and sun exposition and ultraviolet (UV) radiation may exacerbate especially angiofibromas, it is important to instruct the patient to use a cream with UV-filter during the spring and summer [29–31].
2. *Topical mTOR inhibitors (sirolimus, everolimus)*—topical use of an ointment with sirolimus was reported as beneficial, especially for *angiofibromas*—it decreased the size of the lesions and erythema, sometimes resulted in the almost complete resolution [31, 32]. Therapy for AFs is more effective for smaller ones and in younger patients. Therefore, it should be implemented in the early stages of angiofibromas. However, they may re-grow after the discontinuation of the therapy.

For *fibrous cephalic plaques,* an improvement after the use of 1% local sirolimus was reported in 50% of patients [33].

Although *hypomelanotic macule*s usually do not require treatment, the topical mTOR inhibitors may also improve them. Therefore, a therapy may be considered when they located on the face [7, 32].

On the other hand, treatment of *shagreen patches* and *periungual fibromas* with topical sirolimus was less effective. Nevertheless, it may be considered as an option when lesions require treatment and other therapies cannot be used [32, 33].

Topical use of mTOR inhibitors is characterized by a good safety profile and adverse effects are usually not severe, such as mild skin irritation. Moreover, in conducted studies, a blood concentration of sirolimus was undetectable [7, 29, 33]. However, at present, there is no standard dose of sirolimus or everolimus for topical use or optimal base for the ointment. Most studies reported the use of the ointment or gel with a concentration of sirolimus of 0,1–1% [31–33]. A lipid base is preferred considering lipophilic properties of sirolimus.

1. *Systemic mTOR inhibitors*—are currently recommended to treat subependymal giant cell astrocytomas, renal angiomyolipomas, and lymphangioleiomyomatosis. Although skin lesions may improve, systemic therapy with mTOR inhibitors for dermatological manifestations as the only indication is not recommended due to the risk of adverse effects and unfavorable benefit-risk ratio [27, 29]. However, in case of extensive skin lesions causing medical risks, such as extensive angiofibromas resulting in bleeding or obstructed nasal breathing that cannot be treated surgically, a systemic mTOR inhibitor may be an option [29].
2. *Surgical treatment*—may be a therapeutic option for e.g. facial *angiofibromas* or *periungual fibromas*, especially in case of bleeding, pain, impaired function (e.g. obstruction of nasal breathing), irritation, and disfigurement [29, 30].

Laser therapy—pulse-dye laser with or without 5-aminolevulinic acid blue light photodynamic therapy has been recommended to treat flat *angiofibromas* in preschool and school-aged children [30]. Ablative lasers may be an option in the adolescence. However, laser therapy is associated with a risk of hypo- or hyperpigmentation, scarring, cobblestone skin and re-growth of the lesions [29].

Other surgical methods include: shave excision, dermabrasion, electrosurgery, and cryosurgery.

Nevertheless, currently, there is insufficient data to recommend a particular treatment option for dermatological lesions [27].

Treatment of cardiologic manifestation

Cardiac tumors usually do not require treatment, as they rarely cause clinical symptoms and tend to regress over time [34]. However, in some patients, they may result in cardiac arrhythmias, heart failure or even sudden death [19, 20]. Therefore, anti-arrhythmic drugs or surgical treatment may be required in some patients. There are also case reports of the use of mTOR inhibitors to treat and promote natural regression of cardiac rhabdomyoma in TSC infants, which may be an option to support an anti-arrhythmic treatment and as an alternative to the surgery [35].

Prognosis

One of the most deteriorating comorbidity in daily life for TSC patients and families is epilepsy, which affects 70–90% of patients and is associated with seizures and cognitive impairment. However, recent studies have suggested that early, preventative antiepileptic treatment in TSC children, before clinical seizures, may improve neurological and cognitive outcome by decreasing the number of children with epilepsy and developmental delay [25].

Some of the dermatological manifestations tend to progress with advancing age but usually do not cause severe clinical consequences, except possible esthetical discomfort that may result in lower self-esteem and depression, especially related to facial angiofibromas. Fortunately, topical use of mTOR inhibitors is effective in the treatment of AF.

In most cases, a prognosis of cardiological manifestations of TSC is good. In most patients, cardiac tumors are asymptomatic and tend to decrease or even regress over time. However, they may re-growth during the adolescence. Therefore, TSC patients also require cardiological surveillance.

References

1. Curatolo P, Bombardieri R, Jóźwiak S. Tuberous Sclerosis. Lancet. 2008;372(9639):657–68. https://doi.org/10.1016/S0140-6736(08)61279-9.
2. Henske EP, Jóźwiak S, Kingswood JC, et al. Tuberous Sclerosis Complex. Nat Rev Dis Primers 26;2:16035. 2016; https://doi.org/10.1038/nrdp.2016.35.

3. Słowińska M, Jóźwiak S, Peron A, et al. Early diagnosis of tuberous sclerosis complex: a race against time. How to make the diagnosis before seizures? Orphanet J Rare Dis. 2018;13(1):25. https://doi.org/10.1186/s13023-018-0764-z.
4. Northrup H, Krueger DA, International Tuberous Sclerosis Complex Consensus Group. Tuberous sclerosis complex diagnostic criteria update: recommendations of the 2012 International Tuberous Sclerosis Complex Consensus Conference. Pediatr Neurol. 2013;49(4):243–54. https://doi.org/10.1016/j.pediatrneurol.2013.08.001.
5. Cardis MA, DeKlotz CMC. Cutaneous manifestations of tuberous sclerosis complex and the paediatrician's role. Arch Dis Child. 2017;102(9):858–63. https://doi.org/10.1136/archdischild-2016-312001.
6. van Geel N, Speeckaert M, Chevolet I, et al. Hypomelanoses in children. J Cutan Aesthet Surg. 2013;6(2):65–72. https://doi.org/10.4103/0974-2077.112665.
7. Lee BW, Schwartz RA, Hercogová J, et al. Vitiligo road map. Dermatol Ther. 2012;25(Suppl 1):44–56. https://doi.org/10.1111/dth.12006.
8. Schwartz RA, Fernández G, Kotulska K, et al. Tuberous sclerosis complex: advances in diagnosis, genetics, and management. J Am Acad Dermatol. 2007;57:189–202.
9. Wataya-Kaneda M, Tanaka M, Yang L, et al. Clinical and Histologic Analysis of the Efficacy of Topical Rapamycin Therapy Against Hypomelanotic Macules in Tuberous Sclerosis Complex. JAMA Dermatol. 2015;151(7):722–30. https://doi.org/10.1001/jamadermatol.2014.4298.
10. Fitzpatrick TB, Szabó G, Hori Y, et al. White Leaf-Shaped Macules Earliest Visible Sign of Tuberous Sclerosis. Arch Dermatol. 1968;98(1):1–6.
11. Ullah F, Schwartz RA. Nevus depigmentosus: a mark of distinction. Int J Dermatol. 2019; https://doi.org/10.1111/ijd.14393.
12. Józwiak S, Schwartz RA, Janniger CK, et al. Usefulness of diagnostic criteria of tuberous sclerosis complex in pediatric patients. J Child Neurol. 2000;15(10):652–9.
13. Elwood HR. Angiofibroma. 2016. PathologyOutlines.com. http://www.pathologyoutlines.com/topic/skintumornonmelanocyticangiofibroma.html. Accessed 2 Feb 2019.
14. John A, Schwartz RA. Basal cell naevus syndrome: an update on genetics and treatment. Br J Dermatol. 2016;174:68–76. https://doi.org/10.1111/bjd.14206.
15. Orphanet. Rare Disease Platform. 2019. Paris. https://www.orpha.net Accessed 2 Feb 2019.
16. Jóźwiak S, Schwartz RA, Janniger CK, et al. Skin lesions in children with tuberous sclerosis complex: their prevalence, natural course, and diagnostic significance. Int J Dermatol. 1998;37(12):911–7.
17. Bongiorno MA, Nathan N, Oyerinde O, et al. Clinical characteristics of connective tissue nevi in tuberous sclerosis complex with special emphasis on shagreen patches. JAMA Dermatol. 2017;153(7):660–5. https://doi.org/10.1001/jamadermatol.2017.0298.
18. Ma D, Darling T, Moss J, et al. Histologic Variants of Periungual Fibromas in Tuberous Sclerosis Complex. J Am Acad Dermatol. 2011;64(2):442–4.
19. Słowińska M, Kotulska-Jóźwiak K, Sadowski K, et al. Multiple cardiac tumours as a biomarker of tuberous sclerosis complex in children below two years of age. Pediatr Pol. 2018;94(2):137–43. https://doi.org/10.5114/polp.2018.76248.
20. Jóźwiak S, Kotulska K, Kasprzyk-Obara J, et al. Clinical and genotype studies of cardiac tumors in 154 patients with tuberous sclerosis complex. Pediatrics. 2006;118(4):e1146–51.
21. Tworetzky W, McElhinney DB, Margossian R, et al. Association between cardiac tumors and tuberous sclerosis in the fetus and neonate. Am J Cardiol. 2003;92(4):487–9.
22. Sciacca P, Giacchi V, Mattia C, et al. Rhabdomyomas and tuberous sclerosis complex: our experience in 33 cases. BMC Cardiovasc Disord. 2014;9(14):66. https://doi.org/10.1186/1471-2261-14-66.
23. Shepherd CW, Gomez MR, Lie JT, et al. Causes of death in patients with tuberous sclerosis. Mayo Clin Proc. 1991;66(8):792–6.
24. Uzun O, Wilson DG, Vujanic GM, et al. Cardiac tumours in children. Orphanet J Rare Dis. 2007;1(2):11.
25. Jóźwiak S, Kotulska K, Domańska-Pakieła D, et al. Antiepileptic treatment before the onset of seizures reduces epilepsy severity and risk of mental retardation in infants with tuber-

ous sclerosis complex. Eur J Paediatr Neurol. 2011;15(5):424–31. https://doi.org/10.1016/j.ejpn.2011.03.010.
26. Curatolo P, Nabbout R, Lagae L, et al. Management of epilepsy associated with tuberous sclerosis complex: Updated clinical recommendations. Eur J Paediatr Neurol. 2018;22(5):738–48. https://doi.org/10.1016/j.ejpn.2018.05.006.
27. Krueger DA, Northrup H, International Tuberous Sclerosis Complex Consensus Group. Tuberous sclerosis complex surveillance and management: recommendations of the 2012 International Tuberous Sclerosis Complex Consensus Conference. Pediatr Neurol. 2013;49(4):255–65. https://doi.org/10.1016/j.pediatrneurol.2013.08.002.
28. French JA, Lawson JA, Yapici Z, et al. Adjunctive everolimus therapy for treatment-resistant focal-onset seizures associated with tuberous sclerosis (EXIST-3): a phase 3, randomised, double-blind, placebo-controlled study. Lancet. 2016;388:2153–63. https://doi.org/10.1016/S0140-6736(16)31419-2.
29. Teng JM, Cowen EW, Wataya-Kaneda M, et al. Dermatologic and dental aspects of the 2012 International Tuberous Sclerosis Complex Consensus Statements. JAMA Dermatol. 2014;150(10):1095–101. https://doi.org/10.1001/jamadermatol.2014.938.
30. Janniger CK, Goldberg DJ. Angiofibromas in tuberous sclerosis: comparison of treatment by carbon dioxide and argon laser. J Dermatol Surg Oncol. 1990;16:317–20.
31. Koenig MK, Bell CS, Hebert AA, et al. Efficacy and safety of topical rapamycin in patients with facial angiofibromas secondary to tuberous sclerosis complex: the TREATMENT randomized clinical trial. TREATMENT Trial Collaborators. JAMA Dermatol. 2018;154:773–80. https://doi.org/10.1001/jamadermatol.2018.0464.
32. Jóźwiak S, Sadowski K, Kotulska K, et al. Topical use of mammalian target of rapamycin (mTOR) inhibitors in tuberous sclerosis complexd a comprehensive review of the literature. Pediatr Neurol. 2016;61:21–7. https://doi.org/10.1016/j.pediatrneurol.2016.04.003.
33. Malissen N, Vergely L, Simon M, et al. Long-term treatment of cutaneous manifestations of tuberous sclerosis complex with topical 1% sirolimus cream: A prospective study of 25 patients. J Am Acad Dermatol. 2017;77(3):464–472.e3. https://doi.org/10.1016/j.jaad.2017.04.005.
34. Lucchesi M, Chiappa E, Giordano F, et al. Sirolimus in infants with multiple cardiac rhabdomyomas associated with tuberous sclerosis complex. Case Rep Oncol. 2018;11(2):425–30. https://doi.org/10.1159/000490662.
35. Dhulipudi B, Bhakru S, Rajan S, et al. Symptomatic improvement using everolimus in infants with cardiac rhabdomyoma. Ann Pediatr Cardiol. 2019;12:45–8. https://doi.org/10.4103/apc.APC_79_18.

Incontinentia Pigmenti

6

Elena Chiticariu and Daniel Hohl

Introduction and Pathophysiology

Incontinentia pigmenti (IP; synonym: Bloch-Sulzberger syndrome, OMIM #308300) is an X-linked dominant multisystem genodermatosis lethal in XY males. The name describes the main pathological finding of pigmentary incontinence in the third stage of the disease. IP associates linear skin lesions and anomalies of the teeth, hair and nails. More than 30% of cases present ocular and neurological manifestations. A minority of cases with cardiac impairment have been reported.

IP is characterized by a high genetic penetrance and variable phenotypic expressivity while environmental factors do not appear to impinge on the phenotype. Most cases are sporadic; only 10–25% of cases are familial. IP is caused by loss-of-function mutations in the IKBKG gene (NEMO, nuclear factor-kappa B essential modulator; OMIM #300248) located on the chromosome Xq28. More than 80% of mutations are deletions of exons 4 to 10 leading to the complete loss of NEMO/IKKγ protein, a subunit of the inhibitor of the IKK complex involved in the activation of the NF-kB pathway, which protects against TNFα-induced apoptosis. The remaining cases show microdeletions, missense, nonsense, frameshift and splice-site mutations [1, 2].

Absence of NEMO explains a pro-apoptotic state translated by the destruction of epidermal cells. In the absence of NF-kB protective activity, endothelial cells undergo apoptosis and over-express chemotactic factors specific for eosinophils leading to hypereosinophilia (found in the blood and skin lesions), and extensive inflammation. NEMO deficiency also leads to loss of endothelial cells and thus vasculopathy and ischemia, causing ophthalmologic and neurologic abnormalities. They are related to disruption of TAK1 (Transforming growth factor beta-activated kinase 1), a kinase upstream of NEMO [3]. Small vessel occlusion generates

E. Chiticariu · D. Hohl (✉)
Service of Dermatology and Venerology, CHUV, FBM-UNIL, Lausanne, Switzerland
e-mail: elena.chiticariu@chuv.ch; daniel.hohl@chuv.ch

C. Salavastru et al. (eds.), *Skin and the Heart*,
https://doi.org/10.1007/978-3-030-54779-0_6

underperfusion, precipitating ischemia. Secondary neovascularization results in additional damage. Pulmonary hypertension has also been related to vasculopathy [4, 5].

Prevalence

Incidence of IP is estimated at 1/143,000 births by orphanet with a female to male ratio of 20:1 It shows variable heterozygous mosaicism, explained by the random inactivation of the chromosome X (lyonization) [6]. By definition, most patients are females. IP is lethal in most males during foetal life. Exceptionally, males with somatic mosaicism or XXY karyotype survive [7].

Dermatological Manifestation

Clinical manifestation Skin changes in IP represent the major findings and evolve through 4 stages.

Stage 1 (vesiculobullous) appears at birth or within the first two weeks of live as tense vesicles, pustules or papules on an erythematous base. The lesions show a linear distribution along the Blaschko lines and thus respect the midline (Fig. 6.1a). They occur anywhere on the body but more on trunk and extremities, sparing the face. Each crop of blisters clears within a few weeks. Complete blood count shows marked leucocytosis with up to 65% eosinophils. In 5% of cases, the vesicular stage is thought to occur in utero before birth [8].

In **stage 2 (verrucous),** the lesions become verrucous, wart-like streaks (between 2 to 6 weeks of age), usually found on distal limbs (Fig. 6.1b). Sometimes this stage gets unnoticed. The verrucous streaks clear completely by age of 6 months, being progressively replaced by lines of reticulated hyperpigmentation.

Stage 3 (pigmentary) is the hallmark of IP but its extent is variable. The hyperpigmentation varies from few lesions to extensive skin involvement. The hyperpigmentary streaks appear sometimes directly after disappearance of blisters and

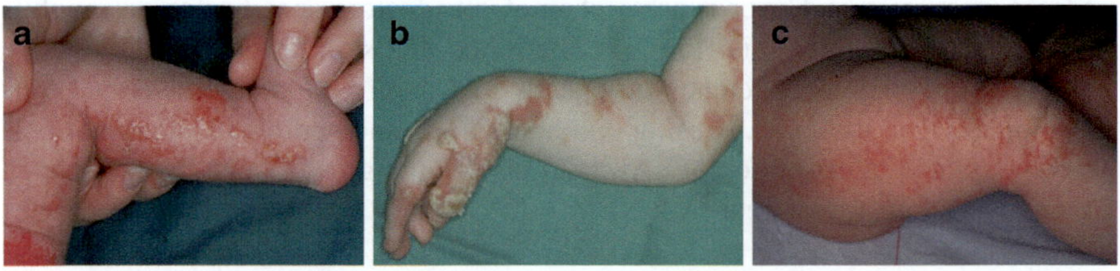

Fig. 6.1 Skin abnormalities in IP: (**a**) vesiculobullous stage: blisters and vesicles on an erythematous base showing a linear distribution on the leg of a new born female; (**b**) verrucous stage: verrucous lesions on a erythematous base on the hand; (**c**) pigmentary stage: the erythematous lesions become progressively hyperpigmented

become progressively darker (Fig. 6.1c). They develop at around 3 months of age and persist usually until early adolescence or adulthood, when they fade slowly and resolve completely by the age of 16. Rarely, lesions persist indefinitely, usually in the groins.

Stage 4 (atrophic/hypopigmented) is characterised by linear macules or patches slightly atrophic and hypopigmented, lacking hair follicles and sweat glands, typically observed on lower legs. They often present before the hyperpigmentation completely disappears. Stage 4 is absent in many patients [9].

IP associates multisystem ectodermal abnormalities which can be present shortly after birth or during childhood [10]. Skin appendages are commonly affected. More than half of patients present hair abnormalities. Cicatricial alopecia on the vertex is seen after the resolution of the blisters but is usually mild and often goes unnoticed, but few patients suffer from severe segmental hair loss. Decreased hair density in children is common. More rarely woolly hair can be identified. Nail dystrophy is found in 40% of patients and ranges from transverse or longitudinal striation and pitting to onychogryphosis and nail disruption. Painful subungual dyskeratotic tumours can be rarely present in adult patients and sometimes are associated with bone deformities of the underlying phalanges [11]. Oral manifestations are found in up to 80% of patients and are characterised by delayed dentition, ano-or hypodontia, conical teeth but also cleft palate, high-arched palate, micrognatia, prognatia or decreased salivary secretion. The dental changes range from mild to severe and occur in 65% of cases [9, 12].

Extracutaneous manifestations include neurologic symptoms in 30% of cases, such as lethargy, seizures and delayed development, associated with local inflammation, ischemia and haemorrhage in the brain [13]. Ocular findings (retinal and non-retinal findings) are common and include proliferative retinopathy, microaneurysms or macular disease [14]. Detachment of the retina and development of vascular retroretineal membrane are common ocular findings, but cataract, nystagmus and optic atrophy were also identified. Skeletal and breast abnormalities may be present [9, 15].

Distinct subtypes. Anhidrotic ectodermal dysplasia associated with immunodeficiency (EDA-ID) is a newly recognized syndrome caused by mutations of the same gene. While the classical IP form is due to amorphic (loss of function) mutations of the IKBKG gene, EDA-ID is induced by milder mutations (hypomorphic) reducing, but not abolishing, NF-kB activation. EDA-ID patients are always males with hemizygous IKBKG mutations. Patients show typical EDA defects (conical teeth, absence of sweat glands, sparse hair, frontal bossing) and a severe immunodeficiency in early childhood. Half of the children die due to severe bacterial infections [16]. Classical IP patients do not show immunodeficiency but a few cases of female patients with **IP and immunodeficiency** have been reported, due to a hypomorphic IKBKG mutation and a delay in X-inactivation skewing [17–19].

Histology. The most specific histological image is obtained in the early inflammatory stage (vesiculobullous), showing spongiosis with intraepidermal vesicles containing eosinophils, and scattered apoptotic keratinocytes (Fig. 6.2). The verrucous stage shows acanthosis with hyperkeratosis and dyskeratosic foci. In the

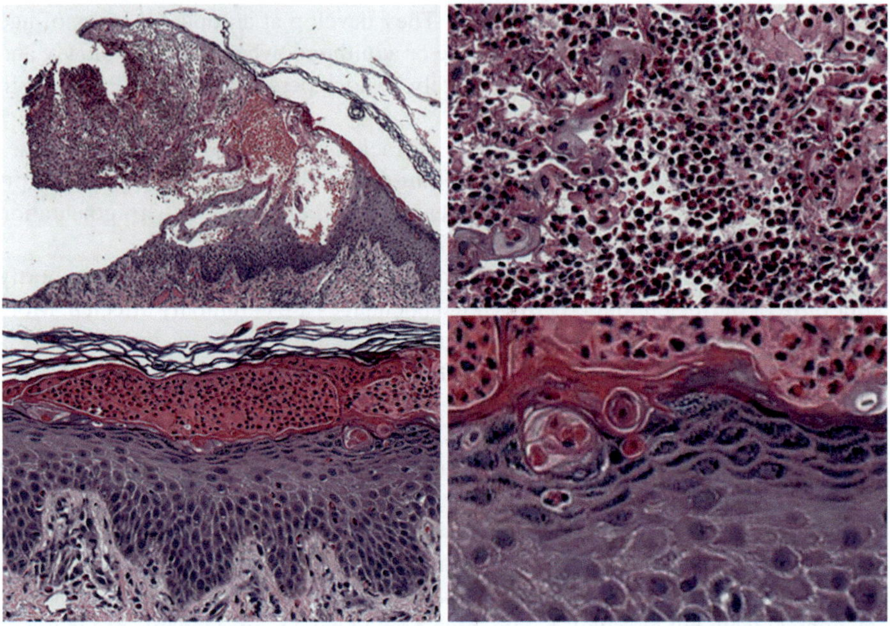

Fig. 6.2 Histology of IP: inflammatory stage, showing spongiosis with intraepidermal vesicles containing a massive eosinophilic infiltrate and scattered apoptotic keratinocytes

hyperpigmented stage the main finding is the pigmentary incontinence, while the fourth stage shown a thin epidermis and the absence of the skin appendages.

Differential diagnosis. IP in the early stage should be differentiated by **infectious diseases** (herpes simplex, varicella, staphylococcal infection) by performing Tznack smears, PCR for HSV and/or Varicella-Zoster virus and bacterial cultures. Differentiation from an **epidermal nevus** in the second stage is done by biopsy. The third stage should be distinguished from **hypomelanosis of Ito (pigmentary mosaicism)**, a skin condition characterized by linear hypo- or hyperpigmentation along the Blaschko lines, not preceded by inflammation. 30% of patients with hypomelanosis of Ito present brain or musculoskeletal abnormalities [20]. **Naegeli-Franceschetti-Jadassohn** syndrome is an autosomal dominant disorder characterized by reticulated hyperpigmentation in association with palmo-plantar keratoderma and hypohidrosis [21] (Table 6.1).

Cardiological Manifestations

Few cases of IP have been reported in association with cardiopulmonary abnormalities, notably a primary pulmonary hypertension (PHTN) of variable severity. Pulmonary hypertension was reported in nine children worldwide [4, 15, 22–28]. The infants develop PHTN shortly after birth, leading to respiratory distress with cyanoses and diminished consciousness, necessitating neonatal intensive care with intubation and mechanical ventilation. Cardiac anomalies such as tricuspid valve

Table 6.1 Differential diagnosis of IP

Stage	Clinical finding	Differential diagnosis
Stage 1 (vesiculobullous)	Vesicles and/or pustules on erythematous base	Impetigo Herpes simplex Varicella
Stage 2 (verrucous)	Wart-like streaks	Linear epidermal nevus X-linked-dominant chondrodysplasia punctate Warts Molluscum contagiosum
Stage 3 (pigmentary)	Hyperpigmentation	Hypomelanosis of Ito Pigmentary mosaicism Naegeli-Franceschetti-Jadassohn syndrome
Stage 4 (atrophic/ hypopigmented)	Hypopigmentation and atrophy	Vitiligo Ectodermal dysplasia

insufficiency, abnormal shunt of the right pulmonary artery to superior vena cava, right ventricular hypertrophy, dilated right ventricle, patent foramen ovale or atrial sept defect, and in most cases neurological and ophthalmological abnormalities are associated [4].

Independent of PHTN, a case of a 32-year old female with IP complicated with endomyocardial fibrosis [27] and tetralogy of Fallot in a 5-year old boy associating IP and a trisomy 14 mosaicism [26] were reported. A case of IP associated with congenital absence of portal vein system and nodular regenerative hyperplasia of the liver has been recently reported [29]. Cardiac complications are rare in IP patients but the prognosis of these patients requires cardiological and pulmonary evaluation in order to recognise such abnormalities.

Diagnosis/Investigations

Diagnostic criteria originally established in 1993 [9] were recently revised [30] (Table 6.2). Clinical diagnostic requires at least two major criteria or one major and one or more minor criteria (see Table 6.2). Eosinophilia supports the diagnosis, occurs in stages I and II and represents up to 65% of total leucocytes. Magnetic resonance imaging of the brain and electroencephalogram should be obtained if neurological symptoms are present. Cardiac echography shows a persistent pulmonary hypertension. In some cases, dilated right ventricle and tricuspid regurgitation can be visualised. Computed tomography (CT) angiogram might show signs of pulmonary artery hypoplasia. Cardiac catheterisation can identify a distal pulmonary artery stenosis [4].

Diagnosis of IP is established by suggestive clinical and histological findings, and confirmed by the demonstration of a IKBKG gene mutation. For most patients, a targeted mutational analysis of DNA extracted from peripheral blood is sufficient to detect the common IKBKG deletion, present in 80% of cases. Targeted mutational analysis detects a 11.7 kb deletion removing exons 4 to 10. Other patients

Table 6.2 Diagnostic criteria for IP after Minc et al. [30]

Major criteria	Minor criteria
Typical stages of skin eruption along Blaschko's lines: 1. Vesiculobullous 2. Verrucous 3. Hyperpigmented 4. Atrophic/hypopigmented	Typical skin histological findings Alopecia Abnormal hair (sparse hair, wooly hair, anomalies of the eyebrows and eyelashes) Dental anomalies Palate anomalies Ocular anomalies CNS anomalies Nipple and breasts anomalies Multiple males miscarriages
In absence of IKBKG data: Two major criteria or one major and one minor In presence of typical IKBKG mutation: Any single major or minor criteria IP in a first degree female relative: a major or at least two minor criteria	

need extensive sequence analysis. In suspected male patients, genetic testing is performed on DNA from lesional skin to detect the mosaicism, together with karyotyping and fluorescence in situ hybridization to identify the XXY aneuploidy. In females, X-chromosome inactivation studies may be performed to identify skewed lyonization. Prenatal diagnosis is possible via multiplex polymerase chain reaction analysis on DNA from tissue obtained by amniocentesis or chronic villus sampling in fetuses with a family history of IP [31].

Treatment

There is currently no treatment for the disease as a whole. Medical care is limited to symptom management and requires a pluridisciplinary approach (dermatologic, genetic, ophthalmologic, neurologic, dental, and cardiologic). Skin lesions initially require gentle wound care and antiseptics to prevent infections and excessive scarring. Topical corticosteroids have been successfully used [32]. Stage two requires emollients. Systemic and topical retinoids could be beneficial [33, 34].

Patients presenting PHTN benefit from diuretics at the beginning. If the child survives, phosphodiesterase-5 inhibitors can be used [4]. Dental malformation benefit from orthodontic care. Retinal neovascularization responsible of ophthalmologic manifestations is treated similarly to retinopathy of prematurity with cryotherapy or laser treatment. Retinal detachment requires surgical repair. Early experimental use of intravitreal anti-vascular endothelial growth factor (VEGF) may be a promising treatment [35].

Prognosis and Complications

Skin lesions lead to hypo-/hyperpigmentation and scarring. Besides the extremely rare cardiological complications, eye and brain are the most affected extracutaneous organs in terms of complications and definitive functional loss. The natural history of retinal impairment leads to retinal detachment. Neurological disease is associated with a considerable morbidity and are often cause of death in IP patients. Prognosis of patients with cardiological manifestations is very poor. Four of reported cases died by age of 5 months because of severe PHTN [22, 23, 25, 28].

References

1. Aradhya S, Woffendin H, Jakins T, Bardaro T, Esposito T, Smahi A, et al. A recurrent deletion in the ubiquitously expressed NEMO (IKK-gamma) gene accounts for the vast majority of incontinentia pigmenti mutations. Hum Mol Genet. 2001;10(19):2171–9.
2. Maubach G, Schmadicke AC, Naumann M. NEMO links nuclear factor-kappaB to human diseases. Trends Mol Med. 2017;23:1138–55. Trends Mol Med 2018;24(7):654
3. Muller K, Courtois G, Ursini MV, Schwaninger M. New insight into the pathogenesis of cerebral small-vessel diseases. Stroke. 2017;48(2):520–7.
4. Alshenqiti A, Nashabat M, AlGhoraibi H, Tamimi O, Alfadhel M. Pulmonary hypertension and vasculopathy in incontinentia pigmenti: a case report. Ther Clin Risk Manag. 2017;13:629–34.
5. Fusco F, Pescatore A, Steffann J, Royer G, Bonnefont JP, Ursini MV. Clinical utility gene card for: incontinentia pigmenti. Eur J Hum Genet. 2013;21:7.
6. Smahi A, Courtois G, Vabres P, Yamaoka S, Heuertz S, Munnich A, et al. Genomic rearrangement in NEMO impairs NF-kappaB activation and is a cause of incontinentia pigmenti. The international Incontinentia Pigmenti (IP) consortium. Nature. 2000;405(6785):466–72.
7. Kenwrick S, Woffendin H, Jakins T, Shuttleworth SG, Mayer E, Greenhalgh L, et al. Survival of male patients with incontinentia pigmenti carrying a lethal mutation can be explained by somatic mosaicism or Klinefelter syndrome. Am J Hum Genet. 2001;69(6):1210–7.
8. Osorio F, Magina S, Nogueira A, Azevedo F. Incontinentia Pigmenti with vesicular stage in utero. Dermatol Online J. 2010;16(10):13.
9. Landy SJ, Donnai D. Incontinentia pigmenti (Bloch-Sulzberger syndrome). J Med Genet. 1993;30(1):53–9.
10. Nelson-Adesokan P, Mallory SB. Name this syndrome. Incontinentia pigmenti Pediatr Dermatol. 1992;9(3):304–8.
11. Young A, Manolson P, Cohen B, Klapper M, Barrett T. Painful subungal dyskeratotic tumors in incontinentia pigmenti. J Am Acad Dermatol. 2005;52(4):726–9.
12. Chun SR, Rashid RM. Delayed onychodystrophy of incontinentia pigmenti: an evidence-based review of epidemiology, diagnosis and management. J Drugs Dermatol. 2010;9(4):350–4.
13. Soltirovska Salamon A, Lichtenbelt K, Cowan FM, Casaer A, Dudink J, Dereymaeker A, et al. Clinical presentation and spectrum of neuroimaging findings in newborn infants with incontinentia pigmenti. Dev Med Child Neurol. 2016;58(10):1076–84.
14. Liu TYA, Han IC, Goldberg MF, Linz MO, Chen CJ, Scott AW. Multimodal retinal imaging in Incontinentia Pigmenti including optical coherence tomography angiography: findings from an older cohort with mild phenotype. JAMA Ophthalmol. 2018;136(5):467–72.
15. Miteva L, Nikolova A. Incontinentia pigmenti: a case associated with cardiovascular anomalies. Pediatr Dermatol. 2001;18(1):54–6.
16. Fusco F, Pescatore A, Conte MI, Mirabelli P, Paciolla M, Esposito E, et al. EDA-ID and IP, two faces of the same coin: how the same IKBKG/NEMO mutation affecting the NF-kappaB pathway can cause immunodeficiency and/or inflammation. Int Rev Immunol. 2015;34(6):445–59.
17. Kosaki K, Shimasaki N, Fukushima H, Hara M, Ogata T, Matsuo N. Female patient showing hypohidrotic ectodermal dysplasia and immunodeficiency (HED-ID). Am J Hum Genet. 2001;69(3):664–6.
18. Martinez-Pomar N, Munoz-Saa I, Heine-Suner D, Martin A, Smahi A, Matamoros N. A new mutation in exon 7 of NEMO gene: late skewed X-chromosome inactivation in an incontinentia pigmenti female patient with immunodeficiency. Hum Genet. 2005;118(3–4):458–65.

19. Ohnishi H, Kishimoto Y, Taguchi T, Kawamoto N, Nakama M, Kawai T, et al. Immunodeficiency in two female patients with Incontinentia Pigmenti with heterozygous NEMO mutation diagnosed by LPS unresponsiveness. J Clin Immunol. 2017;37(6):529–38.
20. Bodemer C. Incontinentia pigmenti and hypomelanosis of Ito. Handb Clin Neurol. 2013;111:341–7.
21. Lugassy J, Itin P, Ishida-Yamamoto A, Holland K, Huson S, Geiger D, et al. Naegeli-Franceschetti-Jadassohn syndrome and dermatopathia pigmentosa reticularis: two allelic ectodermal dysplasias caused by dominant mutations in KRT14. Am J Hum Genet. 2006;79(4):724–30.
22. Godambe S, McNamara P, Rajguru M, Hellmann J. Unusual neonatal presentation of incontinentia pigmenti with persistent pulmonary hypertension of the newborn: a case report. J Perinatol. 2005;25(4):289–92.
23. Hayes IM, Varigos G, Upjohn EJ, Orchard DC, Penny DJ, Savarirayan R. Unilateral acheiria and fatal primary pulmonary hypertension in a girl with incontinentia pigmenti. Am J Med Genet A. 2005;135(3):302–3.
24. Onnis G, Diociaiuti A, Zangari P, D'Argenio P, Cancrini C, Iughetti L, et al. Cardiopulmonary anomalies in incontinentia pigmenti patients. Int J Dermatol. 2018;57(1):40–5.
25. Triki C, Devictor D, Kah S, Roge-Wolter M, Lacroix C, Venencie PY, et al. Cerebral complications of incontinentia pigmenti. A clinicopathological study of a case. Rev Neurol (Paris). 1992;148(12):773–6.
26. Vachvanichsanong P, Jinorose U, Sangnuachua P. Trisomy 14 mosaicism in a 5-year-old boy. Am J Med Genet. 1991;40(1):80–3.
27. Wood AE, Boyle D, O'Hara MD, Cleland J. Mitral annuloplasty in endomyocardial fibrosis: an alternative to valve replacement. Ann Thorac Surg. 1982;34(4):446–51.
28. Yasuda K, Minami N, Yoshikawa Y, Taketani T, Fukuda S, Yamaguchi S. Fatal pulmonary arterial hypertension in an infant girl with incontinentia pigmenti. Pediatr Int. 2016;58(5):394–6.
29. Romano R, Grasso F, Gallo V, Cirillo E, Prencipe R, Mamone G, et al. A case of incontinentia pigmenti associated with congenital absence of portal vein system and nodular regenerative hyperplasia. Br J Dermatol. 2019;180(3):674–5.
30. Minic S, Trpinac D, Obradovic M. Incontinentia pigmenti diagnostic criteria update. Clin Genet. 2014;85(6):536–42.
31. Scheuerle AE, Ursini MV. Incontinentia Pigmenti. In: Adam MP, Ardinger HH, Pagon RA, Wallace SE, LJH B, Stephens K, et al., editors. GeneReviews((R)): Seattle (WA); 1993.
32. Kaya TI, Tursen U, Ikizoglu G. Therapeutic use of topical corticosteroids in the vesiculobullous lesions of incontinentia pigmenti. Clin Exp Dermatol. 2009;34(8):e611–3.
33. Donati P, Muscardin L, Amantea A, Paolini F, Venuti A. Detection of HPV-15 in painful subungual tumors of incontinentia pigmenti: successful topical therapy with retinoic acid. Eur J Dermatol. 2009;19(3):243–7.
34. Malvehy J, Palou J, Mascaro JM. Painful subungual tumour in incontinentia pigmenti. Response to treatment with etretinate. Br J Dermatol. 1998;138(3):554–5.
35. Shah PK, Bachu S, Narendran V, Kalpana N, David J, Srinivas CR. Intravitreal bevacizumab for incontinentia pigmenti. J Pediatr Ophthalmol Strabismus 2013;50 Online:e52–e54.

The Heart in Neurofibromatosis 1

7

Christina Bergqvist and Pierre Wolkenstein

Neurofibromatosis type 1 (NF1) is one of the most common inherited disorders and affects one in 3000 people worldwide. It is a multisystem genetic disorder that is primarily associated with cutaneous, neurologic, and orthopedic manifestations. NF1 is caused by dominant loss-of-function mutations of the tumor suppressor *NF1* (Neurofibromin 1; MIM #613113), which is located at 17q11.2 and contains 60 translated exons over ~280 kb [1]. It is a completely penetrant Mendelian disease marked by an extremely variable clinical expressivity of the major features as well as the less frequent complications [2–4].

The major features of NF1 are multiple neurofibromas, café-au-lait macules, intertriginous freckling, Lisch nodules, tibial pseudarthrosis, and a tendency to develop benign and malignant tumors of the nervous system [5]. NF1 is diagnosed primarily on clinical grounds using the National Institutes of Health (NIH)

C. Bergqvist
Assistance Publique-Hôpital Paris (AP-HP), Hôpital Henri-Mondor, Department of Dermatology, Créteil, France

Université Paris-Est Creteil (UPEC), Faculty of Medicine, Créteil, France

P. Wolkenstein (✉)
Assistance Publique-Hôpital Paris (AP-HP), Hôpital Henri-Mondor, Department of Dermatology, Créteil, France

Université Paris-Est Creteil (UPEC), Faculty of Medicine, Créteil, France

INSERM, Centre d'Investigation Clinique 006, Assistance Publique-Hôpital Paris (AP-HP), Hôpital Henri-Mondor, Referral Center of Neurofibromatosis, Créteil, France

INSERM U955 Neurofibromatosis and Lymphoma Oncogenesis, Créteil, France

C. Salavastru et al. (eds.), *Skin and the Heart*,
https://doi.org/10.1007/978-3-030-54779-0_7

diagnostic criteria [6]. The diagnosis of NF1 requires at least two out of the following seven NIH criteria:

- 6 or more café au lait macules (>0.5 cm in children or >1.5 cm in adults)
- 2 or more cutaneous/subcutaneous neurofibromas or one plexiform neurofibroma
- Intertriginous (axillary or groin) freckling
- Optic pathway glioma
- 2 or more Lisch nodules (iris hamartomas seen on slit lamp examination)
- Bony dysplasia (sphenoid wing dysplasia, bowing of long bone ± pseudarthrosis)
- First degree relative with NF1

By using these criteria, the diagnosis of NF1 can be made based on physical examination and by evaluating the patient's family history. Genetic testing is not necessary if the diagnosis has already been clinically confirmed. These criteria usually appear in the following predictable order: café-au-lait macules (CALMs), axillary freckling, Lisch nodules, and neurofibromas. The characteristic osseous lesions usually develop within the first year of life, and the diagnosis of symptomatic optic glioma appears by 3 years of age [7]. However, these diagnostic criteria emerge in a variable manner, with some patients revealing criteria at a late onset and others never developing certain signs and symptoms. Definitive diagnosis may therefore be delayed by years. Indeed, although the NIH diagnostic criteria are useful for the diagnosis of NF1 in the majority of children at the age of 5 years, they are inadequate for reaching a diagnosis at an earlier age [7, 8]. Ninety-seven percent of NF1 patients meet the NIH criteria by the age of 8 years, and all do so by the age of 20 years [7]. On the other hand, only 50% of children younger than 2 years with sporadic NF1 fulfil a single NIH criterion, leading to delayed diagnosis [7].

Genetic testing is therefore useful for confirming the diagnosis in children who present with an unusual phenotype or those who do not meet the diagnostic criteria. Revising these diagnostic criteria is currently a hot topic in the NF1 community which believes that genetic testing should also be a diagnostic criteria; specially, that a positive genetic test shortens the period of diagnostic uncertainty which entails early appropriate surveillance. Furthermore, the clinical picture may be incomplete in some rare forms in adults, requiring genetic testing to confirm the NF1 diagnosis. Patients with limited and localized clinical features and no family history of NF1 may possibly have segmental NF1 [9].

Café-au-lait macules are large, generally oval, well-defined hyperpigmented macules which are usually present at birth and occur in >90% of patients (Figs. 7.1) [7]. CALMs may increase in number and size in early childhood [5]. They have no malignant potential. The majority of patients with NF1 (around 80%) will have more than 5 CALMs by 1 year of age. They become darker with sun exposure and fade with age or become obscured by numerous neurofibromas. Legius syndrome [10, 11], Noonan syndrome and constitutional mismatch repair-deficiency syndrome [12] are other syndromes which exhibit multiple CALMS [13]. Children with multiple CALMs and no other NF1 clinical feature and no family history of

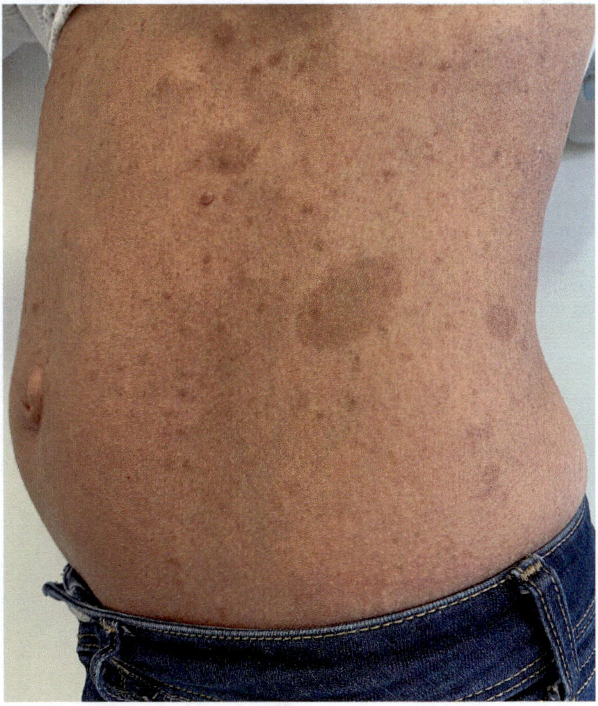

Fig. 7.1 Café-au-lait macules are large, generally oval, well-defined hyperpigmented macules

NF1 might be referred to genetic testing to confirm a diagnosis of NF1. In a study of 71 patients younger than 20 years of age with six or more CALMs and no non-pigmentary criterion, 66.2% were confirmed to have NF1, 8.5% had Legius syndrome and 25.3% harbored no disease causing variant [14].

Neurofibromas (NF) are benign peripheral nerve sheath tumors and are the cardinal feature of NF1.

Cutaneous (or dermal) NFs are flesh-colored or purplish soft nodules that become pedunculated as they grow (Figs. 7.2 and 7.3). They usually start appearing during late adolescence and are found in the vast majority (>95%) of patients with NF1 [15]. They vary in number from a few lesions to thousands [15]. These tumors are benign and have no risk of malignant transformation, but sometimes lead to significant discomfort and cosmetic disfigurement. *Subcutaneous neurofibromas (or peripheral nodular NFs)* are firm discrete rubbery nodules bulging under the skin. They affect at least 20% of NF1 patients and usually develop during adolescence [16]. *Internal (nodular) NFs* are neurofibromas that cannot be felt by physical examination. They are associated with a high-risk phenotype necessitating closer monitoring and management [17]. *Plexiform neurofibromas* are congenital lesions found in 20 to 26% of individuals with NF1 [18]. They present as a subtle enlargement of soft tissue with a "wrinkled" texture or a patch of hyperpigmentation with or without hypertrichosis. A substantial increase in size occurs during the first

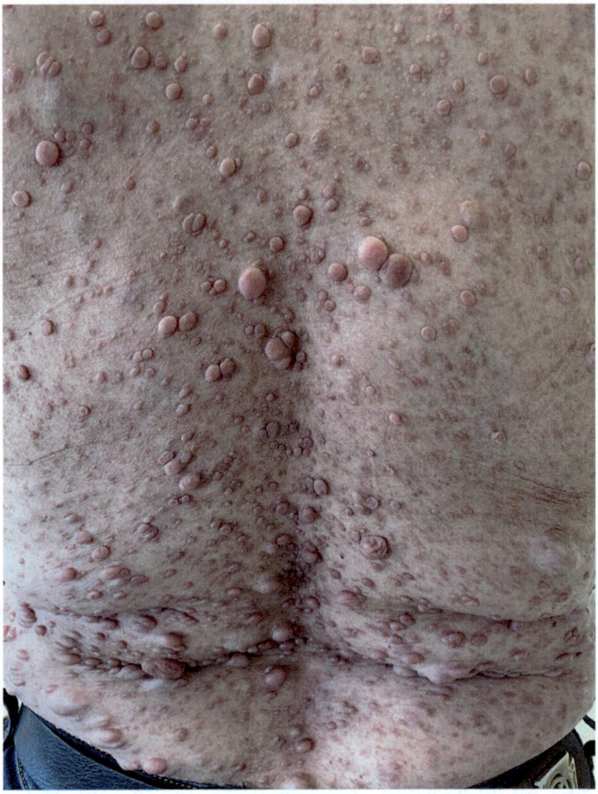

Fig. 7.2 Cutaneous neurofibromas are flesh-colored or purplish pedunculated soft nodules

decade of life and adolescence [19]. These tumors can invade surrounding structures, including muscle and bone which leads to substantial pain and bone destruction [20].

Malignant peripheral nerve sheath tumors (MPNSTs) are a subtype of sarcoma that arise in preexisting plexiform neurofibromas or subcutaneous NF (Fig. 7.4) [21]. The cumulative lifetime risk of developing MPNST in NF1 patients is 8–13% [21–23]. Seventy percent of MPNSTs are high-grade tumors that can metastasize widely and entail a poor prognosis [22]. Symptoms most suggestive of MPNST are a rapid increase in the size of an existing plexiform neurofibroma or alteration in its consistency from soft to hard, persistent or difficult to control pain, or new neurological deficit [22].

Intertriginous freckling is found in >80% of NF1 individuals [5, 15]. They may be found in any area where skinfolds are in apposition, including the axilla, intertriginous area, base of the neck, upper eyelid and under the breasts in women (Figs. 7.5) [24].

Optic pathway gliomas (OPG) are benign tumors seen in 15–20% [25–30] of children with NF1. They are slow growing tumors with a low potential of malignancy and they usually occur within the optic pathway including the optic nerve and optic chiasma [26, 31]. They are often indolent; however, due to their space

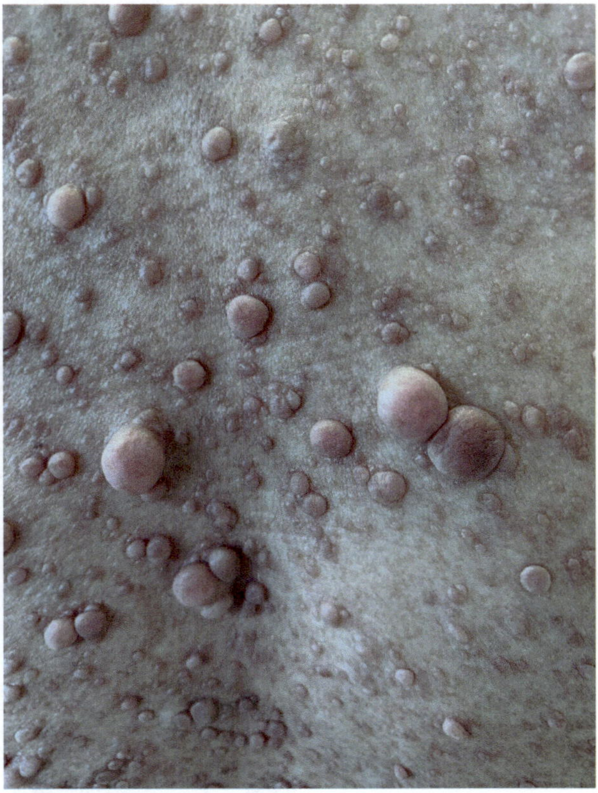

Fig. 7.3 Cutaneous neurofibromas are flesh-colored or purplish pedunculated soft nodules

occupying nature they can be locally invasive and become symptomatic [30, 32–35]. OPG can cause a rapid onset of proptosis leading to moderate-to-severe visual loss in the affected eye [25, 29, 36]. Precocious puberty can occur if the optic pathway tumor impinges on the optic chiasm [29, 37]. Therefore, all children diagnosed with NF1 should have a regular specific pediatric ophthalmological exam.

Lisch nodules are pigmented iris hamartomas that first appear around the age of 3 years and are found in 100% of patients by the age of 30 years [7, 38, 39]. They are asymptomatic 1–2 mm yellow-brown dome shaped papules of the iris; they are best visualized using careful slit-lamp examination of the non-dilated iris.

Congenital dysplasia of the long bones is a classic manifestation of NF1 and occurs in 7.2% of patients [40]. Bowing of long bones leads to a visible deformity and a fragile bone that is susceptible to fracture [41]. Repeated fractures that fail to heal can lead to pseudarthrosis (failure of primary union of the separate bone ends can create a false joint) [40, 42]. Bowing in an NF1 infant necessitates prompt radiographic examination and referral to an orthopedic surgeon.

Sphenoid wing dysplasia is a distinctive feature of NF1 found in a minority of patients (1–7%) [43].

The sphenoid bones comprise multiple ossification centers that fuse to become the important elements of the orbits. Sphenoid wing dysplasia is usually found early

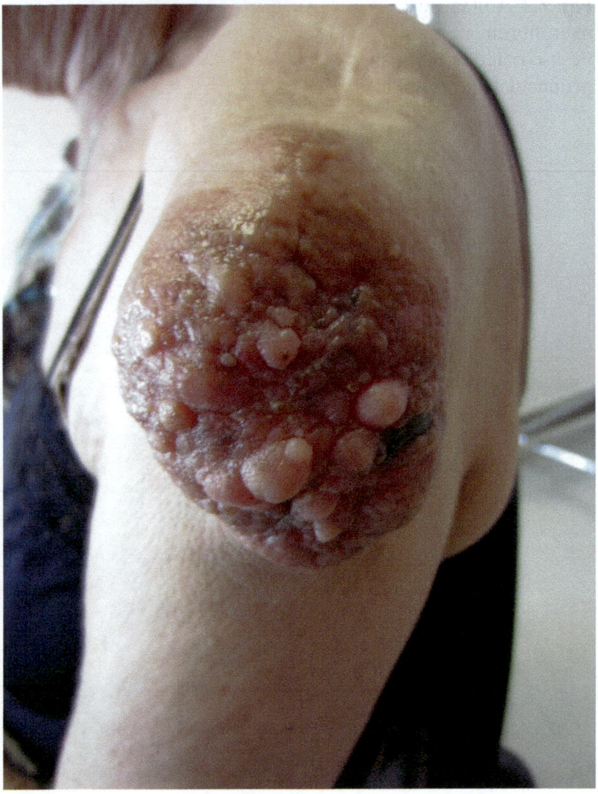

Fig. 7.4 A malignant peripheral nerve sheath tumor (MPNST) over the shoulder

in life, is often unilateral and may progress over time. One complication of sphenoid wing dysplasia is a pulsating exophthalmos without visual loss; and an absent sphenoid wing can lead to herniation of the temporal lobe into the orbit [44]. The treatment of sphenoid wing dysplasia should be carried out by a multidisciplinary team including cranio-facial teams familiar with this complex surgery.

People with NF1 may also develop cardiac disease, however their prevalence, natural history, and pathogenesis have only recently received medical and scientific attention. This chapter focuses on the vast array of cardiac manifestations associated with NF1, including congenital and acquired hearing defects, as well as the role of Neurofibromin 1 in cardiac embryogenesis.

Congenital Heart Defects

The incidence and type of congenital heart defects in individuals with NF1 were long undefined and not well-characterized. The previously reported frequencies of congenital heart defects ranged from 0.4 to 8.6% in 8 large series of NF1 patients

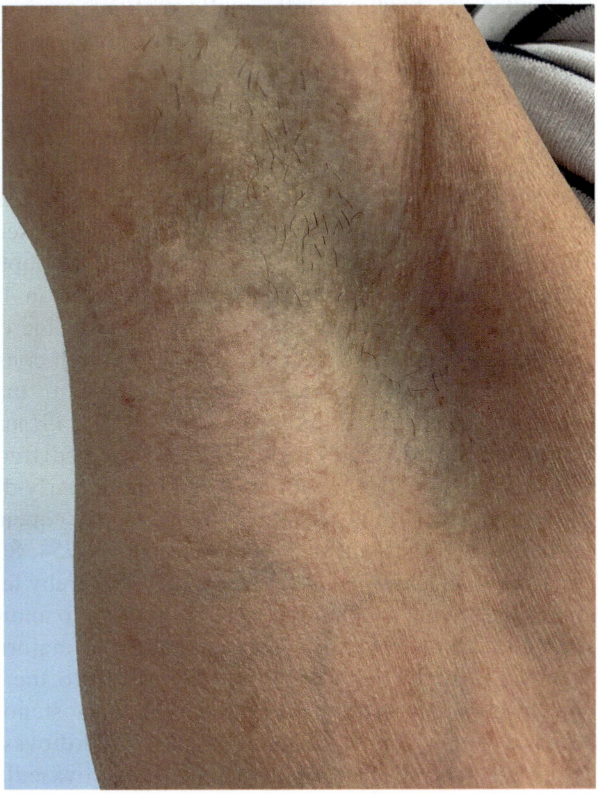

Fig. 7.5 Skinfold freckling of the axilla

[45–52]. However, the diagnosis of both NF1 and congenital heart diseases was not clearly established in these patients and not clearly distinguished from Watson and NF1-Noonan syndromes.

It has been suggested that the seemingly conflicting data concerning the prevalence of cardiovascular malformations in NF1 is attributable to the fact that not all NF1 patients are systematically screened by means of echocardiography, especially that the cardiac defect is often mild and asymptomatic. Tedesco et al. were the first to evaluate the prevalence of cardiovascular abnormalities in patients with NF1 using echocardiography with color Doppler scan and found cardiac abnormalities in 13/ 48 young patients (27%) [53]. The same group later described the cardiac abnormalities in 13 out of a total of 69 young patients (18.8%) with NF1 [54]. This was followed by a study in the Turkish population whereby sixty-five NF1 patients were retrospectively studied, looking specifically at their standard electrocardiography and echocardiography. Congenital cardiac abnormalities were found in 11 patients (15.3%) [55]. However, all of these studies are limited by their small sample size.

Two large series have carefully looked at the cardiovascular malformation in patients with NF1. The first one reviewed the cardiovascular abnormalities, in particular the cardiovascular malformations among 2,322 patients with well-established NF1 in the National Neurofibromatosis Foundation International Database (NNFFID) from 1991–98 [56]. A clear diagnosis of cardiovascular disease was found in 97/2,322 (4.2%) of patients with NF1. Cardiovascular malformations were found in 54/2,322 (2.3%) of these NF1 patients, of whom only two had Watson syndrome and only two had NF1-Noonan syndrome. When excluding patients with the latter syndromes, the overall frequency of cardiovascular malformations among NF1 patients was 2%. The second and more recent large series was a retrospective registry-based total population study conducted in Finland that evaluated the congenital anomalies in 465 children with NF1 [57]. NF1 children were found to have a significantly increased risk of congenital cardiovascular anomalies (adjusted OR 3.35), with congenital heart defects occurring in 1.8% of NF1 patients, a figure similar to that reported in the NNFFID study as well as in the studies by Carey et al. [49] and Schorry et al. [50] All of these data demonstrate a higher than expected frequency of congenital heart defects among patients with NF1, warranting early diagnosis in NF1 children to prevent potential long-term hemodynamic consequences.

In the NNFFID study, the predominant (43/54, 80%) cardiovascular malformations were classified as "flow defects," whereby left or right heart obstruction or simple shunts are thought to be secondary to anomalous embryonic intracardiac hemodynamics [56]. Among these, the majority (25/43) had pulmonary stenosis, usually valvular. When compared to the patients in the Baltimore-Washington Infant Study (BWIS), pulmonary stenosis in NF1 patients constituted a much larger proportion of all cardiovascular malformations than expected. Indeed, the proportion of all cardiovascular malformations that were pulmonary stenosis was 4.3 times greater among NF1 patients. Similarly, individual case reports and smaller series also frequently reported pulmonary stenosis. Fortunately, pulmonary stenosis in patients with NF1 seems to be generally mild and not a source of serious morbidity. It is interesting to note that pulmonary stenosis is also a well-recognized feature of three clinical subtypes of NF1: NF1-Noonan syndrome, Watson syndrome, and individuals with large deletions of the NF1 gene [56, 58]. Pulmonary stenosis should therefore be considered in any NF1 patient with a systolic murmur.

Aortic coarctation was observed in 5/54 of patients in the NNFFID study and was 3.2 times greater among the NF1 patients than in the BWIS population. However, in 3 out of these 5 patients, the coarctation was a fusiform narrowing of the descending thoracic aorta, which is different from the typical juxtaductal shelf usually described [56]; suggesting that aortic coarctation is more of a NF1 vasculopathy rather than a true cardiovascular malformation.

It remains uncertain whether hypertrophic cardiomyopathy (HCM) constitutes a rare manifestation of NF1, or whether their simultaneous occurrence is simply related to chance. None of the reported patients in the NNFFID study had HCM which may have been due to the small sample size and insufficient statistical power to identify this particular association. Lin et al. reviewed the different case reports in the literature: out of the 18 reported patients in the literature at that time, probably 14 had primary HCM (idiopathic hypertrophic subaortic stenosis and left ventricular). None of these patients had molecular analysis for either the NF1 or any of the common HCM mutations [59]. One patient had extrinsic compression by a neurofibroma which resulted in biventricular hypertrophy [60]. In 2 patients, HCM and NF1 were most likely segregating as independent autosomal dominant traits [61]. Histological examination of the myocardium was available in two patients (postmortem examination [62] or biopsy [63]) revealing non-specific changes and fiber disproportion with interstitial fibrosis, respectively. Tedesco et al.'s echocardiography study detected two patients with septal to posterior left ventricular free wall ratio greater than 1.5, suggesting hypertrophic cardiomyopathy [53]. Another case report presented the case of an 18-year-old boy with NF1 with hypertrophic cardiomyopathy diagnosed using echocardiography showing the systolic anteward movement of the anterior leaflet of the mitral valve [64]. Further large series are needed to elucidate whether HCM is truly a rare manifestation of the NF1 mutation or simply a chance incident.

Interestingly, Class I conotruncal defects and Fallot's tetralogy were rare in the NNFFID study, and there were no atrioventricular canal, anomalous pulmonary venous return, complex single ventricle and laterality defects detected [56]. This is in striking contrast to the Nf1 knockout mouse homozygous mutant embryos discussed below [65].

Table 7.1 describes the different congenital cardiac malformations detected in large series.

Table 7.1 Specific congenital cardiac malformations detected in large series found in literature

Authors	Lin et al. [56]	Tedesco e al. [53]	İncecik et al. [55]	Leppävirta et al. [57]
Year	2000	2002	2015	2018
Number of NF1 patients included	2322	48	65	465
Conotruncal, outflow	2			
Tetralogy of Fallot	2			
Pulmonary stenosis	25	1	1	2
Pulmonary valve stenosis	21		1	2
Pulmonary artery stenosis	1	1		
Aortic stenosis	2			1
Aortic valve regurgitation		2	1	1
Mitral valve regurgitation		2	5	
Mitral valve prolapse	1	1		
Tricuspid valve regurgitation			1	

(continued)

Table 7.1 (continued)

Authors	Lin et al. [56]	Tedesco e al. [53]	İncecik et al. [55]	Leppävirta et al. [57]
Secundum atrial septal defect	4	2	2	1
Ventricular septal defect	6		1	1
Patent ductus arteriorsus	1			2
Coarctation thoracic aorta	5	1		
Atrial septal aneurysm		2		
Hypertrophic cardiomyopathy		2		

Genotype–Phenotype Correlation

The majority of NF1 cases result from truncating mutations or whole gene deletions, causing an expected deterioration or absence of the RNA generated from the mutated allele. This leads to the total amount of protein being translated from a single allele only, creating a dosage effect [66].

For patients with intragenic *NF1* mutations which represent over 90% of all NF1 cases, no straightforward genotype–phenotype correlations have been identified except for few exceptions [67].

NF1 and its Related Disorders (NF1-Noonan Syndrome (NFNS) and Watson Syndrome (WS))

Watson syndrome (WS) and NF1–Noonan syndrome (NFNS) were first described clinically and were later shown to be caused by NF1 mutations [68–70]. Over 20 years ago, Watson had described three families with an autosomal dominant inheritance of pulmonary stenosis, multiple café-au-lait macules and lower intelligence [71]. Further studies showed that the Watson phenotype is distinct from that of NF1, as adult patients rarely had neurofibromas, if any [72].

Patients with NFNS, have overlapping features of both NF1 and Noonan syndrome. Although at first thought to be a distinct condition, subsequent clinical [51] and molecular studies have proved that the majority of NFNS patients have NF1 gene mutations only, mostly non-truncating mutations consisting of in-frame deletions as compared to typical NF1 [73, 74].

A recent study investigated whether pulmonary stenosis is related to specific types of NF1 gene mutations in NF1, NFNS and WS. The study examined the frequency of different NF1 mutation types in a cohort of published and unpublished cases with NF1/NFNS/WS and pulmonary stenosis [66].

Compared with NF1 in general, NFNS patients had statistically significant higher rates of pulmonary stenosis (9/35 = 26% vs 25/2322 = 1.1%). Further stratification of NFNS group according to the mutation type showed that the higher pulmonary stenosis rate appears to be affected specifically by non-truncating mutations. Eight out of twelve (66.7%) NFNS cases with non-truncating mutations had pulmonary stenosis compared with only 1.1% pulmonary stenosis frequency in NF1 in general. In contrast, only 6.2% (1/16) of NFNS patients with a truncating mutation had pulmonary stenosis (not significantly different from NF1 patients). Looking specifically at individuals with NF1 and pulmonary stenosis, 8/11 (73%) of them had non-truncating mutations, which is largely higher than expected in the NF1 population (19% reported in NF1 cohorts). As for WS, out of the three available published cases with intragenic mutations, two of them had non-truncating mutations. Therefore, non-truncating mutations seem to play a specific role in pulmonary stenosis in NF1 and its related disorders. The authors postulated that unlike in truncating mutations whereby there is decay or absence of the RNA generated from the mutated allele with resulting dosage effect, non-truncating mutations do not result in loss of the NF1 protein. Instead it might result in an abnormally functioning protein with special cardiac effect. This suggests that the pulmonary stenosis is caused by an additional effect of the mutated protein instead of the common loss-of function effect. This effect may be similar to the cardiac effect of Noonan syndrome and other RAS opathies and may characterize a particular role of these mutations in the Ras–MAPK pathway.

NF1 Microdeletion Syndrome (MIM 613675)

In 5–10% of patients, NF1 results from microdeletions that encompass the entire *NF1* gene and a variable number of flanking genes [75]. Patients carry a heterozygous deletion of 17q11.2 region usually spanning about 1–1.4 Mb [58, 76]. Typically, they present with a more severe phenotype compared with the one observed in NF1 with intragenic mutation [77].

Numerous studies have described cardiac defects in patients with NF1 microdeletions [52, 58, 77–85].

However, the overall frequency of cardiac defects in patients with NF1 microdeletions is still uncertain. Venturin et al. showed a prevalence of cardiovascular malfomations of 18% in the subgroup of patients with NF1 microdeletion [58]. In another study, 8/28 (29%) NF1 microdeletion patients had cardiovascular anomalies [77]. The first thorough investigation of the frequency of heart defects in patients with NF1 microdeletions showed major cardiac abnormalities in 6 of 16 NF1 microdeletion patients whereas none of 16 patients with intragenic NF1 mutations in that study had heart defects [85].

The specific type and frequency of the heart defects described in patients with NF1 microdeletions are quite varied and are shown in Table 7.2.

It is worth mentioning that mitral valve prolapse and aortic dilatation are both associated with connective tissue abnormalities, now generally recognized as a part of NF1 microdeletion syndrome and have been reported in 12% in one series [83].

The higher frequency of cardiovascular malformations in NF1-microdeleted patients is most likely due to the haploinsufficiency of genes lying in the deletion interval, possibly involved in heart morphogenesis. One such gene includes *ADAP2* which encodes a protein belonging to the centaurins protein family. Expression analysis studies showed *ADAP2* murine ortholog expression in heart during

Table 7.2 Literature review of cardiac malformations in patients with NF1 microdeletion syndrome

	Kayes et al. [78]	Upadhyaya et al. [86]	Tonsgard et al. [52]	Wu et al. [79]	Dorschner et al. [80]	Riva et al. [81]	Oktenli et al. [82]	Venturin et al. [58]	Mensink et al. [83]	Nguyen et al. [85]
Pulmonary stenosis			1		2	2				
Aortic stenosis										1
Aortic valve regurgitation					1					1
Mitral valve regurgitation								1		2
Mitral valve prolapse				1			1	1	3	
Atrial septal defect	1				1					
Ventricular septal defect			1					1		1
Patent ductus arteriorsus		1								
Hypertrophic cardiomyopathy								1	1	3
Intracardiac neurofibromas										2

fundamental phases of cardiac morphogenesis [87]. The findings of this study suggested a correlation between ADAP2 haploinsufficiency and the presence of valve defects in NF1-microdeleted patients.

Specific Mutations

A specific mutation consisting of a 3-bp inframe deletion (c.2970–2972 delAAT) in exon 17 of the *NF1* gene has recently been found to be associated with a much milder NF1 phenotype with a lack of dermal neurofibromas, and increased rate of pulmonary stenosis [68].

Another genotype-phenotype correlation with cardiac involvement in NF1 are the missense mutations affecting arginine at position 1809. Patients present with pulmonary stenosis, Noonan-like features and developmental delay, but no external plexiform neurofibromas [88, 89]. Affected amino acids reside outside the GAP-related domain (GRD) domain.

A third and more recent genotype-phenotype correlation involves the constitutional missense mutation affecting one of five neighboring NF1 codons—Leu844, Cys845, Ala846, Leu847, and Gly848—located in the cysteine-serine-rich domain (CSRD).

Cardiovascular abnormalities observed in a studied group included hypertension, pulmonic stenosis, mitral valve stenosis, atrial septal defect, ventricular septal defect, Moyamoya disease, pericarditis carcinomatosa, mitral valve insufficiency, mild pulmonary insufficiency, and hypertrophic cardiomyopathy [90].

Acquired Heart Diseases

In addition to congenital heart defects, there is evidence that individuals with NF1 have an increased risk of developing acquired heart diseases. Diastolic function was evaluated in young patients with NF who were free of structural cardiovascular abnormalities using standard Doppler and Pulsed Doppler tissue imaging (DTI), which is a new technique that allows analysis of myocardial velocities and time intervals throughout the cardiac cycle [53]. The main finding of the study are that certain standard and DTI indexes are abnormal in patients with NF as compared to controls, indicating that patients with NF may have abnormal diastolic function. These findings were found in both mild and severe disease, suggesting that the suspected diastolic functional abnormalities may be independent of the clinical severity of NF1. The authors suggested that this may be attributed to cardiac myofibrillar dysplasia or, they may be secondary to abnormal vascular compliance [91].

The same group later evaluated the cardiac function of NF1 patients looking specifically at hypertension. The study revealed the presence of early cardiac morphologic and functional changes in young NF1 patients with hypertension. NF1 hypertensive patients had thicker myocardial walls, increased left ventricular mass index and increased atrial dimension compared with NF1 normotensive patients and healthy subjects [92]. Using standard Doppler, diastolic function was shown to be significantly more impaired in NF1 hypertensives than normotensive NF1 patients and controls. However, using DTI technique (which detects changes induced by hypertension as well as those independent of blood pressure.), myocardial velocities in NF1 patients were found to be significantly higher than controls regardless of blood pressure. Hence the myocardial abnormalities are an early phenotype in patients with NF1 that presents independently of blood pressure and that can be identified using DTI. The authors here postulated that the high DTI values in NF1 normotensives could be explained by the abnormal sympathetic nerve supply to the heart based on the neural crest origin of NF. Furthermore, the presence of a significant decline in myocardial systolic velocity in NF1 hypertensives, when compared with normotensives, could be used as a measure for the long-term follow-up of those patients, since hypertension has been shown to decrease life expectancy in NF1 patients [93].

To sum up, patients with NF1 require a cardiologic assessment at regular intervals. Serial echocardiograms with standard and DTI measurements could provide important information about cardiac damage in NF1 patients diagnosed with hypertension.

Death from Cardiac Disease

Although heart diseases were found to be slightly lower than expected on death certificates of individuals with NF1 [94], sporadic cases of sudden death in adults

Table 7.3 Literature review of myocardial infarctions with the associated coronary artery anomalies in patients with NF1

Author	Age	Gender	Cardiac event	Pathology
Ruggieri et al. [101]	16	M	Presumed myocardial infarction	Aneurysm of the LAD
Kandarpa et al. [102]	30	M	Myocardial infarction	Coronary artery aneurysm
Daly et al. [96]	39	M	Myocardial infarction	Coronary artery aneurysm
Evrengul et al. [103]	17	F	Myocardial infarction	Coronary artery aneurysm
Fuchi et al. [99]	23	M	Myocardial infarction	Organic stenosis and spasm of LAD
Halper et al. [104]	38	M	Presumed myocardial infarction	Diffuse circumferential thickening of intima of coronary arteries; focal intimal smooth muscle nodules within intima of LAD
Kanter et al. [95]	2	M	Presumed myocardial infarction	Circumferential proliferation of the tunica intima LMCA and LAD
	7	M	Myocardial infarction	Nodular and circumferential proliferations of the tunica intima and tunica media of LMCA and LAD

LAD left anterior descending artery, *LMCA* left main coronary artery with NF1 have been reported secondary to coronary artery involvement, vasospasm and myocardial infarction [95–99].

Cardiac diseases related to vascular lesions in patients with NF1 result mainly from an intrinsic pathology of the vessel walls. The NF1 vasculopathy most commonly affects the renal arteries; however, it has also been described in cardiac diseases. It consists of hyperplasia and luminal narrowing, with the proliferating cell type being smooth myocytes. Lesions have been categorized as pure intimal, advanced intimal, intimal-aneurysmal, and nodular [100]. Coronary imaging should therefore be considered in children and adults with NF1 who present with symptoms of angina such as chest pain and syncope.

Table 7.3 describes the different coronary artery anomalies described in NF1 patients in the literature in the form of case reports.

Molecular Basis of Cardiac Malformation and Dysfunction in NF1

The *Nf1* gene codes for neurofibromin, a large protein of 2800 aa. It includes a Ras-GTPase-activating domain (GAP) capable of accelerating the hydrolysis of GTP-bound Ras, thus down-regulating the activity of *Ras* proto-oncogenes which are important regulators of cell proliferation, growth, and differentiation [65, 105] Hence, mutations that inactivate *Nf1* result in elevated levels of RAS signaling and increased cell proliferation. Further cellular functions for neurofibromin have also been recognized, including modulation of protein kinase A and cyclic adenosine monophosphate pathways [106–108]. The full-length of neurofibromin has been shown to bind to the scaffolding domain of Caveolin 1 [109], whereas the C terminal region of Neurofibromin 1 has been shown to interact with a major class of heparan sulfate proteoglycans [110].

Neurofibromin is a ubiquitous protein [111] and plays a pivotal role in embryogenesis. The role of haploinsufficiency for neurofibromin in heart development and function has been the subject of many studies. Our understanding of the role of *Nf1* in embryogenesis stems from animal studies, essentially targeted mouse mutants and more recently zebrafish studies [65, 112–116]. All of these studies have shown that complex developmental mechanisms including neural crest migration are involved in the cardiac development in NF1.

Surprisingly enough, the earliest studies have shown that *Nf1* heterozygous mice do not exhibit any in utero cardiovascular malformations. However, *Nf1* knockout mouse homozygous mutant embryos have been found to die during midgestation due to outflow tract septation defects (double outlet right ventricle/membranous ventricular septal defect) and concurrent hyperproliferative enlarged endocardial cushions (the precursors of cardiac valves), that could impede forward blood flow [65, 112].

Zebrafish embryos displayed similar cardiovascular abnormalities to those seen in mouse models following transient knockdown of the orthologous *Nf1* genes (abnormal cardiac valves, presence of pericardial effusions, thinned myocardium) [116].

These cardiovascular malformations were previously thought to be due to abnormal migration of ectomesenchymal cells derived from the cranial neural crest [117]. However, more recent studies demonstrated using conditional gene inactivation that ablating the neurofibromin function specifically in neural crest did not cause cardiac defects. On the other hand, endothelial-specific inactivation of Nf1 recapitulated the cardiovascular phenotype observed in *Nf1* knockout embryos: enlarged endocardial cushions, ventricular septal defects, double outlet right ventricle, thinned myocardium and pericardial effusions [113, 114]. These myocardial defects were not reproduced by tissue-specific inactivation of *Nf1*in myocardial cells indicating that signaling between the endocardium and myocardium is vital for proper myocardial development. Furthermore, loss of *Nf1*in the embryonic endocardium of these transgenic mice was then shown to be directly associated with an increase in activated GTP-bound Ras with the resulting stimulation of MAPK signaling leading to the abnormal enlargement of the outflow tract septum. Reconstitution of the neurofibromin GRD in endothelial cells is sufficient to rescue cardiovascular development and midgestational lethality in *Nf1*null embryos; however these mice succumb in the early postnatal period due to overgrowth of neural crest–derived tissues, suggesting that other domains outside the GRD are important for neural crest growth and homeostasis [114].

A more recent study also identified ectopic cardiac blood island formation as a new phenotype that arises in *Nf1*-deficient murine embryos and that this phenotype is a direct result of dysregulation of the Ras signaling pathway [118].

In a further study, neurofibromin was also shown to function as an important Ras-GAP in the myocardium of adult mice. Tissue-specific inactivation of *Nf1* in myocardial cells during mid-gestation led to no distinct phenotype at birth or in young adults, consistent with the aforementioned observations [65, 119]. However, as these cardiac *Nf1* deficient mice aged, they developed progressive cardiac hypertrophy, dilatation, fibrosis, and failure with secondary premature mortality. Reconstitution of the Ras-GAP activity in *Nf1* deficient myocardial cells led to the rescue of Ras activity and its downstream effectors, along with partial improvement of in the cardiac dysfunction and hypertrophy [119].

The role of Ras activation in cardiac hypertrophy is better highlighted when evaluating patients with Noonan, Costello, and Cardio-facial-cutaneous (CFC) syndromes. Each of these syndromes can be caused by activating mutations in components of the Ras-MAPK pathway and they are all strongly associated with cardiovascular defects including hypertrophic cardiomyopathy [120–122].

Parallels have been drawn with Noonan syndrome specifically as the spectrum of heart defects in mouse models of both NF1 and Noonan syndrome is markedly similar, including the enlarged endocardial cushions and double outlet right ventricle [123, 124]. These similarities imply that the in utero cardiovascular manifestations of *Nf1* null mice appear to result from endothelially driven hyperproliferation of the endocardial cushions associated with ERK activation.

Conclusion

Although once thought as a rare manifestation of NF1, cardiac malformations are now known to have a higher than expected frequency among patients with NF1 and occur in 2% of these patients. This warrants early diagnosis in NF1 children to prevent potential long-term hemodynamic consequences. Pulmonary stenosis was found to be the most common cardiac defect and related to non-truncating mutations in the *Nf1* gene. NF1 patients also present with cardiac function anomalies such as abnormal diastolic function which were found to be independent of the clinical severity of NF1. Furthermore, NF1 patients exhibit early cardiac functional changes independent of blood pressure which can be identified using DTI. Therefore, NF1 patients require cardiology assessment at regular intervals. Serial echocardiograms with standard and DTI measurements could provide important information about cardiac damage in NF1 patients, especially those diagnosed with hypertension. Animal studies have helped tremendously in understanding the role of *Nf1* in embryogenesis showing that complex developmental mechanisms are involved in cardiac development. Further experiments are needed to better understand disease pathogenesis of cardiovascular malformations in order to develop potential therapeutic strategies for patients with NF1.

References

1. Gutmann DH, Ferner RE, Listernick RH, Korf BR, Wolters PL, Johnson KJ. Neurofibromatosis type 1. Nat Rev Dis Primers. 2017;3:17004. https://doi.org/10.1038/nrdp.2017.4.
2. Easton DF, Ponder MA, Huson SM, Ponder BA. An analysis of variation in expression of neurofibromatosis (NF) type 1 (NF1): evidence for modifying genes. Am J Hum Genet. 1993;53(2):305–13.
3. Sabbagh A, Pasmant E, Laurendeau I, Parfait B, Barbarot S, Guillot B, et al. Unravelling the genetic basis of variable clinical expression in neurofibromatosis 1. Hum Mol Genet. 2009;18(15):2768–78. https://doi.org/10.1093/hmg/ddp212.
4. Szudek J, Joe H, Friedman JM. Analysis of intrafamilial phenotypic variation in neurofibromatosis 1 (NF1). Genet Epidemiol. 2002;23(2):150–64. https://doi.org/10.1002/gepi.1129.
5. Ferner RE, Huson SM, Thomas N, Moss C, Willshaw H, Evans DG, et al. Guidelines for the diagnosis and management of individuals with neurofibromatosis 1. J Med Genet. 2007;44(2):81–8. https://doi.org/10.1136/jmg.2006.045906.
6. Neurofibromatosis. Conference statement. National Institutes of Health consensus development conference. Arch Neurol. 1988;45(5):575–8.
7. DeBella K, Szudek J, Friedman JM. Use of the national institutes of health criteria for diagnosis of neurofibromatosis 1 in children. Pediatrics. 2000;105(3 Pt 1):608–14.
8. Obringer AC, Meadows AT, Zackai EH. The diagnosis of neurofibromatosis-1 in the child under the age of 6 years. Am J Dis Child (1960). 1989;143(6):717–9.
9. Ruggieri M, Huson SM. The clinical and diagnostic implications of mosaicism in the neurofibromatoses. Neurology. 2001;56(11):1433–43.
10. Brems H, Chmara M, Sahbatou M, Denayer E, Taniguchi K, Kato R, et al. Germline loss-of-function mutations in SPRED1 cause a neurofibromatosis 1-like phenotype. Nat Genet. 2007;39(9):1120–6. https://doi.org/10.1038/ng2113.

11. Pasmant E, Sabbagh A, Hanna N, Masliah-Planchon J, Jolly E, Goussard P, et al. SPRED1 germline mutations caused a neurofibromatosis type 1 overlapping phenotype. J Med Genet. 2009;46(7):425–30. https://doi.org/10.1136/jmg.2008.065243.
12. Wimmer K, Etzler J. Constitutional mismatch repair-deficiency syndrome: have we so far seen only the tip of an iceberg? Hum Genet. 2008;124(2):105–22. https://doi.org/10.1007/s00439-008-0542-4.
13. Roberts AE, Allanson JE, Tartaglia M, Gelb BD. Noonan syndrome. Lancet (London, England). 2013;381(9863):333–42. https://doi.org/10.1016/s0140-6736(12)61023-x.
14. Evans DG, Bowers N, Burkitt-Wright E, Miles E, Garg S, Scott-Kitching V, et al. Comprehensive RNA analysis of the NF1 gene in classically affected NF1 affected individuals meeting NIH criteria has high sensitivity and mutation negative testing is reassuring in isolated cases with pigmentary features only. EBioMedicine. 2016;7:212–20. https://doi.org/10.1016/j.ebiom.2016.04.005.
15. Korf BR. Diagnostic outcome in children with multiple cafe au lait spots. Pediatrics. 1992;90(6):924–7.
16. Duong TA, Bastuji-Garin S, Valeyrie-Allanore L, Sbidian E, Ferkal S, Wolkenstein P. Evolving pattern with age of cutaneous signs in neurofibromatosis type 1: a cross-sectional study of 728 patients. Dermatology. 2011;222(3):269–73. https://doi.org/10.1159/000327379.
17. Sbidian E, Bastuji-Garin S, Valeyrie-Allanore L, Ferkal S, Lefaucheur JP, Drouet A, et al. At-risk phenotype of neurofibromatose-1 patients: a multicentre case-control study. Orphanet J Rare Dis. 2011;6:51. https://doi.org/10.1186/1750-1172-6-51.
18. Darrigo LG Jr, Geller M, Bonalumi Filho A, Azulay DR. Prevalence of plexiform neurofibroma in children and adolescents with type I neurofibromatosis. J Pediatr. 2007;83(6):571–3. https://doi.org/10.2223/JPED.1718.
19. Tucker T, Friedman JM, Friedrich RE, Wenzel R, Funsterer C, Mautner VF. Longitudinal study of neurofibromatosis 1 associated plexiform neurofibromas. J Med Genet. 2009;46(2):81–5. https://doi.org/10.1136/jmg.2008.061051.
20. Mautner VF, Hartmann M, Kluwe L, Friedrich RE, Funsterer C. MRI growth patterns of plexiform neurofibromas in patients with neurofibromatosis type 1. Neuroradiology. 2006;48(3):160–5. https://doi.org/10.1007/s00234-005-0033-4.
21. Evans D, Baser M, McGaughran J, Sharif S, Howard E, Moran A. Malignant peripheral nerve sheath tumours in neurofibromatosis 1. J Med Genet. 2002;39(5):311–4. https://doi.org/10.1136/jmg.39.5.311.
22. Ferner RE, Gutmann DH. International consensus statement on malignant peripheral nerve sheath tumors in neurofibromatosis. Cancer Res. 2002;62(5):1573–7.
23. Ducatman BS, Scheithauer BW, Piepgras DG, Reiman HM, Ilstrup DM. Malignant peripheral nerve sheath tumors. A clinicopathologic study of 120 cases. Cancer. 1986;57(10):2006–21.
24. Friedman JM. Neurofibromatosis 1: clinical manifestations and diagnostic criteria. J Child Neurol. 2002;17(8):548–554. https://doi.org/10.1177/088307380201700802. discussion 71–2, 646–51.
25. Listernick R, Charrow J, Greenwald MJ, Esterly NB. Optic gliomas in children with neurofibromatosis type 1. J Pediatr. 1989;114(5):788–92.
26. Lewis RA, Gerson LP, Axelson KA, Riccardi VM, Whitford RP. von Recklinghausen neurofibromatosis. II. Incidence of optic gliomata. Ophthalmology. 1984;91(8):929–35.
27. Lund AM, Skovby F. Optic gliomas in children with neurofibromatosis type 1. Eur J Pediatr. 1991;150(12):835–8.
28. Prada CE, Hufnagel RB, Hummel TR, Lovell AM, Hopkin RJ, Saal HM, et al. The use of magnetic resonance imaging screening for optic pathway gliomas in children with neurofibromatosis type 1. J Pediatrics. 2015;167(4):851–6.e1. https://doi.org/10.1016/j.jpeds.2015.07.001.
29. Blazo MA, Lewis RA, Chintagumpala MM, Frazier M, McCluggage C, Plon SE. Outcomes of systematic screening for optic pathway tumors in children with Neurofibromatosis Type 1. Am J Med Genet Part A. 2004;127A(3):224–9. https://doi.org/10.1002/ajmg.a.20650.
30. Listernick R, Charrow J, Greenwald M, Mets M. Natural history of optic pathway tumors in children with neurofibromatosis type 1: a longitudinal study. J Pediatr. 1994;125(1):63–6.

31. Molloy PT, Bilaniuk LT, Vaughan SN, Needle MN, Liu GT, Zackai EH, et al. Brainstem tumors in patients with neurofibromatosis type 1: a distinct clinical entity. Neurology. 1995;45(10):1897–902.
32. Slamovits TL. Von Recklinghausen neurofibromatosis: II. Incidence of optic gliomata. Ophthalmology. 1985;92(5):714–5.
33. Kornreich L, Blaser S, Schwarz M, Shuper A, Vishne TH, Cohen IJ, et al. Optic pathway glioma: correlation of imaging findings with the presence of neurofibromatosis. AJNR Am J Neuroradiol. 2001;22(10):1963–9.
34. Deliganis AV, Geyer JR, Berger MS. Prognostic significance of type 1 neurofibromatosis (von Recklinghausen disease) in childhood optic glioma. Neurosurgery. 1996;38(6):1114–8. discussion 8–9
35. Listernick R, Darling C, Greenwald M, Strauss L, Charrow J. Optic pathway tumors in children: the effect of neurofibromatosis type 1 on clinical manifestations and natural history. J Pediatr. 1995;127(5):718–22.
36. Listernick R, Louis DN, Packer RJ, Gutmann DH. Optic pathway gliomas in children with neurofibromatosis 1: consensus statement from the NF1 optic pathway glioma task force. Ann Neurol. 1997;41(2):143–9. https://doi.org/10.1002/ana.410410204.
37. Laue L, Comite F, Hench K, Loriaux DL, Cutler GB Jr, Pescovitz OH. Precocious puberty associated with neurofibromatosis and optic gliomas. Treatment with luteinizing hormone releasing hormone analogue. Am J Dis Child (1960). 1985;139(11):1097–100.
38. Lewis RA, Riccardi VM. Von Recklinghausen neurofibromatosis. Incidence of iris hamartomata. Ophthalmology. 1981;88(4):348–54.
39. Otsuka F, Kawashima T, Imakado S, Usuki Y, Hon-Mura S. Lisch nodules and skin manifestation in neurofibromatosis type 1. Arch Dermatol. 2001;137(2):232–3.
40. Boulanger JM, Larbrisseau A. Neurofibromatosis type 1 in a pediatric population: Ste-Justine's experience. Can J Neurol Sci. 2005;32(2):225–31.
41. Heerva E, Koffert A, Jokinen E, Kuorilehto T, Peltonen S, Aro HT, et al. A controlled register-based study of 460 neurofibromatosis 1 patients: increased fracture risk in children and adults over 41 years of age. J Bone Miner Res Off J Am Soc Bone Miner Res. 2012;27(11):2333–7. https://doi.org/10.1002/jbmr.1685.
42. Ferner RE. Neurofibromatosis 1. Eur J Hum Genet. 2007;15(2):131–8. https://doi.org/10.1038/sj.ejhg.5201676. [pii]
43. Pinson S, Creange A, Barbarot S, Stalder JF, Chaix Y, Rodriguez D et al. Recommendations for the treatment of neurofibromatosis type 1. J Fr Ophtalmol. 2002;25(4):423–33. MDOI-JFO-04-2002-25-4-0181-5512-101019-ART13 [pii].
44. Ferner RE. Neurofibromatosis 1 and neurofibromatosis 2: a twenty first century perspective. The Lancet Neurology. 2007;6(4):340–51. https://doi.org/10.1016/s1474-4422(07)70075-3.
45. Crowe FW, Schull WJ, Nee JV. A clinical, pathological, and genetic study of multiple neurofibromatosis…. Charles C. Thomas: Springfield, IL; 1956.
46. Kaufman R, Hartmann A, McAlister WH. Family studies in congenital heart disease IV: congenital heart disease associated with neurofibromatosis. Birth Defects Orig Artic Ser. 1972;7:92–5.
47. Neiman HL, Mena E, Holt JF, Stern AM, Perry BL. Neurofibromatosis and congenital heart disease. Am J Roentgenol Radium Therapy, Nucl Med. 1974;122(1):146–9.
48. Holt JF. 1977 Edward B. D. Neuhauser lecture: neurofibromatosis in children. AJR Am J Roentgenol. 1978;130(4):615–39. https://doi.org/10.2214/ajr.130.4.615.
49. Carey JC, Laub JM, Hall BD. Penetrance and variability in neurofibromatosis: a genetic study of 60 families. Birth Defects Orig Artic Ser. 1979;15(5B):271–81.
50. Schorry EK, Stowens DW, Crawford AH, Stowens PA, Schwartz WR, Dignan PS. Summary of patient data from a multidisciplinary neurofibromatosis clinic. Neurofibromatosis. 1989;2(2):129–34.
51. Colley A, Donnai D, Evans DG. Neurofibromatosis/Noonan phenotype: a variable feature of type 1 neurofibromatosis. Clin Genet. 1996;49(2):59–64.
52. Tonsgard JH, Yelavarthi KK, Cushner S, Short MP, Lindgren V. Do NF1 gene deletions result in a characteristic phenotype? Am J Med Genet. 1997;73(1):80–6.

53. Tedesco MA, Di Salvo G, Natale F, Caputo S, Calabrese E, Grassia C, et al. Cardiac abnormalities detected by Doppler imaging in patients with neurofibromatosis type 1. Am J Cardiol. 2001;88(10):1198–200.
54. Tedesco MA, Di Salvo G, Natale F, Pergola V, Calabrese E, Grassia C, et al. The heart in neurofibromatosis type 1: an echocardiographic study. Am Heart J. 2002;143(5):883–8.
55. Incecik F, Herguner OM, Alinc Erdem S, Altunbasak S. Neurofibromatosis type 1 and cardiac manifestations. Turk Kardiyol Dern Ars. 2015;43(8):714–6. https://doi.org/10.5543/tkda.2015.27557.
56. Lin AE, Birch PH, Korf BR, Tenconi R, Niimura M, Poyhonen M, et al. Cardiovascular malformations and other cardiovascular abnormalities in neurofibromatosis 1. Am J Med Genet. 2000;95(2):108–17.
57. Leppavirta J, Kallionpaa RA, Uusitalo E, Vahlberg T, Poyhonen M, Peltonen J, et al. Congenital anomalies in neurofibromatosis 1: a retrospective register-based total population study. Orphanet J Rare Dis. 2018;13(1):5. https://doi.org/10.1186/s13023-017-0756-4.
58. Venturin M, Guarnieri P, Natacci F, Stabile M, Tenconi R, Clementi M, et al. Mental retardation and cardiovascular malformations in NF1 microdeleted patients point to candidate genes in 17q11.2. J Med Genet. 2004;41(1):35–41.
59. Coonar AS, McKenna WJ. Molecular genetics of familial cardiomyopathies. Adv Genet. 1997;35:285–324.
60. Pung S, Hirsch EF. Plexiform neurofibromatosis of the heart and neck. AMA Arch Pathol. 1955;59(3):341–6.
61. Wille LE, Forre O, Steffensen RW. A familial syndrome with von Recklinghausen's neurofibromatosis, gammopathy and aorta outflow obstruction. Acta Med Scand. 1980;207(4):297–304.
62. Sachs RN, Buschauer-Bonnet C, Kemeny JL, Amouroux J, Lanfranchi J. Hypertrophic myocardiopathy and von Recklinghausen's disease. Rev Med Interne. 1984;5(2):154–6.
63. Schräder R, Kunkel B, Schneider M, Kaltenbach M. Hypertrophische Kardiomyopathie bei einer Patientin mit Neurofibromatose von Recklinghausen. Med Klin. 1986;81:264–7.
64. Jurko A Jr, Minarik M, Minarikova E, Nagi AS. Neurofibromatosis associated with hypertrophic cardiomyopathy. Saudi Med J. 2010;31(8):935–6.
65. Brannan CI, Perkins AS, Vogel KS, Ratner N, Nordlund ML, Reid SW, et al. Targeted disruption of the neurofibromatosis type-1 gene leads to developmental abnormalities in heart and various neural crest-derived tissues. Genes Dev. 1994;8(9):1019–29.
66. Ben-Shachar S, Constantini S, Hallevi H, Sach EK, Upadhyaya M, Evans GD, et al. Increased rate of missense/in-frame mutations in individuals with NF1-related pulmonary stenosis: a novel genotype-phenotype correlation. Eur J Hum Genet. 2013;21(5):535–9. https://doi.org/10.1038/ejhg.2012.221.
67. Sabbagh A, Pasmant E, Imbard A, Luscan A, Soares M, Blanche H, et al. NF1 molecular characterization and neurofibromatosis type I genotype-phenotype correlation: the French experience. Hum Mutat. 2013;34(11):1510–8. https://doi.org/10.1002/humu.22392.
68. Upadhyaya M, Huson SM, Davies M, Thomas N, Chuzhanova N, Giovannini S, et al. An absence of cutaneous neurofibromas associated with a 3-bp inframe deletion in exon 17 of the NF1 gene (c.2970–2972 delAAT): evidence of a clinically significant NF1 genotype-phenotype correlation. Am J Hum Genet. 2007;80(1):140–51. https://doi.org/10.1086/510781.
69. Tassabehji M, Strachan T, Sharland M, Colley A, Donnai D, Harris R, et al. Tandem duplication within a neurofibromatosis type 1 (NF1) gene exon in a family with features of Watson syndrome and Noonan syndrome. Am J Hum Genet. 1993;53(1):90–5.
70. Upadhyaya M, Shen M, Cherryson A, Farnham J, Maynard J, Huson SM, et al. Analysis of mutations at the neurofibromatosis 1 (NF1) locus. Hum Mol Genet. 1992;1(9):735–40.
71. Watson GH. Pulmonary stenosis, cafe-au-lait spots, and dull intelligence. Arch Dis Child. 1967;42(223):303–7.
72. Allanson JE, Upadhyaya M, Watson GH, Partington M, MacKenzie A, Lahey D, et al. Watson syndrome: is it a subtype of type 1 neurofibromatosis? J Med Genet. 1991;28(11):752–6.

73. De Luca A, Bottillo I, Sarkozy A, Carta C, Neri C, Bellacchio E, et al. NF1 gene mutations represent the major molecular event underlying neurofibromatosis-Noonan syndrome. Am J Hum Genet. 2005;77(6):1092–101. https://doi.org/10.1086/498454.
74. Nystrom AM, Ekvall S, Allanson J, Edeby C, Elinder M, Holmstrom G, et al. Noonan syndrome and neurofibromatosis type I in a family with a novel mutation in NF1. Clin Genet. 2009;76(6):524–34. https://doi.org/10.1111/j.1399-0004.2009.01233.x.
75. Leppig KA, Kaplan P, Viskochil D, Weaver M, Ortenberg J, Stephens K. Familial neurofibromatosis 1 microdeletions: cosegregation with distinct facial phenotype and early onset of cutaneous neurofibromata. Am J Med Genet. 1997;73(2):197–204.
76. Pasmant E, Sabbagh A, Spurlock G, Laurendeau I, Grillo E, Hamel MJ, et al. NF1 microdeletions in neurofibromatosis type 1: from genotype to phenotype. Hum Mutat. 2010;31(6):E1506–18. https://doi.org/10.1002/humu.21271.
77. Mautner VF, Kluwe L, Friedrich RE, Roehl AC, Bammert S, Hogel J, et al. Clinical characterisation of 29 neurofibromatosis type-1 patients with molecularly ascertained 1.4 Mb type-1 NF1 deletions. J Med Genet. 2010;47(9):623–30. https://doi.org/10.1136/jmg.2009.075937.
78. Kayes LM, Burke W, Riccardi VM, Bennett R, Ehrlich P, Rubenstein A, et al. Deletions spanning the neurofibromatosis 1 gene: identification and phenotype of five patients. Am J Hum Genet. 1994;54(3):424–36.
79. Wu BL, Schneider GH, Korf BR. Deletion of the entire NF1 gene causing distinct manifestations in a family. Am J Med Genet. 1997;69(1):98–101.
80. Dorschner MO, Sybert VP, Weaver M, Pletcher BA, Stephens K. NF1 microdeletion breakpoints are clustered at flanking repetitive sequences. Hum Mol Genet. 2000;9(1):35–46.
81. Riva P, Corrado L, Natacci F, Castorina P, Wu BL, Schneider GH, et al. NF1 microdeletion syndrome: refined FISH characterization of sporadic and familial deletions with locus-specific probes. Am J Hum Genet. 2000;66(1):100–9. https://doi.org/10.1086/302709.
82. Oktenli C, Saglam M, Demirbas S, Thompson P, Upadhyaya M, Consoli C, et al. A large deletion (1.5 Mb) encompassing the neurofibromatosis type 1 (NF1) gene in a patient with sporadic NF1 associated with dysmorphism, mental retardation, and unusual ocular and skeletal features. Clin Dysmorphol. 2003;12(3):199–201. https://doi.org/10.1097/01.mcd.0000077565.66911.43.
83. Mensink KA, Ketterling RP, Flynn HC, Knudson RA, Lindor NM, Heese BA, et al. Connective tissue dysplasia in five new patients with NF1 microdeletions: further expansion of phenotype and review of the literature. J Med Genet. 2006;43(2):e8. https://doi.org/10.1136/jmg.2005.034256.
84. De Luca A, Bottillo I, Dasdia MC, Morella A, Lanari V, Bernardini L, et al. Deletions of NF1 gene and exons detected by multiplex ligation-dependent probe amplification. J Med Genet. 2007;44(12):800–8. https://doi.org/10.1136/jmg.2007.053785.
85. Nguyen R, Mir TS, Kluwe L, Jett K, Kentsch M, Mueller G, et al. Cardiac characterization of 16 patients with large NF1 gene deletions. Clin Genet. 2013;84(4):344–9. https://doi.org/10.1111/cge.12072.
86. Upadhyaya M, Roberts SH, Maynard J, Sorour E, Thompson PW, Vaughan M, et al. A cytogenetic deletion, del(17)(q11.22q21.1), in a patient with sporadic neurofibromatosis type 1 (NF1) associated with dysmorphism and developmental delay. J Med Genet. 1996;33(2):148–52.
87. Venturin M, Carra S, Gaudenzi G, Brunelli S, Gallo GR, Moncini S, et al. ADAP2 in heart development: a candidate gene for the occurrence of cardiovascular malformations in NF1 microdeletion syndrome. J Med Genet. 2014;51(7):436–43. https://doi.org/10.1136/jmedgenet-2013-102240.
88. Rojnueangnit K, Xie J, Gomes A, Sharp A, Callens T, Chen Y, et al. High incidence of Noonan syndrome features including Short stature and pulmonic stenosis in patients carrying NF1 missense mutations affecting p.Arg1809: genotype-phenotype correlation. Hum Mutat. 2015;36(11):1052–63. https://doi.org/10.1002/humu.22832.

89. Pinna V, Lanari V, Daniele P, Consoli F, Agolini E, Margiotti K, et al. P.Arg1809Cys substitution in neurofibromin is associated with a distinctive NF1 phenotype without neurofibromas. Eur J Hum Genet. 2015;23(8):1068–71. https://doi.org/10.1038/ejhg.2014.243.
90. Koczkowska M, Chen Y, Callens T, Gomes A, Sharp A, Johnson S, et al. Genotype-phenotype correlation in NF1: evidence for a more severe phenotype associated with missense mutations affecting NF1 codons 844–848. Am J Hum Genet. 2018;102(1):69–87. https://doi.org/10.1016/j.ajhg.2017.12.001.
91. Tedesco MA, Di Salvo G, Ratti G, Natale F, Calabrese E, Grassia C, et al. Arterial distensibility and ambulatory blood pressure monitoring in young patients with neurofibromatosis type 1. Am J Hypertens. 2001;14(6 Pt 1):559–66.
92. Tedesco MA, Di Salvo G, Natale F, Graziano L, Grassia C, Calabro R, et al. Early cardiac morphologic and functional changes in neurofibromatosis type 1 hypertensives: an echocardiographic and tissue Doppler study. Int J Cardiol. 2005;101(2):243–7. https://doi.org/10.1016/j.ijcard.2004.03.028.
93. Zoller M, Rembeck B, Akesson HO, Angervall L. Life expectancy, mortality and prognostic factors in neurofibromatosis type 1. A twelve-year follow-up of an epidemiological study in Goteborg, Sweden. Acta Derm Venereol. 1995;75(2):136–40.
94. Evans DG, O'Hara C, Wilding A, Ingham SL, Howard E, Dawson J, et al. Mortality in neurofibromatosis 1: in north West England: an assessment of actuarial survival in a region of the UK since 1989. Eur J Hum Genet. 2011;19(11):1187–91. https://doi.org/10.1038/ejhg.2011.113.
95. Kanter RJ, Graham M, Fairbrother D, Smith SV. Sudden cardiac death in young children with neurofibromatosis type 1. J Pediatr. 2006;149(5):718–20. https://doi.org/10.1016/j.jpeds.2006.07.046.
96. Daly MP, Rubinstein MN. A case of neurofibromatosis associated with a coronary artery aneurysm and myocardial infarction. Clin Cardiol. 1992;15(8):616–8.
97. Nogami A, Hiroe M, Marumo F. Regional sympathetic denervation in von Recklinghausen's disease with coronary spasm and myocarditis. Int J Cardiol. 1991;32(3):397–400.
98. Hamilton SJ, Allard MF, Friedman JM. Cardiac findings in an individual with neurofibromatosis 1 and sudden death. Am J Med Genet. 2001;100(2):95–9.
99. Fuchi T, Ishimoto N, Kajinami T, Kajinami M, Ohmichi N, Kinoshita M. A 23-year-old patient with neurofibromatosis associated with acute myocardial infarction, vasospasm and a coronary artery ectasis. Intern Med. 1997;36(9):618–23.
100. Hamilton SJ, Friedman JM. Insights into the pathogenesis of neurofibromatosis 1 vasculopathy. Clin Genet. 2000;58(5):341–4.
101. Ruggieri M, D'Arrigo G, Abbate M, Distefano A, Upadhyaya M. Multiple coronary artery aneurysms in a child with neurofibromatosis type 1. Eur J Pediatr. 2000;159(7):477–80.
102. Kandarpa K, Stoll JF, Reiss C, Rutherford JD, Cohn LM. A case of neurofibromatosis associated with a coronary artery aneurysm and myocardial infarction. Cardiovasc Intervent Radiol. 1988;11(3):143–5.
103. Evrengul H, Kilic DI, Zungur M, Alihanoglu YI, Tanriverdi H. Myocardial infarction in a 17-year-old patient due to neurofibromatosis-associated coronary aneurysm. Cardiol Young. 2013;23(3):454–6. https://doi.org/10.1017/S1047951112000984.
104. Halper J, Factor SM. Coronary lesions in neurofibromatosis associated with vasospasm and myocardial infarction. Am Heart J. 1984;108(2):420–2.
105. Downward J. Cell cycle: routine role for Ras. Curr Biol. 1997;7(4):R258–60.
106. Brown JA, Gianino SM, Gutmann DH. Defective cAMP generation underlies the sensitivity of CNS neurons to neurofibromatosis-1 heterozygosity. J Neurosci. 2010;30(16):5579–89. https://doi.org/10.1523/JNEUROSCI.3994-09.2010.
107. The I, Hannigan GE, Cowley GS, Reginald S, Zhong Y, Gusella JF, et al. Rescue of a Drosophila NF1 mutant phenotype by protein kinase a. Science. 1997;276(5313):791–4.
108. Wolman MA, de Groh ED, McBride SM, Jongens TA, Granato M, Epstein JA. Modulation of cAMP and ras signaling pathways improves distinct behavioral deficits in a zebrafish model of neurofibromatosis type 1. Cell Rep. 2014;8(5):1265–70. https://doi.org/10.1016/j.celrep.2014.07.054.

109. Boyanapalli M, Lahoud OB, Messiaen L, Kim B, Anderle de Sylor MS, Duckett SJ, et al. Neurofibromin binds to caveolin-1 and regulates ras, FAK, and Akt. Biochem Biophys Res Commun. 2006;340(4):1200–8. https://doi.org/10.1016/j.bbrc.2005.12.129.
110. Hsueh YP, Roberts AM, Volta M, Sheng M, Roberts RG. Bipartite interaction between neurofibromatosis type I protein (neurofibromin) and syndecan transmembrane heparan sulfate proteoglycans. J Neurosci. 2001;21(11):3764–70.
111. Viskochil D, Buchberg AM, Xu G, Cawthon RM, Stevens J, Wolff RK, et al. Deletions and a translocation interrupt a cloned gene at the neurofibromatosis type 1 locus. Cell. 1990;62(1):187–92.
112. Jacks T, Shih TS, Schmitt EM, Bronson RT, Bernards A, Weinberg RA. Tumour predisposition in mice heterozygous for a targeted mutation in Nf1. Nat Genet. 1994;7(3):353–61. https://doi.org/10.1038/ng0794-353.
113. Gitler AD, Epstein JA. Regulating heart development: the role of Nf1. Cell Cycle. 2003;2(2):96–8.
114. Ismat FA, Xu J, Lu MM, Epstein JA. The neurofibromin GAP-related domain rescues endothelial but not neural crest development in Nf1 mice. J Clin Invest. 2006;116(9):2378–84. https://doi.org/10.1172/JCI28341.
115. Xu GF, Lin B, Tanaka K, Dunn D, Wood D, Gesteland R, et al. The catalytic domain of the neurofibromatosis type 1 gene product stimulates ras GTPase and complements ira mutants of *S. cerevisiae*. Cell. 1990;63(4):835–41.
116. Padmanabhan A, Lee JS, Ismat FA, Lu MM, Lawson ND, Kanki JP, et al. Cardiac and vascular functions of the zebrafish orthologues of the type I neurofibromatosis gene NFI. Proc Natl Acad Sci U S A. 2009;106(52):22305–10. https://doi.org/10.1073/pnas.0901932106.
117. Hutson MR, Kirby ML. Neural crest and cardiovascular development: a 20-year perspective. Birth Defects Res C Embryo Today. 2003;69(1):2–13. https://doi.org/10.1002/bdrc.10002.
118. Yzaguirre AD, Padmanabhan A, de Groh ED, Engleka KA, Li J, Speck NA, et al. Loss of neurofibromin Ras-GAP activity enhances the formation of cardiac blood islands in murine embryos. elife. 2015;4:e07780. https://doi.org/10.7554/eLife.07780.
119. Xu J, Ismat FA, Wang T, Lu MM, Antonucci N, Epstein JA. Cardiomyocyte-specific loss of neurofibromin promotes cardiac hypertrophy and dysfunction. Circ Res. 2009;105(3):304–11. https://doi.org/10.1161/CIRCRESAHA.109.201509.
120. Schubbert S, Zenker M, Rowe SL, Boll S, Klein C, Bollag G, et al. Germline KRAS mutations cause Noonan syndrome. Nat Genet. 2006;38(3):331–6. https://doi.org/10.1038/ng1748.
121. Pandit B, Sarkozy A, Pennacchio LA, Carta C, Oishi K, Martinelli S, et al. Gain-of-function RAF1 mutations cause Noonan and LEOPARD syndromes with hypertrophic cardiomyopathy. Nat Genet. 2007;39(8):1007–12. https://doi.org/10.1038/ng2073.
122. Quezada E, Gripp KW. Costello syndrome and related disorders. Curr Opin Pediatr. 2007;19(6):636–44. https://doi.org/10.1097/MOP.0b013e3282f161dc.
123. Araki T, Mohi MG, Ismat FA, Bronson RT, Williams IR, Kutok JL, et al. Mouse model of Noonan syndrome reveals cell type- and gene dosage-dependent effects of Ptpn11 mutation. Nat Med. 2004;10(8):849–57. https://doi.org/10.1038/nm1084.
124. Arrington DK, Danehy AR, Peleggi A, Proctor MR, Irons MB, Ullrich NJ. Calvarial defects and skeletal dysplasia in patients with neurofibromatosis type 1. J Neurosurg Pediatr. 2013;11(4):410–6. https://doi.org/10.3171/2013.1.peds12409.

Cardiocutaneous Desmosomal Disorders

8

Angela Hernández-Martín and Amalia Tamariz-Martel

Introduction

Epidermal integrity is essential for proper immune response against microbes and exogen allergens, as well as for preventing dehydration. Epidermal cell differentiation and barrier formation are critically dependent upon precise temporal and spatial organization of several intra and intercellular structures, among which are intercellular junctions. There are four main types of intercellular skin junctions: tight junctions, adherens junctions, desmosomes and gap junctions. Desmosomes are important transmembrane structures that are composed of three main protein families called cadherins, armadillo proteins and plakins [1]. In the upper layers of the stratum corneum, desmosomes experience a deep transformation and are called corneodesmosomes [2] (Fig. 8.1). The cadherins desmocollin (DSC) and desmoglein (DSG) are heterodimers with an intercellular domain and an intracellular part that interact with the armadillo proteins plakoglobin (PG) and plakophilin (PKP) which also interact to desmoplakin (DSP), which in turn is attached to the intracellular intermediate filaments. Intermediate intracellular filaments are composed of keratin in the skin and desmin in cardiomyocytes [3]. Desmosomal proteins may have different isoforms (DSC 1–3, DSG1–4, PKP1–3) and are distinctly expressed in the skin and heart, and therefore cardiocutaneous syndromes will appear only when the specific isoform is expressed in both keratinocytes and cardiac myocytes.

A. Hernández-Martín (✉)
Department of Dermatology, Hospital Infantil Niño Jesús, Madrid, Spain
e-mail: ahernandez@aedv.es

A. Tamariz-Martel
Department of Cardiology, Hospital Infantil Niño Jesús, Madrid, Spain
e-mail: amalia.tamarizmartel@salud.madrid.org

C. Salavastru et al. (eds.), *Skin and the Heart*,
https://doi.org/10.1007/978-3-030-54779-0_8

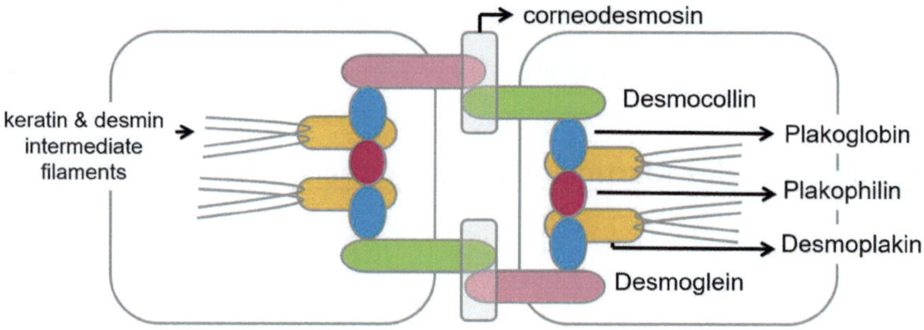

Fig. 8.1 Desmosome structure. Schematic representation of desmosomal intercellular plaque and intermediate filaments

Desmosomes and Heart

Desmosomes are essential for the heart to endure mechanical stresses caused by the contractile cycle and participate in intercellular signaling cascades whose perturbation may contribute to Arrhythmogenic cardiomyopathy (ACM) [4]. ACM is a rare, primary heart muscle disorder, presenting with increased risk for ventricular arrhythmias and sudden cardiac death. Histologically, ACM is characterized by loss of myocardial tissue and its replacement by fibrofatty tissue. ACM affects approximately one in 2000–5000 individuals and is considered one of the major causes of arrhythmic sudden cardiac death in the young and athletes. The disorder was originally termed 'arrhythmogenic right ventricular dysplasia' suggesting the dysplastic nature of the disease. ACM patients have a structurally normal heart at birth and develop the cardiomyopathy changes later in life. It was later named 'arrhythmogenic right ventricular cardiomyopathy' as it was believed that the disease predominantly affects the right ventricle (RV). This is only true for classic disease subtypes and the recognition of other forms, that is predominant left-sided or biventricular cardiomyopathy, has led to the adoption of the broader term 'arrhythmogenic cardiomyopathy'[5].

ACM is most commonly inherited autosomal dominantly, with incomplete penetrance and variable expressivity, but it can also be recessively inherited [6]. Fifty percent of patients with ACM display a mutation in the JUP, DSP, DSC2 and PKP2 and DSG2 genes encoding the desmosomal proteins plakoglobin, desmoplakin, desmocollin 2, plakophilin 2, and desmoglein 2, respectively [7, 8]. Mutations in at least ten additional genes encoding for non-desmosomal proteins have been reported in ACM so far [9]. ACM is fully penetrant in adolescence and its clinic varies from a few ventricular premature contractions and cardiac failure to cardiac arrest and sudden death. 2010 Task Force Criteria for ACM diagnosis are available [7, 8]. The diagnosis relies on the demonstration, by MRI and 2-dimensional echocardiography, of structural, functional, and electrophysiological abnormalities that are caused by or reflect the underlying histological changes [10]. The histological hallmark of ACM is the substitution of cardiac myocytes by fibrofatty tissue; this tissue replacement primarily occurs in the epicardium extending transmurally into the endocardium, which results in thinning of the right ventricular walls [11].

Desmosomes and Skin

Desmosomes do not only attach cell to cell providing tissue integrity but participate in cellular signaling, differentiation, inflammation and even carcinogenesis. They are involved in relevant cutaneous diseases such as autoimmune disorders including pemphigus vulgaris and foliaceous, toxin-mediated diseases (staphylococccal scalded skin syndrome), epithelial cancers (where desmosomal proteins seem to be downregulated facilitating malignant cell progression), and in genetic skin and heart diseases [1]. Desmosomes are essential not only for mechano-resilience of cutaneous barrier but also seem to have a key role in hair follicle biology, and their abnormality results in erythroderma, skin fragility, keratoderma and hair abnormalities. All these clinical manifestations can appear isolate or in association, giving rise to several autosomal dominant and recessive syndromes grouped under the umbrella term of desmosomopathies (Fig. 8.2). While the lack of phenotypic and genotypic correlation can make it difficult differential diagnosis among desmosomopathies, knowing the causative gene is extremely important because it allows not only predicting potential cardiological involvement but providing genetic counselling. As the only desmosomal proteins encompassing both cardiac and cutaneous abnormalities are plakoglobin and desmoplakin, in this chapter we will only comment on desmosomopathies involving them specifically.

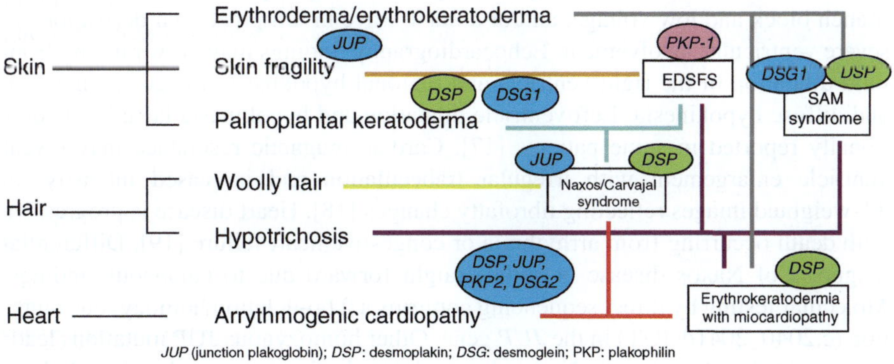

Fig. 8.2 Main desmosomopathies. The scheme shows skin, hair and heart findings and their underlying genetic basis. Note the absence of phenotype and genotype correlation

Cardiocutaneous Desmosomopathies Secondary to *JUP* Mutations

Plakoglobin (PG) is 83 kDa cytoplasmatic protein and a constituent of both desmosomes and adherens junctions, regulating the crosstalk between both types of intercellular junctions. The PG protein contains a central domain with 12 arm repeats flanked by distinct amino- and carboxy-terminal domains [2, 12]. The central domain interacts with DSP, which tethers intermediate filaments to the desmosomal plaque [13]. Plakoglobin is encoded by *JUP* (junction plakoglobin), which maps to chromosome 17q21 [14].

Heterozygous *JUP* mutations are responsible for 1–2% of all desmosomal ACM but only biallelic mutations produce cardiocutaneous syndromes [15].

Naxos Syndrome (also Naxos-Carvajal Syndrome)

Naxos syndrome was described in the island of Naxos (Greece) in 1986 [16]. Apart from the Greek island of Naxos, where the prevalence of the disease can be as high as 1 in 1000 individuals, only anecdotal cases have been reported in other countries. Naxos syndrome is caused by a biallelic homozygous 2pb-deletion mutation in *JUP* [14]. Woolly or curly hair is usually apparent from birth whereas PPK develops later in life, it is non-transgrediens and shows striata, diffuse or focal morphology. Pathology shows non-epidermolytic keratoderma [17]. ACM may be present since early in life but usually presents in adolescence with syncope and/or sustained ventricular tachycardia which may result in sudden death. Cardiac involvement initially begins from a localized region of the right ventricle, progressively affects the entire right ventricle and then the left ventricle. Electrocardiography often shows an inverted T wave in V1-V3, wide QRS complex in V1-V3, epsilon wave, right bundle branch block and low voltage, and/or a flat T wave in left precordial derivations in severe ventricular involvement. Echocardiography findings may vary, ranging from mild dilatation of the right ventricle and regional hypokinesia to severe dilatation and diffuse hypokinesia. Left ventricle dilatation and hypokinesia have been additionally reported in some patients [17]. Cardiac magnetic resonance may reveal ventricle enlargement with irregular trabeculation and increased intensity on T1-weighted images reflecting fibrofatty changes [18]. Heart disease is progressive with death occurring from arrhythmia or congestive heart failure [19]. Differential diagnosis of Naxos disease is quite straight forward due to cutaneous findings. Molecular testing by direct sequencing confirms a 2 bp-deletion homozygous mutation (c.2040_2041delGT) in the *JUP* gene. Other homozygous JUP mutations leading to a similar phenotype to Naxos disease have also been reported, although these patients show alopecia rather than woolly hair [20]. In addition, bi-allelic *JUP* mutations may result in skin fragility without heart disease [21, 22] or a lethal form of epidermolysis bullosa [23]. Heterozygous JUP mutations carriers do not show skin or hair abnormalities but ~25% have heart involvement [24] Exceptional cases of Naxos disease due to *DSC2* homozygous mutations have also been reported exceptionally [25]. The Carvajal variant of Naxos disease is due to desmoplakin mutations (see below).

The primary objective of treatment is the prevention of prolonged arrhythmia attacks and sudden cardiac deaths. Treatment options include antiarrhythmic therapy, medical therapy for congestive heart failure, cardioverter defibrillator (ICD) implantation and even cardiac transplantation [26]. Regarding cutaneous disease, PPK may benefit from topical keratolytics and oral retinoids. Prognosis is ominous if progressive myocardiopathy is left untreated. As in all desmosomopathies, genetic testing is mandatory to confirm diagnosis, prevent cardiac lethality and provide genetic counselling before future pregnancies.

Cardiocutaneous Desmosomopathies Secondary to *DSP* Mutations

DSP is a 2871 amino acid plakin protein consisting of six spectrin repeats (SRs) at its N terminus and three tandem plakin repeat regions at the C-terminus. The N-terminus of DSP interacts with the PKPs and PG, and the C-terminus mediates binding to intermediate keratin and desmin intermediate filaments in the epithelium and myocytes respectively [27]. DSP has to isoforms, DSP I and DSP II, and it is encoded by the *DSP* gene, which is mapped to chromosome 6p24 [28].

Both recessive and dominant *DSP* mutations can produce cardiocutaneous syndromes. Interestingly, bi-allelic and heterozygous mutations may result in a similar phenotype such is the case of the Carvajal variant of Naxos-Carvajal disease and autosomal dominant DSP mutations with ACM, woolly hair and PPK [29]. Cutaneous involvement in autosomal dominant *DSP* mutations varies from mild to moderate woolly hair and PPK to severe generalized involvement with erythroderma. Notably mutations within SR6 cause three autosomal dominant disorders with overlapping clinical features: erythrokeratodermia with cardiomyopathy (EKC), DSP-related SAM (severe dermatitis, allergies and metabolic wasting) and dilated myopathy with woolly hair, keratoderma and tooth agenesia.

Carvajal Syndrome (or Carvajal Variant of Naxos-Carvajal Syndrome)

The so-called Carvajal variant of Naxos syndrome was described in Ecuador in 1998 [30] and a few years later known to be due to homozygous mutations in the *DSP* gene resulting in a premature stop codon in the C-terminal tail domain and a truncated protein [31]. Autosomal recessive *DSP* mutations are associated with ACM, woolly hair and PPK, a phenotype alike Naxos syndrome. Heart disease usually presents at a younger age and has more pronounced left ventricular involvement [31] (see below). Despite being caused by two different genes, patients with Naxos and Carvajal syndromes are now considered a single entity (Naxos-Carvajal syndrome). Interestingly, heterozygous carriers of such mutations do not show cardiocutaneous disease [29].

ACM, Woolly Hair and PPK in Autosomal Dominant *DSP* Mutations

Heterozygous autosomal dominant *DSP* mutations may also result in ACM, woolly hair and a variable degree of PPK [29] (Br J D_2018). Unlike autosomal recessive *DSP* mutations in patients with Naxos-Carvajal syndrome, this group of patients display mutations in the N-terminal domain, either in the head [32] or in an in-frame duplication [29]. In a recent study of six unrelated families carrying loss of function (nonsense/frameshift) *DSP* mutations, curly hair was a highly sensitive and specific indicator of carriership status in the N -terminal mutation -carrier families, while PPK was mild and its presence seemed related to more severe cardiac symptoms [29]. Heart involvement shows incomplete penetrance and variable phenotypic expression hampering its diagnosis even with the scoring system stablished in the 2010 Task Force Criteria [7, 8]. In the above mentioned study, 40% of patients fulfilled the 2010 TFC for ACM diagnosis, and fibrofatty infiltration was observed by magnetic resonance in 30% [29].

Erythrokeratodermia with Cardiomyopathy Syndrome (EKC)/ Severe dermatitis, multiple Allergies and Metabolic wasting (SAM) Syndrome

ECK is an extremely rare condition first described in 2016 [33]. It is due to autosomal dominant *DSP* gene mutations and since the initial report of three unrelated children, very few additional cases have been published [34]. The characteristic clinical triad includes erythrokeratodermia, hypotrichosis and myocardiopathy. Erythroderma (or erythrokeratodermia) presents congenitally or early in life and may be accompanied by widespread fissures and cracks and pustular flares [34]. Severe intractable pruritus is a prominent feature. Eyebrows, eyelashes and scalp hair are sparse and there is dystrophy of all twenty nails. Teeth abnormalities include absence of secondary teeth, enamel defects and widespread caries (Fig. 8.3). Children show failure to thrive and may have recurrent sepsis. Other findings include hoarse voice, spasticity, mild developmental delay and transient pigmentary lesions histologically consistent with postinflammatory hyperpigmentation (Fig. 8.4). Cardiac phenotype in EKC seems to affect primarily the left ventricle. Echocardiogram shows left ventricle dilation in all three patients, progressing to right atrial involvement in one case and leading to congestive heart failure and death in another one [33] (Fig. 8.5). Pathology shows psoriasiform hyperplasia, parakeratosis, reduced granular layer, and intraepidermal neutrophils (Fig. 8.6). Differential diagnosis includes other causes of congenital erythroderma. Erythroderma, pruritus, failure to thrive, recurrent sepsis and psoriasiform histology are highly suggestive of Netherton's syndrome, which can be easily ruled out by immunochemistry showing negative Lekti immunostaining. Molecular testing also helps to exclude Netherton syndrome as well as DITRA, Ommen syndrome and erythrodermic congenital ichthyosis. Heterozygous *de novo DSP* gene mutations were present in all

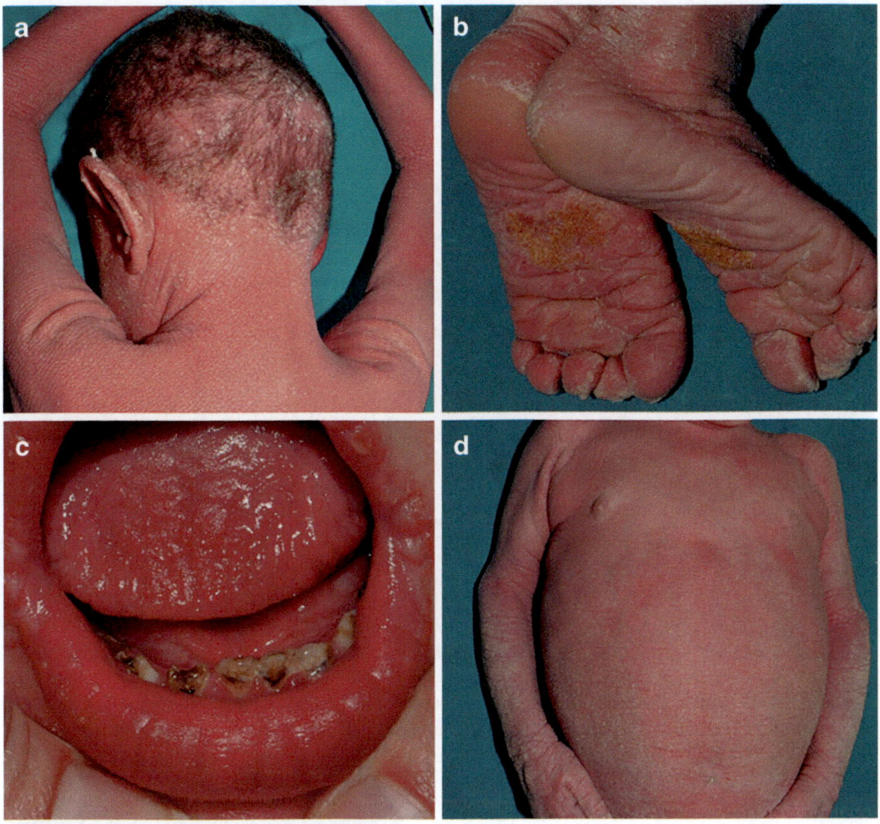

Fig. 8.3 Clinical findings in EKC. Erythema and desquamation on the cephalic pole and diffuse scalp alopecia (**a**). Warty hypekeratosis on the feet (**b**) Dental anomalies with caries in all teeth, dentine exposure and inflammation of the gingival margin. Note also everted lips with creases. (**c**) Erythrokeratodermia on the anterior trunk and upper limbs (**d**)

patients. Missense mutations were clustered in exon 14 within a short segment of SR6 and produced a consistent substitution of proline for the native residue suggesting a unique and specific pathobiology.

Severe dermatitis, multiple allergies and metabolic wasting (SAM) syndrome was first reported in 2013 [35] and it is due either to *DSG1* biallelic mutations [35] or heterozygous mutations in *DSP* [36] (Fig. 8.7). Although patients with autosomal dominant *DSP* mutations are meant to have cardiac abnormalities, the heart was normal in the only case reported to date. However, considering that the patient was 6 years old at that time, cardiomyopathy might have appeared later in life. This patient presented with erythroderma since the first weeks of life, generalized scaling, nail dystrophy, PPK and diffuse hypotrichosis. Pruritus was severe and intractable. He suffered recurrent infections and severe metabolic wasting in infancy and early childhood, pustular flares, mild global developmental delay and keratitis. Patients with SAM syndrome, both with DSG1 and DSP mutations, may show

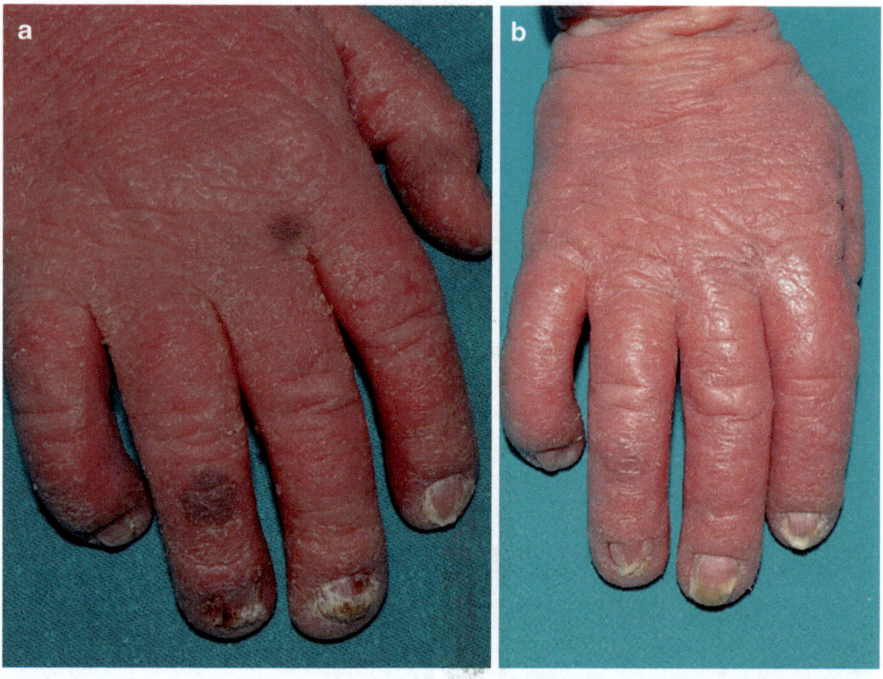

Fig. 8.4 Well-limited round to oval hyperpigmented patches on the dorsum of the fourth finger and dorsum of the hand (**a**). Note that theses lesiones faded-away spontaneously 3 years later (**b**)

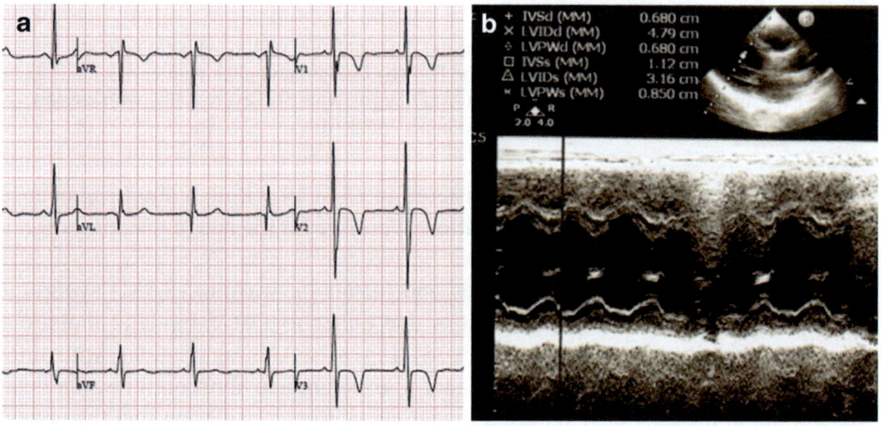

Fig. 8.5 Cardiac anomalies in EKC syndrome. Electrocardiogram shows biventricular enlargement (negative T waves from V1 to V3) (**a**). Echocardiogram showing left ventricular enlargement with normal contractility (**b**)

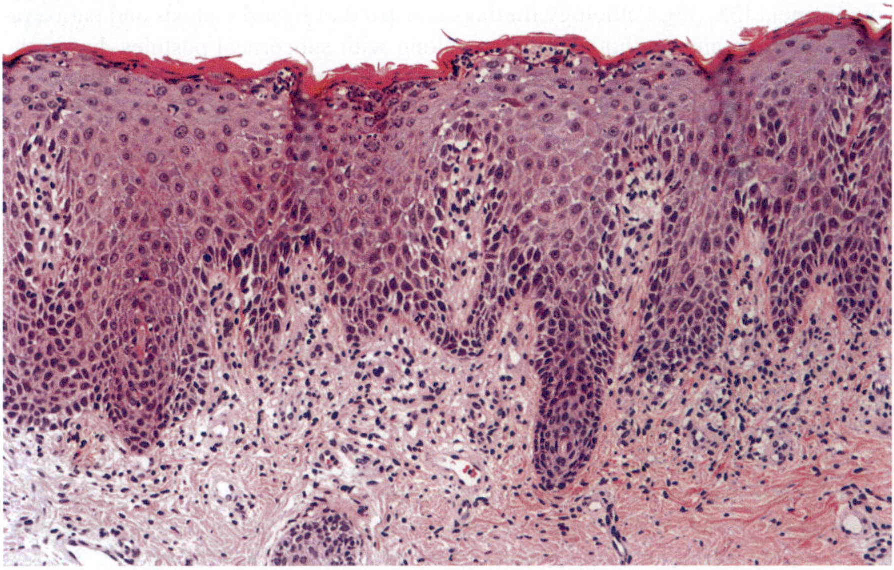

Fig. 8.6 Pathology findings showing epidermal psoriasiform hyperplasia, parakeratosis, reduced granular layer and subcorneal pustules. There is widening of the intercellular spaces between keratinocytes and mixed inflammatory infiltrates within the dermis (Fig. 8.6)

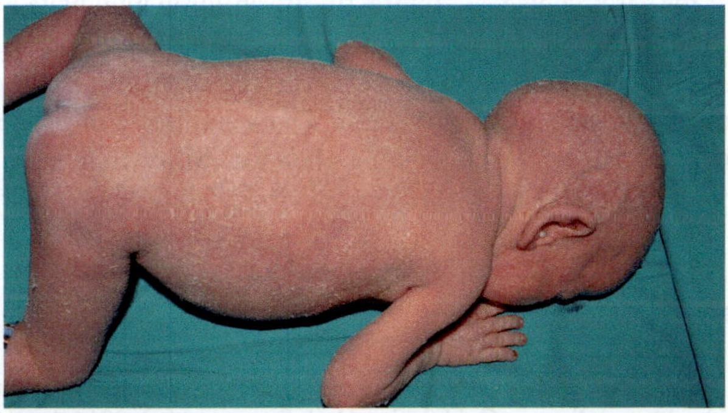

Fig. 8.7 Baby with DSG1-related SAM syndrome showing severe erythroderma, alopecia and failure to thrive (22 months of age when the picture was taken)

multiple food allergies, eosinophilia and raised IgE levels as well as esophageal involvement [35, 36]. Pathology findings consisted of hyperkeratosis and parakeratosis overlying an acanthotic epidermis along with subcorneal pustules during the pustular flares. Mixed superficial inflammatory infiltrate was present in the upper dermis. Molecular testing showed a *de novo* point mutation c.1757A>C in *DSP*. This mutation is located in the SR6 of exon 14, near but not exactly in the same area than EKC syndrome and also produces a heterozygous proline substitution. The similarities between EKC and *DSP*-related SAM syndrome are so striking that we, along with other authors, think that these two conditions are within the spectrum of the same disease [34]. Additional cases showing heterozygous SR6 *DSP* without transition to proline have been reported; all patients had cardiomyopathy and a mild to severe cutaneous involvement [34, 37].

Therapy should be addressed by a multidisciplinary team both in EKC and SAM syndrome. Recurrent sepsis and failure to thrive in infancy pose these patients´ lives at risk and should be adequately addressed. Heart disease must be monitored and properly treated. Cutaneous treatment is largely unsatisfactory and consists of symptomatic therapy with emollients and keratolytics. Pruritus is unresponsive to antihistamines and hardly improves with other sedative agents. Systemic retinoids and a variety of immunosuppressant agents have little to no efficacy [33, 34, 36]. Biologics such as ustekinumab have shown promising results in some patients [34], and a patient with SAM-like phenotype has been successfully treated secukinumab [38].

A thorough genetic testing and close follow-up is mandatory in all patients in which a desmosomopathy is suspected both to provide genetic counselling and early treatment for cardiac disease. Interestingly, children may have normal heart in infancy and childhood and develop heart disease over the years. Also, there are patients whose clinical findings but are completely superimposable to SAM syndrome in whom no desmosomal molecular abnormalities can be detected after a thorough genetic testing [38], suggesting the possibility that there are involved genes or molecular mechanisms yet to be described.

References

1. Johnson JL, Najor NA, Green KJ. Desmosomes: regulators of cellular signaling and adhesion in epidermal health and disease. Cold Spring Harb Perspect Med. 2014;4:a015297.
2. Garrod D, Chidgey M. Desmosome structure, composition and function. Biochim Biophys Acta. 2008;1778:572–87.
3. Kottke MD, Delva E, Kowalczyk AP. The desmosome: cell science lessons from human diseases. J Cell Sci. 2006;119:797–806.
4. Broussard JA, Getsios S, Green KJ. Desmosome regulation and signaling in disease. Cell Tissue Res. 2015;360:501–12.
5. Karmouch J, Protonotarios A, Syrris P. Genetic basis of arrhythmogenic cardiomyopathy. Curr Opin Cardiol. 2018;33:276–81.
6. Herren T, Gerber PA, Duru F. Arrhythmogenic right ventricular cardiomyopathy/dysplasia: a not so rare “disease of the desmosome” with multiple clinical presentations. Clin Res Cardiol. 2009;98:141–58.

7. Marcus F, Basso C, Gear K, Sorrell VL. Pitfalls in the diagnosis of arrhythmogenic right ventricular cardiomyopathy/dysplasia. Am J Cardiol. 2010a;105:1036–9.
8. Marcus FI, McKenna WJ, Sherrill D, Basso C, Bauce B, Bluemke DA, Calkins H, Corrado D, Cox MG, Daubert JP, Fontaine G, Gear K, Hauer R, Nava A, Picard MH, Protonotarios N, Saffitz JE, Sanborn DM, Steinberg JS, Tandri H, Thiene G, Towbin JA, Tsatsopoulou A, Wichter T, Zareba W. Diagnosis of arrhythmogenic right ventricular cardiomyopathy/dysplasia: proposed modification of the task force criteria. Circulation. 2010b;121:1533–41.
9. Vimalanathan AK, Ehler E, Gehmlich K. Genetics of and pathogenic mechanisms in arrhythmogenic right ventricular cardiomyopathy. Biophys Rev. 2018;10:973–82.
10. Miles C, Finocchiaro G, Papadakis M, Gray B, Westaby J, Ensam B, Basu J, Parry-Williams G, Papatheodorou E, Paterson C, Malhotra A, Robertus JL, Ware JS, Cook SA, Asimaki A, Witney A, Ster IC, Tome M, Sharma S, Behr ER, Sheppard MN. Sudden death and left ventricular involvement in Arrhythmogenic cardiomyopathy. Circulation. 2019;139:1786–97.
11. Sen-Chowdhry S, Syrris P, McKenna WJ. Genetics of right ventricular cardiomyopathy. J Cardiovasc Electrophysiol. 2005;16:927–35.
12. Huber AH, Nelson WJ, Weis WI. Three-dimensional structure of the armadillo repeat region of beta-catenin. Cell. 1997;90:871–82.
13. Smith EA, Fuchs E. Defining the interactions between intermediate filaments and desmosomes. J Cell Biol. 1998;141:1229–41.
14. McKoy G, Protonotarios N, Crosby A, Tsatsopoulou A, Anastasakis A, Coonar A, Norman M, Baboonian C, Jeffery S, McKenna WJ. Identification of a deletion in plakoglobin in arrhythmogenic right ventricular cardiomyopathy with palmoplantar keratoderma and woolly hair (Naxos disease). Lancet. 2000;355:2119–24.
15. Basso C, Pilichou K, Bauce B, Corrado D, Thiene G. Diagnostic criteria, genetics, and molecular basis of Arrhythmogenic cardiomyopathy. Heart Fail Clin. 2018;14:201–13.
16. Protonotarios N, Tsatsopoulou A, Patsourakos P, Alexopoulos D, Gezerlis P, Simitsis S, Scampardonis G. Cardiac abnormalities in familial palmoplantar keratosis. Br Heart J. 1986;56:321–6.
17. Protonotarios N, Tsatsopoulou A. Naxos disease. Indian Pacing Electrophysiol J. 2005;5:76–80.
18. Mavrogeni S, Bratis K, Protonotarios N, Tsatsopoulou A, Papadopoulos G. Cardiac magnetic resonance can early assess the presence and severity of heart involvement in Naxos disease. Int J Cardiol. 2012;154:e19–20.
19. Schonberger J, Seidman CE. Many roads lead to a broken heart: the genetics of dilated cardiomyopathy. Am J Hum Genet. 2001;69:249–60.
20. Erken H, Yariz KO, Duman D, Kaya CT, Sayin T, Heper AO, Tekin M. Cardiomyopathy with alopecia and palmoplantar keratoderma (CAPK) is caused by a JUP mutation. Br J Dermatol. 2011;165:917–21.
21. Cabral RM, Liu L, Hogan C, Dopping-Hepenstal PJ, Winik BC, Asial RA, Dobson R, Mein CA, Baselaga PA, Mellerio JE, Nanda A, Boente Mdel C, Kelsell DP, McGrath JA, South AP. Homozygous mutations in the 5′ region of the JUP gene result in cutaneous disease but normal heart development in children. J Invest Dermatol. 2010;130:1543–50.
22. Oktem A, Doolan BJ, Akay BN, Onoufriadis A, Okcu Heper A, Kocak O, Ersoy-Evans S, McGrath JA. Autosomal recessive mutations in plakoglobin and risk of cardiac abnormalities, vol. 45. Clin Exp: Dermatol; 2020. p. 654–7.
23. Pigors M, Kiritsi D, Krumpelmann S, Wagner N, He Y, Podda M, Kohlhase J, Hausser I, Bruckner-Tuderman L, Has C. Lack of plakoglobin leads to lethal congenital epidermolysis bullosa: a novel clinico-genetic entity. Hum Mol Genet. 2011;20:1811–9.
24. Ishida-Yamamoto A, Igawa S. Genetic skin diseases related to desmosomes and corneodesmosomes. J Dermatol Sci. 2014;74:99–105.
25. Simpson MA, Mansour S, Ahnood D, Kalidas K, Patton MA, McKenna WJ, Behr ER, Crosby AH. Homozygous mutation of desmocollin-2 in arrhythmogenic right ventricular cardiomyopathy with mild palmoplantar keratoderma and woolly hair. Cardiology. 2009;113:28–34.
26. Corrado D, Wichter T, Link MS, Hauer RN, Marchlinski FE, Anastasakis A, Bauce B, Basso C, Brunckhorst C, Tsatsopoulou A, Tandri H, Paul M, Schmied C, Pelliccia A, Duru F,

Protonotarios N, Estes NM 3rd, McKenna WJ, Thiene G, Marcus FI, Calkins H. Treatment of Arrhythmogenic right ventricular cardiomyopathy/dysplasia: an international task force consensus statement. Circulation. 2015;132:441–53.
27. Green KJ, Parry DA, Steinert PM, Virata ML, Wagner RM, Angst BD, Nilles LA. Structure of the human desmoplakins. Implications for function in the desmosomal plaque. J Biol Chem. 1990;265:11406–7.
28. Arnemann J, Spurr NK, Wheeler GN, Parker AE, Buxton RS. Chromosomal assignment of the human genes coding for the major proteins of the desmosome junction, desmoglein DGI (DSG), desmocollins DGII/III (DSC), desmoplakins DPI/II (DSP), and plakoglobin DPIII (JUP). Genomics. 1991;10:640–5.
29. Maruthappu T, Posafalvi A, Castelletti S, Delaney PJ, Syrris P, O'Toole EA, Green KJ, Elliott PM, Lambiase PD, Tinker A, McKenna WJ, Kelsell DP. Loss-of-function desmoplakin I and II mutations underlie dominant arrhythmogenic cardiomyopathy with a hair and skin phenotype. Br J Dermatol. 2019;180:1114–22.
30. Carvajal-Huerta L. Epidermolytic palmoplantar keratoderma with woolly hair and dilated cardiomyopathy. J Am Acad Dermatol. 1998;39:418–21.
31. Norgett EE, Hatsell SJ, Carvajal-Huerta L, Cabezas JC, Common J, Purkis PE, Whittock N, Leigh IM, Stevens HP, Kelsell DP. Recessive mutation in desmoplakin disrupts desmoplakin-intermediate filament interactions and causes dilated cardiomyopathy, woolly hair and keratoderma. Hum Mol Genet. 2000;9:2761–6.
32. Norgett EE, Lucke TW, Bowers B, Munro CS, Leigh IM, Kelsell DP. Early death from cardiomyopathy in a family with autosomal dominant striate palmoplantar keratoderma and woolly hair associated with a novel insertion mutation in desmoplakin. J Invest Dermatol. 2006;126:1651–4.
33. Boyden LM, Kam CY, Hernandez-Martin A, Zhou J, Craiglow BG, Sidbury R, Mathes EF, Maguiness SM, Crumrine DA, Williams ML, Hu R, Lifton RP, Elias PM, Green KJ, Choate KA. Dominant de novo DSP mutations cause erythrokeratodermia-cardiomyopathy syndrome. Hum Mol Genet. 2016;25:348–57.
34. Paller AS, Czarnowicki T, Renert-Yuval Y, Holland K, Huynh T, Sadlier M, McAleer MA, Tran G, Geddes GC, Irvine AD, Guttman-Yassky E. The spectrum of manifestations in desmoplakin gene (DSP) spectrin repeat 6 domain mutations: Immunophenotyping and response to ustekinumab. J Am Acad Dermatol. 2018;78(498–505):e2.
35. Samuelov L, Sarig O, Harmon RM, Rapaport D, Ishida-Yamamoto A, Isakov O, Koetsier JL, Gat A, Goldberg I, Bergman R, Spiegel R, Eytan O, Geller S, Peleg S, Shomron N, Goh CSM, Wilson NJ, Smith FJD, Pohler E, Simpson MA, McLean WHI, Irvine AD, Horowitz M, McGrath JA, Green KJ, Sprecher E. Desmoglein 1 deficiency results in severe dermatitis, multiple allergies and metabolic wasting. Nat Genet. 2013;45:1244–8.
36. McAleer MA, Pohler E, Smith FJ, Wilson NJ, Cole C, MacGowan S, Koetsier JL, Godsel LM, Harmon RM, Gruber R, Crumrine D, Elias PM, McDermott M, Butler K, Broderick A, Sarig O, Sprecher E, Green KJ, McLean WH, Irvine AD. Severe dermatitis, multiple allergies, and metabolic wasting syndrome caused by a novel mutation in the N-terminal plakin domain of desmoplakin. J Allergy Clin Immunol. 2015;136:1268–76.
37. Vakkilainen S, Puhakka L, Klemetti P, Heiskanen K, Seppanen M, Muona M, Posseme C, Duffy D, Vaisanen T, Elomaa O, Palomaki M, Saxen H, Ranki A, Hannula-Jouppi K. Novel DSP Spectrin 6 region variant causes neonatal erythroderma, failure to thrive, severe herpes simplex infections and brain lesions. Acta Derm Venereol. 2019;99:789–96.
38. Hernandez-Martin A, Kennedy-Batalla R, Canedo E, Bernaldo-de-Quiros E, Carazo-Gallego B, Vera A, Torrelo A, Noguera-Morel L, Gonzalez-Sarmiento R, Bolling M, Martinez-Bonet M, Pion M, Correa-Rocha R. Imbalance in T-helper 17 cells and targeted therapy in an infant with SAM-like syndrome. N Engl J Med. 2019;381:2176–8.

Part III

Inflammatory Diseases

Lupus Erythematosus, Scleroderma and Dermatomyositis

9

Branka Marinović, Marijan Pašalić, Anamaria Balić, and Zrinka Bukvić Mokos

Lupus Erythematosus

Lupus erythematosus (LE) is an autoimmune connective tissue disease that can affect different organs. LE includes three entities i.e. cutaneous lupus erythematosus (CLE), subacute cutaneous lupus erythematosus (SCLE) and systemic lupus erythematosus (SLE). All three usually involve the skin [1].

As this book concerns changes of the skin and the heart in different diseases the predominant focus of this chapter is the skin and the heart in systemic lupus erythematosus.

Systemic lupus erythematosus (SLE) is a typical example of an autoimmune disorder with multiorgan involvement and a wide variety of clinical manifestations. The autoimmune nature of SLE is marked by production of different non-organ-specific humoral autoantibodies, which develop due to the loss of tolerance and failure of homeostatic immunological mechanisms (either as a consequence of polyclonal B-cell activation or specific antigenic drive). In SLE, autoantibodies are directed against intracellular targets (antinuclear antibodies (ANA), anti-double-strand DNA (anti dsDNA), anti-Smith (anti-Sm), anti-Ro, anti-La) are markers and

B. Marinović (✉) · A. Balić · Z. B. Mokos
Department of Dermatology and Venereology, University Hospital Centre Zagreb, School of Medicine University of Zagreb, Zagreb, Croatia
e-mail: branka.marinovic@kbc-zagreb.hr

M. Pašalić
Department of Cardiovascular Diseases, University Hospital Centre Zagreb, School of Medicine University of Zagreb, Zagreb, Croatia

C. Salavastru et al. (eds.), *Skin and the Heart*,
https://doi.org/10.1007/978-3-030-54779-0_9

are not necessarily the primary pathogens causing the disease itself. However, these autoantibodies have been associated with various systemic manifestations and are believed to be a reflection of the multiorgan nature of SLE. In the light of this complex interaction, specific autoantibody-linked clinical syndromes have been identified. Among these the most notable are: anti-dsDNA form of SLE with severe glomerulonephritis, anti-Ro subacute cutaneous lupus erythematosus (presenting with cutaneous vasculitis), anti-U1 ribonucleoprotein antibody mediated mixed CTDs and SLE presenting with APS antibodies [1–3].

Cutaneous Involvement

The skin is one of the major organs involved in LE. Skin manifestations of lupus erythematosus, according classification made by Gilliam in 1977 are divided in LE-specific skin diseases (acute cutaneous lupus erythematosus (ACLE), subacute cutaneous lupus erythematosus (SCLE) and chronic cutaneous lupus erythematosus (CCLE)), as well as LE-nonspecific cutaneous diseases (calcinosis cutis, sclerodactily, cutaneous vasculitis, rheumatoid nodules etc.). Cutaneous lupus can occur as a part of systemic lupus erythematosus or as a disease *per se* [4] (Table 9.1).

Patients with systemic disease can have a broad spectrum of cutaneous and systemic manifestations. The skin is affected in 80% of SLE cases out of which in 20–25% of the patients', the skin is the initial disease symptom. Most commonly SLE patients have a clinical picture of acute cutaneous lupus erythematosus, but

Table 9.1 Modified Gillian classification of cutaneous manifestations of lupus erythematous

Acute cutaneous lupus erythematosus (ACLE)
- Localized ACLE
- Generalized ACLE
- Toxic epidermal necrolysis-like ACLE

Subacute cutaneous lupus erythematosus (SCLE)
- Annular SCLE
- Papulosquamous SCLE
- Drug-induced SCLE
- Less common variants: erythrodermic, poikilodermatous, erythema multiforme-like (Rowell syndrome) and vesiculobullous annular SCLE

Chronic cutaneous lupus erythematosus (CCLE)
- Discoid lupus erythematous (DLE)
  - Localized DLE
  - Generalized DLE
  - Hypertrophic DLE
- Lupus erythematosus tumidus
- Lupus profundus
- Chilblain lupus erythematosus
- Lichenoid cutneeous lupus erythematosus-lichen planus overlap sndrome

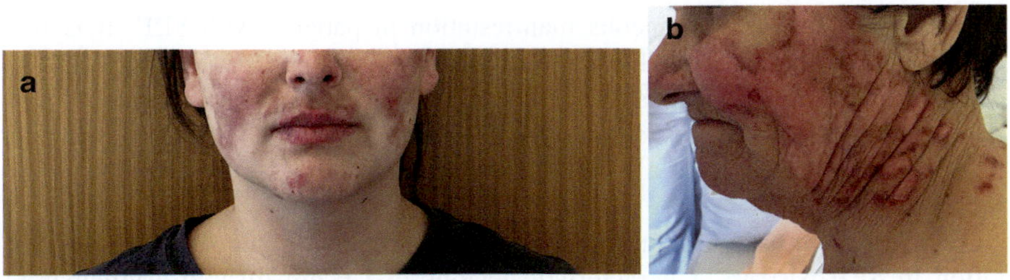

Fig. 9.1 (**a**, **b**) Skin lesions on the face of SLE patients

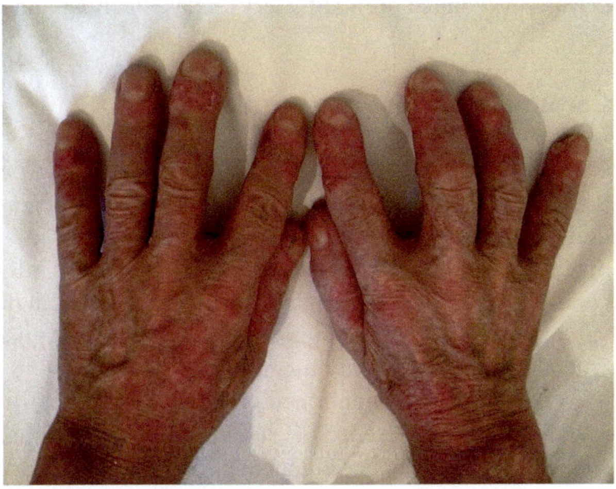

Fig. 9.2 Lesions on the hands in SLE patients

they can have also manifestations of subacute and chronic cutaneous subset. The most typical feature of ACLE is a butterfly or malar rash (localized ACLE). Less commonly lesions can also be generalized, and rarely patients can have toxic epidermal necrolysis-like presentation. Beside ACLE, patients can have clinical picture of SCLE, DLE, or lupus profundus (Figs. 9.1a, b and 9.2). In some patients more than one of cutaneous manifestation can be present. Beside mentioned manifestations, SLE patients can have oral ulcerations and alopecia.

Malar rash can precede other manifestations of SLE for more than a year. The clinical picture is of typical erythema and edema of the skin of the cheeks and the bridge of the nose (butterfly rash). Lupus erythematosus is an extremely photosensitive disease, so photoexposure can aggravate or trigger the disease. In cases with generalized ACLE patients have erythematous maculopapular eruption not only on photoexposed skin. Sometimes acute SLE can present with EM-like lesions (Rowell syndrome).

SCLE is a frequent cutaneous manifestation in patients with SLE. It is well known that patients with SCLE more commonly develop SLE (in about 50% of cases). Clinical manifestations of SCLE are characterized by psoriasiform or annular plaques. Lesions are most commonly on the shoulders, neck forearms and upper torso. Although SCLE is a highly photosensitive disorder, the face is commonly spared.

CCLE is the most common form of LE, but an uncommon cutaneous manifestation in SLE patients. Characteristic lesions of LE are discoid erythematous lesions usually on the face and neck, with follicular plugging and they heal with atrophy.

Lesions should be clinically differentiated from rosacea, sunburn, seborrheic dermatitis, contact dermatitis, erysipelas, flushing and dermatomyositis [1–4].

Cardiovascular Involvement

Cardiovascular manifestations (CVMs) are common in SLE (affecting over 50% of patients) and of notable prognostic significance (increased both morbidity and mortality), but only pericarditis and pericardial effusion are included into the current diagnostic criteria set. However, apart from pericardial inflammatory syndromes, cardiovascular involvement also includes myocardial dysfunction, valvular disease, vasculopathy, coronary artery disease and arrhythmias, all of which may have a crucial impact on patient outcome.

Whether various mentioned clinical and laboratory phenotypes represent separate diseases or different SLE subtypes remains an unsettled issue. In addition, it is still unresolved whether cutaneous lupus erythematosus (DLE) and SLE are variants of the same disease or separate entities. Be that as it may, SLE is a very diverse entity, with both cutaneous and CVMs shaping a significant portion of its clinical spectrum [5, 6].

Pericardial disease is the most prevalent CVMs of SLE, affecting between one quarter and one half of all patients. Although generally accompanied by other organ involvement, pericarditis can precede all the usual manifestations of SLE. Patients commonly present with acute (or recurrent) pericarditis or with pericardial effusion without hemodynamic compromise. They are often asymptomatic, but can exhibit constitutional symptoms, (mostly fever) and chest pain. Pericardial friction, signs of pleural effusions and ascites may be detected during clinical examination. Albeit rare, cardiac tamponade (due to voluminous effusions) and (effusive-) constrictive pericarditis do occur in SLE. These patients present with symptoms and signs of global heart failure and even hemodynamic compromise (including cardiogenic shock). Differential diagnosis of pericarditis in patients with SLE includes myocarditis, pleuritis, ischemic heart disease and pulmonary embolism.

Myocarditis is another relevant CVM of SLE, affecting up to one quarter of all patients and occurring more often in patients of African-American ethnicity. Acute myocarditis is the most common presentation (frequently accompanied by pericarditis), while subacute and chronic forms of myocarditis (characterized by extensive myocardial fibrosis and progression towards dilated cardiomyopathy) are seldom seen in SLE. Usually patients are asymptomatic, however, depending on the degree of systolic and diastolic myocardial dysfunction, they can exhibit symptoms and signs of both left-sided (dyspnea, orthopnea, exercise intolerance) and right-sided heart failure (peripheral oedema, ascites, jugular vein distention). Clinical presentation is frequently a mild one, but in rare cases it can be marked by fulminant heart failure, pulmonary oedema, and cardiogenic shock, especially when systolic function has been severely compromised. Differential diagnosis envelops myocarditis and cardiomyopathies of other etiologies occurring in SLE patients, such as viral myocarditis, drug-induced cardiomyopathy (due to cyclophosphamide, antimalarial, or phenothiazine therapy), postpartum cardiomyopathy and infiltrative heart disease (due to coexisting sarcoidosis or amyloidosis). In patients with SLE and symptomatic heart failure alternative causes of myocardial dysfunction, such as ischemic heart disease, valvular disease and arterial hypertension, also should be considered [7–9].

Valvular involvement is very common in SLE, presenting as either valve thickening, mitral valve prolapse (MVP) or nonbacterial thrombotic endocarditis (NBTE, also known as marantic or Libman-Sacks or verrucous endocarditis). Thickening of valve leaflets (as a result of valvulitis and fibrosis) occurs in up to 50% of patients with SLE, valvular vegetations (consisting of sterile platelet-thrombi) in up to 40% and MVP in up to 20%. Left-sided heart valves are most frequently affected, predominantly the mitral valve, which is affected in up to two thirds of cases. Also, vegetations are often localized on the atrial side of the mitral valve and arterial side of the aortic valve. Valvular lesions can develop at any stage of SLE and do not correlate with the disease activity. Interestingly, NBTE is found to be more prevalent among patients with elevated levels of APS antibodies (which has been shown for both lupus anticoagulant and IgG anticardiolipin antibodies). Thickened valve leaflets and NBTE usually do not cause significant valvular dysfunction, with vegetations even being prone to complete resolution. Nevertheless, valve fibrosis and tissue retraction may lead to substantial regurgitation, while valve vegetations may cause considerable orifice stenosis. On rare occasions, rapidly progressing valve dysfunction can occur due to severe valvulitis, valve tissue destruction and fenestration formation. In patients with SLE and MVP, incidence of significant mitral regurgitation is up to 20%. Important feature of NBTE (particularly when compared to infective endocarditis) is its tendency to embolize and cause extensive infarctions. This is thought to be due to easy dislodgement of vegetations in NBTE because of little inflammatory reaction at the site of attachment. Although most patients with valve involvement are asymptomatic, up to 30% of them can present with embolic phenomena. Common sites of embolization include the spleen, kidney, skin, extremities, central nervous system and coronary arteries. Patients with symptomatic embolization present with flank pain, hematuria, rash, stroke, myocardial infarction and limb ischemia. Despite cardiac murmurs being noted in half of these patients, only a minority of them will present with heart failure due to significant valvular dysfunction (i.e. aortic regurgitation). When considering the differential diagnoses of a patient with NBTE, infective endocarditis has to be taken into account. Also, as previously mentioned, in all patients with SLE and symptomatic heart failure, myocarditis and alternative causes of myocardial dysfunction should be considered [5, 7–9].

When compared to the general population, patients with SLE have a higher incidence of cardiovascular disease (CVD: ischemic heart disease—IHD, cerebrovascular disease, peripheral vascular disease), which also constitutes a substantial cause of their mortality and morbidity. Traditional risk factors (TRF: hypertension, hyperlipidemia, diabetes, obesity, cigarette smoking, family history), glucocorticoid use, disease duration and disease activity are all associated with increased CVD risk. Interestingly, younger SLE patients were found to have the highest relative CVD risk when compared with healthy controls, but the absolute risk was higher in older SLE patients. IHD presents both as acute coronary syndrome (ACS: unstable angina—UA, non-ST elevation myocardial infarction—NSTEMI, ST elevation myocardial infaction—STEMI) and stable coronary artery disease (SCAD). Cerebrovascular disease usually presents with transient ischemic attacks (TIA) and stroke (CVI). Peripheral vascular disease typically presents either as chronic or acute limb ischemia, but can also manifest as mesenterial ischemia and renovascular disease. The most common cause of CVD in SLE is accelerated atherosclerosis, the pathogenesis of which is not completely understood. Be that as it may, an important role in this process is attributed to the TRF. Not only that these are prevalent in patients with SLE per se, but also, various drugs used in treatment of SLE (predominantly NSAIDs and glucocorticoids) are associated with much higher incidence of TRF. NSAIDs are found to exacerbate arterial hypertension, heart failure, renal failure and antagonize the beneficial effects of aspirin, as well as promote thrombosis. Glucocorticoids are found to worsen diabetes, dyslipidemia and arterial hypertension, and can potentially lead to development of metabolic syndrome. Nevertheless, SLE itself confers an additional increase in CVD risk (even beyond previously mentioned role of TRF). Rapidly progressive atherosclerosis in SLE is thought to be due to systemic inflammation, that accelerates plaque formation and subsequent rupture. The following mechanisms promote autoimmune vascular injury: excessive oxidative stress, dysfunctional proinflammatory high-density lipoprotein cholesterol, type I interferon, neutrophil extracellular trap and APS antibodies. It is noteworthy that certain autoimmune disorders (including SLE) are considered as independent CVD risk factors, and are incorporated into different CVD risk scores. Regarding clinical presentation, IHD typically manifests as exertional chest pain (angina pectoris) or chest pain at rest (in ACS). Other atypical manifestations include chest discomfort, dyspnea, diaphoresis etc. In extensive myocardial infarctions, patient can present with heart failure and cardiogenic shock. TIA and stroke present with a wide variety of neurologic deficits, while peripheral vascular disease with claudication, limb pain at rest and gangrene. When considering differential diagnosis of atherosclerotic CVD in SLE, coronary arteritis must be taken into account. Although a rare manifestation, it can rapidly progress and cause a fulminant clinical presentation (e.g. as a massive myocardial infarction). Also, acute ischemic events can develop due to NBTE embolization and APS-related-thrombosis, which is why these entities have to be bared in mind when diagnosing extensive embolic myocardial infarctions, strokes and acute limb ischemia in SLE [5–7, 9].

Despite pulmonary artery hypertension (PAH) being a common finding, it is rarely a clinically significant condition in SLE. It can be caused by thromboembolic disease (in patients with APS, WHO class V), intimal proliferation of the pulmonary artery (WHO class I) and in rare instances by arteritis of pulmonary vessels. While usually presenting without symptoms, patients can also present with different degrees of (exertional) dyspnea, cough, fatigue and chest pain. Severe and chronic PAH can precipitate right heart failure, which is associated with a poor prognosis. Differential diagnosis of PAH in SLE includes pulmonary embolism, myocarditis and valvular dysfunction. It is noteworthy that the latter two conditions cause secondary-postcapillary PAH (WHO class II).

Both tachyarrhythmias and bradyarrhythmias occasionally occur in patients with SLE. While tachyarrhythmias are a common finding in myocarditis and occult pulmonary embolism, bradyarrhythmias are a consequence of inflammation and fibrotic scarring of the conduction system caused by the disease itself. Among tachyarrhythmias, sinus tachycardia and atrial fibrillation are the most common ones, with a prevalence of up to 20% and 10% respectively. QT interval prolongation is a frequent finding in patients with SLE, occurring in around 15% of patients. Bradyarrhythmias presenting as AV node block also occur, mostly as first-degree AV block, with higher degrees being a seldom manifestation. The presence of anti-Ro and anti-La antibodies has been associated with complete AV block in infants. While this seems to be a rare phenomenon, pregnant women with systemic autoimmune disease should undergo regular ultrasound studies to detect fetal conduction abnormalities.

APS is a special entity associated with SLE that exhibits a prominent cardiovascular involvement. It is defined as presence of antiphospholipid and anticardiolipin antibodies that lead to recurrent venous and arterial thrombosis and miscarriages. APS occurs in up to 30% of patients with SLE, but can also accompany other autoimmune and infectious diseases, or present in the absence of an underlying systemic disease (as primary APS). The most common clinical manifestation is the venous thromboembolic disease, usually occurring in deep veins of the legs (deep vein thrombosis—DVT) and embolizing to the lungs (pulmonary embolism—PE). Stroke is the most frequent result of arterial thrombosis, which can also affect a wide range of other locations (i.e. coronary arteries). In addition, cardiac manifestations of APS include intracardiac thrombi and NBTE. As mentioned above, PAH secondary to chronic thromboembolic disease can occur as well. Hemolytic anemia, thrombocytopenia and livedo reticularis are also present in patients with APS. Thrombotic thrombocytopenic purpura, idiopathic thrombocytopenic purpura, and occult neoplasia should all be taken into account when considering the differential diagnosis of APS [5–9].

Diagnostic Approach

Diagnostic procedure always starts with clinical picture and the history of the disease. Very important data in the history are those about sun exposure, drug intake. Classical histopathological findings of ACLE are consistent with interface dermatitis with apoptotic keratinocytes and vacuolization of the basal cells of the epidermis. In dermis lymphohistiocytic infiltrate as well as dermal mucin can be found. In direct immunofluorescence linear deposits of IgG and C3 fraction of complement are found along the basement membrane zone (lupus band test). In some patient with extensive cutaneous manifestations phototesting can be used.

Basic laboratory findings (complete blood count and blood urea nitrogen) and immunologic analysis (ANA, anti-dsDNA, anti-Sm, anti-Ro, anti-La titers and C3, C4, CH50 complement levels) are of high importance when diagnosing a patient with SLE [2, 3].

Besides standard evaluation necessary to diagnose SLE, patients with potential cardiovascular involvement have to undergo additional cardiovascular diagnostics. Although not sensitive nor specific enough, medical history and clinical examination are fundamental in the initial evaluation of every patient. Constitutional symptoms occur frequently and can be associated with different CVMs (mostly pericarditis, myocarditis, endocarditis). Chest pain occurs in patients with pericarditis, myocarditis, IHD (due to various causes), pulmonary hypertension and pulmonary embolism. Dyspnea and signs of left-sided heart failure can occur in myocarditis, large pericardial effusions, severe IHD, severe valvular dysfunction caused by NBTE, and tachyarrhythmias. As previously mentioned, severe reduction in systolic function of the left ventricle can cause pulmonary oedema and cardiogenic shock. PAH and pulmonary embolism also can cause dyspnea. Right-sided heart failure can occur in severe myocarditis, constrictive pericarditis, chronic PAH and IHD affecting the right ventricle. Palpitations and syncope can occur due to various arrhythmias.

Determining titers of antiphospholipid autoantibodies is crucial in detecting APS (and its manifestations: deep vein thrombosis and pulmonary embolism). It may also prove to be beneficial in diagnosing NBTE (especially in asymptomatic patients). D-dimer levels are an important tool in the diagnostic algorithm of various APS (and NBTE) related thromboembolic complications. NT-proBNP is a very precise marker of heart failure, that can be used in patients presenting with myocarditis, valvular dysfunction, PAH and severe IHD. High-sensitivity cardiac troponin assays are very accurate in detecting even minor myocardial necrosis, and can be used in patients with suspected IHD and myocarditis. Blood cultures are a standard part of diagnostic algorithm in patients with NBTE. Additional laboratory workup can envelop the analysis of ascites, pleural and (rarely) pericardial effusions. Pericardial, as well as pleural fluid and ascites, generally show neutrophil predominance, elevated protein levels, low or normal glucose concentration, and low complement levels. ANA, phagocytic cells with nuclei (lupus erythematosus cells), and immune complexes can also be detected. All these findings are nonspecific, which is why, when accounting for the elevated risk of complications, routine diagnostic pericardiocentesis is not recommended. However, it may be considered when trying to exclude potentially life-threatening forms of pericarditis, such as purulent, tuberculous, or neoplastic pericarditis (all of which mostly occur in immunosuppressed patients).

Electrocardiography (ECG) is a useful tool in detection of myocardial ischemia (changes in ST-T segment) and myocardial scarring (q waves), therefore being important in evaluating patients with IHD. Signs of ventricular hypertrophy can be detected in patients with arterial hypertension, valvular dysfunction and PAH. Although certain ECG changes can be detected in myocarditis, pericarditis and pulmonary embolism, these are usually of low sensitivity and specificity, thus requiring further diagnostic tests to confirm or rule out these diagnoses. ECG and Holter ECG monitor are crucial in diagnosing arrhythmias.

Non-invasive cardiac imaging methods, including echocardiography (Figs. 9.3 and 9.4), MRI (Fig. 9.5) of the heart, MSCT coronary angiography, and myocardial perfusion SPECT study, are essential in diagnosing and evaluating various cardiac manifestations of SLE. Echocardiography is the most widely used cardiac imaging modality, that can provide extensive information on all heart structures and determine their function. Dimensions of all heart cavities, systolic and diastolic function

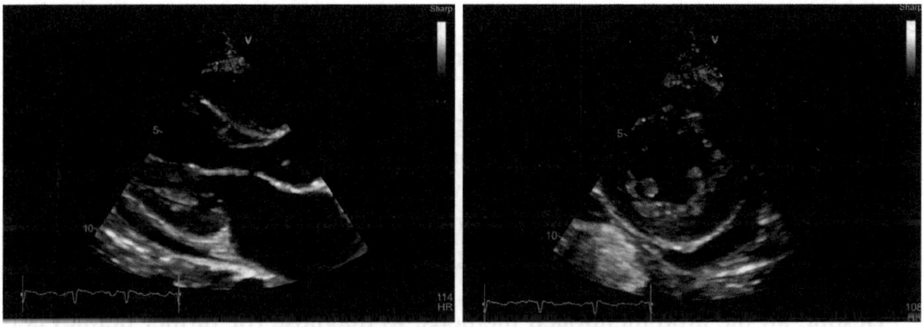

Fig. 9.3 Echocardiography of the patient with pericardial effusion

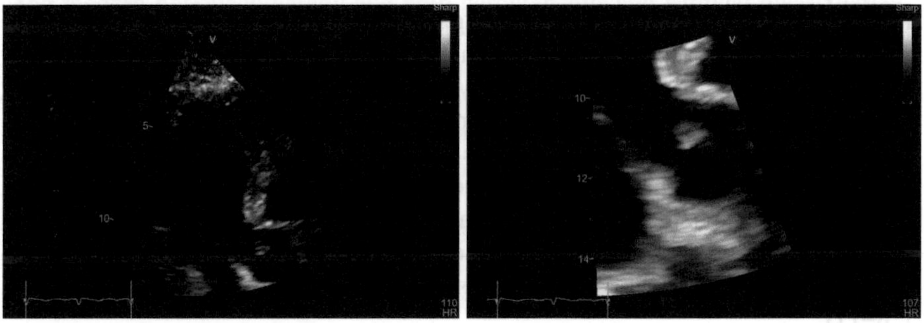

Fig. 9.4 Echocardiography of the patient with endocarditis of aortal valve

PAH present with exertional dyspnea, fatique, chest pain and cough. Depending on the severity of condition symptomatic right-sided heart failure can also occur.

Renal crisis is a vascular manifestation of scleroderma, occurring in around 10% of patients with systemic sclerosis. It is caused by microangiopathy, with renin-angiotensin axis having a central role in the etiopathogenesis. Renal crisis can present with severe hypertension, laboratory findings suggestive of renal failure, thrombocytopenia and left-sided heart failure. Although usually associated with hypertension, up to 10% of patients can have a normal blood pressure. Clinical features of renal crisis include headache, dyspnea, fatigue and syncope [14–16].

Diagnostic Approach

Diagnosis starts with clinical picture and history of the diseases. In histopathology of the early lesions there is swelling of collagen fibers and the infiltrate of plasma cells and eosinophils around vessels. In sclerotic form in histopathology there are few cells but thickened collagen bundles parallel to epidermis

As already mentioned, patient history and clinical examination are not sensitive nor specific enough to diagnose different cardiovascular manifestations of CTDs. Most of clinical features (such as constitutional symptoms, chest pain, fatigue, palpitations and heart failure) can accompany a wide spectrum of conditions and diseases. Therefore, additional testing is warranted to establish an appropriate diagnosis. Among a variety of laboratory findings, complete blood count and blood urea nitrogen can be used to determine certain manifestations of renal crisis, high-sensitivity troponin can be used to determine myocardial necrosis in coronary artery disease, and NT-proBNP can be used to confirm heart failure in myocardial dysfunction and pulmonary artery hypertension. Routine diagnostic pericardiocentesis and analysis of the pericardial fluid in scleroderma is not recommended due to non-specific findings. Curiously enough, pericardial fluid in scleroderma is of noninflammatory nature (defined by the absence of autoantibodies and immune complexes). As previously mentioned, ECG changes in pericarditis, myocarditis, and PAH are usually of no real diagnostic value. However, ECG and Holter monitor are essential in diagnosing different arrhythmias. Echocardiography is the most important tool in evaluating patients with scleroderma and cardiac involvement (including pericardial diseases, myocardial dysfunction, and PAH). It can be used to assess systolic and diastolic function of both ventricles, regional myocardial contractility, pulmonary artery pressure, presence and hemodynamic significance of pericardial effusion. MRI of the heart can complement echocardiography and be useful in analysing myocardial fibrosis and making the diagnosis of myocarditis. Myocardial perfusion SPECT study can also give an insight into the localization and extent of myocardial fibrosis. Heart catheterization and invasive hemodynamic studies are particularly useful when evaluating patients with myocardial dysfunction and PAH. As mentioned above, endomyocardial biopsy is indicated when myocarditis and infiltrative cardiomyopathy are suspected. Coronary angiography is performed when clinical features and non-invasive tests point towards coronary artery disease [12–16].

Treatment

Before starting therapy it is very important to determine disease subset, and organ involvement. In patients with Raynaud's phenomenon it is very important to avoid cold exposure and to adapt lifestyle of the patient (including cessation of smoking). Physical therapy can be helpful. In patients with ulcerations, different topical measures which can support wound healing should be used. In some patients useful is phototherapy (specially PUVA-bath therapy) to reduce fibrosis. . Systemic corticosteroids, methotrexate, azathioprine, and cyclophosphamide can be given to control inflammation.

As is the case with SLE, specific CVMs of scleroderma are to be managed on an individual basis. Pericarditis should be treated using NSAIDs, with close monitoring of renal function. Glucocorticoids and immunosuppressive therapy may be considered in cases of pericarditis with large pericardial effusions and in cases of myocarditis presenting with severe heart failure. It is important to bare in mind that steroid therapy may increase the risk of developing recurrent pericarditis and scleroderma associated renal crises. In cases of cardiac tamponade pericardiocentesis is warranted. In patients with myocardial fibrosis and preserved systolic function, calcium-channel blockers and ACE inhibitors should be considered, because of their beneficial effects on myocardial perfusion. Patients with extensive myocardial fibrosis, reduced systolic function and symptomatic heart failure, are to be managed according to the appropriate guidelines (drugs such as ACE-inhibitors, beta-blockers, mineralocorticoid receptor antagonists, diuretics can be considered). Arrhythmias and conduction abnormalities should be managed as they would be in the absence of scleroderma. Treatment of patients with PAH and scleroderma should follow the same algorithm as in idiopathic PAH according to the appropriate guidelines. Renal crisis should be managed with ACE inhibitors and other antihypertensive medications, in order to achieve rapid control of blood pressure in the low-to-normal range [12–16].

Dermatomyositis

Dermatomyositis is autoimmune disease primarily affecting the skin and striated muscles. Disease can predominantly affect either the skin or the muscles or both can be involved. Disease is usually divided in juvenile form and adult form with or without malignancy

Lungs and the heart are usually the only visceral organs affected in dermatomyositis. Interstitial lung disease is the most important lung manifestation, and myocarditis is the most relevant cardiac manifestation. Both of these are inclined to worsen the mortality of patients with dermatomyositis. Causes and mechanisms leading towards the occurrence of disease itself are unknown, however inflammation and humoral autoimmune response seem to play a significant role [1, 17].

Cutaneous Involvement

Characteristic features of the disease is poikiloderma (atrophy, telangiectasias, hyper- and hypopigmentation on the face, around the eyes and on the back of the fingers. With evolution of these lesions clinical picture of heliotrope eyelids and Gottron papules develop which are most pathognomonic cutaneous signs of the disease [17].

Cardiovascular Involvement in Dermatomyositis

Myocarditis with localized or generalized myocardial dysfunction is a common manifestation in dermatomyositis. Patients are typically asymptomatic, but can present with both left-sided and right-sided heart failure. On rare occasions acute heart failure, pulmonary oedema and cardiogenic shock can occur, mostly due to severe reduction in ventricular systolic function.

Conduction abnormalities and tachyarrhythmias also occur frequently in patients with dermatomyositis. Atrioventricular blocks are the most common conduction abnormalities, while premature atrial and ventricular beats are the most common arrhythmias. Atrial tachycardia, ventricular tachycardia, and atrial fibillation also occur in dermatomyositis. Palpitations are the most prevalent clinical feature of arrhythmias.

In line with other CTDs, patients with dermatomyositis are prone to progressive atherosclerosis, and have an increased CVD risk (irrespective of TRF). Therefore they are also at a high risk for developing coronary artery disease and myocardial infarction. Clinical presentation does not differ between patients with dermatomyositis and general population.

PAH in patients with dermatomyositis occurs as a consequence of interstitial lung disease. These patients exhibit the same symptoms as they would in the absence of dermatomyositis [18, 19].

Diagnostic Approach

In histopathology there is epidermal atrophy with degeneration of the basal layer keratinocytes producing vacoular interface dermatitis. Under the microscope dermatomyositic seems very similar to LE. Muscle biopsy is much more useful.

Medical history and clinical examination are essential in the early evaluation of a patient with myocarditis and dermatomyositis. NT-proBNP and high-sensitivity troponin serve as biomarkers of heart failure and myocardial necrosis. ECG and Holter monitoring are useful for detecting of different arrhythmias. Echocardiography is the principal diagnostic tool in evaluation of these patients. MRI of the heart is useful in analysing myocardial fibrosis and confirming the diagnosis of myocarditis. Myocardial perfusion SPECT study can be used to evaluate myocardial viability and ischemia in patients with suspected coronary artery disease. Heart catheterization and invasive measurements can provide important hemodynamic data for patients with myocarditis and severe heart failure. Endomyocardial biopsy can also contribute to making the diagnosis of myocarditis. As previously mentioned, coronary angiography is performed when clinical features and non-invasive tests point towards coronary artery disease [17–19].

Treatment of Cardiovascular Manifestations of Dermatomyositis

Although there is not enough evidence to guide the treatment, in patients with dermatomyositis and symptomatic myocarditis, high doses of glucocorticoids and immunosuppressive therapy (e.g. with cyclosporine, tacrolimus, methotrexate, azathioprine) should be considered. Furthermore, symptomatic heart failure should be treated according to the appropriate guidelines. Local treatment of skin lesions include topical corticosteroids and topical immunomodulators [17–19].

References

1. Bolognia J, Schaffer J, Cerroni L. Dermatology. 4th ed. Philadelphia, PA: Elsevier; 2018.
2. Fanouriakis A, Mostopoulou M, Alunno A, et al. 2019 update of EULAR recommendations for the management of systemic lupus erythematous. Ann Rheum Dis. 2019;78:736–45.
3. Aringer M, Costenbader K, Daikh D, et al. 2019 European league against rheumatism/American college of rheumatology classification criteria for systemic lupus erythematosus. Arthritis Rhematol. 2019;71:1400–12.
4. Lee HJ, Sinha AA. Cutaneous lupus erythematosus: understanding of clinical features, genetic basis, and pathobiology of disease guides therapeutic strategies. Autoimmunity. 2006;39:433–44.
5. Villa-Forte A, Mandell BF. Rheumatic diseases and the cardiovascular system. In: Bonow RO, Mann DL, Zipes DP, Libby P, editors. Braunwald's heart disease: a textbook of cardiovascular medicine. 9th ed. Philadelphia PA: Elsevier Saunders; 2012. p. 1876–92.
6. Hochberg MC, Silman AJ, Smolen JS, Weinblatt ME, Weisman MH. Rheumatology. 5th ed. Philadelphia PA: Mosby Elsevier; 2011.
7. Doria A, Iaccarino L, Sarzi-Puttini P, et al. Cardiac involvement in systemic lupus erythematosus. Lupus. 2005;14:683.
8. Tincani A, Rebaioli CB, Taglietti M, Shoenfeld Y. Heart involvement in systemic lupus erythematosus, anti-phospholipid syndrome and neonatal lupus. Rheumatology (Oxford). 2006 Oct;45(Suppl 4):iv8–13.
9. Miner JJ, Kim AH. Cardiac manifestations of systemic lupus erythematosus. Rheum Dis Clin North Am. 2014;40:51.
10. Asanuma Y, Oeser A, Shintani AK, et al. Premature coronary-artery atherosclerosis in systemic lupus erythematosus. N Engl J Med. 2003;349:2407.
11. Roman MJ, Shanker BA, Davis A, et al. Prevalence and correlates of accelerated atherosclerosis in systemic lupus erythematosus. N Engl J Med. 2003;349:2399.
12. Knobler R, Moinzadeh P, Hunzelmann N, et al. European Dermatology Forum S1-guideline on the diagnosis and treatment of sclerosing diseases of the skin, Part 1: localized scleroderma, systemic sclerosis and overlap syndromes. J Eur Acad Dermatol Venereol. 2017;31:1401–24.
13. Kahan A, Allanore Y. Primary myocardial involvement in systemic sclerosis. Rheumatology (Oxford). 2006;45(Suppl 4):iv14.

14. Desai CS, Lee DC, Shah SJ. Systemic sclerosis and the heart: current diagnosis and management. Curr Opin Rheumatol. 2011;23:545.
15. Lambova S. Cardiac manifestations in systemic sclerosis. World J Cardiol. 2014 Sep 26;6(9):993–1005.
16. Parks JL, Taylor MH, Parks LP, Silver RM. Systemic sclerosis and the heart. Rheum Dis Clin North Am. 2014;40:87.
17. Callen JP. Cutaneous manifestations of dermatomyositis and their management. Curr Rheumatol Rep. 2010;12:192–7.
18. Lundberg IE. The heart in dermatomyositis and polymyositis. Rheumatology (Oxford). 2006;45(Suppl 4):iv18.
19. Rai SK, Choi HK, Sayre EC, Aviña-Zubieta JA. Risk of myocardial infarction and ischaemic stroke in adults with polymyositis and dermatomyositis: a general population-based study. Rheumatology (Oxford). 2016;55:461.

Vasculitis

10

Birgül Özkesici Kurt and Erkan Alpsoy

Abbreviations

AAV	Antineutrophil cytoplasmic antibody associated vasculitis
ANCA	Antineutrophil cytoplasmic antibodies
anti-GBM	Anti-glomerular basement membrane
CHCC	International Chapel Hill Consensus Conference Nomenclature system
CSVV	Cutaneous small vessel vasculitis
CT	Computed tomography
CTA	Computed tomography angiography
CV	Cryoglobulinemic vasculitis
D-CHCC	Dermatologic Addendum to the 2012 Revised International Chapel Hill Consensus Conference Nomenclature of Vasculitides
DIF	Direct immunofluorescence
EED	Erythema elevatum et diutinum
EGPA	Eosinophilic granulomatosis with polyangiitis
FDG-PET	Fluoro-2-deoxyglucose positron-emission tomography
GCA	Giant cell arteritis
GPA	Granulomatosis with polyangiitis
HBV	Hepatitis B virus
HCV	Hepatitis C virus
HUV	Hypocomplementemic urticarial vasculitis
Ig	Immunoglobulin

B. Ö. Kurt
Clinic of Dermatology and Venereology, Adıyaman University Training and Research Hospital, Adıyaman, Turkey

E. Alpsoy (✉)
Department of Dermatology and Venereology, Akdeniz University School of Medicine, Antalya, Turkey
e-mail: ealpsoy@akdeniz.edu.tr

C. Salavastru et al. (eds.), *Skin and the Heart*,
https://doi.org/10.1007/978-3-030-54779-0_10

IgAV	IgA vasculitis
KD	Kawasaki disease
MPA	Microscopic polyangiitis
MRA	Magnetic resonance angiography
MRI	Magnetic resonance imaging
PAN	Polyarteritis nodosa
TAK	Takayasu arteritis

Introduction and Pathophysiology of Disease

Vasculitis refers to a wide spectrum of diseases characterized by inflammation and destruction of blood vessel walls. It can occur in any organ system of the body. Systemic vasculitis is a multi-system disorder of blood vessels that affects at least one organ in addition to the skin. Nonspecific signs or symptoms of systemic inflammation, such as elevated acute phase reactants, or arthralgia, are not sufficient evidence of systemic vasculitis. Cutaneous vasculitis may be a single-organ vasculitis of the skin, or a cutaneous component of systemic vasculitis, or a skin-limited or skin-dominant expression or variant of systemic vasculitis [1].

Vasculitis can affect any size of vessels of the arterial and/or venous system. The first categorization level is based on the predominant vessel size affected; large, medium and small vessel vasculitis. Small vessels are intraparenchymal arteries, arterioles, capillaries, postcapillary venules, and veins. Small vessels are located within the superficial and the mid-dermis of the skin. Medium-sized vessels are the main visceral arteries and veins and their initial branches which are located within the deep dermis or subcutis of the skin. Large vessels include the aorta, its major branches, and the analogous veins. Large vessels are not located in the skin. Cutaneous involvement is predominantly seen with vasculitis of small and medium-sized arteries [1, 2].

Large vessel vasculitis affects large arteries more often than other vasculitides. Medium vessel vasculitis affects predominantly medium arteries. Small vessel vasculitis affects predominantly small vessels. But, vasculitis of all three major categories can affect any size artery. Medium vessel vasculitis and even large vessel vasculitis can affect small arteries. Variable vessel vasculitis can affect any type of vessel, from the aorta to veins [1, 2].

The pathogenesis of vasculitis is not fully elucidated. In particular, the initial event/events are unknown. Environmental factors, infections, dysregulation in both the innate and adaptive immunity, certain medications and altered autoantigen presentation might contribute to the development of vasculitis in genetically susceptible individuals. Malignancies, connective tissue disease, and inflammatory bowel diseases are also suggested in the pathogenesis of vasculitis [3]. The association with the human leukocyte antigen (HLA) complex and the increased incidence of some type of vasculitis in some populations indicate the role of a genetic component [4]. Hepatitis B virus (HBV) is the best-identified trigger in the pathogenesis of vasculitis, in polyarteritis nodosa (PAN). In the pathogenesis of HBV-associated PAN, injury on the vessel wall might be induced by viral replication directly or, immune complexes that activate the complement cascade, and thus attracts and activates neutrophils might result in vascular lesions [5]. Hepatitis C virus (HCV) is another infectious agent that is strictly associated with cryoglobulinemic vasculitis (CV) [6]. Antineutrophil cytoplasmic antibodies (ANCA) has a central role in the pathogenesis of ANCA-associated vasculitis (AAV) [7]. Eosinophils possibly have a role in the development of eosinophilic granulomatosis with polyangiitis (EGPA) directly or through their granule degradation products [8]. In the pathogenesis of IgA vasculitis (IgAV) (Henoch-Schönlein) IgA system plays a central role.

The major nomenclature systems are the 2012 revised International Chapel Hill Consensus Conference Nomenclature system (CHCC2012) which is the revised form of the first CHCC published in 1994 and Nomenclature of Cutaneous Vasculitides which is a Dermatologic addendum to the CHCC2012 (D-CHCC) (Table 10.1) [1, 2, 9]. CHCC is a nomenclature system which provides names and

Table 10.1 Nomenclature of vasculitis by the 2012 revised International Chapel Hill Consensus Conference Nomenclature system (CHCC2012) and Dermatologic addendum to the CHCC2012 (D-CHCC) [1, 2]

CHCC2012	D-CHCC (Skin-limited or skin dominant variant)
Large vessel vasculitis (MVV)	
Takayasu arteritis (TAK)	None
Giant cell arteritis (GCA)	None
Medium vessel vasculitis (MVV)	
Polyarteritis nodosa (PAN)	Cutaneous arteritis (cutaneous PAN)
Kawasaki disease (KD)	None
Small vessel vasculitis (SVV)	
Antineutrophil cytoplasmic antibody (ANCA)-associated vasculitis (AAV)	ANCA-associated vasculitis limited to the skin (not further specified)
Microscopic polyangiitis (MPA)	Skin-limited MPA (including drug-induced skin-limited MPA)
Granulomatosis with polyangiitis (Wegener's) (GPA)	Skin-limited GPA (including drug-induced skin-limited GPA)
Eosinophilic granulomatosis with polyangiitis (Churg-Strauss) (EGPA)	Skin-limited EGPA (including drug-induced skin-limited EGPA)
Immune complex SVV	Skin-limited immune complex vasculitis
Anti-glomerular basement membrane (anti-GBM) disease	None
Cryoglobulinemic vasculitis (CV)	Skin-limited CV, without systemic vasculitis
IgA vasculitis (Henoch-Schönlein) (IgAV)	Skin-limited IgA vasculitis, without systemic vasculitis
Hypocomplementemic urticarial vasculitis (HUV) (anti-C1q vasculitis)	Skin-limited HUV, without systemic vasculitis

(continued)

Table 10.1 (continued)

CHCC2012	D-CHCC (Skin-limited or skin dominant variant)
Variable vessel vasculitis (VVV)	
Behçet's disease (BD)	Skin-limited (muco)cutaneous vasculitis in absence of systemic vasculitis (Behçet's disease with skin-limited vasculitis)
Cogan's syndrome (CS)	None
Vasculitis associated with systemic disease	
Lupus vasculitis Rheumatoid vasculitis Sarcoid vasculitis Others	Cutaneous vasculitis, without systemic vasculitis (the name should be, e.g., skin-limited rheumatoid vasculitis, etc.)
Vasculitis associated with probable etiology	
Hepatitis C virus–associated cryoglobulinemic vasculitis Hepatitis B virus–associated vasculitis Syphilis-associated aortitis Drug-associated immune complex vasculitis Drug-associated ANCA-associated vasculitis Cancer-associated vasculitis Others	Cutaneous vasculitis, without systemic vasculitis (e.g., septic vasculitis of the skin)
Single-organ vasculitis (SOV) Cutaneous leukocytoclastic angiitis Cutaneous arteritis Primary central nervous system vasculitis Isolated aortitis Others	**(Not in D-CHCC)**
(Not in CHCC)	**Single-organ vasculitis (SOV)** Cutaneous IgM/IgG immune complex vasculitis Nodular cutaneous vasculitis (erythema induratum of Bazin) Erythema elevatum et diutinum (EED) Recurrent macular vasculitis in hypergammaglobulinemia (hypergammaglobulinemic purpura of Waldenström) Normocomplementemic urticarial vasculitis (NUV) (non–anti-C1q vasculitis)

definitions. These are neither a classification nor a diagnostic system and represents an expert consensus rather than being data-driven. The use of CHCC2012 in combination with D-CHCC will be more useful in understanding vasculitis. This review is based on these two studies. Although Degos disease (malignant atrophic papulosis) is a vasculopathy of small and medium-sized arteries, it has been included in this review even though it is not included in CHCC.

Prevalence/Population Affected

Epidemiological studies on vasculitis have some challenges. It is difficult to obtain accurate epidemiological data in rare diseases. In addition, a reliable classification system and well-defined population are the requirements of high-quality epidemiology researches. In general, vasculitis is a rare disease. The overall annual incidence of biopsy-proven cutaneous vasculitis is 38.6/million [10]. Cutaneous vasculitis may affect both genders and all age groups. But, it is much more common in adults than in children [11]. IgAV is the most common vasculitis in children, affecting 10–20 children per 100.000 per year [12, 13]. The epidemiological studies on vasculitis in the literature are based on hospital records. Therefore, the data in the literature needs to be evaluated cautiously.

Cardiac involvement is most common in Takayasu arteritis (TAK), PAN, and EGPA. The heart is affected 5–55% of patients with TAK, 28–49% of patients with EGPA and 10–40% of patients with PAN [14].

Dermatological Manifestations

Clinical

The skin is one of the most frequently affected organs in vasculitis. Dermatological manifestations might occur as a result of vasculitis of vessels in the skin, or vasculitis of extracutaneous arteries that feed the skin or the mucosa [e.g. giant cell arteritis (GCA)], or extravascular nonvasculitic granulomatous inflammation (e.g. GCA, EGPA), or nonvasculitic mucocutaneous lesions with an unknown mechanism [e.g. Kawasaki disease (KD)]. Cutaneous vasculitis presents with a wide range of elementary lesions, mainly occuring on lower extremities. In vasculitis associated with systemic disease, lesions occur diffusely without a predilection site. Palpable purpura is the most common cutaneous manifestation of vasculitis. At the beginning, purpura is often non-palpable. Some lesions become papular, nodular, bullous, erosive, or ulcerative in course of time. Urticarial lesions are also a common cutaneous manifestation of vasculitis. These are often long-lasting lesions, persist more than 24 h and often associated with pain or burning rather than pruritus. The lesions may resolve with some residual hyperpigmentation or ecchymosis. Other cutaneous manifestations include papules, nodules, plaques, pustules, vesiculo-bullae, ulcers, and necrotic and livedoid lesions. Raynaud phenomenon, erythema multiforme-like lesions, pyoderma gangrenosum-like lesions, superficial thrombophlebitis, and gangrene are also seen as a cutaneous manifestation of vasculitis. While small vessel involvement usually presents with palpable purpura and petechia, macular purpura, urticarial lesions, vesiculo-bullous lesions, and pustules; medium-sized vessel involvement is usually associated with subcutaneous nodules, livedo, retiform purpura, ulcers, and digital necrosis [3, 15–17].

Large Vessel Vasculitis

Cutaneous vasculitic lesions have not been reported in TAK, although non-vasculitic dermatoses such as pyoderma gangrenosum-like ulcerations and Raynaud's phenomenon may occur. In GCA bullae, ulcers or massive necrosis on the scalp, glossitis, tongue necrosis, distal gangrene might occur as a result of occlusive vasculitis of extracutaneous arteries [18–20]. A very rare involvement of small arteries in the panniculus is reported [21]. Classically, the skin over the temporal, occipital or facial arteries is tender and red, and tender nodules might be palpable [22]. Skin-limited or skin-dominant variant of TAK and GCA are not present [1].

Medium Vessel Vasculitis

Mucocutaneous lesions in Kawasaki disease are nonvasculitic, and skin-limited or skin-dominant variant are not present [1]. This title has been discussed in detail in Chap. 12. Cutaneous manifestations might be seen up to 60% of patients with systemic PAN. And, it might be the first manifestation of the disease in one-third of the cases [23]. Cutaneous or subcutaneous nodules are the characteristic presentation of the disease. Palpable purpura, livedoid lesions, and nodules are the most common cutaneous manifestations of the systemic PAN [20, 24]. Skin lesions are mainly on the lower extremities. Less common manifestations include urticarial lesions, transient erythema, superficial phlebitis, splinter hemorrhage, distal necrosis and necrotic ulcers (Fig. 10.1) [23, 24]. Cutaneous lesions are more common in idiopathic PAN than HBV-associated PAN [25]. The skin-limited variant of PAN is cutaneous PAN (cutaneous arteritis). It is commonly presented with painful subcutaneous nodules, livedo, macules, cutaneous necrosis and ulcerations [26, 27].

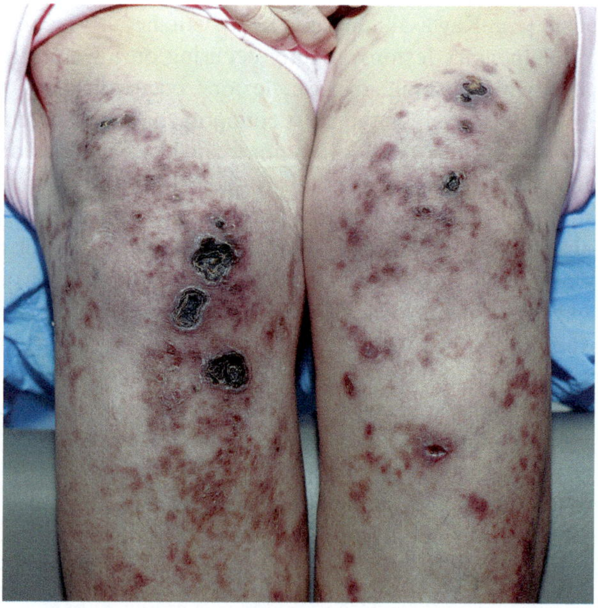

Fig. 10.1 PAN; Livedo rasemoza, palpable purpura, nodules, and ulcers some of which are covered with ectimatoid crusts on the knee and tibia

Retiform purpura that occurs by a complete blockage of blood flow in the dermal and subcutaneous vasculature, can be the first manifestation of the disease [28]. Atrophie blanche can also be a manifestation of cutaneous PAN. Other skin manifestations include palpable purpura and peripheral gangrene. The cutaneous lesions are mainly located on the lower extremities [29]. And, most of the cases are confined to the extremities [30].

Small Vessel Vasculitis

Cutaneous involvement is seen approximately 50% of patients with granulomatosis with polyangiitis (GPA) [8, 31, 32]. Palpable purpura is the most common cutaneous manifestation [14, 33]. Papules, tender subcutaneous nodules, vesicles, blisters, segmentary edema, urticarial lesions, genital ulcer, and necrotic-ulcers with livedo reticularis are the other cutaneous presentations. Cutaneous lesions most commonly occur on the lower extremities [3]. However, papulonecrotic lesions occur particularly on the elbows and it can also affect the face and scalp. Ulcerations and gangrene of the digits and penis might rarely develop [31]. Pyoderma gangrenosum-like ulcerative lesions have also been reported in patients with GPA [33–35]. Oral mucosa involvement is common, presented with nonspecific erosive and ulcerative lesions. Strawberry gingivitis is a rare mucosal manifestation which is nearly pathognomonic for GPA [36, 37]. Skin involvement is seen up to 60% of patients with microscopic polyangiitis (MPA). Palpable purpura is the most common manifestation [8, 23, 31, 33]. Other manifestations include segmentary edema, livedo reticularis, nodules, urticarial lesions, and necrotic skin ulcers [23, 33]. Skin lesions most commonly occur on the lower extremities and usually appear at an early stage of MPA [38]. Neutrophilic dermatosis such as erythema elevatum et diutinum (EED) and Sweet syndrome is also reported in patients with MPA [35]. Skin involvement is seen approximately 80% of patients with EGPA. Cutaneous findings occur typically during the third phase of the disease. Palpable purpura is the most common cutaneous manifestation of EGPA [8, 31, 33]. Segmentary edema, nodules, vesicles, aseptic pustules, livedo reticularis, urticarial lesions, necrotic purpura, and necrotic ulcers are the other cutaneous presentations [31, 33, 39]. Erythema multiforme-like eruptions and Sweet syndrome have also been described [33, 40].

AAV limited to the skin is mostly drug-induced cutaneous AAV. It may be further defined as skin limited GPA, MPA or EGPA [1].

All categories of immune complex vasculitis have cutaneous features of systemic vasculitis and skin-limited variant, except anti-glomerular basement membrane (anti-GBM) disease [1]. Palpable purpura is one of the classic tetrads of IgAV and it is usually the initial presentation [41]. Gravity-dependent areas and pressure point, especially lower extremities and buttocks, are the predilection site of cutaneous lesions. Palpable purpura is mostly symmetric and localized especially around the ankles (Fig. 10.2). Purpura may be bullous hemorrhagic or necrotic in adults. Erythematous macules, ecchymoses, petechia, and urticarial wheals may also occur in patients with IgAV [13]. Persistent urticarial lesions, that may be accompanied with petechiae or postinflammatory hyperpigmentation is the characteristic cutaneous manifestation of hypocomplementemic urticarial vasculitis (HUV). Livedo

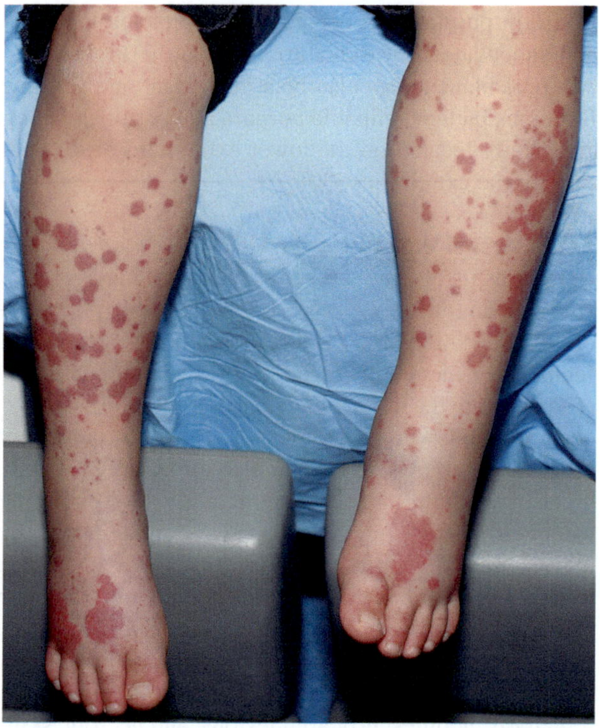

Fig. 10.2 IgA vasculitis; left ankle arthritis with numerous palpable purpuric lesions

reticularis, papules, nodules, bullae, and necrotic ulcerative lesions may occur [3]. Cutaneous manifestations are one of the most frequent symptoms in patients with CV. Purpura is one of the typical clinical triads of CV. Purpura located on the lower extremities, Reynaud's phenomenon and acrocyanosis are the cutaneous presentations of CV.

Variable Vessel Vasculitis

Behçet's disease has cutaneous features of systemic vasculitis and skin-limited form. This title has been discussed in detail in Chap. 11. Cogan's syndrome has cutaneous features of systemic vasculitis. Skin-limited or skin-dominant variant is not present [1].

Vasculitis Associated with Systemic Disease

Systemic diseases have cutaneous features of systemic vasculitis and skin-limited form. Rheumatoid vasculitis is a late complication of rheumatoid arthritis [42]. Skin is one of the most commonly involved organs in rheumatoid vasculitis. Common cutaneous manifestations of rheumatoid vasculitis include palpable purpura, cutaneous ulcers, digital ischemia/gangrene, nail fold infarcts, and pyoderma gangrenosum with a predilection of the lower extremities. Ulcers on the lower extremities characteristically occur on the dorsum of the foot [43, 44]. Pyoderma gangrenosum has a well-documented association with both systemic lupus erythematosus and rheumatoid arthritis [3].

Single Organ Vasculitis

In dermatology, cutaneous small vessel vasculitis (CSVV) is the most common type of vasculitis. Palpable purpura is the major cutaneous manifestation of CSVV. Other cutaneous manifestations include papules, nodules, plaques, pustules, vesiculo-bullae, ulcers, and urticarial lesions. Skin lesions mainly occur on legs, particularly the lower legs [3].

Nodular cutaneous vasculitis (erythema induratum of Bazin) is characterized by recurrent violaceous nodules and plaques that usually occur on the lower legs, especially the calves. Nodules tend to ulceration. Resolution of lesions with postinflammatory hyperpigmentation occurs [45, 46].

The typical cutaneous lesions of EED are persistent, symmetrical, firm, red to reddish brown or purple papules and nodules, plaques or nodules. Acral and periarticular areas, in particular, the extensor surfaces of the fingers, hands, elbows, ankles, and knees are the predilection sites of EED [47].

Others

Degos disease has cutaneous features of systemic vasculitis and skin-limited form. Cutaneous lesions appear initially as small erythematous papules. After a few days, characteristic cutaneous lesions occur that are large papules with an atrophic porcelain-white center and an erythematous, telangiectatic rim. The appearance of the lesions is similar to atrophie blanche. The lesions are mostly located on the trunk and the upper extremities, and cutaneous involvement typically precedes systemic manifestations [48, 49].

Histological Manifestation

Histopathology is the "gold standard" for the diagnosis of cutaneous vasculitis. Timing and appropriate sampling of skin biopsy is crucial to increase diagnostic yield. Vasculitis is a dynamic process and the inflammatory infiltrate changes within time. The optimal time for skin biopsy is between 24 and 48 h after the appearance of lesion for histopathological examination. Ideally, skin lesions should be biopsied within the first 24 h of appearance for direct immunofluorescence (DIF) examination. In general, for the diagnosis of small vessel vasculitis punch biopsies are adequate while an incisional or excisional biopsy is required to diagnose vasculitis of larger vessels [15].

The main histopathological pattern of cutaneous vasculitis (e.g. PAN, AAV, immune complex vasculitis, CSVV, rheumatoid vasculitis, lupus vasculitis, septic vasculitis, EED) in skin biopsy is leukocytoclastic vasculitis with fibrinoid necrosis, neutrophilic infiltration of the vessel walls and nuclear dust [3]. The neutrophils undergo degeneration (leukocytoclasis) with the formation of nuclear dust. In older lesions, mononuclear cells predominate, particularly lymphocytes. In addition, palisaded and neutrophilic granulomatous dermatitis, also known as Winkelman's granuloma, can be seen in GPA, EGPA, and rheumatoid vasculitis. While the presence of eosinophils and flame figures with such granulomas is in favor of EGPA, the presence of neutrophils and nuclear dust favors GPA and rheumatoid vasculitis. Additional histopathologic patterns such as vacuolar interface dermatitis in lupus vasculitis, or subepidermal and intraepidermal neutrophilic abscesses in infection-related vasculitis, may be helpful in the diagnosis of cutaneous vasculitis [50].

Presence of lesions at all stages of development, representing different stages of the inflammatory process is a characteristic feature of PAN [3, 51]. And, PAN always affects arteries, not involve veins. AAV affects cutaneous postcapillary venules, small veins and arterioles, and small arteries [1]. Granulomatous inflammation that is observed in biopsy specimens taken from internal organ infiltrates, is uncommonly demonstrated in skin lesions of GPA and EGPA. Numerous eosinophils in the inflammatory infiltrate are diagnostic for EGPA. Although, AAV is pauci-immune (mean no or minimal immune deposits) vasculitis, DIF on skin lesions might demonstrate immunoglobulin (Ig), particularly IgM and complement C3 deposits around the wall of small vessels in the dermis. DIF positivity is most common in patients with GPA, and least common in patients with MPA [3, 52]. Deposition of IgM and complement C3 can be demonstrated in all cases of cutaneous vasculitis and it is nonspecific. CV, IgAV, HUV, and CSVV mainly affect postcapillary venules. IgA depositions in dermal vessel walls are characteristic for IgAV [13]. DIF studies reveal of IgM, IgG and/or complement C3 perivascular deposits in CV, urticarial vasculitis and CSVV [3]. Vasculitis associated with systemic disease mainly affects small and medium-sized vessels. Skin biopsy specimen in sarcoidosis may demonstrate the histopathological pattern of leukocytoclastic vasculitis or granulomatous vasculitis [1, 53]. The primary histopathological pattern in nodular cutaneous vasculitis is lobular panniculitis, with varying combinations of granulomatous inflammation, vasculitis, and septal fibrosis [45]. Histopathologically, the characteristic finding of EED is angiocentric and storiform fibrosis with leukocytoclastic vasculitis and is known as fibrosing vasculitis. Skin lesions of Degos disease are characterized by wedge-shaped necrosis with a sparse perivascular lymphohistiocytic infiltrate at the edge of the necrotic area and an atrophic epidermis, histologically. Necrosis occurs due to thrombotic occlusion of the small arteries [48].

Differential

Cutaneous vasculitis presents with a wide range of elementary lesions, but none of them is specific for vasculitis. Clinical differential diagnosis of cutaneous vasculitis is summarized in Table 10.2 according to most common cutaneous manifestations.

Table 10.2 Clinical differential diagnosis of cutaneous vasculitis

Purpuric papules/ plaques/ macules/ patches	**Hemorrhage** • Trauma • Solar/senile purpura • Arthropod bites • Medication-related (e.g. aspirin, topical or systemic corticosteroids) • Thrombocytopenia and platelet dysfunction • Coagulopathies • Viral exanthems (e.g. parvovirus B19) • Scurvy • Pigmented purpuric dermatosis • Primary systemic amyloidosis • Ehler Danlos syndrome • Gardner-Diamond syndrome **Thromboses** • Hypercoagulable state (e.g. antiphospholipid antibody, protein S and protein C deficiency) • Livedoid vasculopathy • Purpura fulminans • Heparin necrosis • Warfarin necrosis • Thrombocythemia • Thrombotic thrombocytopenic purpura • Hemolytic uremic syndrome • Paroxysmal nocturnal hemoglobinuria • Calcyphylaxis **Dysproteinemia** • Cryoglobulinemia • Cryofibrinogenemia • Hypergammaglobulinemic purpura of Waldenström **Emboli** • Cholesterol • Cardiac (infective endocarditis, atrial myxoma) • Fibrinocruroric emboli • Other (e.g. fat, air, neoplastic)
Urticarial lesions	• Urticaria • Arthropod bites and papular urticaria • Urticaria multiforme • Erythema multiforme • Serum sickness-like reaction • Viral exanthems • Sweet syndrome • Urticarial phase of bullous pemphigoid • Urticarial drug eruptions • Autoinflammatory diseases (e.g. periodic fevers) • Cryopyrin- associated periodic syndromes (e.g. Muckle-Wells syndrome) • Schnitzler syndrome • Adult-onset Still disease

(continued)

Table 10.2 (continued)

Ulcers ± atrophie blanche	**Physical** • Pressure • Burns (chemical, thermal, electrical) • Factitial • Cold injury • Radiation • Trauma **Vascular diseases** • Arterial (e.g. atherosclerotic) • Venous (e.g. stasis), • Lymphedema **Infections** • Bacterial (e.g. ecthyma, ecthyma gangrenosum) • Mycobacterial and treponemal infections • Fungal • Protozoal (e.g. leishmaniasis) **Drugs** • Heparin necrosis • Warfarin necrosis • Halogenodermas **Vasculopathies** • Livedoid vasculopathy • Buerger disease **Hematologic diseases** • Hemoglobinopathies (e.g. Sickle cell anemia, Thalassemia, Hereditary spherocytosis) • Thrombocytosis • Hypercoagulable states (e.g. antiphospholipid antibodies, protein S and protein C deficiency) **Others** • Pyoderma gangrenosum • Calciphylaxis • Lucio phenomenon (leprosy)

Cardiological Manifestations

Clinical

Cardiologic involvement can occur almost all primary vasculitis, and any cardiac tissue can be involved. Although the overall percentage of cardiologic involvement in patients with vasculitis is less than 10%, it can occur in half of the patients with EGPA and TAK [14, 54]. Cardiac manifestations in primary vasculitis includes pericarditis, myocarditis, coronary arteritis, valvulopathy and intracavitary cardiac thrombosis [54]. A significant proportion of patients with cardiac involvement might be asymptomatic.

In TAK cardiologic involvement is common. It can occur in approximately half of the patients [55]. Aortic regurgitation is the most common cardiac manifestation

[14]. Pericarditis, myocarditis, coronary arteritis, and intracavitary cardiac thrombosis are the other cardiac manifestations [56]. Dilated cardiomyopathy, congestive heart failure, ischemic heart disease, arrhythmia, and sudden death might be the cardiac presentations.

In GCA cardiac involvement is rare. Coronary arteritis, pericarditis, myocarditis and aortic regurgitation are the disease-specific cardiac manifestations.

KD is the leading cause of acquired pediatric heart disease in developed countries [57]. Coronary artery abnormalities are the most characteristic and clinically significant complication of KD which may vary from asymptomatic coronary artery dilatation to giant aneurysms. This title has been discussed in detail in Chap. 12.

In PAN, myocardial involvement is the main cardiac involvement which is secondary to vasculitis of the coronary arteries or uncontrolled hypertension. Congestive heart failure is the main clinical feature and acute myocardial infarction is a rare entity [14, 58]. Coronary arteritis, fibrinous pericarditis, and rarely myocarditis are the inflammatory cardiac manifestations [54, 59].

Cardiac involvement occurs in up to 46% of patients with GPA [60–62]. However, symptomatic cardiac involvement is rare. Pericarditis and arrhythmias are the most common cardiac manifestations [54, 63]. Pericardial effusion is usually mild, and pericarditis is usually asymptomatic. Cardiac arrhythmias in patients with GPA is typically supraventricular tachyarrhythmias. Myocarditis, endocarditis, coronary arteritis, cardiac thrombus, and conduction system disturbances are less frequent manifestations [54, 63, 64]. Cardiac valvular involvement is uncommon, and the most frequent valvular presentation is aortic regurgitation followed by mitral insufficiency [63, 65]. Intracardiac atrial and ventricular masses are also uncommon [66].

Cardiac involvement is uncommon in MPA. Data on cardiac involvement in MPA remains limited. Heart failure, pericarditis, pericardial effusion, cardiomyopathy, aortic incompetence and rhythm disturbances are cardiac manifestations of MPA [67, 68].

Cardiac involvement is the most common in EGPA in AAV and it occurs up to 50% of patients with EGPA [8, 69, 70]. It is usually an early manifestation [54, 70]. Vasculitis-related ischemia and eosinophilic cytotoxicity are the main mechanisms in the development of cardiac involvement in patients with EGPA. The most common cardiac manifestations are arrhythmia, pericarditis, and myocarditis with cardiomyopathy and heart failure. Valvular involvement is frequently asymptomatic [71, 72]. Cardiomyopathy is more common in childhood than in adult patients [73]. Coronary vasculitis, heart block, intraventricular thrombus formation, and sudden cardiac death might also be seen as a cardiac manifestation [54, 74]. Dilated cardiomyopathy has been reported [75]. Patients with negative ANCA test results are more likely to have cardiac involvement [54, 63]. An important proportion of patients with cardiac involvement are asymptomatic [72]. Cardiac involvement might be detected in the absence of clinical symptoms and major electrocardiography (ECG) abnormalities [71]. All patients with GPA and EPGA should be evaluated with both ECG and echocardiography. If any abnormality is detected, cardiac Magnetic resonance imaging (MRI) should be performed [54, 74].

Pericarditis and coronary vasculitis are the cardiac manifestations of CV [54, 76]. Cardiac involvement in IgAV and HUV is very rare.

Pericarditis, valvulopathy and coronary vasculitis are the main cardiac manifestations of Behçet's disease. This title has been discussed in detail in Chap. 11.

In Cogan syndrome, cardiovascular manifestations include aortitis with aortic insufficiency, Takayasu-like stenotic vascular lesions, and coronary artery involvement [77]. Aortitis can be asymptomatic or associated with severe aortic regurgitation [78].

Cardiac involvement in Degos disease is limited to case reports. In the literature, approximately 200 Degos diseases were reported and cardiac involvement was obtained in 20% of patients [49].

Investigations

Cardiac investigations in patients with vasculitis include laboratory tests, ECG, echocardiography, MRI, multislice computed tomography (CT), coronary angiography, fluoro-2-deoxyglucose positron-emission tomography (FDG-PET) and endomyocardial biopsy. Endomyocardial biopsy is not always possible and none of the other investigations are completely sensitive and specific for the diagnosis of vasculitis. The diagnosis of cardiac involvement often requires high suspicion.

In a laboratory test, elevated cardiac biomarkers such as troponin T and natriuretic peptides can be seen due to myocardial ischemia. Patients can also have rhythm and conduction defects, ischemic changes in ECG. Echocardiography is the primary imaging modality and an important tool for the diagnosis and follow-up of cardiac involvement in vasculitis. Coronary artery abnormalities, cardiac chamber enlargement, systolic and diastolic left ventricular dysfunction, valve dysfunction, pericarditis, and cardiac thrombus might be detected with transthoracic echocardiography. For a detailed evaluation of myocardial systolic and diastolic dysfunction, two-dimensional speckle tracking strain, strain rate, and rotation analysis might be used. A normal echocardiogram does not always exclude cardiac involvement [57, 71]. Cardiac MRI might be the most sensitive imaging modality for the detection of an early lesion and follow-up of cardiac involvement [79]. The assessment of the whole myocardium of all cardiac chambers and pericardial involvement can be demonstrated [80]. It is a "gold standard" imaging modality in the assessment of the right ventricle. Delayed contrast enhancement on cardiac MRI is associated with myocardial damage such as active myocarditis or endomyocardial fibrosis [81, 82]. FDG-PET might help to distinguish between fibrosis or active inflammation [83]. Endomyocardial biopsy is the gold standard for the diagnosis of myocardial damage, but is also liable to sampling error. Multislice CT has a diagnostic role in the evaluation of coronary arteries for calcification, stenosis and also for tissue characterization of the atherosclerotic plaque.

Coronary angiography may demonstrate focal or diffuse areas of stenosis, occlusions, and aneurysms. The characteristic pattern of "beads on a string" may also be seen with coronary angiography in PAN. But, it does not sufficiently define the inflammatory or noninflammatory nature of coronary lesions. And, coronary angiography may be totally normal in the isolated microvascular involvement [54].

Multimodality imaging might be helpful to detect subclinical cardiac involvement [62].

Diagnosis/Investigations

The diagnosis of vasculitis based on the combination of clinical features, results of imaging studies, histopathologic findings, and some laboratory tests such as ANCA. The demonstration of vascular inflammation in the histopathological examination is "gold standard" in the diagnosis of vasculitis. A biopsy should always be considered to confirm the diagnosis and exclude mimics [84]. Skin biopsy is the most frequently preferred and it is the most convenient to perform. Other organs such as lung, liver, kidney, nerve, upper respiratory tract or muscle might be considered when needed and if there is involvement. Kidney and liver biopsies are not preferred because of the risk of hemorrhage from rupturing in PAN.

In laboratory investigations, acute-phase reactants such as erythrocyte sedimentation rate and C-reactive protein, are commonly elevated during the active disease in systemic vasculitis [26]. Nonspecific test results such as chronic anemia and leukocytosis might be observed. Laboratory tests can help to demonstrate organ involvement and to determine the extent of involvement. And, laboratory test also valuable to diagnose and to exclude differential diagnosis [85]. Serological tests such as ANCA, anti-GBM antibodies, complement assays (C3, C4, C1q, CH50), C1q antibodies, cryoglobulins are diagnostic parameters in vasculitis. Peripheral blood eosinophilia (more than 10% on differential white blood cell count or more than 1500/μl) is the characteristic laboratory finding of EGPA. Laboratory tests can also help to identify etiologic factors such as HBV, HCV to diagnose viral-associated vasculitis and such as rheumatoid factors, antinuclear antibodies, anti-ds-DNA to diagnose vasculitis associated with systemic disease.

Conventional angiography remains the gold standard imaging modality for the diagnosis of systemic vasculitis. The detection of typical angiographic findings is crucial in the diagnosis of some vasculitis (e.g. PAN). When characteristic angiographic findings are detected, the diagnosis of PAN can be established, even in absence of histologic confirmation [14, 85, 86]. Magnetic resonance angiography (MRA) and computed tomography angiography (CTA) are increasingly being used. MRA and CTA can be substituted for catheter-based conventional angiography in the diagnosis and follow-up. CTA and MRA are non-invasive imaging modalities and end-organ changes might be evaluated in addition to the arterial changes [87–89]. FDG-PET has the potential to recognize early vessel wall inflammation [90]. Chest X-ray and/or CT scan should be performed for all types of AAV to evaluate pulmonary involvement. Sinus X-ray and/or CT scan should be performed for GPA and EGPA.

CSVV can occur as part of systemic vasculitis such as GPA, EGPA or PAN. CSVV is a diagnosis of exclusion [1, 3].

Treatment

Vasculitis includes many subtypes that are different in terms of clinical course from self-limited skin-limited form to potentially life-threatening systemic multiorgan involved disease. The choice of treatment depends on involved organs and disease progression. Firstly, if there is an underlying or associated disease or triggering agents such as a drug or infection are identified, they should be removed or treated [91, 92]. Treatment of self-limiting vasculitis is often symptomatic. Systemic glucocorticoids, in combination with or without immunosuppressants (primarily cyclophosphamide), are the cornerstone of systemic vasculitis treatment [92–94]. Generally, specific treatment for the cutaneous manifestations of systemic vasculitis is not necessary. They are usually responsive to immunosuppressive agents that are given to control systemic disease. If skin involvement is a single-organ vasculitis of the skin or a skin-limited variant of systemic vasculitis, the course of the disease is usually self-limiting, and first-line treatment is usually symptomatic [27, 95].

Treatment of cardiac involvement depends on cardiac manifestations and the activity of the disease. Pericarditis is usually not an important clinical problem. It can be treated with nonsteroidal anti-inflammatory drugs, colchicine or low dose corticosteroids while treatment of myocarditis and coronary arteritis is much more aggressive than pericarditis. High dose glucocorticoids, frequently in combination with immunosuppressive agents, are required for the treatment of myocarditis and coronary vasculitis. Valvulopathy, intracavitary cardiac thrombus, coronary arteriopathy often need surgical interventions. Therapies for heart failure and ischemia should also be added to the treatment when indicated [54].

Prognosis/Complications

The prognosis of vasculitis is also quite variable according to the involved organ and the course of the disease. Adverse events from therapy also have an important role on mortality and morbidity.

Subclinical cardiac involvement is common in vasculitis [54, 96]. Clinically significant pericarditis is a rare complication. However, myocarditis, coronary arteritis and valvular disease are poor prognostic cardiac involvements [54].

Cardiac involvement is one of the major causes of morbidity and mortality in TAK [97, 98]. It is the leading cause of stenotic aorto-arteriopathy in childhood [99]. Myocardial ischemia and aortic valve disease are the main causes of death from cardiac involvement in TAK [97].

The French Vasculitis Study Group (FVSG) suggested the Five Factor Score (FFS) as a prognosis index at diagnosis of PAN, MPA, GPA, and EGPA. FFS is developed to predict mortality, not for relapse or long-term morbidity. Cardiac insufficiency based only on the presence of its clinical symptoms (e.g. pulmonary edema), is a poor prognostic factor in FFS and cardiac involvement is the first cause of death in patients with EGPA [100]. Cardiovascular diseases are also an important cause of morbidity in patients with AAV.

Coronary artery abnormalities are the most common cause of morbidity and mortality in patients with KD. This title has been discussed in detail in Chap. 12.

References

1. Sunderkötter CH, Zelger B, Chen KR, Requena L, Piette W, Carlson JA, et al. Nomenclature of cutaneous vasculitis: dermatologic addendum to the 2012 Revised international Chapel Hill consensus conference nomenclature of vasculitides. Arthritis and Rheumatology. 2018;70(2):171–84.
2. Jennette JC, Falk R, Bacon P, Basu N, Cid M, Ferrario F, et al. 2012 revised international chapel hill consensus conference nomenclature of vasculitides. Arthritis Rheum. 2013;65(1):1–11.
3. Marzano AV, Vezzoli P, Berti E. Skin involvement in cutaneous and systemic vasculitis. Autoimmun Rev. 2013;12(4):467–76.
4. López-Mejías R, Carmona FD, Castañeda S, Genre F, Remuzgo-Martínez S, Sevilla-Perez B, et al. A genome-wide association study suggests the HLA Class II region as the major susceptibility locus for IgA vasculitis. Sci Rep. 2017;7(1):5088.
5. De Virgilio A, Greco A, Magliulo G, Gallo A, Ruoppolo G, Conte M, et al. Polyarteritis nodosa: a contemporary overview. Autoimmun Rev. 2016;15(6):564–70.
6. Ferri C, Sebastiani M, Giuggioli D, Cazzato M, Longombardo G, Antonelli A et al., editors. Mixed cryoglobulinemia: demographic, clinical, and serologic features and survival in 231 patients. Seminars in arthritis and rheumatism; 2004. Elsevier.
7. Gou S-J, Yuan J, Chen M, Yu F, Zhao M-H. Circulating complement activation in patients with anti-neutrophil cytoplasmic antibody–associated vasculitis. Kidney Int. 2013;83(1):129–37.
8. Pagnoux C. Updates in ANCA-associated vasculitis. European Journal of Rheumatology. 2016;3(3):122.
9. Jennette JC, Falk RJ, Andrassy K, Bacon PA, Churg J, Gross WL, et al. Nomenclature of systemic vasculitides. Arthritis and Rheumatism: Official Journal of the American College of Rheumatology. 1994;37(2):187–92.
10. Watts R, Jolliffe V, Grattan C, Elliott J, Lockwood M, Scott D. Cutaneous vasculitis in a defined population--clinical and epidemiological associations. J Rheumatol. 1998;25(5):920–4.
11. Blanco R, Martínez-Taboada VM, Rodríguez-Valverde V, García-Fuentes M. Cutaneous vasculitis in children and adults. Associated diseases and etiologic factors in 303 patients. Medicine. 1998;77(6):403–18.
12. González-Gay MA, García-Porrúa C. Epidemiology of the vasculitides. Rheum Dis Clin. 2001;27(4):729–49.
13. Hetland CE, Susrud KS, Lindahl KH, Bygum A. Henoch-Schönlein purpura: a literature review. Acta Derm Venereol. 2017;97(8–9):1160–6.
14. Ponte C, Águeda A, Luqmani R. Clinical features and structured clinical evaluation of vasculitis. Best Pract Res Clin Rheumatol. 2018;32(1):31–51.
15. Kluger N, Francès C. Cutaneous vasculitis and their differential diagnoses. Clin Exp Rheumatol. 2009;27(1):S124.
16. Pina T, Blanco R, González-Gay MA. Cutaneous vasculitis: a rheumatologist perspective. Curr Allergy Asthma Rep. 2013;13(5):545–54.
17. Khetan P, Sethuraman G, Khaitan BK, Sharma VK, Gupta R, Dinda AK, et al. An aetiological & clinicopathological study on cutaneous vasculitis. Indian J Med Res. 2012;135(1):107.
18. Kinmont P, McCallum D. Skin manifestations of giant-cell Arteritis. Br J Dermatol. 1964;76(7):299–308.
19. Currey J. Scalp necrosis in giant cell arteritis and review of the literature. Rheumatology. 1997;36(7):814–6.
20. Chasset F, Francès C. Cutaneous manifestations of medium-and large-vessel vasculitis. Clin Rev Allergy Immunol. 2017;53(3):452–68.

21. Cuvelier C, Kremer B, Kawski H, Guichard J, Maurier F, editors. Subcutaneous nodules of the head and neck heralding giant cell arteritis. Annales de dermatologie et de venereologie; 2014.
22. Hitch JM. Dermatologic manifestations of giant-cell (temporal, cranial) arteritis. Arch Dermatol. 1970;101(4):409–15.
23. Kluger N, Pagnoux C, Guillevin L, Frances C, Group FVS. Comparison of cutaneous manifestations in systemic polyarteritis nodosa and microscopic polyangiitis. Br J Dermatol. 2008;159(3):615–20.
24. Pagnoux C, Seror R, Henegar C, Mahr A, Cohen P, Le Guern V, et al. Clinical features and outcomes in 348 patients with polyarteritis nodosa: a systematic retrospective study of patients diagnosed between 1963 and 2005 and entered into the French Vasculitis Study Group Database. Arthritis Rheum. 2010;62(2):616–26.
25. Gonzalez-Gay MA, Garcia-Porrua C, Guerrero J, Rodriguez-Ledo P, Llorca J. The epidemiology of the primary systemic vasculitides in northwest Spain: implications of the Chapel Hill Consensus Conference definitions. Arthritis Care Res. 2003;49(3):388–93.
26. Sag E, Batu ED, Ozen S. Childhood systemic vasculitis. Best Pract Res Clin Rheumatol. 2017;31(4):558–75.
27. Morgan AJ, Schwartz RA. Cutaneous polyarteritis nodosa: a comprehensive review. Int J Dermatol. 2010;49(7):750–6.
28. Wysong A, Venkatesan P. An approach to the patient with retiform purpura. Dermatol Ther. 2011;24(2):151–72.
29. Daoud M, Hutton K, Gibson L. Cutaneous periarteritis nodosa: a clinicopathological study of 79 cases. Br J Dermatol. 1997;136(5):706–13.
30. Criado PR, Marques GF, Morita TCAB, de Carvalho JF. Epidemiological, clinical and laboratory profiles of cutaneous polyarteritis nodosa patients: report of 22 cases and literature review. Autoimmun Rev. 2016;15(6):558–63.
31. Marzano AV, Raimondo MG, Berti E, Meroni PL, Ingegnoli F. Cutaneous manifestations of ANCA-associated small vessels vasculitis. Clin Rev Allergy Immunol. 2017;53(3):428–38.
32. Francès C, Piette J-C, Saada V, Boisnic S, Wechsler B, Blétry O, et al. Wegener's granulomatosis: dermatological manifestations in 75 cases with clinicopathologic correlation. Arch Dermatol. 1994;130(7):861–7.
33. Frumholtz L, Laurent-Roussel S, Aumaître O, Maurier F, Le Guenno G, Carlotti A, et al. Clinical and pathological significance of cutaneous manifestations in ANCA-associated vasculitides. Autoimmun Rev. 2017;16(11):1138–46.
34. Tashtoush B, Memarpour R, Johnston Y, Ramirez J. Large pyoderma gangrenosum-like ulcers: a rare presentation of granulomatosis with polyangiitis. Case Rep Rheumatol. 2014;2014
35. De Boysson H, Silva NM, De Moreuil C, Néel A, De Menthon M, Meyer O, et al. Neutrophilic dermatoses in antineutrophil cytoplasmic antibody-associated vasculitis: a French multicenter study of 17 cases and literature review. Medicine. 2016;95(11):e2957.
36. Ruokonen H, Helve T, Arola J, Hietanen J, Lindqvist C, Hagstrom J. "Strawberry like" gingivitis being the first sign of Wegener's granulomatosis. Eur J Intern Med. 2009;20(6):651–3.
37. Stewart C, Cohen D, Bhattacharyya I, Scheitler L, Riley S, Calamia K, et al. Oral manifestations of Wegener's granulomatosis: a report of three cases and a literature review. J Am Dent Assoc. 2007;138(3):338–48.
38. Kawakami T, Soma Y, Saito C, Ogawa H, Nagahuchi Y, Okazaki T, et al. Cutaneous manifestations in patients with microscopic polyangiitis: two case reports and a minireview. Acta Derm Venereol. 2006;86(2):144–7.
39. Decleva I, Marzano AV, Barbareschi M, Berti E. Cutaneous manifestations in systemic vasculitis. Clin Rev Allergy Immunol. 1997;15(1):5–20.
40. Greco A, Rizzo MI, De Virgilio A, Gallo A, Fusconi M, Ruoppolo G, et al. Churg–Strauss syndrome. Autoimmun Rev. 2015;14(4):341–8.

41. Trapani S, Micheli A, Grisolia F, Resti M, Chiappini E, Falcini F et al., editors. Henoch Schonlein purpura in childhood: epidemiological and clinical analysis of 150 cases over a 5-year period and review of literature. Seminars in arthritis and rheumatism; 2005: Elsevier.
42. Makol A, Crowson CS, Wetter DA, Sokumbi O, Matteson EL, Warrington KJ. Vasculitis associated with rheumatoid arthritis: a case–control study. Rheumatology. 2014;53(5):890–9.
43. Makol A, Matteson EL, Warrington KJ. Rheumatoid vasculitis: an update. Curr Opin Rheumatol. 2015;27(1):63–70.
44. Kishore S, Maher L, Majithia V. Rheumatoid vasculitis: a diminishing yet devastating menace. Curr Rheumatol Rep. 2017;19(7):39.
45. Mascaró JM Jr, Baselga E. Erythema induratum of Bazin. Dermatol Clin. 2008;26(4):439–45.
46. Magalhães TS, Dammert VG, Samorano LP, Litvoc MN, Nico MMS. Erythema induratum of Bazin: epidemiological, clinical and laboratorial profile of 54 patients. J Dermatol. 2018;45(5):628–9.
47. Gibson LE, el-Azhary RA. Erythema elevatum diutinum. Clin Dermatol. 2000;18(3):295–9.
48. Theodoridis A, Makrantonaki E, Zouboulis CC. Malignant atrophic papulosis (Köhlmeier-Degos disease) - a review. Orphanet J Rare Dis. 2013;8(1):10.
49. Theodoridis A, Konstantinidou A, Makrantonaki E, Zouboulis C. Malignant and benign forms of atrophic papulosis (Köhlmeier–Degos disease): systemic involvement determines the prognosis. Br J Dermatol. 2014;170(1):110–5.
50. Carlson JA, Chen K-R. Cutaneous vasculitis update: small vessel neutrophilic vasculitis syndromes. Am J Dermatopathol. 2006;28(6):486–506.
51. Lie J. Systemic and isolated vasculitis. A rational approach to classification and pathologic diagnosis. Pathol Annu. 1989;1:25–114.
52. Seishima M, Oyama Z, Makiko O. Skin eruptions associated with microscopic polyangiitis. Eur J Dermatol. 2004;14(4):255–8.
53. Mizuno K, Nguyen CTH, Ueda-Hayakawa I, Okamoto H. Annular lesions of cutaneous sarcoidosis with granulomatous vasculitis. J Cutan Pathol. 2017;44(5):494–6.
54. Miloslavsky E, Unizony S. The heart in vasculitis. Rheum Dis Clin. 2014;40(1):11–26.
55. Bicakcigil M, Aksu K, Kamali S, Ozbalkan Z, Ates A, Karadag O, et al. Takayasu's arteritis in Turkey-clinical and angiographic features of 248 patients. Clin Exp Rheumatol. 2009;27(1):S59.
56. Mathew AJ, Goel R, Kumar S, Danda D. Childhood-onset Takayasu arteritis: an update. Int J Rheum Dis. 2016;19(2):116–26.
57. McCrindle BW, Rowley AH, Newburger JW, Burns JC, Bolger AF, Gewitz M, et al. Diagnosis, treatment, and long-term management of Kawasaki disease: a scientific statement for health professionals from the American Heart Association. Circulation. 2017;135(17):e927–e99.
58. Bletry O, Godeau P, Charpentier G, Guillevin L, Herreman G. Cardiac manifestations of periarteritis nodosa. Incidence of non-hypertensive cardiomyopathy. Archives des maladies du coeur et des vaisseaux. 1980;73(9):1027.
59. Holsinger DR, Osmundson PJ, Edwards JE. The heart in periarteritis nodosa. Circulation. 1962;25(4):610–8.
60. Grant S, Levy R, Venning M, Ward C, Brooks N. Wegener's granulomatosis and the heart. Heart. 1994;71(1):82–6.
61. McGeoch L, Carette S, Cuthbertson D, Hoffman GS, Khalidi N, Koening CL, et al. Cardiac involvement in granulomatosis with polyangiitis. J Rheumatol. 2015;42(7):1209–12.
62. Hazebroek M, Kemna M, Schalla S, Sanders-van Wijk S, Gerretsen S, Dennert R, et al. Prevalence and prognostic relevance of cardiac involvement in ANCA-associated vasculitis: eosinophilic granulomatosis with polyangiitis and granulomatosis with polyangiitis. Int J Cardiol. 2015;199:170–9.
63. Życińska K, Borowiec A. Cardiac manifestations in antineutrophil cytoplasmic autoantibody (ANCA)-associated vasculitides. Kardiologia Polska (Polish Heart J). 2016;74(12):1470–6.
64. Colin GC, Vancraeynest D, Hoton D, Jonard P, Gerber B. Complete heart block caused by diffuse pseudotumoral cardiac involvement in granulomatosis with polyangiitis. Circulation. 2015;132(17):e207–e10.

65. Lacoste C, Mansencal N, Ben m'rad M, Goulon-Goeau C, Cohen P, Guillevin L, et al. Valvular involvement in ANCA-associated systemic vasculitis: a case report and literature review. BMC Musculoskelet Disord. 2011;12(1):50.
66. Herbst A, Padilla MT, Prasad AR, Morales MC, Copeland JG. Cardiac Wegener's granulomatosis masquerading as left atrial myxoma. Ann Thorac Surg. 2003;75(4):1321–3.
67. Guillevin L, Durand-Gasselin B, Cevallos R, Gayraud M, Lhote F, Callard P, et al. Microscopic polyangiitis: clinical and laboratory findings in eighty-five patients. Arthritis Rheum. 1999;42(3):421–30.
68. Shuai Z, Lv Y, Zhang M, Hu Z. Clinical analysis of patients with myeloperoxidase antineutrophil cytoplasmic antibody-associated vasculitis. Genet Mol Res. 2015;14(2):5296–303.
69. Moosig F, Bremer JP, Hellmich B, Holle JU, Holl-Ulrich K, Laudien M, et al. A vasculitis centre based management strategy leads to improved outcome in eosinophilic granulomatosis and polyangiitis (Churg–Strauss, EGPA): monocentric experiences in 150 patients. Ann Rheum Dis. 2013;72(6):1011–7.
70. Vinit J, Bielefeld P, Muller G, Pfitzenmeyer P, Bonniaud P, Lorcerie B, et al. Heart involvement in Churg–Strauss syndrome: retrospective study in French Burgundy population in past 10 years. Eur J Intern Med. 2010;21(4):341–6.
71. Neumann T, Manger B, Schmid M, Kroegel C, Hansch A, Kaiser WA, et al. Cardiac involvement in Churg-Strauss syndrome: impact of endomyocarditis. Medicine. 2009;88(4):236–43.
72. Dennert RM, van Paassen P, Schalla S, Kuznetsova T, Alzand BS, Staessen JA, et al. Cardiac involvement in Churg-Strauss syndrome. Arthritis Rheum. 2010;62(2):627–34.
73. Calatroni M, Oliva E, Gianfreda D, Gregorini G, Allinovi M, Ramirez GA, et al. ANCA-associated vasculitis in childhood: recent advances. Ital J Pediatr. 2017;43(1):46.
74. Szczeklik W, Miszalski-Jamka T. Cardiac involvement in eosinophilic granulomatosis with polyangitis (Churg Strauss)(RCD code: I-3A. 7a). J Rare Cardiovasc Dis. 2014;1(3):91–5.
75. Jeong HC, Kim KH, Cho JY, Song JE, Yoon HJ, Seon HJ, et al. Cardiac involvement of churg-strauss syndrome as a reversible cause of dilated cardiomyopathy. J Cardiovasc Ultrasound. 2015;23(1):40–3.
76. Gorevic PD, Kassab HJ, Levo Y, Kohn R, Meltzer M, Prose P, et al. Mixed cryoglobulinemia: clinical aspects and long-term follow-up of 40 patients. Am J Med. 1980;69(2):287–308.
77. Haynes BF, Kaiser-Kupfer MI, Mason P, Fauci AS. Cogan syndrome: studies in thirteen patients, long-term follow-up, and a review of the literature. Medicine. 1980;59(6):426–41.
78. Gelfand ML, Kantor T, Gorstein F. Cogan's syndrome with cardiovascular involvement: aortic insufficiency. Bull N Y Acad Med. 1972;48(4):647.
79. Marmursztejn J, Vignaux O, Cohen P, Guilpain P, Pagnoux C, Gouya H, et al. Impact of cardiac magnetic resonance imaging for assessment of Churg-Strauss syndrome: a cross-sectional study in 20 patients. Clin Exp Rheum. 2009;27(1):S70.
80. Mavrogeni S, Manoussakis M, Karagiorga T, Douskou M, Panagiotakos D, Bournia V, et al. Detection of coronary artery lesions and myocardial necrosis by magnetic resonance in systemic necrotizing vasculitides. Arthritis Care Res. 2009;61(8):1121–9.
81. Mahrholdt H, Goedecke C, Wagner A, Meinhardt G, Athanasiadis A, Vogelsberg H, et al. Cardiovascular magnetic resonance assessment of human myocarditis: a comparison to histology and molecular pathology. Circulation. 2004;109(10):1250–8.
82. Keenan NG, Mason JC, Maceira A, Assomull R, O'hanlon R, Chan C, et al. Integrated cardiac and vascular assessment in Takayasu arteritis by cardiovascular magnetic resonance. Arthritis Rheum. 2009;60(11):3501–9.
83. Marmursztejn J, Guillevin L, Trebossen R, Cohen P, Guilpain P, Pagnoux C, et al. Churg–Strauss syndrome cardiac involvement evaluated by cardiac magnetic resonance imaging and positron-emission tomography: a prospective study on 20 patients. Rheumatology. 2012;52(4):642–50.
84. Yates M, Watts R. ANCA-associated vasculitis. Clin Med. 2017;17(1):60–4.
85. Hernández-Rodríguez J, Alba MA, Prieto-González S, Cid MC. Diagnosis and classification of polyarteritis nodosa. J Autoimmun. 2014;48:84–9.

86. Albert DA, Rimon D, Silverstein MD. The diagnosis of polyarteritis nodosa. Arthritis Rheum. 1988;31(9):1117–27.
87. Singhal M, Gupta P, Sharma A, Lal A, Rathi M, Khandelwal N. Role of multidetector abdominal CT in the evaluation of abnormalities in polyarteritis nodosa. Clin Radiol. 2016;71(3):222–7.
88. Stanson AW, Friese JL, Johnson CM, McKusick MA, Breen JF, Sabater EA, et al. Polyarteritis nodosa: spectrum of angiographic findings. Radiographics. 2001;21(1):151–9.
89. Schmidt WA. Use of imaging studies in the diagnosis of vasculitis. Curr Rheumatol Rep. 2004;6(3):203–11.
90. Andrews J, Mason J. Takayasu's arteritis—recent advances in imaging offer promise. Rheumatology. 2006;46(1):6–15.
91. Sunderkötter C, Bonsmann G, Sindrilaru A, Luger T. Management of leukocytoclastic vasculitis. J Dermatol Treat. 2005;16(4):193–206.
92. Mukhtyar C, Guillevin L, Cid MC, Dasgupta B, de Groot K, Gross W, et al. EULAR recommendations for the management of primary small and medium vessel vasculitis. Ann Rheum Dis. 2009;68(3):310–7.
93. Mukhtyar C, Guillevin L, Cid MC, Dasgupta B, de Groot K, Gross W, et al. EULAR recommendations for the management of large vessel vasculitis. Ann Rheum Dis. 2009;68(3):318–23.
94. Dasgupta B, Borg FA, Hassan N, Alexander L, Barraclough K, Bourke B, et al. BSR and BHPR guidelines for the management of giant cell arteritis. Rheumatology. 2010;49(8):1594–7.
95. Lotti T, Ghersetich I, Comacchi C, Jorizzo JL. Cutaneous small-vessel vasculitis. J Am Acad Dermatol. 1998;39(5):667–90.
96. Pagnoux C, Guillevin L. Cardiac involvement in small and medium-sized vessel vasculitides. Lupus. 2005;14(9):718–22.
97. Soto M, Espinola N, Flores-Suarez L, Reyes P. Takayasu arteritis: clinical features in 110 Mexican Mestizo patients and cardiovascular impact on survival and prognosis. Clin Exp Rheum. 2008;26(3):S9.
98. Cong X-L, Dai S-M, Feng X, Wang Z-W, Lu Q-S, Yuan L-X, et al. Takayasu's arteritis: clinical features and outcomes of 125 patients in China. Clin Rheumatol. 2010;29(9):973–81.
99. Russo RAG, Katsicas MM. Takayasu arteritis. Front Pediatr. 2018;6:265.
100. Guillevin L, Pagnoux C, Seror R, Mahr A, Mouthon L, Le Toumelin P. The Five-Factor Score revisited: assessment of prognoses of systemic necrotizing vasculitides based on the French Vasculitis Study Group (FVSG) cohort. Medicine. 2011;90(1):19–27.

Behçet's Disease

11

Erkan Alpsoy

Introduction and Pathophysiology of Disease

Behçet's disease (BD) is a chronic, relapsing and debilitating systemic vasculitis of unknown etiology with the clinical features of mucocutaneous lesions, ocular, vascular, articular, neurologic, gastrointestinal, urogenital, pulmonary, and cardiac involvement. The disease usually starts around the third decade of life. The gender distribution is roughly equal. However, severe organ involvement such as neurologic, large vessel, cardiac involvement, and eye disease are more frequent in males [1].

BD shares some standard features with autoimmune, autoinflammatory, or spondyloarthropathies (MHC-I-opathies) and involves more than one pathogenic pathway triggered by environmental factors such as infectious agents in genetically predisposed subjects [2]. The interplay between a complex genetic background and both the innate and adaptive immune systems is related to the BD clinical features. Genetic factors have been investigated extensively, and several recent genome-wide association studies (GWAS) have confirmed that HLA-B*51 is the most critical genetic susceptibility factor. However, new susceptibility loci both on other HLA Class I regions and on non-HLA genes such as endoplasmic reticulum aminopeptidase 1 (ERAP1), IL-23 receptor (IL-23R), IL-23R/IL-12RB2, IL-10, and STAT have also been identified [3, 4]. In general, BD-associated gene polymorphisms have been found in genes that respond to microorganisms and in genes encoding cytokines and adhesion molecules. Polymorphisms in these genes may affect their function and may be associated with disease susceptibility. Infectious agents *(S. sanguinis*, etc.) or the differences in salivary or gut microbiome composition can be considered to trigger both innate-derived inflammation and adaptive immune

E. Alpsoy (✉)
Department of Dermatology and Venereology, Akdeniz University School of Medicine, Antalya, Turkey
e-mail: ealpsoy@akdeniz.edu.tr

C. Salavastru et al. (eds.), *Skin and the Heart*,
https://doi.org/10.1007/978-3-030-54779-0_11

responses. Neutrophils are the key elements of innate immunity, and BD is regarded as a neutrophilic vasculitis. There is an intense neutrophil infiltration in the early stage of inflammation in organs affected by the disease. In adaptive immunity pathway, epistatic interactions between HLA-B*51 and ERAP1 variants seems to cause T cell homeostasis perturbation. Altered trimming of microbial and/or endogenous peptides by ERAP1, presented by HLA-B*51, may play a key role in BD pathogenesis, causing an alteration in T cell balance with downregulation of Tregs and expansion of Th1 and Th17 [3]. HLA-B*51 association and increased IL-17 response are thought to play a role in neutrophil activation. Vessel-based neutrophilic reactions and vasculitis are considered to develop in patients with BD as a result of all these processes [3, 4].

Prevalence/Population Affected

BD is much more frequent in populations along the ancient 'Silk Route' extending from Eastern Asia to countries in the Middle East and the Mediterranean, compared with Western countries. The prevalence of the disease is 14–20 per 100,000 along the "Silk route" [1]. Turkey has the highest prevalence. Azizlerli et al. from Istanbul reported the prevalence of the disease to be nearly 1/250 of the population aged 12 or older [5]. The condition is rarely seen in other European countries; Reported frequency ranges from 0.3 to 7.5, per 100,000. There is a general south-to-north decreasing frequency in Europe. This marked geographic variation of BD can be explained by the genetic basis of the disease and environmental triggers [6]. Cardiac involvement is rarely seen in BD. Sometimes it can be the presenting sign of the disease. Geri et al. reported cardiac involvement in 6% (n: 52) of 807 patients with BD. The majority of patients with cardiac involvement were male patients (86%) [7]. Vascular involvement, especially large vessel involvement such as pulmonary artery aneurysm, deep venous thrombosis is more common in these patients [8–10].

Dermatological Manifestations

Clinical

Mucocutaneous lesions figure prominently in the presentation and diagnosis and may be considered the hallmarks of BD. Mucocutaneous lesions often precede other manifestations. Therefore, their recognition may permit earlier diagnosis and treatment with good results. Oral ulcers (OU) (92–100%), genital ulcers (GU) (57–93%), cutaneous lesions (38–99%) together with ocular (29–100%) and articular involvements (16–84%) are the most common features of the disease in all countries. Erythema nodosum (EN)-like lesions (15–78%) and papulopustular lesions (PPL) (28–96%) are the most commonly observed cutaneous lesions [6].

Oral Ulcers are characterized by recurrent and usually painful ulcerations of the oral mucosa. The most common sites of the lesions are the mucous membranes of the lips, the buccal mucosa, the undersurface of the tongue and the floor of the mouth. Patients may have single or multiple ulcers which often subside spontaneously after a couple of weeks and recur at intervals from days to months. They are identical to aphthae in appearance, but they tend to be more frequent and multiple [11]. The lesions start as an erythematous, slightly raised area evolving into an oval or round ulcer within 48 hours with rolled or overhanging borders and a grayish-yellow necrotic base. An erythematous halo of inflamed mucosa surrounds the ulcer (Fig. 11.1) [1, 6].

Genital Ulcers are similar in appearance and course to OU, but may not recur as often and can have a scarring tendency. They are usually deeper than the OU, and a papulopustular lesion or a tender nodule can precede their appearance. GU are generally painful or, occasionally asymptomatic, especially in female patients. The scrotum is the most frequently involved site in males (Fig. 11.2), and the labia, in females [1, 6].

Cutaneous Lesions are varied and include EN-like lesions, PPL, superficial thrombophlebitis, extragenital ulcerations, reactivity of the skin to needle prick or injection (pathergy reaction) and other cutaneous vasculitic lesions e.g. Sweet's syndrome-like, pyoderma gangrenosum-like, erythema multiforme-like lesions, palpable purpura, subungual infarctions, hemorrhagic bullae, furuncles, and abscesses [6].

Papulopustular Lesions (PPL) the most common type of cutaneous lesions in BD, are sterile, folliculitis or acne-like lesions on an erythematous base which appear as a papule and in the course of 24–48 h become a pustule. Trunk and the lower limbs (Fig. 11.3) are the most common locations [12].

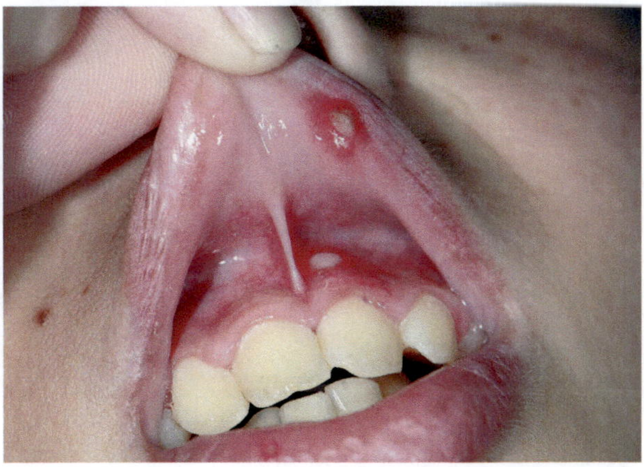

Fig. 11.1 Oral ulcer. Oval-round ulcers with grayish-yellow necrotic base and erythematous halo on the upper lip mucosa and gingiva

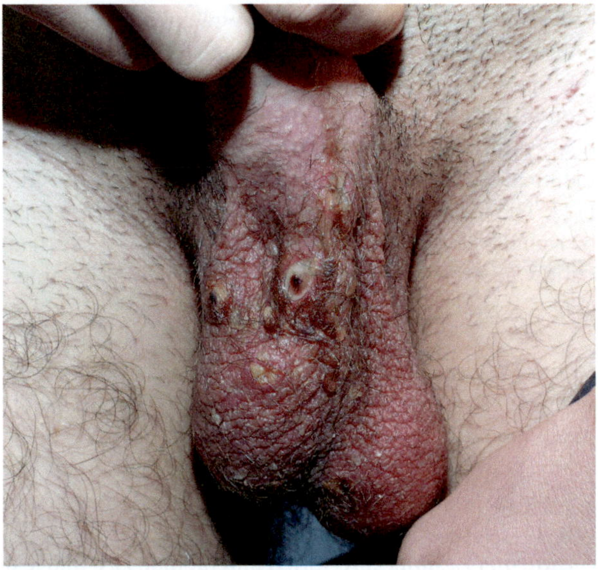

Fig. 11.2 Genital ulcer. Oval-round ulcers with a grayish-yellow necrotic base on the scrotum

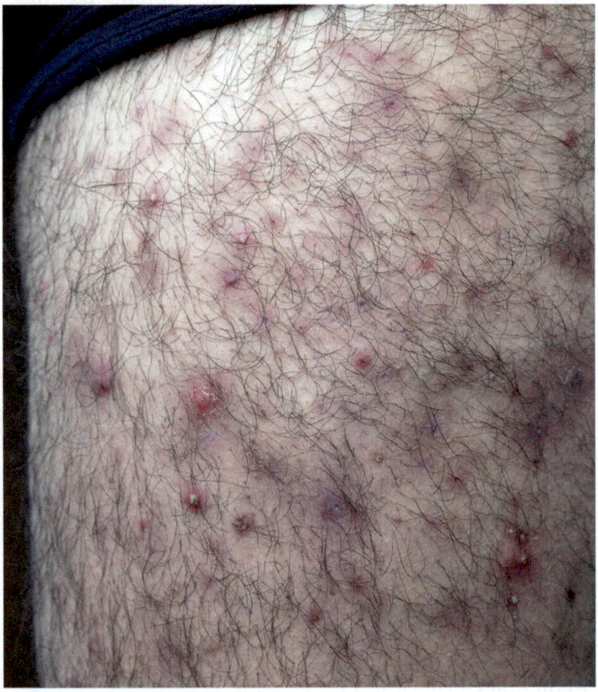

Fig. 11.3 Papulopustular lesions. Sterile, follicular or non-follicular papulopustular lesions on an erythematous base on the leg

Erythema Nodosum (EN)-like Lesions are mostly seen in females and occur in about one-third of all patients. They have a typical clinical presentation with bilateral, pretibial, painful and hot, erythematous nodules. EN-like lesions, sometimes, can be localized to the face, neck, and buttocks. The lesions do not ulcerate and resolve spontaneously within 2–3 weeks, in pigmented ethnic groups with residual pigmentation, but recurrence is frequent (Fig. 11.4) [13].

Superficial Thrombophlebitis is frequently confused with EN-like lesions. The patients usually present with erythematous, tender subcutaneous nodules arranged linearly. The subcutaneous venules of the extremities, especially in male patients, tend to develop thrombosis leading to sclerosis. The small vein can be palpated as a string-like hardening of the subcutaneous tissue with reddening of the overlying skin (Fig. 11.5). The location of nodules shows a tendency to change from day to day because multiple segments of the vein might be involved, resembling migrating

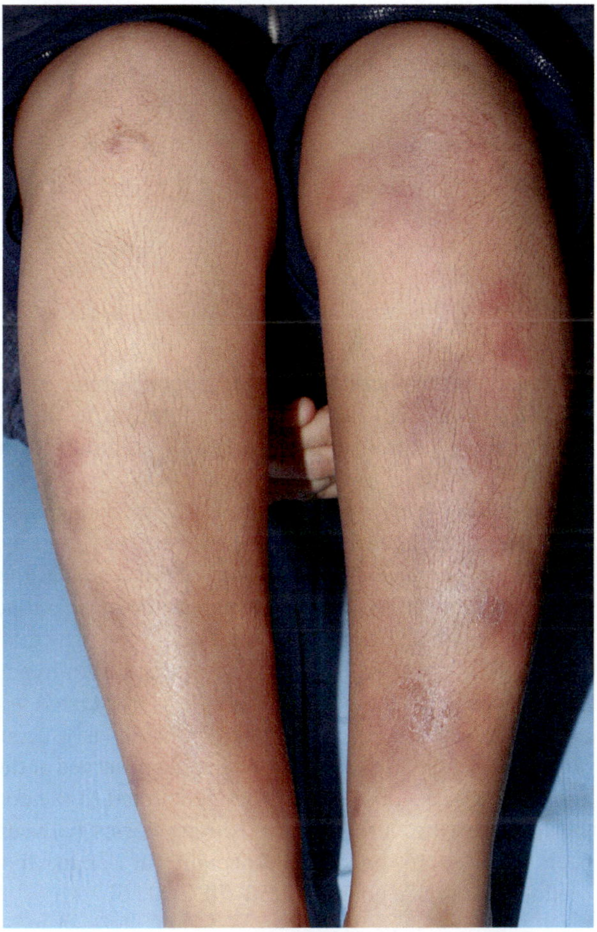

Fig. 11.4 Erythema nodosum-like lesions. Bilateral, pretibial, painful and hot, erythematous nodules and postinflammatory hyperpigmentation

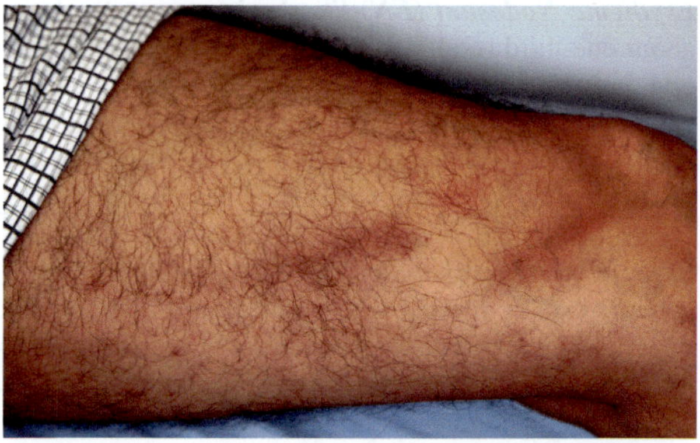

Fig. 11.5 Superficial thrombophlebitis. erythematous, tender subcutaneous nodules arranged linearly on the leg. The affected vein can be palpated as a string-like hardening of the subcutaneous tissue

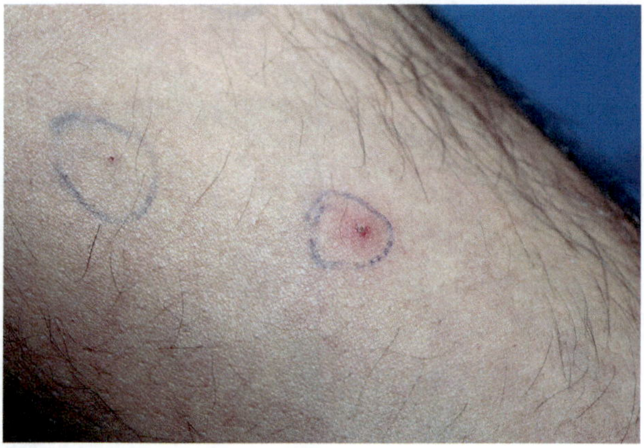

Fig. 11.6 The skin pathergy test. Papulopustular lesions on an erythematous base at the needle-prick site 48 h after application of a sterile needle. Please note that the negative result on the upper needle-prick site on the forearm

obliterative thrombophlebitis. Thrombophlebitis is clinically important since it could frequently be associated with other forms of vascular disease, deep venous thrombosis and dural sinus thrombosis in central nervous system [14].

Extragenital Ulcers are relatively common cutaneous lesions and clinically resemble other aphthous lesions of the disease. They are recurrent and usually heal with scarring. In our series, the frequency of this lesion is approximately 6%. The lesions can be seen in various locations such as the legs, axillae, breast, interdigital skin of the foot, inguinal region, and neck [1].

The Skin Pathergy Test is a nonspecific skin hyper-reactivity, induced by needle prick or intracutaneous injection. It is associated with a papule or pustule on an erythematous base, similar to the spontaneously occurring PPL of BD. The test positivity is defined as at least one papule observed at the needle-prick site 48 h after application of a sterile needle that penetrated to the corium of an avascular site on the forearm (Fig. 11.6). Test positivity varies between geographic areas and has been reported to be high, especially in Japan, the Middle Eastern, and the Mediterranean Sea countries (50–70%) [1, 6].

Histological

In 2012 Revised International Chapel Hill Consensus Conference, BD is defined as variable vessel vasculitis which means the disease can affect vessels of any size (small, medium, and large) and type (arteries, veins, and capillaries) [15]. In a recent study, Sunderkötter et al. prepared a dermatologic addendum to the 2012 Chapel Hill consensus conference nomenclature to address vasculitides affecting the skin. The main aim was to standardize names and definitions for cutaneous vasculitis. There was a broad consensus among experts in BD that the early stages of cutaneous lesions are vessel-based neutrophilic reactions with leukocytoclasia and endothelial swelling, and sometimes vasculitis with fibrinoid necrosis. Larger thrombosed vessels often present with vasculitis of vasa vasorum [16]. Histopathological features may vary according to the clinical features of cardiac involvement. For example, in the case of intracardiac thrombosis, organized thrombus containing mononuclear cells is seen.

Differential

Relapsing OU and GU are the most common and characteristic features of the disease. They are often the presenting symptoms, and powerfully evocative of BD. Conditions to consider in the differential diagnosis of OU and/or GU are those that produce recurrent ulcers on the oral mucosa and/or genital area. Herpes simplex, recurrent aphthous stomatitis (RAS), some cases of erythema multiforme and fixed drug eruption have a recurrent course. Herpes simplex presents with grouped, small, shallow ulcers. It is wise to remember that herpetiform lesions can also be seen in the course of conventional RAS and BD. A Tzanck smear should be performed in all cases with such lesions. If multinucleated acantholytic cells are seen, the diagnosis is herpes simplex. However, herpes simplex virus-PCR is more reliable. Target lesions mainly on the acral and periorificial areas indicate erythema multiforme and a nummular erythematous base and a history of recurrence of erosions at the same site after each intake of the causative drug, fixed drug eruption. RAS may be a part of BD, besides MAGIC syndrome, Reiter's syndrome and Sweet's syndrome, or maybe secondary to anemia due to deficiency of iron, vitamin B12 or folic acid or inflammatory bowel diseases (Crohn's disease and ulcerative colitis). Complex aphthosis, first described by Jorizzo et al., or malignant aphthosis, first defined by Tourraine (1941) are the terms used to describe patients who have almost constant multiple (>3) OU or recurrent OU and GU without systemic manifestations of BD [17]. Differentiation of BD from the complex (malignant) aphthosis might be problematic since the initial clinical presentation of BD is often confined to oral and genital ulcers. In our opinion, patients with complex aphthosis must be monitored at intervals using clinical criteria for evolution into BD.

Cardiological Manifestations

Clinical

Cardiac involvement may be endocarditis, myocarditis, pericarditis, intracardiac thrombus, endomyocardial fibrosis, coronary arteritis, myocardial infarction, and valve diseases [8–10]. Interatrial septum aneurysm, mitral valve prolapse, mitral regurgitation, and sinus Valsalva dilatations are rarely seen [8]. Geri et al., in a large cohort of 52 BD patients with cardiac involvement reported that pericarditis (38%) was the most common clinic which was followed by endocarditis (26%), intracardiac thrombus (19%), myocardial infarction (17%), endomyocardial fibrosis (7%) and myocardial aneurysm (2%). Arterial and venous involvement was reported more common in patients with cardiac involvement than in patients without cardiac involvement [7].

Clinical presentation of pericardial involvement may include acute pericarditis, hemorrhagic pericardial tamponade, constrictive pericarditis, recurrent pericarditis, or even a small, asymptomatic pericardial effusion [18–21]. Endomyocardial involvement typically occurs as endomyocardial fibrosis [19]. Intracardiac thrombus is one of the most serious cardiac complications of BD patients with cardiac involvement and may present with pulmonary embolism. Intracardiac thrombus may also cause cerebral embolism by passing through the patent foramen ovale. Most often, the right ventricle is involved [22, 23].

Koç et al. reported that left ventricular diastolic function was impaired in patients with BD. Also, P wave abnormalities were detected, and a significant relationship was found between P wave dispersion and diastolic dysfunction [24]. Disruption of left ventricular diastolic function may be due to small vessel involvement in the myocardium and may be an early sign of cardiac involvement [25]. Turkolmez et al. conducted a study to identify silent myocardial ischemia in patients with BD using treadmill exercise test and thallium-201 myocardial perfusion single-photon emission computed tomography. They found that the frequency of silent myocardial ischemia was higher in patients with BD than in the control group. Coronary angiography showed no significant coronary stenosis in the BD patients with a diagnosis of silent myocardial ischemia. These results indicate that small vessel vasculitis is common in the myocardium of patients with BD [26]. This supports the results of the previous study [25]. Aktürk et al. showed left atrium volume, and its mechanical functions were inadequate in patients with BD compared to healthy controls. The authors suggested that these changes may be an early form of subclinical cardiac involvement in BD patients who have no clinical evidence for cardiac disease [27].

Studies have shown that ventricular arrhythmia incidence and sudden cardiac death is higher in patients with BD than in the normal population. The cause and mechanism of sudden cardiac death in BD are not fully understood. However, this is thought to be associated with asymptomatic cardiac involvement [28]. QT dispersion may increase, and heart rate variability may be impaired in patients with BD [29, 30]. Pulmonary embolism, dissecting aortic aneurysm rupture, coronary artery disease, cardiac failure, cardiomyopathies, and left ventricular hypertrophy may also be among the causes of sudden death [31, 32].

The prevalence of coronary artery involvement in BD was reported to be 0.5% [33]. Histopathologically, inflammatory occlusive endarteritis of the vasa vasorum is detected. The inflammatory process causes destruction of the media and subsequent development of fibrosis weakens the arterial wall and facilitates aneurysm formation [34]. Stenosis and occlusion may also be seen in coronary artery involvement [18].

In a recent systematic review and meta-analysis of a total of 1624 BD patients with cardiac involvement from 22 studies, Aslam et al. reported a significant increase in diastolic dysfunction in patient group compared to controls. Significantly larger left atrial dimension, greater aortic diameter, and reduced ejection fraction was observed in the patient group. Also, significant prolongation of mitral deceleration time, lower E /A ratio (decrease in transmitral early filling peak velocity (E)/transmitral late filling peak velocity (A)), and increase in isovolumetric relaxation time were observed [10].

Investigations

A good anamnesis and physical examination are the first steps to be taken in the investigation of these patients. Since cardiac involvement is rare in BD, it is often neglected by the physician and cardiac complaints are not questioned. Additionally, symptoms of cardiac involvement are often not sufficiently diagnostic. Therefore, most patients can be diagnosed late. Depending on the location and severity of the involvement, the patient may present with complaints of chest pain, palpitations, pericardial friction rub, murmur, dyspnea, cough, fever, hemoptysis, symtoms of right or left heart failure. Since the prognosis is usually not good, patients should be carefully monitored for cardiac involvement. Patients with suspected cardiac involvement should be referred to an experienced cardiologist. Electrocardiogram, chest X-ray, transthoracic echocardiogram, computed tomography (CT) scan, magnetic resonance imaging (MRI), scintigraphy, coronary angiography can be planned according to the anamnesis and physical examination findings [7].

Balta et al. [35] found that serum endocan levels were significantly higher in BD patients compared to controls. Also, they found serum endocan levels to be correlated with C-reactive protein, erythrocyte sedimentation rate, and disease activity. In another study, Kul et al. [36] observed a positive correlation between serum endocan levels and VEGF and TNF-α levels, both of which play an essential role in the pathogenesis of BD. In conclusion, the expression of the endocan in vascular endothelial cells may be a marker for systemic inflammatory vasculitis characterized by endothelial dysfunction such as BD and can be used to determine the risk of cardiovascular disease.

Diagnosis/Investigations

The diagnosis is based on clinical criteria as there is as yet no pathognomonic test. The International Study Group for Behçet's Disease developed in 1990, internationally agreed, criteria which depend on the presence of recurrent oral ulcers, relapsing at least three times in 12 months, plus any two of recurrent genital ulcers, typical eye lesions, typical cutaneous lesions or a positive pathergy test [37]. This diagnostic criteria have been widely accepted among experts and are still the most widely used criteria worldwide [1].

Treatment

The treatment of BD has become much more effective in recent years, because of advances in understanding the pathogenesis of the disease, and availability of a wide spectrum of therapeutic agents. Although several effective treatments currently exist, none of them result in a cure of the disease, and some are associated with significant side effects. The choice of treatment is generally based on the clinical presentation and the area affected. However, the main aim of the treatment should be the prevention of irreversible organ damage, especially during the early, active phase of the disease. Close monitoring and appropriate treatment may control and change the course of the disease [1].

The treatment of patients with cardiac involvement is not entirely satisfactory, and the treatment of these patients is predominantly based on the clinical experience of experts in this field. Since cardiac involvement is rare, there are no high-quality, controlled studies in the literature. There is no standard protocol for remission and maintenance therapy. Treatment options vary depending on the type and severity of cardiac involvement.

Pericarditis is usually treated with aspirin and immunosuppressive agents. Geri et al. [7] reported good results with colchicine (1 mg/day) and aspirin (100 mg/day). Different treatment options, including corticosteroids, immunosuppressants (azathioprine), anticoagulation, and surgery, are used for intracardiac thrombus. Surgical treatment is generally not recommended. Further studies are needed to determine the ideal treatment option for this life-threatening complication of BD. Percutaneous coronary revascularization or surgical revascularisation seem to be the main therapeutic approaches in the acute myocardial infarction treatment [7, 19]. Myocardial involvement is almost always associated with endomyocarditis. Good results have been reported with both surgical and medical treatment (corticosteroids, colchicine, intravenous cyclophosphamide) in endomyocardial fibrosis [7, 38]. In cardiac failure, high-dose prednisolone and azathioprine may be used in combination with routine cardiac failure treatment. Cardiac functions have improved in some patients with these drugs [19, 39]. The coronary aneurysm can be treated with a combined approach of immunosuppression and endovascular non-surgical intervention [19, 34].

Some authors do not recommend the use of anticoagulants because they can cause bleeding in patients with thrombotic complications [20]. Kwon et al. reported that anticoagulants such as coumadin might cause aneurysm formation and growth in BD [40].

Prognosis/Complications

The disease generally runs a chronic course with unpredictable exacerbations and remissions. Male sex and a younger age of onset are associated with more severe disease. Each or any combination of mucocutaneous, articular, and ocular symptoms of the disease may have significant pain or loss in function, or both. Besides considerable morbidity, the disease confers increased mortality, mainly because of pulmonary as well as large vessel involvement, neurologic, cardiac involvement, and a bowel perforation.

The prognosis of patients with cardiac involvement is generally poor. Geri et al. found that the 5-year survival rate in BD patients with cardiac involvement was significantly lower than in patients without cardiac involvement (83.6% and 95.8%, respectively). Eight deaths were observed in the patient group followed up for an average of 3 years, and three of these were directly related to cardiac involvement. Oral anticoagulants, immunosuppressants, and colchicine treatment were found to be associated with remission of cardiac involvement in the same study [7].

References

1. Alpsoy E. Behçet's disease: a comprehensive review with a focus on epidemiology, etiology and clinical features, and management of mucocutaneous lesions. J Dermatol. 2016;43(6):620–32.
2. McGonagle D, Aydin SZ, Gul A, Mahr A, Direskeneli H. 'MHC-I-opathy'-unified concept for spondyloarthritis and Behcet disease. Nat Rev Rheumatol. 2015;11(12):731–40.
3. Leccese P, Alpsoy E. Behçet's disease: an overview of etiopathogenesis. Front Immunol. 2019;5(19):1067.
4. Salmaninejad A, Gowhari A, Hosseini S, Aslani S, Yousefi M, Bahrami T, et al. Genetics and immunodysfunction underlying Behçet's disease and immunomodulant treatment approaches. J Immunotoxicol. 2017;14:137–51.
5. Azizlerli G, Kose AA, Sarica R, Gül A, Tutkun IT, Kulaç M, et al. Prevalence of Behcet's disease in Istanbul, Turkey. Int J Dermatol. 2003;42:803–6.
6. Alpsoy E, Zouboulis CC, Ehrlich CE. Mucocutaneous lesions of Behçet's disease. Yonsei Med J. 2007;48:573–85.
7. Geri G, Wechsler B, Thi Huong du L, Isnard R, Piette JC, Amoura Z, et al. Spectrum of cardiac lesions in behçet disease: a series of 52 patients and review of the literature. Medicine (Baltimore). 2012;91(1):25–34.
8. Heper G, Polat M, Yetkin E, Senen K. Cardiac findings in Behçet's patients. Int J Dermatol. 2010;49(5):574–8.
9. Gurgun C, Ercan E, Ceyhan C, Yavuzgil O, Zoghi M, Aksu K, et al. Cardiovascular involvement in Behcet's disease. Jpn Heart J. 2002;43(4):389–98.
10. Aslam F, Bandeali SJ, Crowson C, Alam M. Cardiac function and diastolic dysfunction in Behcet's disease: a systematic review and meta-analysis. Int J Rheumatol. 2016;2016:9837184.

11. Oh S, Han EC, Lee JH, Bang DT. Comparison of the clinical features of recurrent aphthous stomatitis and Behçet's disease. Clin Exp Dermatol. 2009;34:e208–12.
12. Alpsoy E, Aktekin M, Er H, Durusoy C, Yilmaz E. A randomized, controlled and blinded study of papulopustular lesions in Turkish Behcet's patients. Int J Dermatol. 1998;37:839–43.
13. Kim B, LeBoit PE. Histopathologic features of erythema nodosum-like lesions in Behcet disease: a comparison with erythema nodosum focusing on the role of vasculitis. Am J Dermatopathol. 2000;22:379–90.
14. Tunc R, Saip S, Siva A, Yazici H. Cerebral venous thrombosis is associated with major vessel disease in Behçet's syndrome. Ann Rheum Dis. 2004;63:1693–4.
15. Jennette JC, Falk RJ, Bacon PA, Basu N, Cid MC, Ferrario F, et al. 2012 revised international Chapel Hill consensus conference nomenclature of vasculitides. Arthritis Rheum. 2013;65:1–11.
16. Sunderkötter CH, Zelger B, Chen KR, Requena L, Piette W, Carlson JA, et al. Nomenclature of cutaneous vasculitis: dermatologic addendum to the 2012 revised international Chapel Hill consensus conference nomenclature of vasculitides. Arthritis Rheumatol. 2018;70(2):171–84.
17. Jorizzo JL, Taylor RS, Schmalstieg FC, Solomon AR Jr, Daniels JC, Rudloff HE, et al. Complex aphthosis: a forme fruste of Behçet's syndrome? J Am Acad Dermatol. 1985;13:80–4.
18. Bletry O, Mohattane A, Wechsler B, Beaufils P, Valère P, Petit J, et al. Cardiac manifestations of Behcet's disease. 12 cases. Presse Med. 1988;17:2388–91.
19. Demirelli S, Degirmenci H, Inci S, Arisoy A. Cardiac manifestations in Behcet's disease. Intractable Rare Dis Res. 2015;4(2):70–5.
20. Kwon CM, Lee SH, Kim JH, Lee KH, Kim HD, Hong YH, et al. A case of Behcet's disease with pericarditis, thrombotic thrombocytopenic purpura, deep vein thrombosis and coronary artery pseudo aneurysm. Korean J Intern Med. 2006;21:50–6.
21. Okcun B, Baran T, Babalik E, Kücükoglu S. Multichamber masses and constrictive pericarditis in Behcet's disease. Clin Exp Rheumatol. 2003;21:55.
22. Darie C, Knezinsky M, Demolombe-Rague S, Pinède L, Périnetti M, Ninet JF, Ninet J. Cardiac pseudotumor revealing Behcet's disease. Rev Med Interne. 2005;26:420–4.
23. Fekih M, Fennira S, Ghodbane L, Zaouali RM. Intracardiac thrombosis: unusual complication of Behcet's disease. Tunis Med. 2004;82:785–90.
24. Koc F, Koc S, Yuksek J, Vatankulu MA, Ozbek K, Gul EE, et al. Is diastolic dysfunction associated with atrial electrocardiographic parameters in Behçet's disease? Acta Cardiol. 2011;66(5):607–12.
25. Gemici K, Baran I, Güllülü S, Kazazoglu AR, Cordan J, Ozer Z. Evaluation of diastolic dysfunction and repolarization dispersion in Behcet's disease. Int J Cardiol. 2000 Apr 28;73(2):143–8.
26. Turkolmez S, Gokcora N, Alkan M, Gorer MA. Evaluation of myocardial perfusion in patients with Behçet's disease. Ann Nucl Med. 2005 May;19(3):201–6.
27. Aktürk E, Yağmur J, Kurtoğlu E, Ermis N, Acikgoz N, Sener S, et al. Left atrial volume and function in patients with Behcet's disease assessed by realtime three-dimensional echocardiography. Eur Heart J Cardiovasc Imaging. 2012;13(8):650–5.
28. Rolland JM, Bical O, Laradi A, Robinault J, Benzidia R, Vanetti A, et al. False aneurysm of the left ventricle and coronary aneurysms in Behcet disease. Arch Mal Coeur Vaiss. 1993;86(9):1383–5.
29. Aksoyek S, Aytemir K, Ozer N, Ozcebe O, Oto A. Assessment of autonomic nervous system function in patients with Behcet's disease by spectral analysis of heart rate variability. J Auton Nerv Syst. 1999;77(2-3):190–4.
30. Aytemir K, Ozer N, Aksoyek S, Ozcebe O, Kabakcı G, Oto A. Increased QT dispersion in the absence of QT prolongation in patients with Behçet's disease and ventricular arrhythmias. Int J Cardiol. 1998;67(2):171–5.
31. Morshedi-Meibodi A, Larson MG, Levy D, O'Donnell CJ, Vasan RS. Heart rate recovery after treadmill exercise testing and risk of cardiovascular disease events (The Framingham Heart Study). Am J Cardiol. 2002;90(8):848–52.
32. Marshall SE. Behcet's disease. Best Pract Res Clin Rheumatol. 2004;18(3):291–311.

33. Le Thi HD, Wechsler B, Papo T, Piette JC, Bletry O, Vitoux JM, et al. Arterial lesions in Behcet's disease. A study in 25 patients. J Rheumatol. 1995;22(11):2103–13.
34. Ozeren M, Dogan OV, Dogan S, Yucel E. True and pseudo aneurysms of coronary arteries in a patient with Behçet's disease. Eur J Cardiothorac Surg. 2004;25(3):465–7.
35. Balta I, Balta S, Koryurek OM, Demirkol S, Mikhailidis DP, Celik T, et al. Serum endocan levels as a marker of disease activity in patients with Behçet disease. J Am Acad Dermatol. 2014;70(2):291–6.
36. Kul A, Ateş O, Alkan Melikoğlu M, Uğur M, Öztürk N, Erkayhan G, et al. Endocan measurement for active Behçet disease. Arch Rheumatol. 2017 Mar 24;32(3):197–202.
37. International Study Group for Behçet's Disease. Criteria for diagnosis of Behçet's disease. Lancet. 1990;335:1078–180.
38. Ozatli D, Kav T, Haznedaroglu IC, Büyükaşik Y, Koşar A, Ozcebe O, et al. Cardiac and great vessel thrombosis in Behcet's disease. Intern Med. 2001;40:68–72.
39. Kaatz M, Görnig M, Bocker T, Zouboulis CC, Wollina U. Late manifestation of a fatal Behcet's disease with cardiac involvement and lethal outcome. Dtsch Med Wochenschr. 1998;123:217–22.
40. Espinosa G, Cervera R, Reverter JC, Tassies D, Font J, Ingelmo M. Vascular involvement in Behçet's disease. Isr Med Assoc J. 2002;4:614–6.

12 Kawasaki Disease

Vasu D. Gooty, Kavita Sharma, and Tarique Hussain

Introduction and Pathophysiology

Kawasaki disease (KD) is an acute systemic vasculitis syndrome of unknown etiology occurring in infants and children. It primarily affects small-medium sized arteries, especially coronary arteries [1] and was originally described in Japan by Dr. Tomisaki Kawasaki in 1967 [2]. It is one of the leading causes of ischemic heart disease in infants and children from thrombosis in coronary artery aneurysms secondary to coronary arteritis. Although, several theories including role of pathogens, genetic markers, environmental factors have shown to be associated with KD, the true cause of KD still remains unknown.

Epidemiology

KD is markedly more prevalent in Japan with an annual incidence of 264.8 per 100,000 in 2012. The estimated incidence of KD in North America is 25 cases per 100,000 children who are less than 5 years of age per year [3]. Although KD has

V. D. Gooty (✉)
University of Tennessee Heath Science Center, LeBonheur Children's Hospital, Memphis, TN, USA
e-mail: vgooty@uthsc.edu

K. Sharma
Department of Pediatrics, UT Southwestern Medical Center, Office: Children's Medical Center, Dallas, TX, USA
e-mail: kavitha.sharma@UTSouthwestern.edu

T. Hussain
Department of Pediatrics, UT Southwestern Medical Center, Director of Congenital Cardiac MR Service, Office: Children's Medical Center, Dallas, TX, USA
e-mail: mohammad.hussain@UTSouthwestern.edu

C. Salavastru et al. (eds.), *Skin and the Heart*,
https://doi.org/10.1007/978-3-030-54779-0_12

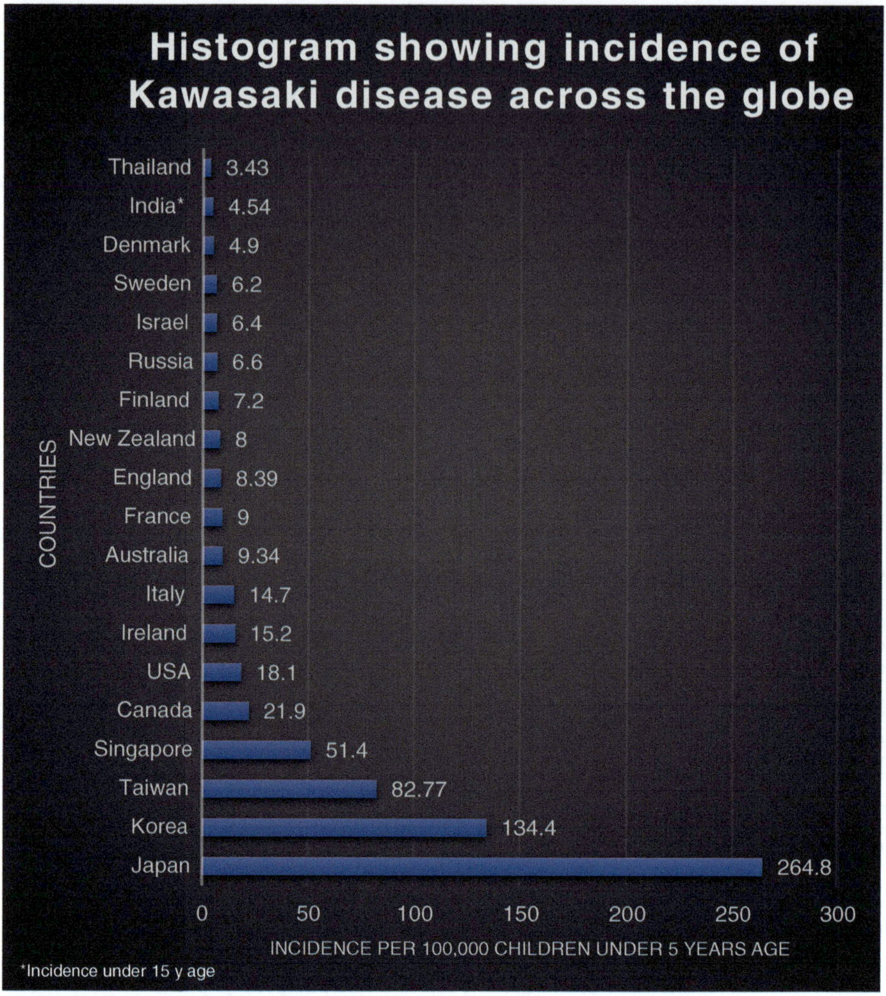

Fig. 12.1 Histogram showing incidence of KD across the globe

been well described in developed countries, it is increasingly recognized in many developing or resource limited countries. The incidence in Europe and Australia is approximately 6–9/100,000 [4–6]. The global incidence of KD is shown in Fig. 12.1 [7].

KD is more common during winter and early spring in the extratropical northern hemisphere, with the lowest number of cases in late summer and fall. However, there is a lack of seasonal variation in the tropics and the extratropical southern hemisphere [8]. The highest relative risk is seen in Asian children, especially those of Japanese ancestry. Boys are slightly more affected than girls with ratio of 1.5–1.7:1 of affected children <5 y [9–11]. The recurrence rate of KD is ~3.5% in Japan, Asians, Pacific Islanders. In United States, the rate of recurrence is quite low at 1.7% [11] occurring at a median age of 1.5 y after initial episode [12], increasing the risk for development of coronary artery sequelae [13]. After a first case in the family, the incidence of KD in a sibling has approximately ten-fold higher relative risk and of these, 50% will develop within 10 days of the first case [14]. This risk is higher in identical twins, which could likely be secondary to genetic predisposition that interacts with exposure to similar pathogenic agent in the environment [15, 16]. It is important to note that the peak mortality usually occurs 15–45 days after the onset of fever, this is secondary to coronary vasculitis, elevation in platelet count and hypercoagulable state [17]. Sudden death in children and adults occur later in life and has been shown to be secondary to myocardial infarction from aneurysm and stenosis of the coronary arteries [18].

Pathology

KD causes systemic vasculitis of medium sized arteries and inflammation of various organs during the acute febrile phase. Apart from coronary artery involvement, it can also cause myocarditis, pericarditis, valvulitis and extracardiac involvement leading to hepatitis, interstitial pneumonitis, abdominal pain, vomiting, diarrhea, gall bladder hydrops, aseptic meningitis, irritability, pyuria, pancreatitis and lymphadenopathy.

The primary pathology involves following three process:

1. **Necrotizing arteritis:** Self-limiting neutrophilic process leading to progressive destruction of arterial wall into adventitia, causing aneurysms, vasculitis and perivasculitis of microvessels causing edema and inflammation. This lasts for 2 weeks after fever onset.
2. **Subacute/chronic vasculitis:** Subacute process beginning 2 weeks after fever onset leading to infiltration of lymphocytes, plasma cells, eosinophils and may continue for several months.
3. **Luminal myofibroblastic proliferation (LMP):** This is an active proliferative process that begins in first few weeks after fever onset and leads to arterial stenosis of the coronary arteries [19–23]. This stage is characterized myofibroblastic proliferation process consisting of myoblasts and inflammatory cells which may persist for months to years.

The pathological outcomes of involvement of coronary artery damage depends on the severity of lesions. Mildly dilated arteries usually return to normal size soon. Large sized aneurysms usually lose their intima, media and elastica which cannot be regenerated. Fusiform aneurysms can thrombose or develop progressive stenosis. Large aneurysms may resolve when the lumen size decreases because of layered mural thrombi or myofibroblastic proliferation. Giant aneurysms generally lose all the media, with only a rim of adventitia remaining that leads to successive layers of thrombi, with organization and calcification of the oldest thrombi. Giant aneurysms may rupture in the first 2 to 3 weeks after fever onset but rarely do so thereafter. Myocardial infarction can occur from acute or progressive thrombosis or from stenosis [24].

Etiology

Etiological factors for KD have not been well confirmed, although several factors have been described including preceding respiratory illness, or an autoimmune process. Other epidemiological studies have correlated the incidence of KD cases in Japan, Hawaii and western United States with tropospheric wind currents originating in Northeastern China suggesting a wind-borne agent trigger. The high incidence of KD in Asian children especially in Japan, China, Korea and Taiwan strongly supports the hypothesis that genetic susceptibility determines host response to the KD pathogen. Several genes and signaling pathways have been shown to have association with aneurysm formation and host susceptibility [25, 26].

KD also has clinical similarities to scarlet fever and Staphylococcus toxic shock syndrome (SSS), both of which are caused by toxin producing bacteria, causing release of superantigens. However, KD differs markedly from SSS, in that there is a lack of acute vasculitis in SSS [27–30].

Clinical Features and Diagnosis

The clinical features and diagnosis of KD is made based on clinical criteria (Table 12.1, Fig. 12.2). Patients who meet the definition based on the primary findings are said to have complete KD or typical KD or classical KD. Patients who do not have sufficient clinical findings are known to have incomplete or atypical KD. In the absence of a specific diagnostic test, other clinical, laboratory and echocardiographic findings can support the diagnosis of incomplete KD without meeting the classical definition [3].

The principal diagnostic criteria used for classical/typical KD are:

- Persistent fever >5 days
- Conjunctival injection
- Oropharynx changes
- Peripheral extremity changes
- Diffuse erythematous rash
- Cervical lymphadenopathy

The diagnosis of classical KD can be made based on the presence of ≥5 days of fever and presence of ≥4 of the 5 principal clinical features (Table 12.1 and Fig. 12.3). In the presence of >4 principal clinical criteria, particularly when redness and swelling of the hands and feet are present, the diagnosis may be made with only 4 days of fever.

Fever is typically high spiking (>39 °C – 40 °C) and continues for 1–3 weeks. After the IVIG infusion, the fever usually resolves within 36 hours. However, if the fever does not resolve in that time frame, the patient is considered to have resistance to IVIG (discussed later in the chapter).

Table 12.1 Diagnosis of classical Kawasaki disease

Classical or typical KD is diagnosed by presence of fever for at least 5 days (the day of fever onset is taken to be the first day of fever) along with at least 4 of 5 principal clinical features:
1. Erythema and cracking of lips, strawberry tongue, and/or erythema of oral and pharyngeal mucosa
2. Bilateral bulbar conjunctival injection without exudate
3. Rash: Any of the following form: Maculopapular, diffuse erythroderma, erythema multiforme-like
4. Erythema and edema of the hands and feet in acute phase and/or periungual desquamation in subacute phase (usually after 1–2 weeks of fever onset)
5. Unilateral cervical lymphadenopathy ≥1.5 cm diameter
Patients who lack full clinical features of classical KD, may be diagnosed as incomplete or atypical KD
Laboratory test findings in such cases:
1. Normal or elevated white blood cell count
(a) Neutrophil predominance
2. Elevated acute phase reactants – during acute phase
(a) C-reactive protein (b) Erythrocyte sedimentation rate (ESR)
3. Low serum sodium
4. Low albumin level
5. Elevated liver enzymes
6. Sterile pyuria
7. In the second week after fever onset, thrombocytosis is common

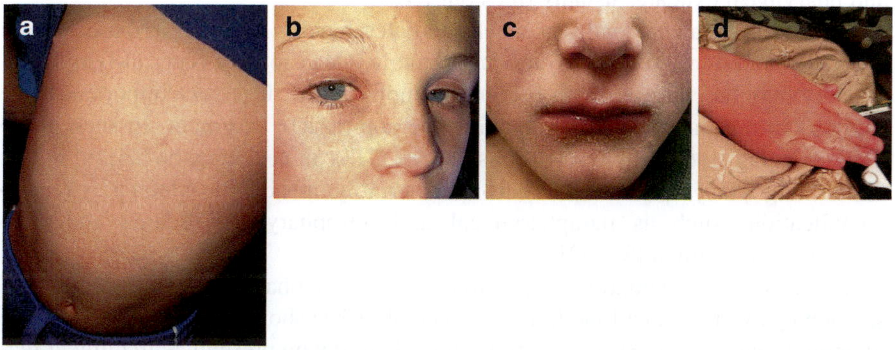

Fig. 12.2 Clinical features of classic Kawasaki disease. (**a**) Diffuse maculopapular rash on the trunk or erythema multiforme-like, (**b**) Bulbar conjunctival injection without exudate, (**c**) Erythema and cracking of lips, (**d**) Palmar erythema with swelling in acute phase

In the early phase, painful erythema of the palms and soles may occur. Within 2–3 weeks after the onset of fever, desquamation of the fingers and toes occurs, which may extend into palms and soles in about two thirds of all patients.

A diffuse erythematous maculopapular rash usually appears within 5 days of fever onset and is extensive, primarily involving the trunk and extremities with early

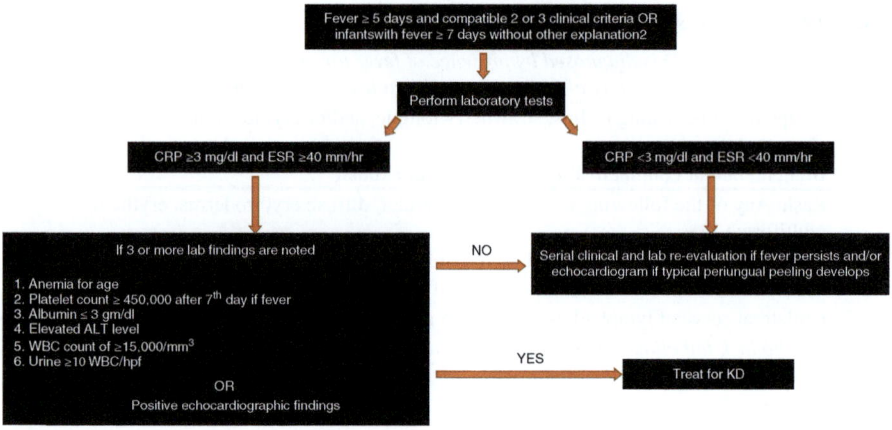

Fig. 12.3 Evaluation algorithm of incomplete or atypical Kawasaki disease presentation

desquamation. Other common findings include scarlatiniform erythroderma and erythema multiforme-like lesions. Bullous, vesicular and petechial rashes are not consistent with KD; hence the doctor should search for alternative diagnosis. Bilateral non-exudative bulbar conjunctivitis begins shortly after fever onset and is limbus sparing. Changes of lips and oral cavity including erythema, dryness, fissuring, peeling, cracking and bleeding of the lips, strawberry tongue and diffuse erythema of the oropharyngeal mucosa are classical for KD. Presence of oral ulcers and pharyngeal exudates usually rules out KD.

Cervical lymphadenopathy is usually unilateral and is ≥1.5 cm in diameter and is usually noted in the anterior cervical triangle. Occasionally cervical lymphadenopathy may be confused with bacterial lymphadenitis. It is very important to be cautious in misdiagnosing and delaying the appropriate treatment. In such situations, imaging studies including ultrasound or CT scan neck may be helpful in differentiating KD lymphadenopathy from bacterial lymphadenitis which may lead to complications such as parapharyngeal and retropharyngeal edema and non-suppurative phlegmon [31, 32].

The presence of exudative conjunctivitis, exudative pharyngitis, oral ulcerations, splenomegaly and vesiculobullous or petechial rashes should prompt consideration of another diagnosis [33]. In a nonimmunized child who presents with clinical features, measles should always be considered as one of the diagnoses. Detection of a virus such as respiratory syncytial virus, metapneumovirus, coronavirus, parainfluenza or influenza virus doesn't necessarily exclude the diagnosis of KD as there may be concurrent viral infections during the winter seasons [34–36]. In children with clinical features of KD and a positive rapid test or culture for group-A streptococcus without improvement after 24–48 hours of effective antibiotic therapy, the diagnosis of KD should be reconsidered.

Incomplete/Atypical KD

The diagnosis of incomplete KD should be considered in any infant or child with prolonged, unexplained fever and have less than 4 of the principal clinical criteria along with lab and echo findings (Fig. 12.3) [37].

Hence it is important to include KD as one of the differential diagnosis in infants <6 months of age who present with prolonged fever and irritability, and unresponsive to antibiotic therapy.

Other Clinical and Lab Findings

Other than involvement of coronary arteries, KD may also cause features of neurological irritability, diarrhea, vomiting, abdominal pain, gallbladder hydrops, urethritis, arthritis or interstitial pneumonia.

Lab findings include leukocytosis during acute stage of illness, with a predominance of immature and mature granulocytes. Leukopenia and lymphocyte predominance usually suggest an alternate diagnosis. Presence of normocytic normochromic anemia is common and usually resolves with resolution of inflammation. Acute phase reactants such as ESR and CRP are elevated during the acute phase and is universal in the diagnosis of KD. The CRP usually normalizes more quickly than the ESR during resolution of inflammation, however, the ESR is elevated with IVIG therapy as well. Hence, monitoring of CRP trend is a useful marker of inflammation after treatment of acute inflammation.

Thrombocytosis is an important finding and it generally doesn't occur until the second week, peaking in the third week and normalizing by 4–6 weeks after its onset. Thrombocytopenia is rare but may occur in the first 1–2 weeks of illness. Other lab findings may include elevation in serum transaminases or gamma glutamyl transpeptidase (GGT) [38, 39], hypoalbuminemia, and B-type natriuretic peptide (NT-pro-B-NP; which is indicative of myocardial involvement may be elevated in some patients with KD but may non-specific in diagnosing KD [40, 41].

Cardiovascular Manifestation

During the acute phase, most importantly, coronary arteries may be inflamed due to arteritis. However, in certain cases, the whole heart may be affected including pericardium, myocardium, endocardium and the valves. The clinical manifestation during acute phase may include tachycardia, hyperdynamic precordium, innocent murmur, gallop rhythm. Presence of pericardial effusion is a common echocardiographic finding, but a precordial rub or tamponade may be rarely found. Most commonly mitral valve may be involved in up to 25% of patients. Aortic root dilation may be noticed in ~10% of patients during the acute illness [42]. Involvement of the sinus node and AV node can lead to arrhythmias and prolonged PR interval. Non-specific ST-T changes with abnormal ventricular repolarization may also be noted.

Since the introduction of gamma globulin in 1992, there has been a significant decline in the incidence of transient dilation and aneurysm formation of the coronary arteries. Historically, most of these patients received Aspirin as a part of anti-platelet therapy. Use of IVIG has significantly reduced the prevalence of coronary artery abnormalities [43, 44]. These landmark studies have led to the initiation of IVIG therapy as a primary standard of therapy for KD.

Occasionally myocarditis may be seen and can be transient in nature leading to myocardial dysfunction in a few children. They respond well to anti-inflammatory therapy. Certain subsets of patients may develop Kawasaki disease shock syndrome (KDSSS) associated with shock like presentation requiring inotropic support and may develop greater risk for coronary artery abnormalities, mitral regurgitation and have prolonged course of myocardial dysfunction [45].

Involvement of Coronary Arteries

Coronary artery involvement may lead to mild dilation to giant aneurysms in both proximal and distal arteries. Most of the patients with significant coronary artery dilatation may have baseline dilatation within the first 10 days of illness. Up to 50% of patients may develop mild dilatation of coronary arteries that will resolve within 4–8 weeks, patients with extensive or giant aneurysm may be asymptomatic unless they present with myocardial ischemia. Rarely, patients may develop aneurysms of other medium sized blood vessels such as axillary, subclavian, brachial, femoral, iliac, splanchnic and mesenteric arteries usually near the branching points [24, 46] with similar pathology as the involvement of coronary arteries during acute phase of illness.

Resolution of acute inflammatory process may be followed by chronic vasculitis and luminal myofibroblastic proliferation (LMP) which may normalize eventually but this may eventually increase the risk for stenosis of the arteries.

Echocardiography is considered as the primary imaging modality in the assessment of KD both during acute phase of illness as well as during follow-up period. It is non-invasive and has high sensitivity and specificity to detect abnormalities of proximal coronary artery segments. In the acute phase of illness, echo should be performed for diagnosis of KD. However, unavailability of echocardiography or technical limitations should not delay the treatment for patients. Presence of normal initial echocardiogram during the first week of illness does not completely rule out diagnosis of KD. The initial echocardiogram establishes a baseline for long-term follow-up for many patients, hence in an uncooperative or irritable patient, sedation may be needed.

In addition to standard anatomic and physiological imaging windows, the 2D imaging should focus on left main coronary artery, left circumflex, left anterior descending, right coronary artery and posterior descending artery. Maximal efforts must be made to visualise complete coronary arteries from multiple imaging planes (Fig. 12.4). The most common sites of coronary artery aneurysms are proximal left anterior descending, proximal right coronary artery, left main coronary artery and left circumflex coronary artery.

Coronaries may show diffuse ectasia or aneurysms (Figs. 12.5 and 12.6). The aneurysms may be described based on the morphology as saccular or fusiform. The use of z-score is shown to better evaluate the coronary artery dimension by correcting for body surface area (BSA). The coronary artery luminal dimensions are

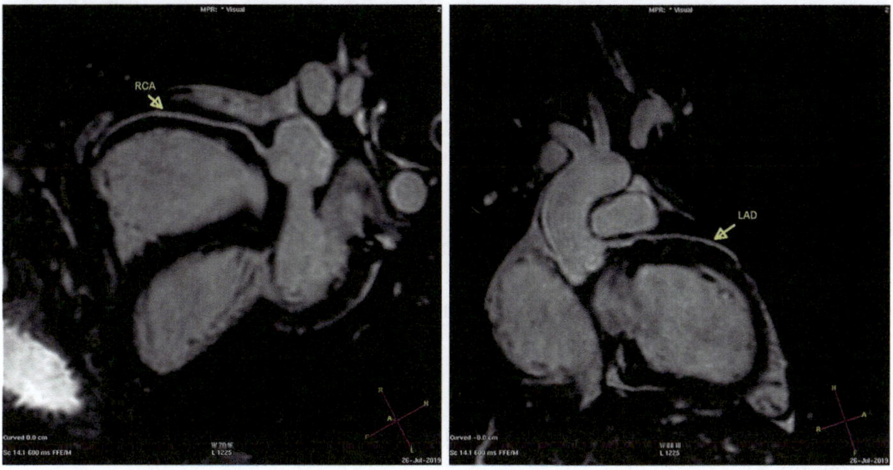

Fig. 12.4 Multiplanar reconstruction of a normal right and left anterior descending coronary artery

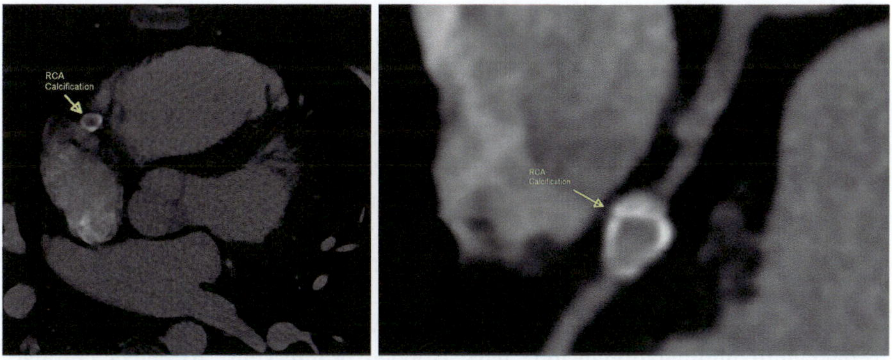

Fig. 12.5 Follow-up cardiac CT in patient with Kawasaki disease presenting with areas of calcification within the aneurysm of the right coronary artery

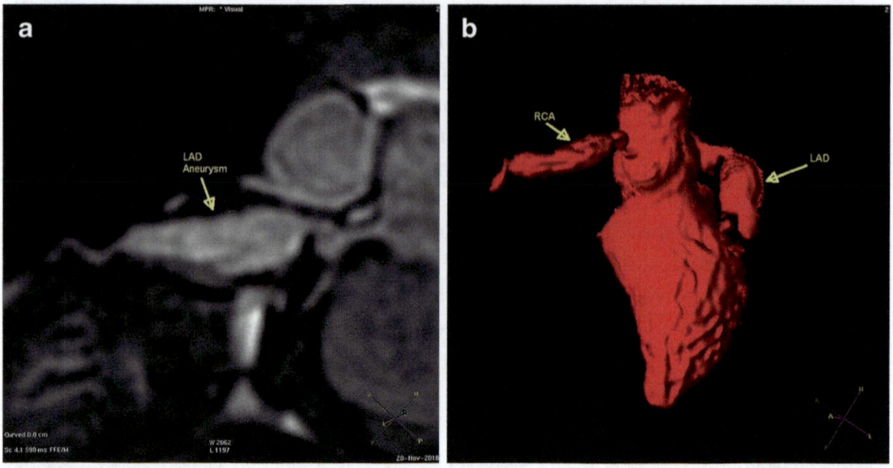

Fig. 12.6 (**a**) Cardiac MRI of a patient with multiplanar reconstruction showing severe aneurysm of left anterior descending (LAD) coronary artery; (**b**) Multiplanar 3D reconstruction of same patient with diffuse aneurysms of LAD and right coronary artery

classified based on the z-score and relative or absolute dimension of coronary lumen as follows [47]:

Following z-score classification is broadly used for assessment of coronary abnormalities:

1. **No involvement:** Always <2
2. **Dilation only:** 2 to <2.5; or if initially <2, a decrease in Z score during follow-up ≥1
3. **Small aneurysm:** ≥2.5 to <5
4. **Medium aneurysm:** ≥5 to <10, and absolute dimension <8 mm
5. **Large or giant aneurysm:** ≥10, or absolute dimension ≥8 mm

Echocardiography is an excellent tool for diagnosis and follow up of the size, thrombus, stenosis or aneurysm as well, it is also helpful in assessment of the aortic root, detection of ventricular wall motion abnormalities, pericardial effusion, valvar regurgitation. Use of other advance imaging modalities such as computed tomographic angiography (CTA), cardiac magnetic resonance imaging (MRI) or invasive angiography may be helpful in making decisions in further management of these patients over long-term course of the disease process.

In uncomplicated patients, echo should be repeated within 1 to 2 weeks, and 4–6 weeks after the initial treatment. For those patients who have coronary artery involvement with z-score > 2.5, at least weekly echocardiography should be performed until luminal dimensions have stopped progressing. To detect coronary artery thrombosis, it may be reasonable to perform echo in rapidly expanding large or giant aneurysms at least twice a week (or more frequently while the dimension is increasing) until 3 months after the illness onset.

Treatment

Acute Treatment

The primary goal of starting immediate therapy is to reduce the coronary artery inflammation and arterial damage to prevent thrombosis in the coronary artery abnormalities. The mainstay of therapy for both complete and incomplete KD is a single high dose of IVIG along with acetyl salicylic acid (ASA) (Table 12.2).

Table 12.2 Medications used in Kawasaki disease

Initial management		
IVIG 2 gm/kg	Given as single IV dose for 10–12 hours within first 10 days of onset	Additional dose of IVIG 2 gm/kg may be given 24 hours after first dose if fever doesn't subside
Aspirin 80–100 mg/kg/day divided every 6 hours	Given until the child is afebrile for 48–72 hours	After fever subsides continue with low dose 3–5 mg/kg until patient has no evidence of coronary artery changes by 6–8 weeks
Clopidogrel 0.2–1.0 mg/kg/day	Thromboprophylaxis given together with ASA for complex coronary artery aneurysms including giant aneurysms where dual antiplatelet therapy is warranted	
Adjunct therapies		
IVIG + Prednisolone: 2 mg/kg/day divided every 8 hours followed by oral taper over 2–3 weeks		
Infliximab: IV 3 mg/kg/day divided every 12 hours Or Oral 4–8 mg/kg/day divided every 12 hours		
Alternative therapies		
Cyclosporine: IV: 3 mg/kg/day divided every 12 hours Oral: 4–8 mg/kg/day divided every 12 hours		
Anakinra: 2–6 mg/kg/day given subcutaneous		
Cyclophosphamide: 2 mg/kg/day IV		
Plasma exchange		

(continued)

Table 12.2 (continued)

Initial management		
Antithrombotic therapy		
Low Molecular Weight Heparin (LMWH)	Monitored by Anti-factor Xa level 0.5–1.0 U/ml	
Enoxaparin: Given every 12 hours subcutaneous <2 mo. age: 1.5 mg/kg per dose >2 mo. age: 1.0 mg/kg/dose	Titrate to anti-factor Xa target range	
Warfarin: Load with 0.2 mg/kg/day, followed by 0.1 mg/kg/day, titrate the dose to INR target level	INR target level 2–3	
Thrombolytic therapy		
Tissue plasminogen activator – Alteplase: Following dosing regimen may be used: 0.1–0.6 mg/kg/hr. IV for 6 hours Or 0.2 mg/kg IV bolus (max 15 mg), followed by 0.75 mg/kg over 30 min (max 50 mg), followed by 0.5 mg/kg over 60 min (max 35 mg) for total max dose of 100 mg	Monitor closely for bleeding	Reassess for thrombus after completion of the infusion by echocardiogram

All patients meeting the AHA diagnostic criteria for KD should be treated as soon as possible in the course of illness. IVIG should be started as early as possible within first 10 days of onset of fever. IVIG should also be started in patients with delayed diagnosis (>10 days of fever) if they have ongoing elevation in the ESR, CRP along with associated coronary artery aneurysms (z-score > 2.5).

IVIG has been shown to reduce new coronary artery abnormalities in several studies. All patients should be started treatment with IVIG 2 gm/kg as a single infusion given over 10–12 hours period along with ASA [48]. As IVIG is a biological product made from pooled donor plasma, rare complications may develop such as aseptic meningitis without any neurological sequelae. Children receiving IVIG should defer measles, mumps, varicella immunizations after receiving high dose IVIG. However, children in whom risk of exposure to measles is high may receive vaccination earlier and then be reimmunized at least 11 months after IVIG administration if they have inadequate serological response.

Standard treatment during the acute phase of illness consists of administering high dose ASA of 80–100 mg/kg/day every 6 hours in North America, 50 mg/kg/day in Japan and western Europe. The high dose is transitioned to low dose aspirin of 3–5 mg/kg/day after the patient is afebrile for 48–72 hours. The low dose aspirin is continued until the patient has no evidence of coronary artery changes by 6–8 weeks after the onset of illness.

Use of high dose ASA for prolonged period of time when there is active influenza or varicella infection is associated with Reye's syndrome [49–51]. Hence in patients presenting with active influenza and KD, in addition to starting IVIG, alternative antipyretics such as acetaminophen should be considered for a minimum of 2 weeks. Ibuprofen antagonizes the irreversible platelet inhibition by ASA, hence ibuprofen should be avoided in patients with coronary aneurysms for the antiplatelet effects [52].

7% of patients develop KD shock syndrome (KDSS) [45, 53] defined by the presence of shock, hypotension requiring initiation of volume expanders, infusion of vasoactive agents or transfer to intensive care unit for the management. It is critical to recognize early signs of KD during KDSS presentation so that IVIG therapy can be initiated promptly to reduce coronary complications.

Adjunct Therapy for KD

A combination of corticosteroids along with IVIG as an initial treatment in high risk KD patients is associated with reduction in the coronary artery abnormalities [54]. Another drug, Infliximab which is a chimeric monoclonal antibody that binds with high affinity to TNF-alpha may be used as a rescue therapy in patients resistant to IVIG therapy [55, 56]. Adding infliximab to the initial therapy along with IVIG does not necessarily prevent recrudescent fever.

IVIG Resistance

Although most of the patients are responsive to IVIG within first 24–48 hours, ~10—20% of patients with KD develop recrudescence or persistence of fever [57–59]. The presence of fever at least 36 hours after the end of IVIG infusion is known as IVIG resistant KD. The mechanism of resistance is poorly understood and may be associated with host genetic factors or polymorphisms in the receptors. Patients who are resistant to initial IVIG dose are at a higher risk of developing coronary artery abnormalities [60–62].

In case of resistance to IVIG treatment, a second dose or retreatment with IVIG 2 gm/kg may be given. Administration of high-dose pulse steroids such as IV methylprednisolone 20–30 mg/kg IV for 3 days with or without a subsequent course and taper of oral prednisone may be considered as an alternative to second infusion of IVIG. Other adjunct therapies including infliximab (5 mg/kg) may be used as an alternative to a secondary infusion of IVIG or corticosteroids for this subset of patients. Patients who do not respond either to second dose of IVIG, steroids or infliximab, will require additional therapy to control inflammation. Plasma exchange or Cyclosporine may also be used as another adjunct therapy.

A newer drug, Anakinra is a recombinant, non-glycosylated form of human IL-1 receptor antagonist and may be used for treatment of highly refractory KD [63, 64].

Thrombus Management

Antiplatelet therapy is considered as the standard therapy for patients with coronary artery aneurysms. For patients with small coronary artery aneurysms, monotherapy with low dose ASA therapy is sufficient for prophylaxis of thrombosis. In patients with moderate size aneurysms, ASA therapy along with a Thienopyridine such as Clopidogrel may be used, due to the superior efficacy of this regimen when compared to ASA alone [65–68].

Patients with large or giant aneurysms, with internal luminal diameter z-score $\geq$ 10 or absolute dimension $\geq$8 mm, are at particularly high risk for coronary artery thrombosis and eventually development of stenosis. In such patients, treatment should be initiated with an antiplatelet and anticoagulant therapy, most commonly low-dose ASA together with warfarin therapy (to maintain INR ratio target 2.0–3.0) or with low molecular weight heparin (LMWH).

Transition from LMWH to warfarin may be considered once aneurysms have stopped expanding and the patient is stable. More aggressive therapies may be used in patients with exceptionally high risk for coronary artery thrombosis. Infants and children requiring thrombolysis for coronary artery thrombosis may be maintained for a limited time on 3 agents such as ASA, Clopidogrel and an anticoagulant therapy. Ibuprofen and other NSAIDs with known or potential involvement of cyclooxygenase pathway may be harmful in patients taking ASA for its antiplatelet actions.

For the therapy of acute coronary syndrome with thrombosis, the goal is to reestablish coronary artery flow, patency, salvage the myocardium and overall reduce morbidity and mortality. The coronary artery thrombosis of adult coronary artery disease is caused by plaque rupture or inflammation, with exposure of lipids and extracellular matrix to the coagulation system. However, this is different in KD as the pathology is due to abnormal flow characteristics leading to thrombus formation. Therapy for coronary thrombus rarely requires use of thrombolytic therapy such as tissue-type plasminogen activator (t-PA). It is used in acute occlusive or near-occlusive thrombosis in infants and children.

Long-term Outcomes and Management

Long term management begins at the end of acute illness which is 4–6 weeks after fever onset. The primary goals of long-term management are to prevent thrombosis and myocardial ischemia which can be achieved by thromboprophylaxis and careful surveillance of coronary artery stenosis and myocardial ischemia respectively along with maintenance of optimal long-term cardiovascular health.

KD can also lead to long term vascular changes including systemic arterial dysfunction and increasing arterial stiffness and intima-media thickness and thus overall vascular health is affected.

The long-term risk stratification is assessed by the use of echocardiographic coronary artery body surface area (BSA) adjusted z-score measurements. Risk stratification may help in specific recommendations for medical therapy, thromboprophylaxis, physical activity and reproductive health.

Only in patients without coronary artery involvement, ASA is stopped after 6–8 weeks. However, those with coronary artery involvement, low dose ASA (3–5 mg/kg) is continued. Addition of anticoagulation including warfarin or LMWH along with dual antiplatelet therapy (ASA + Clopidogrel) may be used depending on the extent of coronary artery aneurysm involvement. Additional therapies including statin and beta-blocker may be use in those with higher risk including small-medium aneurysms.

Long Term Follow-up

Assessment of patients during follow-up period includes history and physical examination, electrocardiography, echocardiography. Patients without coronary artery involvement and those with z-score < 2 are discharged from the cardiology care after echo surveillance at 4–6 weeks. It is unlikely to develop new coronary artery dilation after 4–6 weeks after acute treatment [69–72].

Ongoing cardiology follow-up is recommended in patients with aneurysm of any size (Table 12.3). Patients with small to medium size aneurysms often regress

Table 12.3 Long-term medication management and indications

Coronary artery involvement	ASA low dose (3–5 mg/kg/day)	Dual antiplatelet therapy (ASA + Clopidogrel)	Warfarin or LMWH	Statin
No involvement (z-score < 2)	6–8 weeks, then discontinue	Not indicated	Not indicated	Not indicated
Dilatation only (z-score 2 to <2.5)	May continue after 6–8 weeks	Not indicated	Not indicated	Not indicated
Small aneurysm (≥2.5 to <5)	Continue	Not indicated	Usually not indicated	Empiric therapy may be considered
Medium aneurysm (≥5 to <10, or < 8 mm diameter)	Continue	May be considered	Usually not indicated	Empiric therapy may be considered
Large and giant aneurysm (≥10, or ≥ 8 mm diameter)	Continue	May be considered	Indicated	Empiric therapy may be considered

towards normal luminal dimensions most quickly during first year after acute treatment. However, large or giant aneurysms take longer and fewer of them regress back to normal luminal dimension. As this slow regression happens over a period of time, these aneurysms are associated with increased risk of stenosis and obstruction. For routine surveillance, historically, only invasive coronary angiography was used for follow-up. However, other modalities are currently being used such as use of physiological and pharmacological stress imaging including nuclear medicine (NM) scintigraphy stress imaging, Positron Emission Tomography (PET) and cardiac MRI for assessment of myocardial perfusion imaging (MPI). Physiological exercise stress echocardiography is found to be superior to exercise stress electrocardiography alone in the detection of ischemia, the major limitation is the rapid return of the heart rate back to normal rate in young patients and that younger children cannot optimally perform on treadmills. Hence alternatives include Dobutamine stress echocardiography. Patients with inducible myocardial ischemia on testing should eventually undergo invasive coronary angiography.

Cardiac MRI considered as a useful for the assessment in long term imaging of KD patients and has an advantage of avoiding radiation exposure [73]. Myocardial stress cardiac MRI is a promising new technique where it can be used for risk stratification of patients. In a recent study by Bratis et al., the authors demonstrated an inducible perfusion defect and myocardial scar in patients and they showed significant impaired myocardial perfusion reserve when compared to control subjects suggesting the presence of microvascular dysfunction in these patients [74].

Cardiac CT angiogram can provide 3-D visualization of the coronary artery tree and may identify regions of stenosis more optimally than cardiac MRI. It can also provide detailed view of the presence of thrombus in the coronary arteries as well. However, the radiation exposure may be significant and may limit its use. Newer CT scan systems with lower levels of radiation exposure could increase the utility and safety of this modality.

Invasive angiography is considered as the "gold standard" for coronary artery assessment, although it is invasive. It provides detail coronary anatomy, luminal diameter and structure. Fractional flow reserve (FFR) measured during angiography is useful in determination of ischemia causing areas in patients affected by KD. Intravascular ultrasound (IVUS) has also been used to demonstrate vascular pathology in patients where coronary artery abnormalities are noted.

Important Long-term Cardiovascular Health

Patients with KD has a different pattern or susceptibility to CVD risk factors than general population. Due to their increased risk for coronary artery disease (CAD) in KD patients, it warrants more aggressive management and lifestyle modifications to reduce CVD risk factors such as cholesterol levels, adiposity, vascular health.

Empiric use of hydroxy methylglutaryl coenzyme-A (HMG-CoA) reductase inhibitors (Statins) is the cornerstone of therapy for the primary and secondary prevention of atherosclerotic cardiovascular events in adults [75, 76]. Statins have shown to lower the low-density lipoprotein (LDL) cholesterol and have potential benefits by its pleotropic effects on inflammation, endothelial function, oxidative stress, platelet aggregation and coagulation. Hence empiric therapy with low-dose statin may be considered in KD patients with past or current aneurysms, regardless of age or sex as a long-term therapy.

For antiplatelet action, most commonly Aspirin is used. However, in patients with Aspirin allergy, other types of antiplatelet therapy may be considered. For anticoagulation, most common medication used is Warfarin. However, dosing based on the levels may be problematic especially for monitoring levels for few patients and in such cases, LMWH may be an alternative.

Since KD is an illness of childhood, most of the early education and care is directed towards parents. Hence it is important to educate and involve the child (patient) during the transition of care discussion starting as early as 12 years [77]. Patients who never had coronary artery involvement or aneurysms, long term cardiology follow-up is not recommended in such cases. Due to the ongoing need for long term management, both pediatric and adult cardiologist should collaborate together for optimal transition and long-term care of these patients.

Effect of COVID-19 Pandemic

A special emphasis is deserved during the COVID-19 pandemic era caused by the virus, SARS-CoV-2. Several pediatric cases of a Kawasaki-like disease have been reported, with clusters of children and adolescents requiring admission to intensive care units who are presenting with atypical Kawasaki disease or acute toxic shock like syndrome. This Multisystem Inflammatory Syndrome in children (MIS-C) is been reported across the world, predominantly in Europe [78] and other countries [79–82]. The proposed hypothesis and mechanism for lung and myocardial injury from SARS-CoV-2 is due to a “cytokine storm” from the proinflammatory and regulatory T cells [83].

The World Health Organization (WHO) currently has a preliminary case definition which is similar to atypical KD criteria, which includes: fever for ≥3 days and a constellation of clinical and lab features of KD in addition to positive COVID-19 testing or contact with a COVID-19 positive patient [84]. Although the WHO clinical data platform is being updated constantly, of the reported cases, almost all patients present with significant myocardial dysfunction leading to hypotension or shock requiring inotropic support in the ICU setting. Coronary artery involvement is seen in 17% of cases in one of the multiinstitutional studies [78] as opposed to 50% in classical KD. Gastrointestinal symptoms such as diarrhea and vomiting is in several children in addition to a -purulent bilateral conjunctivitis, lymphadenopathy, skin rash, and cracked lips have been described. Due to the overlap with atypical KD symptoms, several children are being treated with IVIG in addition to inotropic support (as indicated). Although several children have had relatively short hospital stays with near recovery [78], the long-term implications of MIS-C needs to be studied in children post-discharge.

Global recognition of MIS-C is imperative during this time period, since the early recognition of these clinical findings is important to avoid delaying treatment with IVIG and other KD related adjunctive therapies.

References

1. Kato H, Koike S, Yamamoto M, Ito Y, Yano E. Coronary aneurysms in infants and young children with acute febrile mucocutaneous lymph node syndrome. J Pediatr. 1975;86(6):892–8.
2. Kawasaki T. Acute febrile mucocutaneous syndrome with lymphoid involvement with specific desquamation of the fingers and toes in children. Arerugi. 1967;16(3):178–222.
3. McCrindle BW, Rowley AH, Newburger JW, Burns JC, Bolger AF, Gewitz M, et al. Diagnosis, Treatment, and Long-Term Management of Kawasaki Disease: A Scientific Statement for Health Professionals From the American Heart Association. Circulation. 2017;135(17):e927–e99.
4. Yim D, Curtis N, Cheung M, Burgner D. Update on Kawasaki disease: epidemiology, aetiology and pathogenesis. J Paediatr Child Health. 2013;49(9):704–8.
5. Tacke CE, Breunis WB, Pereira RR, Breur JM, Kuipers IM, Kuijpers TW. Five years of Kawasaki disease in the Netherlands: a national surveillance study. Pediatr Infect Dis J. 2014;33(8):793–7.
6. Salo E. Epidemiology of Kawasaki disease in Northern Europe. Prog Clin Biol Res. 1987;250:67–70.
7. Singh S, Vignesh P, Burgner D. The epidemiology of Kawasaki disease: a global update. Arch Dis Child. 2015;100(11):1084–8.
8. Burns JC, Herzog L, Fabri O, Tremoulet AH, Rodo X, Uehara R, et al. Seasonality of Kawasaki disease: a global perspective. PLoS One. 2013;8(9):e74529.
9. Chang RK. The incidence of Kawasaki disease in the United States did not increase between 1988 and 1997. Pediatrics. 2003;111(5 Pt 1):1124–5.
10. Holman RC, Curns AT, Belay ED, Steiner CA, Schonberger LB. Kawasaki syndrome hospitalizations in the United States, 1997 and 2000. Pediatrics. 2003;112(3 Pt 1):495–501.
11. Maddox RA, Holman RC, Uehara R, Callinan LS, Guest JL, Schonberger LB, et al. Recurrent Kawasaki disease: USA and Japan. Pediatr Int. 2015;57(6):1116–20.
12. Chahal N, Somji Z, Manlhiot C, Clarizia NA, Ashley J, Yeung RS, et al. Rate, associated factors and outcomes of recurrence of Kawasaki disease in Ontario. Canada Pediatr Int. 2012;54(3):383–7.
13. Nakamura Y, Oki I, Tanihara S, Ojima T, Yanagawa H. Cardiac sequelae in recurrent cases of Kawasaki disease: a comparison between the initial episode of the disease and a recurrence in the same patients. Pediatrics. 1998;102(6):E66.
14. Fujita Y, Nakamura Y, Sakata K, Hara N, Kobayashi M, Nagai M, et al. Kawasaki disease in families. Pediatrics. 1989;84(4):666–9.
15. Quasney MW, Bronstein DE, Cantor RM, Zhang Q, Stroupe C, Shike H, et al. Increased frequency of alleles associated with elevated tumor necrosis factor-alpha levels in children with Kawasaki disease. Pediatr Res. 2001;49(5):686–90.
16. Yanagawa H, Yashiro M, Nakamura Y, Kawasaki T, Kato H. Epidemiologic pictures of Kawasaki disease in Japan: from the nationwide incidence survey in 1991 and 1992. Pediatrics. 1995;95(4):475–9.
17. Burns JC, Glode MP, Clarke SH, Wiggins J Jr, Hathaway WE. Coagulopathy and platelet activation in Kawasaki syndrome: identification of patients at high risk for development of coronary artery aneurysms. J Pediatr. 1984;105(2):206–11.
18. Burns JC, Shike H, Gordon JB, Malhotra A, Schoenwetter M, Kawasaki T. Sequelae of Kawasaki disease in adolescents and young adults. J Am Coll Cardiol. 1996;28(1):253–7.
19. Fujiwara H, Hamashima Y. Pathology of the heart in Kawasaki disease. Pediatrics. 1978;61(1):100–7.
20. Amano S, Hazama F, Hamashima Y. Pathology of Kawasaki disease: I. Pathology and morphogenesis of the vascular changes. Jpn Circ J. 1979;43(7):633–43.

21. Naoe S, Takahashi K, Masuda H, Tanaka N. Kawasaki disease. With particular emphasis on arterial lesions. Acta Pathol Jpn. 1991;41(11):785–97.
22. Landing BH, Larson EJ. Pathological features of Kawasaki disease (mucocutaneous lymph node syndrome). Am J Cardiovasc Pathol. 1987;1(2):218–29.
23. Sasaguri Y, Kato H. Regression of aneurysms in Kawasaki disease: a pathological study. J Pediatr. 1982;100(2):225–31.
24. Orenstein JM, Shulman ST, Fox LM, Baker SC, Takahashi M, Bhatti TR, et al. Three linked vasculopathic processes characterize Kawasaki disease: a light and transmission electron microscopic study. PLoS One. 2012;7(6):e38998.
25. Onouchi Y, Ozaki K, Burns JC, Shimizu C, Terai M, Hamada H, et al. A genome-wide association study identifies three new risk loci for Kawasaki disease. Nat Genet. 2012;44(5):517–21.
26. Onouchi Y, Gunji T, Burns JC, Shimizu C, Newburger JW, Yashiro M, et al. ITPKC functional polymorphism associated with Kawasaki disease susceptibility and formation of coronary artery aneurysms. Nat Genet. 2008;40(1):35–42.
27. Larkin SM, Williams DN, Osterholm MT, Tofte RW, Posalaky Z. Toxic shock syndrome: clinical, laboratory, and pathologic findings in nine fatal cases. Ann Intern Med. 1982;96(6 Pt 2):858–64.
28. Paris AL, Herwaldt LA, Blum D, Schmid GP, Shands KN, Broome CV. Pathologic findings in twelve fatal cases of toxic shock syndrome. Ann Intern Med. 1982;96(6 Pt 2):852–7.
29. Mancia L, Wahlstrom J, Schiller B, Chini L, Elinder G, D'Argenio P, et al. Characterization of the T-cell receptor V-beta repertoire in Kawasaki disease. Scand J Immunol. 1998;48(4):443–9.
30. Pietra BA, De Inocencio J, Giannini EH, Hirsch R. TCR V beta family repertoire and T cell activation markers in Kawasaki disease. J Immunol. 1994;153(4):1881–8.
31. Kanegaye JT, Van Cott E, Tremoulet AH, Salgado A, Shimizu C, Kruk P, et al. Lymph-node-first presentation of Kawasaki disease compared with bacterial cervical adenitis and typical Kawasaki disease. J Pediatr. 2013;162(6):1259–63. 63.e1–2
32. Kato H, Kanematsu M, Kato Z, Teramoto T, Kondo N, Hoshi H. Computed tomographic findings of Kawasaki disease with cervical lymphadenopathy. J Comput Assist Tomogr. 2012;36(1):138–42.
33. Burns JC, Mason WH, Glode MP, Shulman ST, Melish ME, Meissner C, et al. Clinical and epidemiologic characteristics of patients referred for evaluation of possible Kawasaki disease. United States Multicenter Kawasaki Disease Study Group. J Pediatr. 1991;118(5):680–6.
34. Kim JH, Yu JJ, Lee J, Kim MN, Ko HK, Choi HS, et al. Detection rate and clinical impact of respiratory viruses in children with Kawasaki disease. Korean J Pediatr. 2012;55(12):470–3.
35. Benseler SM, McCrindle BW, Silverman ED, Tyrrell PN, Wong J, Yeung RS. Infections and Kawasaki disease: implications for coronary artery outcome. Pediatrics. 2005;116(6):e760–6.
36. Turnier JL, Anderson MS, Heizer HR, Jone PN, Glode MP, Dominguez SR. Concurrent Respiratory Viruses and Kawasaki Disease. Pediatrics. 2015;136(3):e609–14.
37. Minich LL, Sleeper LA, Atz AM, McCrindle BW, Lu M, Colan SD, et al. Delayed diagnosis of Kawasaki disease: what are the risk factors? Pediatrics. 2007;120(6):e1434–40.
38. Tremoulet AH, Jain S, Chandrasekar D, Sun X, Sato Y, Burns JC. Evolution of laboratory values in patients with Kawasaki disease. Pediatr Infect Dis J. 2011;30(12):1022–6.
39. Eladawy M, Dominguez SR, Anderson MS, Glode MP. Abnormal liver panel in acute kawasaki disease. Pediatr Infect Dis J. 2011;30(2):141–4.
40. Dahdah N, Siles A, Fournier A, Cousineau J, Delvin E, Saint-Cyr C, et al. Natriuretic peptide as an adjunctive diagnostic test in the acute phase of Kawasaki disease. Pediatr Cardiol. 2009;30(6):810–7.
41. Lin KH, Chang SS, Yu CW, Lin SC, Liu SC, Chao HY, et al. Usefulness of natriuretic peptide for the diagnosis of Kawasaki disease: a systematic review and meta-analysis. BMJ Open. 2015;5(4):e006703.
42. Printz BF, Sleeper LA, Newburger JW, Minich LL, Bradley T, Cohen MS, et al. Noncoronary cardiac abnormalities are associated with coronary artery dilation and with laboratory inflammatory markers in acute Kawasaki disease. J Am Coll Cardiol. 2011;57(1):86–92.
43. Newburger JW, Takahashi M, Burns JC, Beiser AS, Chung KJ, Duffy CE, et al. The treatment of Kawasaki syndrome with intravenous gamma globulin. N Engl J Med. 1986;315(6):341–7.

44. Newburger JW, Takahashi M, Beiser AS, Burns JC, Bastian J, Chung KJ, et al. A single intravenous infusion of gamma globulin as compared with four infusions in the treatment of acute Kawasaki syndrome. N Engl J Med. 1991;324(23):1633–9.
45. Kanegaye JT, Wilder MS, Molkara D, Frazer JR, Pancheri J, Tremoulet AH, et al. Recognition of a Kawasaki disease shock syndrome. Pediatrics. 2009;123(5):e783–9.
46. Hoshino S, Tsuda E, Yamada O. Characteristics and Fate of Systemic Artery Aneurysm after Kawasaki Disease. J Pediatr. 2015;167(1):108–12.e1-2.
47. Guidelines for diagnosis and management of cardiovascular sequelae in Kawasaki disease (JCS 2008)–digest version. Circ J. 2010;74(9):1989–2020.
48. Oates-Whitehead RM, Baumer JH, Haines L, Love S, Maconochie IK, Gupta A, et al. Intravenous immunoglobulin for the treatment of Kawasaki disease in children. Cochrane Database Syst Rev. 2003;4:Cd004000.
49. Lee JH, Hung HY, Huang FY. Kawasaki disease with Reye syndrome: report of one case. Zhonghua Minguo xiao er ke yi xue hui za zhi [Journal] Zhonghua Minguo xiao er ke yi xue hui. 1992;33(1):67–71.
50. Takahashi M, Mason W. Kawasaki syndrome, Reye syndrome, and aspirin. Pediatrics. 1986;77(4):616–7.
51. Takahashi M MW, Thomas D, Sinatra F. Reye syndrome following Kawasaki syndrome confirmed by liver histopathology. Kawasaki Disease: Proceedings of the 5th International Kawasaki Disease Symposium; 1995 22–25 May 1995; Fukuoka, Japan. New York, NY: Elsevier; 1995.
52. Catella-Lawson F, Reilly MP, Kapoor SC, Cucchiara AJ, DeMarco S, Tournier B, et al. Cyclooxygenase inhibitors and the antiplatelet effects of aspirin. N Engl J Med. 2001;345(25):1809–17.
53. Dominguez SR, Friedman K, Seewald R, Anderson MS, Willis L, Glode MP. Kawasaki disease in a pediatric intensive care unit: a case-control study. Pediatrics. 2008;122(4):e786–90.
54. Chen S, Dong Y, Yin Y, Krucoff MW. Intravenous immunoglobulin plus corticosteroid to prevent coronary artery abnormalities in Kawasaki disease: a meta-analysis. Heart. 2013;99(2):76–82.
55. Weiss JE, Eberhard BA, Chowdhury D, Gottlieb BS. Infliximab as a novel therapy for refractory Kawasaki disease. J Rheumatol. 2004;31(4):808–10.
56. Burns JC, Best BM, Mejias A, Mahony L, Fixler DE, Jafri HS, et al. Infliximab treatment of intravenous immunoglobulin-resistant Kawasaki disease. J Pediatr. 2008;153(6):833–8.
57. Newburger JW, Sleeper LA, McCrindle BW, Minich LL, Gersony W, Vetter VL, et al. Randomized trial of pulsed corticosteroid therapy for primary treatment of Kawasaki disease. N Engl J Med. 2007;356(7):663–75.
58. Tremoulet AH, Best BM, Song S, Wang S, Corinaldesi E, Eichenfield JR, et al. Resistance to intravenous immunoglobulin in children with Kawasaki disease. J Pediatr. 2008;153(1):117–21.
59. Bar-Meir M, Kalisky I, Schwartz A, Somekh E, Tasher D. Prediction of Resistance to Intravenous Immunoglobulin in Children With Kawasaki Disease. Journal of the Pediatric Infectious Diseases Society. 2018;7(1):25–9.
60. Burns JC, Capparelli EV, Brown JA, Newburger JW, Glode MP. Intravenous gamma-globulin treatment and retreatment in Kawasaki disease. US/Canadian Kawasaki Syndrome Study Group. Pediatr Infect Dis J. 1998;17(12):1144–8.
61. Durongpisitkul K, Soongswang J, Laohaprasitiporn D, Nana A, Prachuabmoh C, Kangkagate C. Immunoglobulin failure and retreatment in Kawasaki disease. Pediatr Cardiol. 2003;24(2):145–8.
62. Uehara R, Belay ED, Maddox RA, Holman RC, Nakamura Y, Yashiro M, et al. Analysis of potential risk factors associated with nonresponse to initial intravenous immunoglobulin treatment among Kawasaki disease patients in Japan. Pediatr Infect Dis J. 2008;27(2):155–60.
63. Shafferman A, Birmingham JD, Cron RQ. High dose Anakinra for treatment of severe neonatal Kawasaki disease: a case report. Pediatr Rheumatol Online J. 2014;12:26.
64. Cohen S, Tacke CE, Straver B, Meijer N, Kuipers IM, Kuijpers TW. A child with severe relapsing Kawasaki disease rescued by IL-1 receptor blockade and extracorporeal membrane oxygenation. Ann Rheum Dis. 2012;71(12):2059–61.

65. Mehta SR, Yusuf S. The Clopidogrel in Unstable angina to prevent Recurrent Events (CURE) trial programme; rationale, design and baseline characteristics including a meta-analysis of the effects of thienopyridines in vascular disease. Eur Heart J. 2000;21(24):2033–41.
66. Albers GW, Amarenco P. Combination therapy with clopidogrel and aspirin: can the CURE results be extrapolated to cerebrovascula patients? Stroke. 2001;32(12):2948–9.
67. Gerschutz GP, Bhatt DL. The Clopidogrel in Unstable Angina to Prevent Recurrent Events (CURE) study: to what extent should the results be generalizable? Am Heart J. 2003;145(4):595–601.
68. Peters RJ, Mehta SR, Fox KA, Zhao F, Lewis BS, Kopecky SL, et al. Effects of aspirin dose when used alone or in combination with clopidogrel in patients with acute coronary syndromes: observations from the Clopidogrel in Unstable angina to prevent Recurrent Events (CURE) study. Circulation. 2003;108(14):1682–7.
69. Senzaki H. Long-term outcome of Kawasaki disease. Circulation. 2008;118(25):2763–72.
70. McCrindle BW. Kawasaki disease: a childhood disease with important consequences into adulthood. Circulation. 2009;120(1):6–8.
71. Manlhiot C, Niedra E, McCrindle BW. Long-term management of Kawasaki disease: implications for the adult patient. Pediatr Neonatol. 2013;54(1):12–21.
72. Holve TJ, Patel A, Chau Q, Marks AR, Meadows A, Zaroff JG. Long-term cardiovascular outcomes in survivors of Kawasaki disease. Pediatrics. 2014;133(2):e305–11.
73. Prsa M, Hussain T, McCrindle BW, Grosse-Wortmann L. Comprehensive evaluation of a patient with Kawasaki disease and giant coronary aneurysms with cardiac magnetic resonance. Congenit Heart Dis. 2014;9(6):E195–8.
74. Bratis K, Chiribiri A, Hussain T, Krasemann T, Henningsson M, Phinikaridou A, et al. Abnormal myocardial perfusion in Kawasaki disease convalescence. J Am Coll Cardiol Img. 2015;8(1):106–8.
75. Stone NJ, Robinson JG, Lichtenstein AH, Bairey Merz CN, Blum CB, Eckel RH, et al. ACC/AHA guideline on the treatment of blood cholesterol to reduce atherosclerotic cardiovascular risk in adults: a report of the American College of Cardiology/American Heart Association Task Force on Practice Guidelines. J Am Coll Cardiol. 2014;63(25 Pt B):2889–934.
76. Stone NJ, Robinson JG, Lichtenstein AH, Bairey Merz CN, Blum CB, Eckel RH, et al. 2013 ACC/AHA guideline on the treatment of blood cholesterol to reduce atherosclerotic cardiovascular risk in adults: a report of the American College of Cardiology/American Heart Association Task Force on Practice Guidelines. Circulation. 2014;129(25 Suppl 2):S1–45.
77. Kovacs AH, McCrindle BW. So hard to say goodbye: transition from paediatric to adult cardiology care. Nat Rev Cardiol. 2014;11(1):51–62.
78. Belhadjer Z, Meot M, Bajolle F, Khraiche D, Legendre A, Abakka S, et al. Acute heart failure in multisystem inflammatory syndrome in children (MIS-C) in the context of global SARS-CoV-2 pandemic. Circulation. 2020;
79. DeBiasi RL, Song X, Delaney M, Bell M, Smith K, Pershad J, et al. Severe COVID-19 in Children and Young Adults in the Washington. DC Metropolitan Region J Pediatr. 2020;
80. Jones VG, Mills M, Suarez D, Hogan CA, Yeh D, Bradley Segal J, et al. COVID-19 and Kawasaki Disease: novel Virus and Novel Case. Hosp Pediatr. 2020;
81. Riphagen S, Gomez X, Gonzalez-Martinez C, Wilkinson N, Theocharis P. Hyperinflammatory shock in children during COVID-19 pandemic. Lancet (London, England). 2020.
82. Liu W, Zhang Q, Chen J, Xiang R, Song H, Shu S, et al. Detection of Covid-19 in Children in Early January 2020 in Wuhan. China N Engl J Med. 2020;382(14):1370–1.
83. Mehta P, McAuley DF, Brown M, Sanchez E, Tattersall RS, Manson JJ, et al. COVID-19: consider cytokine storm syndromes and immunosuppression. Lancet (London, England). 2020;395(10229):1033–4.
84. Organization WH. Multisystem inflammatory syndrome in children and adolescents temporally related to COVID-19 2020 Available from: https://www.who.int/news-room/commentaries/detail/multisystem-inflammatory-syndrome-in-children-and-adolescents-with-covid-19.

Part IV

Infectious

COVID-19

13

Atula Gupta, Dedee F. Murrell, James Otton, and Mohamad Goldust

Introduction

The new corona virus (COVID-19) or severe acute respiratory syndrome coronavirus 2 (SARS–CoV-2) infection which initially appeared to present with predominantly respiratory symptoms has now been found to have a wide range of clinical features, from mild self-limiting disease to complications involving several organ systems including acute respiratory distress syndrome, cardiac failure, gastrointestinal disease, cutaneous, hepatic, renal and nervous system involvement. Pre-existing cardiovascular disease and related comorbidities are vital determinants of susceptibility, severity, and mortality in this condition. Various skin manifestations from maculopapular rashes, urticarial lesions, vesicular and vasculitic lesions have been identified in various studies. One of the most critical effects of COVID-19 are those on the cardiovascular system. Myocardial infection can arise from multiple mechanisms, perhaps related to the expression of ACE 2, the receptor for the spike protein of COVID-19, in the heart, although the exact mechanism leading to cardiac

A. Gupta
Department of Dermatology, Skin-Aid Clinic, Gurugram, Haryana, India

D. F. Murrell
Faculty of Medicine, Department of Dermatology, St George Hospital, University of New South Wales, Sydney, NSW, Australia
e-mail: d.murrell@unsw.edu.au

J. Otton
Department of Cardiology, Liverpool Hospital, University of New South Wales, Sydney, NSW, Australia

M. Goldust (✉)
University of Rome G. Marconi, Rome, Italy

Department of Dermatology, University Hospital Basel, Basel, Switzerland
e-mail: mohamad.goldust@usb.ch

C. Salavastru et al. (eds.), *Skin and the Heart*,
https://doi.org/10.1007/978-3-030-54779-0_13

failure is unclear. It is evident that COVID-19 may thus affect extrapulmonary systems such as the skin and heart separately or together in the form of a multiorgan disease.

COVID-19 in Children

COVID-19 infection in children has been found to have a much lower mortality than in adults [1, 2]. Previous data had shown that the pediatric age group had less than 2% of positive cases in population below age 20 years [3]. A study of 731 COVID-19 positive children, identified 90% to have asymptomatic or mild illness [2]. Common pediatric manifestations of COVID-19 include fever, malaise, cough, sore throat, and difficulty in breathing. Severe cases may present with gastrointestinal symptoms, respiratory distress, coagulation disturbances and shock. Contrary to several preliminary studies from different countries which had suggested that critical disease and mortality due to COVID-19 among children is rare [4] whether it be reduced vulnerability to infection among children [5] or similar susceptibility but higher number of cases with asymptomatic disease, [6] recent emerging data has revealed the occurrence of a Kawasaki-like disease in the pediatric age group affected by this illness [7].

The relationship of Kawasaki disease (KD) to COVID-19 may be due to the SARS-C0V-2 infection triggering an inflammatory syndrome in some children. In one study, a 6-month-old infant tested positive for COVID-19, had features of classic KD and improved after treatment with intravenous immunoglobulin (IVIG) [8]. Cases of KD were also identified in Bergamo province in Italy [7]. This preliminary data has hinted towards a plausible association between COVID-19 and KD. Vasculitic lesions initiated by post viral immunological reactions have also been seen in COVID-19 confirmed cases in adults [9, 10].

Kawasaki Disease

Kawasaki disease (KD) is a severe vasculitic inflammation of the blood vessel walls occurring in children commonly under 5 years of age [11]. It is a self-limiting, acute inflammation of the medium and small sized vessels which in severe form manifest with symptoms such as persistent fever, lymphadenopathy, conjunctival injection, cutaneous lesions, mucosal lesions and coronary artery aneurysm as the major cardiac complication [12, 13]. KD is a diagnosis made on the basis of a defined laboratory and clinical criteria. In Japan, the incidence of children under 4 years of age affected with KD is 300 per 100,000 children versus 25 per 100,000 children less than 5 years of age in North America [14]. KD also known as "mucocutaneous lymph node syndrome" is named after Dr. Tomisacu Kawasaki who first established a correlation between a childhood disease with multiorgan involvement with an outbreak of coronavirus rhinitis. A study conducted in 2005 by Esper et al. further confirmed that coronavirus positive nasal swabs were identified in 8 out of 11 children diagnosed with KD [15].

Table 13.1 Diagnostic criteria of kawasaki disease

Classic KD	
Lymphadenopathy	Unilateral cervical lymphadenopathy >1.5 cm
Mucosal changes	Mucosal or oropharyngeal erythema Strawberry tongue seen as glossitis with hyperplastic papillae Fissured erythematous lips
Extremity changes	Acute phase: Induration and erythema of feet and hands Subacute phase: Periungual desquamation
Cutaneous changes	Maculopapular rash
Conjunctiva	Non exudative painless bilateral conjunctival injection
Incomplete or atypical KD	Fever for ≥5 days plus 2 or 3 below mentioned criteria: Elevated C-reactive protein (CRP) or erythrocyte sedimentation rate (ESR) values or both, thrombocytosis, hypoalbuminaemia, leucocytosis, sterile pyuria, echocardiogram showing coronary aneurysms or cardiac dysfunction (left ventricular function depression, mitral valve regurgitation, or pericardial effusion) [16].

KD is a clinical diagnosis based on the following criteria [16]:

Diagnostic criteria—Four of the five mentioned in Table 13.1 plus fever of more than 5 days duration.

If only aneurysms of the coronary arteries are found without the other features of a classic KD, this may be termed as incomplete or atypical KD [17].

Etiology of Kawasaki Disease

Several respiratory viruses have previously been associated with KD [18]. While various studies have identified a correlation between seasonal coronavirus and KD [19], few studies have disputed a link between respiratory viruses and KD [20]. Winter and spring are common months for epidemics of KD [21]. Infections with human coronaviruses HCOV-229E and HCoV- 0C43 are known to occur in spring and winter. It is known that an abnormal response to an infectious agent triggers a clonal expansion of CD8 + T cells in the host leading to the vasculitic features of KD thereby confirming the that certain hosts may be more predisposed than others [21]. (Fig. 13.1).

Cardiac Complications of COVID-19 Related Kawasaki Disease

COVID-19 associated KD has similar cardiovascular manifestations as those described in classic KD [22]. Coronary artery aneurysm (CAA) is one of the major complications of KD [23]. Kawasaki disease shock syndrome (KDSS) is a rare but critical presentation which may arise due to an associated myocarditis during the illness [24, 25]. KDSS is characterized by KD associated with a reduction in basal systolic blood pressure of at least 20%, or evident signs of decreased peripheral blood flow [24]. The initial phase of KD is characterized by mild myocarditis identified in cardiac biopsies [26] and it improves mostly as inflammation subsides [26].

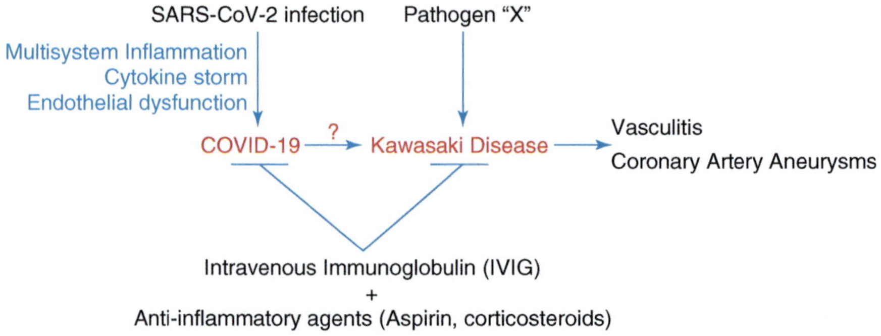

Fig. 13.1 Relationship between COVID-19 and Kawasaki disease

KDSS has an incidence of 1.5 to 7% of KD patients with reduced percentage in Asia than in western countries [27].The pathogenesis of KDSS involves a combination of myocardial dysfunction along with reduced peripheral vascular resistance. Treatment involves IV fluids with administration of inotropic and vasoactive agents. Shock seen in KD may result due to a raised level of pro-inflammatory cytokines such as CRP and IL-6 in circulation [28]. Long lasting diastolic dysfunction is the most recognized feature and left ventricular systolic dysfunction is encountered in only a third of the patients [29].Multisystem inflammatory syndrome in children (MIS-C) is a newly described term for a syndrome linked to possible previous exposure to SARS-CoV-2. MIS-C has myocardial involvement just like atypical KD but cardiac failure in MIS-C is a result of myocardial edema rather than inflammatory myocardial changes. MIS-C also presents with cardiogenic shock in which left ventricular systolic dysfunction and low systolic blood pressure is identified in all patients [28]. MIS-C can also present with fever, skin rash, diarrhea, and lymphadenopathy, similar to KD. It is questionable whether MIS-C is a separate entity or SARS-CoV-2 induced KD. Coronary artery aneurysms may also lead to clot formation in some children with COVID-19 [30]. The pathogenesis of CAA is related to an endothelial dysfunction caused by an increased accumulation of endothelial inflammatory cells and ACE2 after SARS-CoV-2 infection [31]. Up to 25% children with KD may develop CAA.

Treatment

Intravenous immune globulin (IVIG) is an adjunctive therapy in KD. IVIG exerts an anti-inflammatory action on monocytes and macrophages. IVIG administration should be done within 7 days of KD onset until the patient recovers from symptoms and tests negative for COVID-19. Early diagnosis of SARS-CoV-2 associated KD or MIS-CIS is essential in preventing left ventricular dysfunction and acute heart failure in children. A rapid NT Pro B type Natriuretic Peptide (BNP) should be performed for urgent evaluation of children manifesting with symptoms of COVID-19 associated KD. Treating the cytokine storm by targeting the IL-6 receptor is another potential management approach [27].

Myocarditis, and Myocardial Injury

Myocarditis, ranging from mild to life-threatening, has frequently been reported in association with COVID-19. ECG characteristics may simulate ST elevation myocardial infarction, and imaging may show reduced ventricular function, and classic T2 hyper-intensity and late gadolinium enhancement on cardiac MRI.

The cause of this phenomenon is unclear. Although myocytes contain ACE2 receptors, it appears likely that myocarditis manifests from secondary immune effects, the so-called 'cytokine storm' and possibly hypoxia related to microvascular damage and thrombosis [32]. The presence of myocarditis and elevated troponin levels is associated with greatly increased COVID-19 mortality [33].

Myocardial Infarction, Pulmonary Embolism and Right Heart Failure

Myocardial infarction has been frequently reported in association with COVID-19. It is thought that direct vascular injury and pro-thrombotic state may increase the susceptibility towards myocardial infarction, particularly in those with substantial risk factors and pre-existing coronary disease [29] Likewise, type-2 myocardial infarction related to cytokine storm, increased cardiac output or afterload changes may occur in COVID-19. Pulmonary embolism or thrombosis and associated right heart strain is significantly associated with late mortality [34] Typical right ventricular strain on ECG, right ventricular dilatation on echocardiography and troponin elevation may occur after pulmonary embolism.

Cutaneous Vascular Changes Seen in COVID-19

Recent data has revealed ischemic changes like blisters, cyanosis, and asymmetric chilblain like lesions in fingers and toes of patients diagnosed with COVID-19 [35]. An inflammatory thrombogenic vasculopathy with disseminated intravascular coagulation [36], targetoid lesions [36], livedo like signs with necrotic areas have all been reported. [9]

Drug associated Cardiac and Cutaneous Adverse Effects Used in Management of COVID-19

Chloroquine (CQ) and hydroxychloroquine (HCQ) are drugs that were initially trialled for the treatment of COVID-19. A rare but serious cutaneous adverse effect of both CQ and HCQ is toxic epidermal necrolysis (TEN) [37]. Cardiac complications including QT interval prolongation manifesting as ventricular fibrillations have been well described in various studies [38–40]. Proximal myopathy associated with respiratory failure are other complications of CQ or HCQ [39–43]. Both CQ and HCQ have also been shown to cause biventricular dilated or restrictive cardiomyopathy. [44–46]

Conclusion

Heart diseases may be a vital determinant of susceptibility, severity, and mortality in COVID-19. Emerging studies from different countries have suggested an association between SARS-COV2 infection and KD. Establishing an exact pathomechanism in the causation of COVID-19 associated KD requires sero epidemiological and histopathological investigations. Understanding the immune mechanisms and genetic susceptibility of this disease will enable prevention of the severe and fatal manifestations of this condition.

References

1. Castagnoli R, Votto M, Licari A, et al. Severe acute respiratory syndrome coronavirus 2 (SARS-CoV-2) infection in children and adolescents: a systematic review. JAMA Pediatr. 2020; https://doi.org/10.1001/jamapediatrics.2020.1467.
2. Dong Y, Mo X, Hu Y, et al. Epidemiology of COVID-19 among children in China. Pediatrics. 2020;145:e20200702.
3. Wu Z, McGoogan JM. Characteristics of and important lessons from the coronavirus disease 2019 (COVID-19) outbreak in China: summary of a report of 72314 cases from the Chinese Center for Disease Control and Prevention. JAMA. 2020;323:1239.
4. Docherty AB, Harrison EM, Green CA, et al. Features of 16,749 hospitalised UK patients with COVID-19 using the ISARIC WHO Clinical Characterisation Protocol. medRxiv. 2020; Published online April 28; https://doi.org/10.1101/2020.04.23.20076042.
5. Zhang J, Litvinova M, Liang Y, et al. Changes in contact patterns shape the dynamics of the COVID-19 outbreak in China. Science. 2020;368(6498):1481–6. Published online April 29
6. Bi Q, Wu Y, Mei S, et al. Epidemiology and transmission of COVID-19 in 391 cases and 1286 of their close contacts in Shenzhen, China: a retrospective cohort study. Lancet Infect Dis. 2020; https://doi.org/10.1101/2020.03.03.20028423. Published online April 27
7. Verdoni L, Mazza A, Gervasoni A, et al. An outbreak of severe Kawasakilike disease at the Italian epicentre of the SARS-CoV-2 epidemic: an observational cohort study. Lancet. 2020;395:10239. Published online May 13
8. Jones VG, Mills M, Suarez D, et al. COVID-19 and Kawasaki disease: novel virus and novel case. Hosp Pediatr. 2020;10:537–40. https://doi.org/10.1542/hpeds.2020-0123.
9. Galvan Casas C, Catala A, Carretero Hernandez G, et al. Classification of the cutaneous manifestations of COVID-19: a rapid prospective nationwide consensus study in Spain with 375 cases. Br J Dermatol. 2020;183:71–7.
10. Bouaziz JD, Duong T, Jachiet M, et al. Vascular skin symptoms in COVID-19: a French observational study. J Eur Acad Dermatol Venereol. 2020; https://doi.org/10.1111/jdv.16544.
11. McCrindle BW, Rowley AH, Newburger JW, et al. Treatment, and long-term Management of Kawasaki Disease: a scientific statement for health professionals from the American Heart Association. Circulation. 2017;135(17):e927–99.
12. Dietz SM, van Stijn D, Burgner D, et al. Dissecting Kawasaki disease: a state-of-the-art review. Eur J Pediatr 2017; 176: 995–1009. 9 McCrindle BW, Rowley AH, Newburger JW, et al. Diagnosis, treatment, and long-term management of Kawasaki disease: a scientific statement for health professionals from the American Heart Association. Circulation. 2017;135:e927–99.
13. Kawasaki T, Kosaki F, Okawa S, et al. A new infantile acute febrile mucocutaneous lymph node syndrome (MLNS) prevailing in Japan. Pediatrics. 1974;54:271–6.
14. Makino N, Nakamura Y, Yashiro M, et al. Nationwide epidemiologic survey of Kawasaki disease in Japan, 2015-2016. Pediatr Int. 2019;61(4):397–403.
15. Esper F, Shapiro ED, Weibel C, et al. Association between a novel human coronavirus and Kawasaki disease. J Infect Dis. 2005;191:499–502. https://doi.org/10.1086/428291.

16. American Academy of Pediatrics. 2000 Red book: report of the Committee on Infectious Diseases. 25th ed. Elk Grove Village, IL: American Academy of Pediatrics; 2000.
17. Rosenfeld EA, Corydon KE, Shulman ST. Kawasaki disease in infants less than one year of age. J Pediatr. 1995;126:524–9.
18. Turnier JL, Anderson MS, Heizer HR, et al. Concurrent respiratory viruses and Kawasaki disease. Pediatrics. 2015;136(3):e609–14.
19. Chang LY, Lu CY, Shao PL, et al. Viral infections associated with Kawasaki disease. J Formos Med Assoc. 2014;113(3):148–54.
20. Lehmann C, Klar R, Lindner J, et al. Kawasaki disease lacks association with human coronavirus NL63 and human bocavirus. Pediatr Infect Dis J. 2009;28(6):553–4.
21. Yanagawa H, Nakamura Y, Kawasaki T, Shigematsu I. Nationwide epidemic of Kawasaki disease in Japan during winter of 1985–86. Lancet. 1986;2:1138–9.
22. Dadlani GH, Gingell RL, Orie JD. Coronary artery calcifications in the long-term follow-up of Kawasaki disease. Am Heart J. 2005;150:1016.
23. Harada M, Yokouchi Y, Oharaseki T, et al. Histopathological characteristics of myocarditis in acute-phase Kawasaki disease. Histopathology. 2012;61(6):1156–67.
24. Kanegaye JT, Wilder MS, Molkara D, et al. Recognition of a Kawasaki disease shock syndrome. Pediatrics. 2009;123(5):e783–9.
25. Li Y, Zheng Q, Zou L, et al. Kawasaki disease shock syndrome: clinical characteristics and possible use of IL-6, IL-10 and IFN-gamma as biomarkers for early recognition. Pediatr Rheumatol Online J. 2019;17(1):1.
26. Yutani C, Go S, Kamiya T, et al. Cardiac biopsy of Kawasaki disease. Arch Pathol Lab Med. 1981;105(9):470–3.
27. Harahsheh AS, Dahdah N, Newburger JW, et al. Missed or delayed diagnosis of Kawasaki disease during the 2019 novel coronavirus disease (COVID-19) pandemic. J Pediatr. 2020;222:261–2. https://doi.org/10.1016/j.jpeds.2020.04.052.
28. Riphagen S, Gomez X, Gonzalez-Martinez C, Wilkinson N, Theocharis P. Hyperinflammatory shock in children during COVID-19 pandemic. Lancet. 2020 May 7;395(10237):1607–8.
29. Richardson S, Hirsch JS, Narasimhan M, et al. Presenting characteristics, comorbidities, and outcomes among 5700 patients hospitalized with COVID-19 in the New York City area. JAMA. 2020;323(20):2052–9. https://doi.org/10.1001/jama.2020.6775.
30. Gale J. Coronavirus causes damaging blood clots from brain to toes. Bloomberg News. 2020 https://www.bloomberg.com/news/articles/2020-05-04/coronavirus-causes-blood-clots-harming-organs-from-brain-to-toes [Internet], May 4. [Google Scholar].
31. Varga Z, Flammer AJ, Steiger P, et al. Endothelial cell infection and endotheliitis in COVID-19. Lancet. 2020;395(10234):1417–8.
32. Cappannoli L, Scacciavillani R, Iannaccone G, Anastasia G, Di Giusto F, Loria V, Aspromonte N. Novel-coronavirus: cardiovascular insights about risk factors, myocardial injury, therapy and clinical implications. Chron Dis Trans Med. 2019; https://doi.org/10.1016/j.cdtm.2020.06.002.
33. Vrsalovic M, Vrsalovic PA. Cardiac troponins predict mortality in patients with COVID-19: A meta-analysis of adjusted risk estimates. J Inf Secur. 2020 May 19; https://doi.org/10.1016/j.jinf.2020.05.022. Epub ahead of print. PMID: 32416124; PMCID: PMC7234948
34. Argulian E, Sud K, Vogel B, Bohra C, Garg VP, Talebi S, Lerakis S, Narula J. Right ventricular dilation in hospitalized patients with COVID-19 Infection. JACC Cardiovasc Imaging. 2020 May 15; https://doi.org/10.1016/j.jcmg.2020.05.010. Epub ahead of print. PMID: 32426088; PMCID: PMC7228729
35. Alramthan A, Aldaraji W. A case of COVID-19 presenting in clinical picture resembling chilblains disease. First report from the Middle East. Clin Exp Dermatol. 2020;45:746–8. https://doi.org/10.1111/ced.14243.
36. Magro C, Mulvey JJ, Berlin D, et al. Complement associated microvascular injury and thrombosis in the pathogenesis of severe COVID-19 infection: a report of five cases. Transl Res. 2020; https://doi.org/10.1016/j.trsl.2020.04.007. [Epub ahead of print]
37. Murphy M, Carmichael AJ. Fatal toxic epidermal necrolysis associated with hydroxychloroquine. Clin Exp Dermatol. 2001;26:457–8. https://doi.org/10.1046/j.1365-2230.2001.00857-3.x.

38. Chen CY, Wang FL, Lin CC. Chronic hydroxychloroquine use associated with QT prolongation and refractory ventricular arrhythmia. Clin Toxicol (Phila). 2006;44:173–5. https://doi.org/10.1080/15563650500514558.
39. Stas P, Faes D, Noyens P. Conduction disorder and QT prolongation secondary to long-term treatment with chloroquine. Int J Cardiol. 2008;127:e80–2. https://doi.org/10.1016/j.ijcard.2007.04.055.
40. Chorin E, Dai M, Shulman E, et al. The QT interval in patients with SARS-CoV-2 infection treated with hydroxychloroquine/azithromycin. medRxiv. 2020; https://doi.org/10.1101/2020.04.02.20047050.
41. Siddiqui AK, Huberfeld SI, Weidenheim KM, et al. Hydroxychloroquine-induced toxic myopathy causing respiratory failure. Chest. 2007;131:588–90. https://doi.org/10.1378/chest.06-1146.
42. Kwon JB, Kleiner A, Ishida K, et al. Hydroxychloroquine-induced myopathy. J Clin Rheumatol. 2010;16:28–31. https://doi.org/10.1097/RHU.0b013e3181c47ec8.
43. Abdel-Hamid H, Oddis CV, Lacomis D. Severe hydroxychloroquine myopathy. Muscle Nerve. 2008;38:1206–10. https://doi.org/10.1002/mus.21091.
44. Soong TR, Barouch LA, Champion HC, et al. New clinical and ultrastructural findings in hydroxychloroquine-induced cardiomyopathy—a report of 2 cases. Hum Pathol. 2007;38:1858–63. https://doi.org/10.1016/j.humpath.2007.06.013.
45. Cotroneo J, Sleik KM, Rodriguez ER, Klein AL. Hydroxychloroquine-induced restrictive cardiomyopathy: correlation between clinical, echocardiographic and pathologic findings. Eur J Echocardiogr. 2007;8:247–51. https://doi.org/10.1016/j.euje.2006.02.002.
46. Muthukrishnan P, Roukoz H, Grafton G, et al. Hydroxychloroquine-induced cardiomyopathy: a case report. Circ Heart Fail. 2011;4:e7–8. https://doi.org/10.1161/circheartfailure.110.959916.

Lyme Disease

14

Jana Třešňák Hercogová and Eliza Cinteza

Lyme borreliosis is a common, systemic anthropozoonosis, caused by *Borrelia burgdorferi* sensu lato complex and transmitted by *Ixodes ricinus* ticks. Skin manifestations include erythema migrans (EM) (Fig. 14.1), borrelial lymphocytoma (BL) (Fig. 14.2) and acrodermatitis chronica atrophicans (ACA) (Fig. 14.3). Systemic manifestations could be neurological, cardiovascular, rheumatic, ophthalmologic etc. Annular EM and BL on the ear lobe in a child are pathognomic for Lyme borreliosis.

History

The first description of ACA was made by Buchvald under the name "idiopatic skin atrophy" in 1883. The first EM case was published by Arvid Afzelius in 1909. BL was named "lymphadenosis benigna cutis" by Bäferstedt in 1944. In the nineteen-seventies, Alan Steere described a new nosological disease transmitted by ticks. Direct proof of Borreliae in the blood was made by Benach in 1983. Four years later, the new nosological entity has been settled under the name Lyme disease. Eva Asbrink isolated Borrealiae for the first time from skin lesions of EM in 1985 [1–3].

J. Třešňák Hercogová (✉)
Department of Dermatovenereology, 2nd Medical Faculty, Charles University Prague and Na Bulovce Hospital, Prague, Czech Republic

Department of Dermatovenereology, Institute for Clinical and Experimental Medicine, Prague, Czech Republic

Department of Dermatovenereology, Prague, Czech Republic

E. Cinteza
Cardiology Department "Marie Curie" Emergency Children's Hospital, Pediatrics Department "Carol Davila" University of Medicine and Pharmacy, Bucharest, Romania

C. Salavastru et al. (eds.), *Skin and the Heart*,
https://doi.org/10.1007/978-3-030-54779-0_14

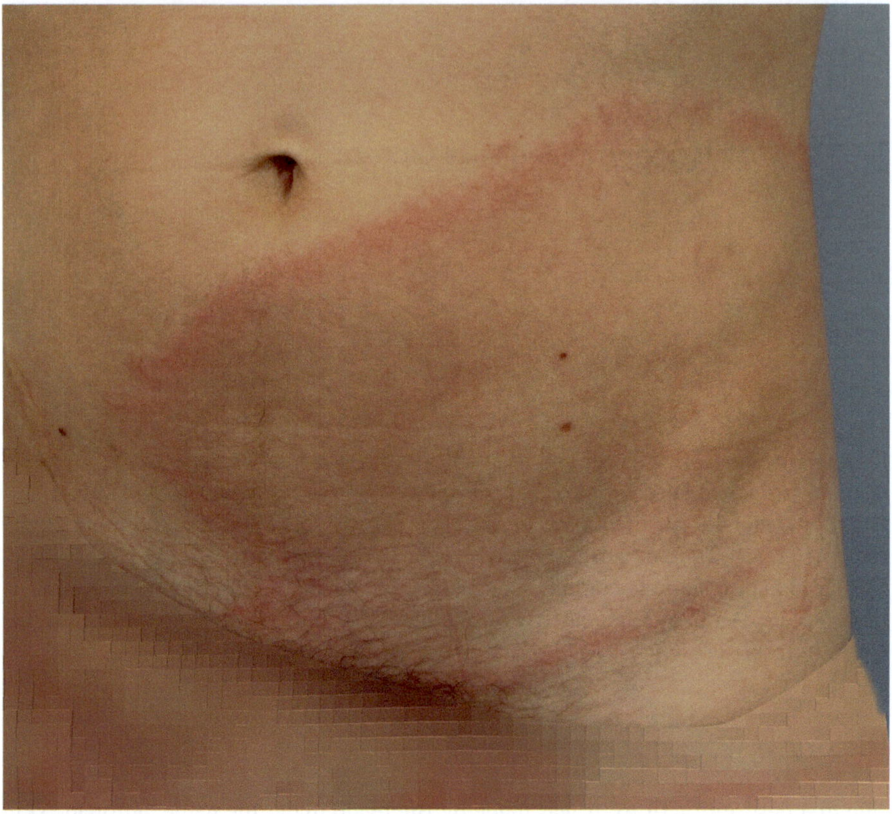

Fig. 14.1 Erythema migrans annulare

Epidemiology

The animal reservoirs of Borreliae include mammals, rodents, birds, and domestic animals. Vectors in Europe are ticks (*Ixodes ricinus, I. ricinus*), and in other continents *I. scapularis, I. pacificus, I. angustus* (North America), *I. persulatus* (Euroasia) *etc.* Infection is transmitted to humans after a long period of tick adherence to the skin surface (approx. 48 h). The infection is asymptomatic in most people who are exposed to infected ticks. The disease is manifest in only about 5% people, in whom either increased levels of antiborrelial antibodies are found (in 3%) or Lyme borreliosis develops (2%).

The incubation period is typically 7–14 days, but it could vary between 2–32 days after the tick bite.

Lyme borreliosis is spread worldwide, and is reported most frequently in Sweden, Austria and Germany (69–111 cases per 100,000 inhabitants in 2016). The disease affects both sexes, ACA is predominant in women. EM appears at any age. BL is typical for children and ACA in elderly. Most skin manifestations of Lyme borreliosis are represented by EM (85%), ACA is present in about 10% and BL in 5% patients [4, 5].

Etiopathogenesis

Borrelia burgdorferi (B. burgdorferi) sensu lato complex is divided into approx. 20 subspecies, but only five subspecies can cause the human disease: *B. afzelii, B. garinii, B. bavariensis, B. burgdorferi* sensu stricto and *B. spielmani*. Borreliae are organotropic. The etiological agents of EM are all five subspecies, ACA is caused by *B. afzelii, B. garinii* and *B. bavariensis* are connected to neuroborreliosis, *B. burgdorferi* sensu stricto is responsible for Lyme arthritis.

Borreliae are spirochetes of the class *Leptospiracae*. They have irregular coils and flagellae under the cell membrane. Borreliae are able to adhere to fibrocyte and Langerhans cell receptors, invade into the cells by a special phagocytosis mechanism, to persist in the cells in forms of cysts. They are also able to digest collagen, fibronectin and laminin, and thus to spread in the skin.

Borrelia superficial antigens, outer surface proteins (OSP) are recognized by the immune system, complement, macrophages, dendritic cells are activated and inflammatory cytokines are induced. Specific immune response (T-helper and B- lymphocytes) and antiborrelial antibodies are produced later. There is no production of neutralizing antibodies after the infection and reinfections may occur.

Some subtypes of Borreliae are considered to be invasive, (i.e. 24 Osp C), the other cause disseminated infections (A, B, I, K typy OspC) and/or some other types are not invading the nervous tissue (OspA 4,7) [5, 6].

Clinical Picture

Skin Manifestations

The illness starts as localized EM (Fig. 14.1) which could be unnoticed by the patient. Hematogenous spreading is characterized by flu-like symptoms, multiple EM or could be asymptomatic. The involvement of systemic organs follows, mainly affecting joints and nerves. The course of the disease could be divided into stages, but to distinguish the early and late infection is more practical. 7–14 days after the tick bite clinical signs and symptoms develop. Skin is affected in 80–90% patients, other organs in 10–20% [2, 6] (Table 14.1).

- Annular erythema migrans (Fig. 14.4)
- Borrelial lymphocytoma on the ear lobe in a child (Fig. 14.2)

Table 14.1 Lyme borreliosis course

Lyme borreliosis stage	Skin symptoms	Systemic involvement
Early localized infection	Erythema migrans Erythema migrans	
Early disseminated infection	Erythemata migrantia Multiple borrelial lymphocytoma	Flu-like symptoms
		Neuroborreliosis • Lymphocytic meningitis • Meningoradiculitis • Cranial neuritis • Myelitis
		Ophthalmological symptoms • Conjunctivitis, photophobia • Iridocyclitis, uveitis, virtitis, diplegia, choroiditis, macular oedema, disc oedema, optic neuritis (very rarely)) and neuroretinitis
		Myositis
		Cardiac symptoms • Acute carditis • AV bloc • Dilate cardiomyopathy
		Acute intermittent monoarthritis
Late infection	Acrodermatitis chronica atrophicans	Periferal neuropathy associated with ACA
		Chronic artritis
		Chronic encephalomyelitis
		Cerebral vasculitis
		Keratitis, episcleritis, orbital myositis

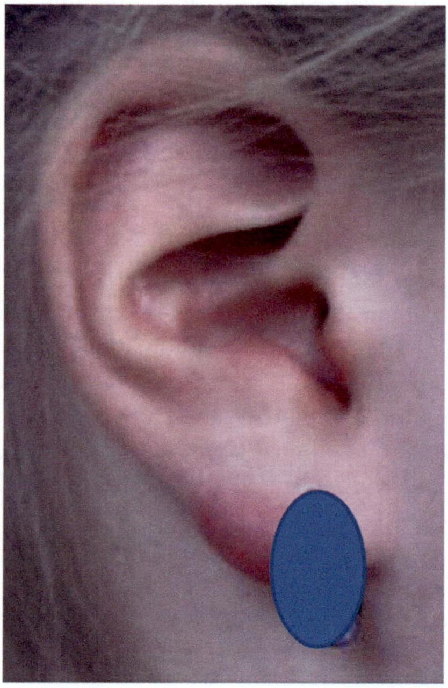

Fig. 14.2 Borrelial lymphocytoma on the ear lobe in a child

Fig. 14.3 Acrodermatitis chronica atrophicans inflammatoria (dorsum of the hand)

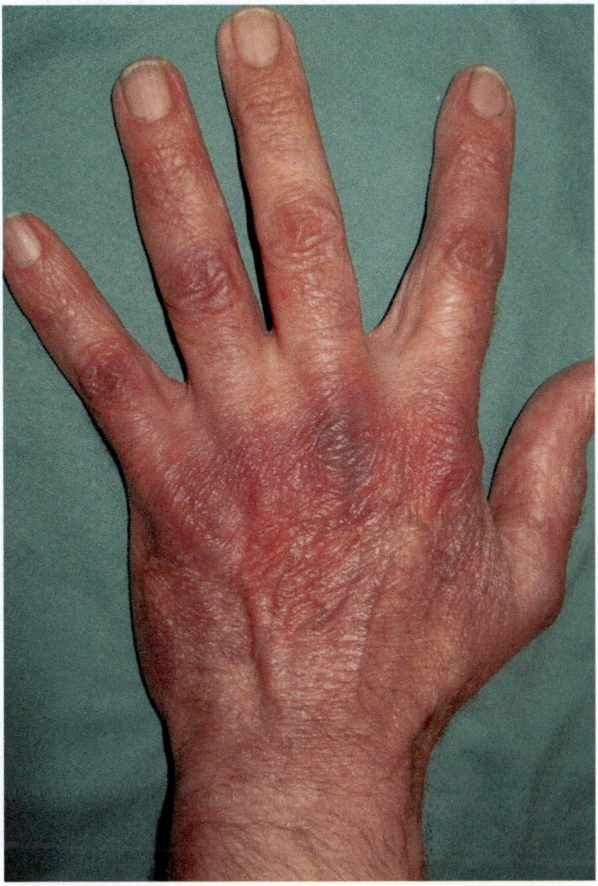

Ist Stage: Early Localized Infection

Erythema Migrans

EM (Figs. 14.1 and 14.4) is a red, smooth macule with a regular shape, more than 5 cm in diameter at the site of insect bite. The asymptomatic period between the tick bite and EM is obviously 7–14 days. EM is localized mainly on the thin skin—beneath the knee, on the lower extremities in adults and on the upper part of the trunk and on the face in children.

EM is asymptomatic or could be slightly pruritic, it is warmer by palpation.

EM could be classified in three subtypes and some more less frequent variants (Table 14.2) [5, 6].

EM is obviously a solitary, it could be also multiple at more body sites after multiple tick bites.

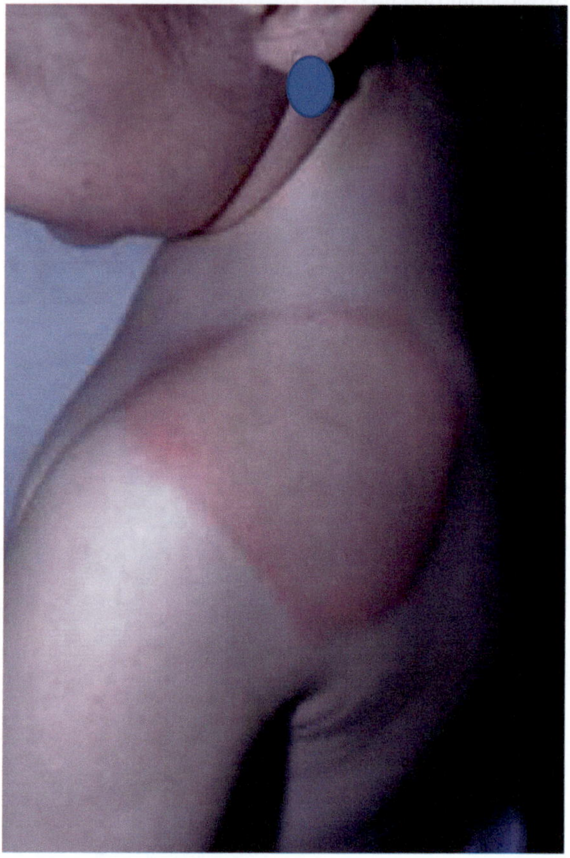

Fig. 14.4 Annular erythema migrans

Table 14.2 Erythema migrans subtypes—variants (Figs. 14.5, 14.6, 14.7, 14.8, 14.9, 14.10, 14.11, 14.12 and 14.13)

Clinical subtype	Characteristics	Example
EM anulare (Figs. 14.1, 14.4, and 14.5)	Macule with the central clearing	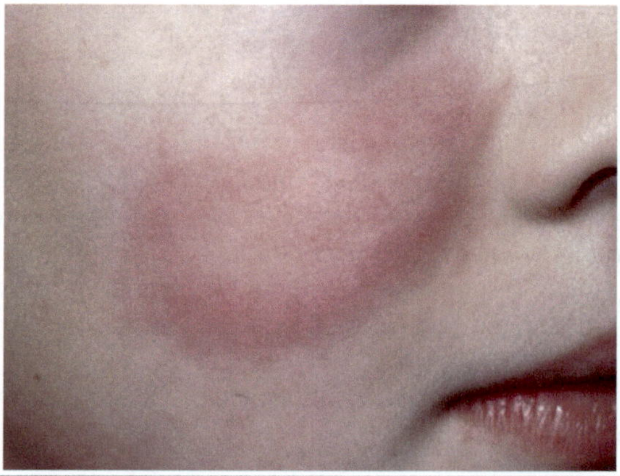

Clinical subtype	Characteristics	Example
EM maculosum (Fig. 14.6)	Homogenous macule	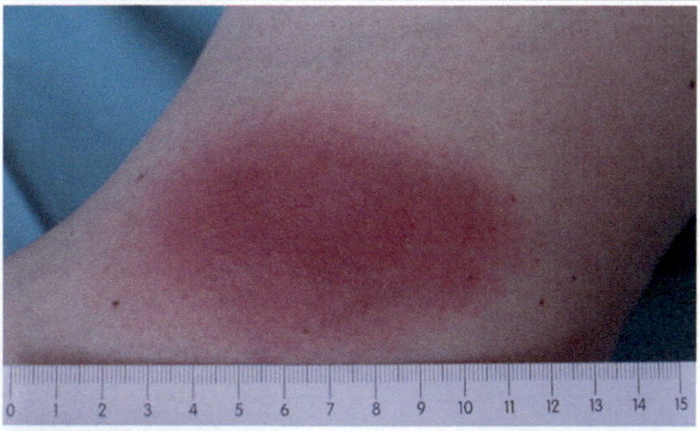
EM concentricum (Fig. 14.7)	Target-like/ iris-like macule	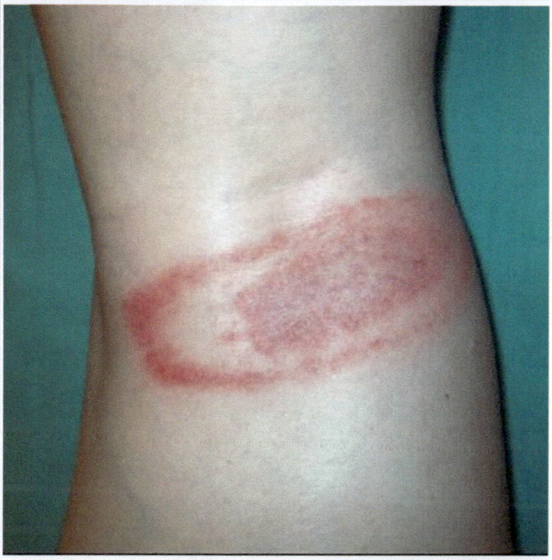
EM infiltrativum (Fig. 14.8)	Plaque	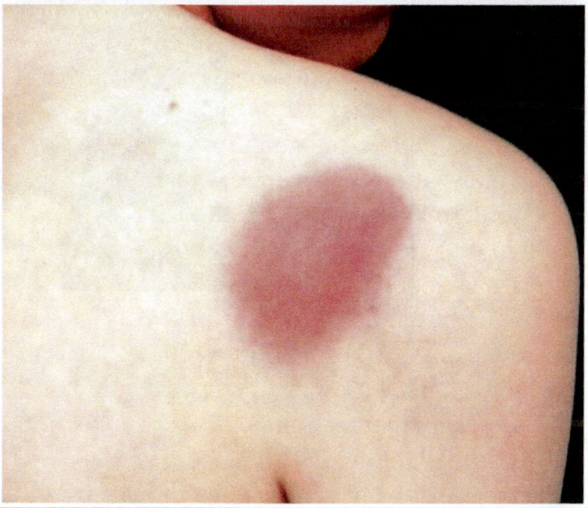

(continued)

Table 14.2 (continued)

Clinical subtype	Characteristics	Example
EM lividum (Fig. 14.9)	Macule with dark red—livid centre	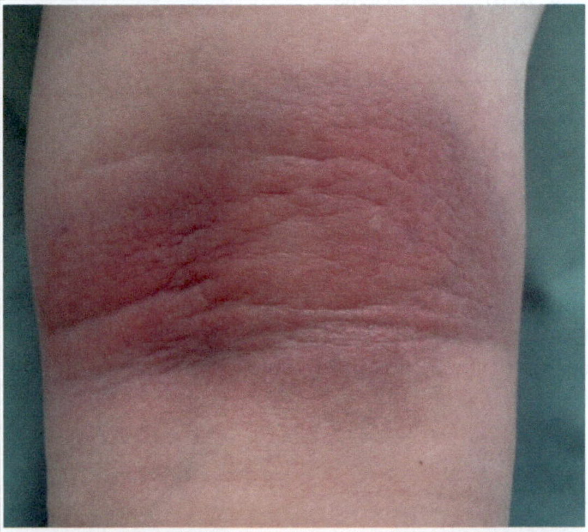
EM vesiculosum (Fig. 14.10)	Macule with vesicules in the center	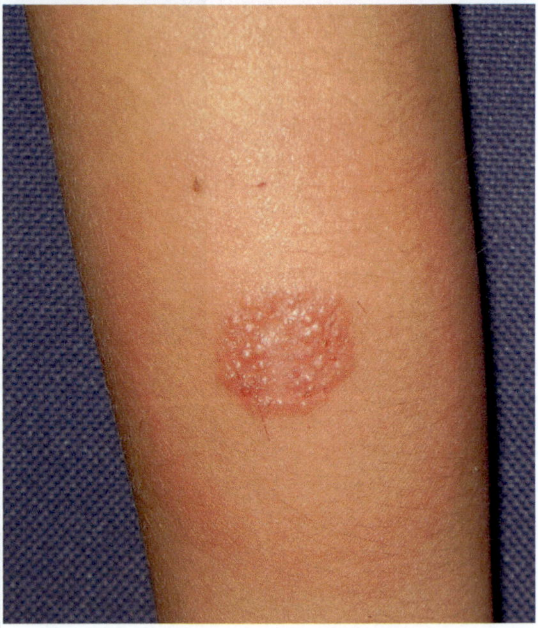

Table 14.2 (continued)

Clinical subtype	Characteristics	Example
EM haemorrhagicum (Fig. 14.11)	Macule with haemorrhagic center	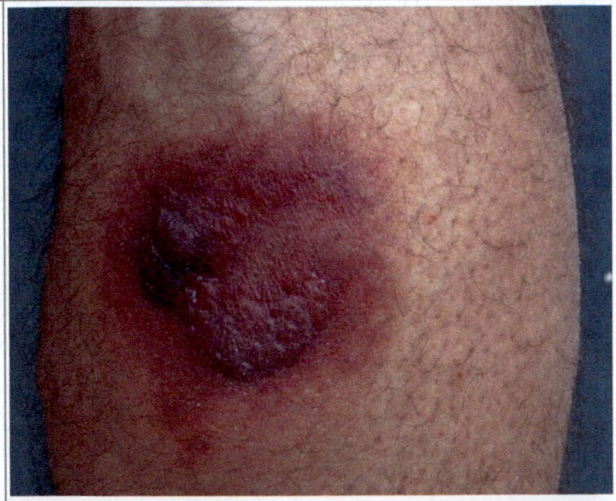
EM irregulare (Fig. 14.12)	Macule with irregular shape	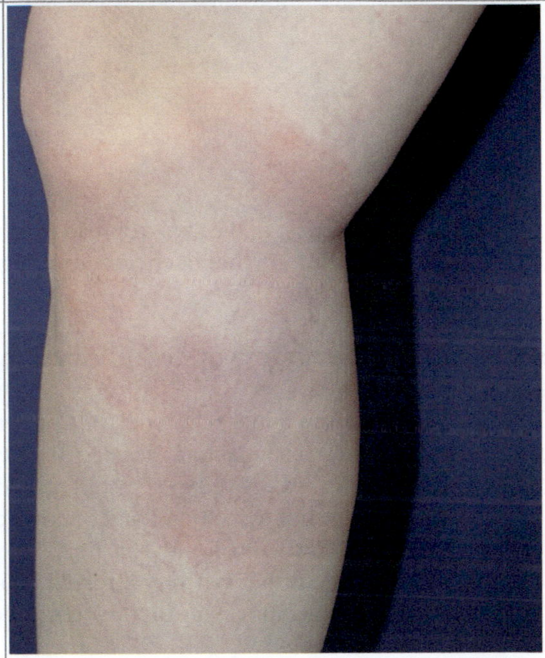

(continued)

Table 14.2 (continued)

Clinical subtype	Characteristics	Example
EM invisibile (Fig. 14.13)	Discrete macule which could be seen after warming	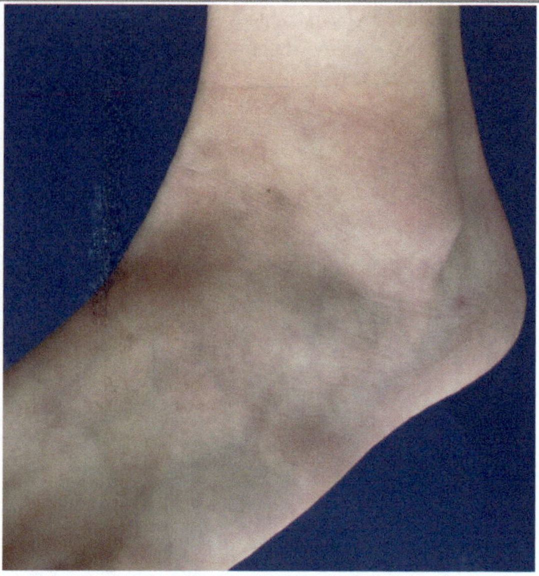

Borreliae could persist in the skin a spread to other organs. If the EM lasts more than 4 weeks it is called **erythema chronicum migrans** (Fig. 14.14).

Borrelial Lymphocytoma or Lymphocytoma Borreliensis

BL (Fig. 14.2) develops at the site of tick bite, as well as EM—which could be still present on the skin as accompanying lesion. BL is typical for children.

BL papulosa (Fig. 14.15a, b, c) is a solitary red papule, roundish, glossy, with the diameter of 1 cm. If it lasts for a longer period of time, it is presented as a dark red plaque (**BL infiltrativa**) (Fig. 14.16a, b).

BL could be also multiple, but very rarely, it could also accompany ACA.

Characteristic localizations of BL are ear lobes, mammilla region, scrotum and nose.

Early Disseminated Infection

Disseminated stage of the disease is the sequelae of Borreliae haematogenic spread. Systemic symptoms could be presented together with skin involvement or separately. The most frequent are flu-like symptoms–fever, arthralgias, myalgias,

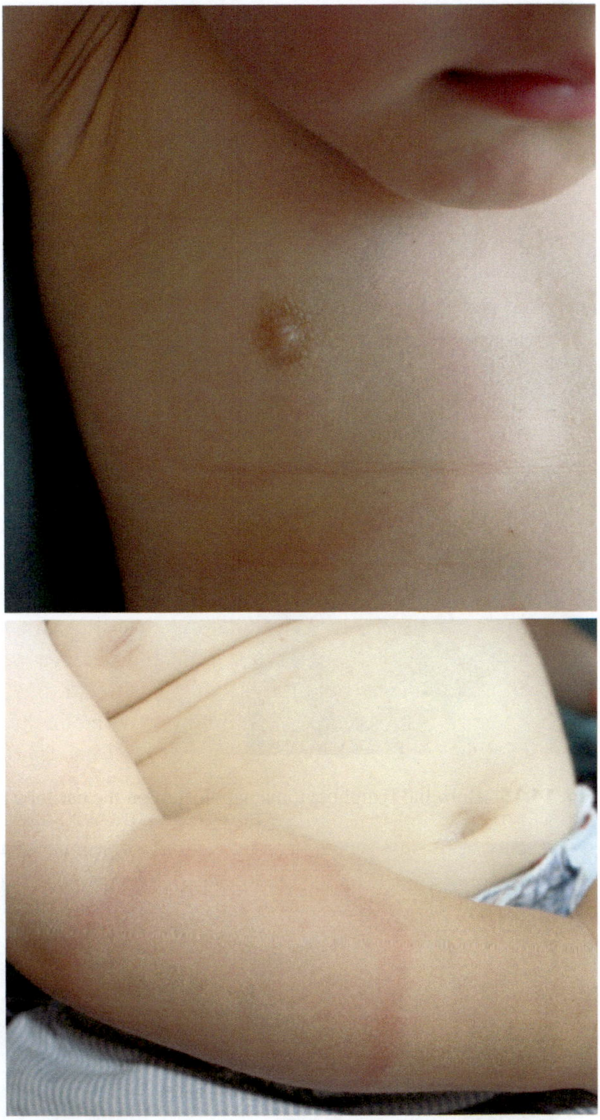

Fig. 14.14 Double erythema migrans—lesion on the upper extremity in the same child

cephalea, lymphadenopathy, nervous system involvement, and cardiovascular ones [4–7].

The skin manifestation during this stage is multiple EM, **erythemata migrantia**. First, EM develops and is followed in one week by smaller macules, obviously of anular or macular subtype. Secondary EM could be localized symmetrically on the face in children. There could be accompanied neurological symptoms (Fig. 14.17a, b, c, d).

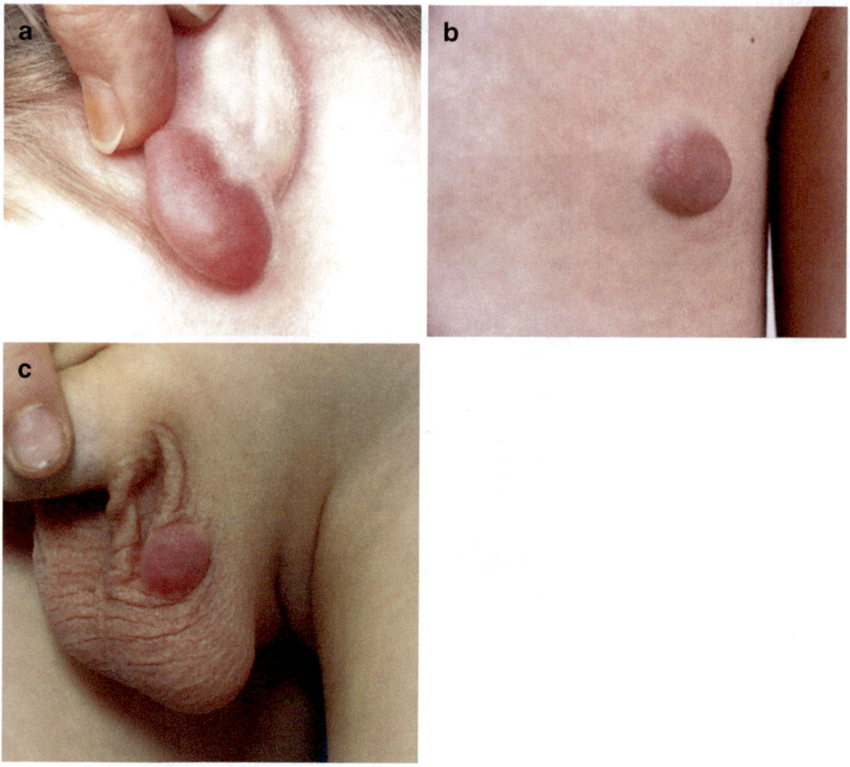

Fig. 14.15 Borrelial lymphocytoma papulosum on the ear lobe (**a**), mammilla (**b**), scrotum (**c**)

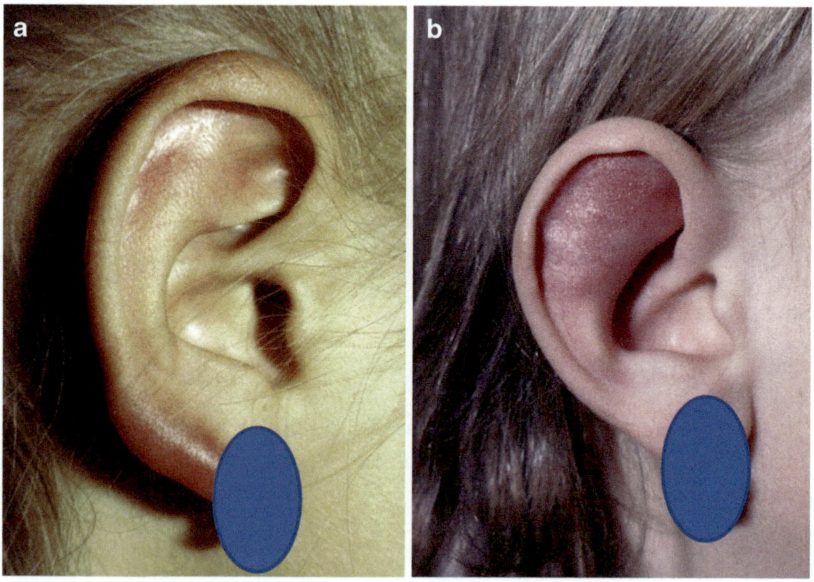

Fig. 14.16 Borrelial lymphocytoma infiltrativum on the helix of the ear (**a**) and the pinna of the ear (**b**)

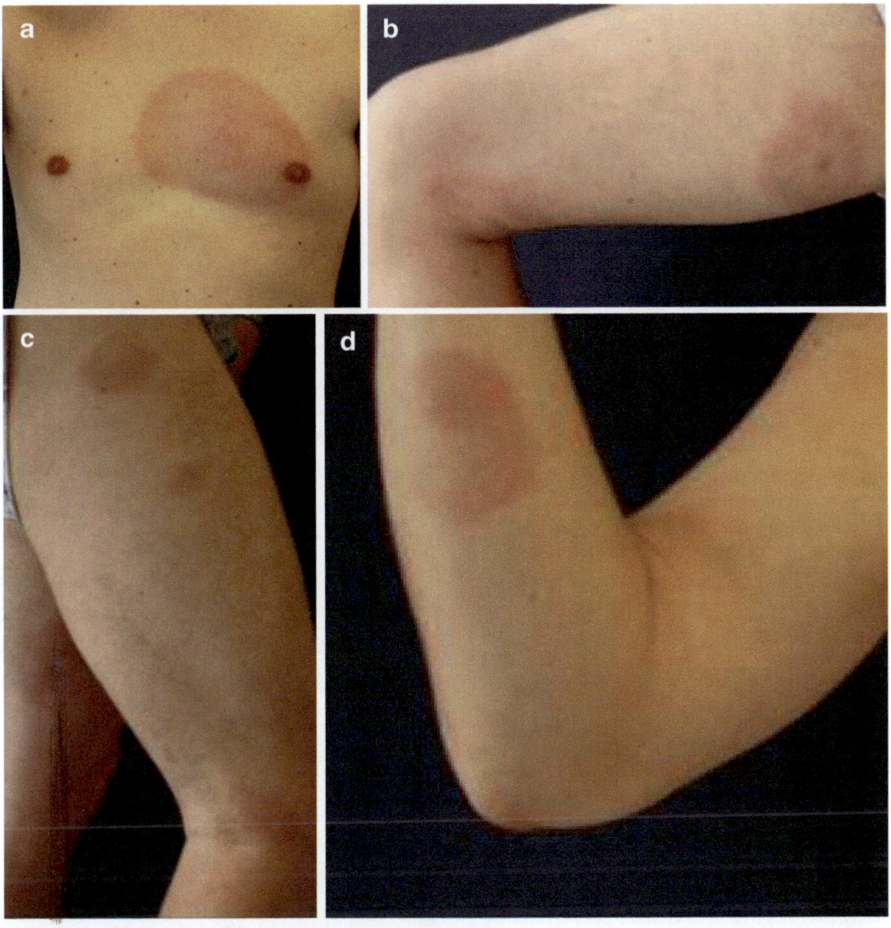

Fig. 14.17 Erythemata migrantia—the first erythema migrans on the trunk (**a**), smaller lesions on extremities one week later (**b, c, d**)

Chronic Skin Manifestations

Chronic Lyme borreliosis is developed after months after the tick bite, it is seen mainly in people who are frequently in contact with ticks (hunters, dog owners, farmers, sportsmen etc.).

Skin manifestation is ACA, mostly accompanied by peripheral neuropathy and/or chronic arthritis. ACA has two phases, an inflammatory and atrophic one.

ACA inflammatory phase (Figs. 14.3, 14.18, 14.19 and 14.20) is acral, dark red, sharply demarcated, irregular erythema with oedema. It is localized typically on the acral parts of the hands and feet, above elbows, ankles, knees. It is mostly on one extremity, but even all four could be involved.

The most affected parts are areas above the joints and bone prominences. In case of prominent oedema, erythema is not predominant and the patient could be examined for oedema of the extremity.

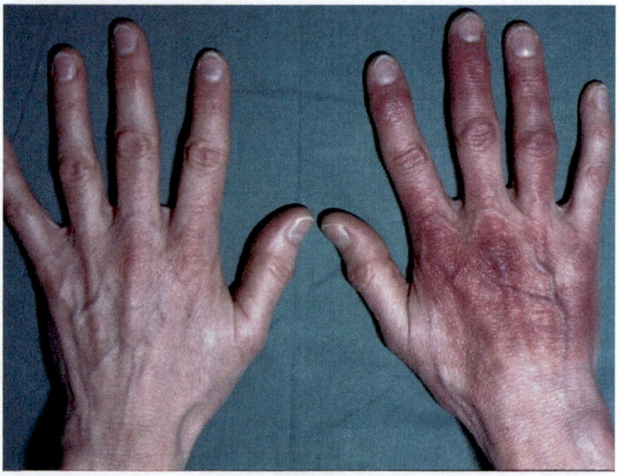

Fig. 14.18 ACA maculosa—right hand is involved

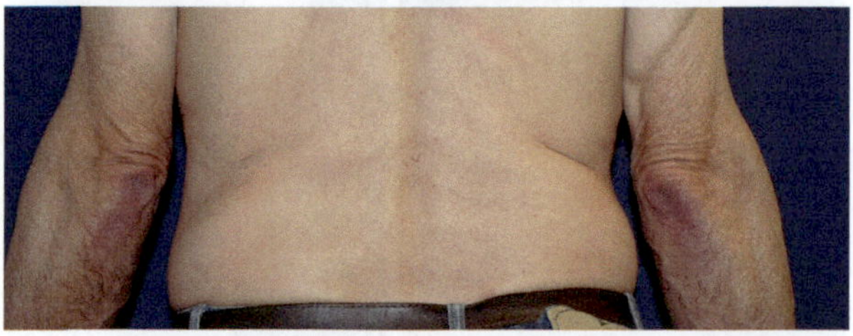

Fig. 14.19 Inflammatory ACA maculosa bilateral involvement of the elbow area

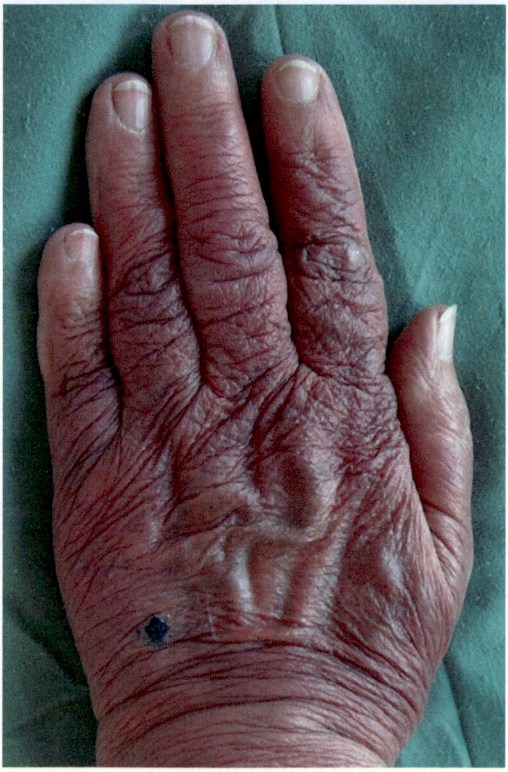

Fig. 14.20 ACA oedematosa

ACA atrophic phase (Figs. 14.21, 14.22, and 14.23,) is hardly recognized and frequently misdiagnosed as the clinical presentation in not unique:

Telangiectatic ACA resembles chronic venous insufficiency, in addition to livid erythema, oedema above joints, Achille tendon and heel, there are telangiectasias.

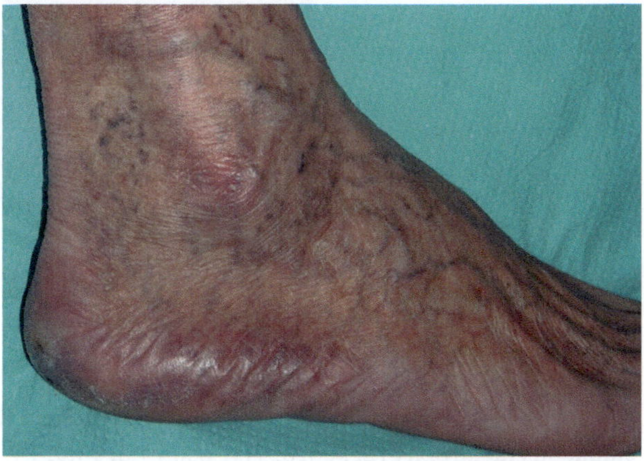

Fig. 14.21 ACA teleangiectatica

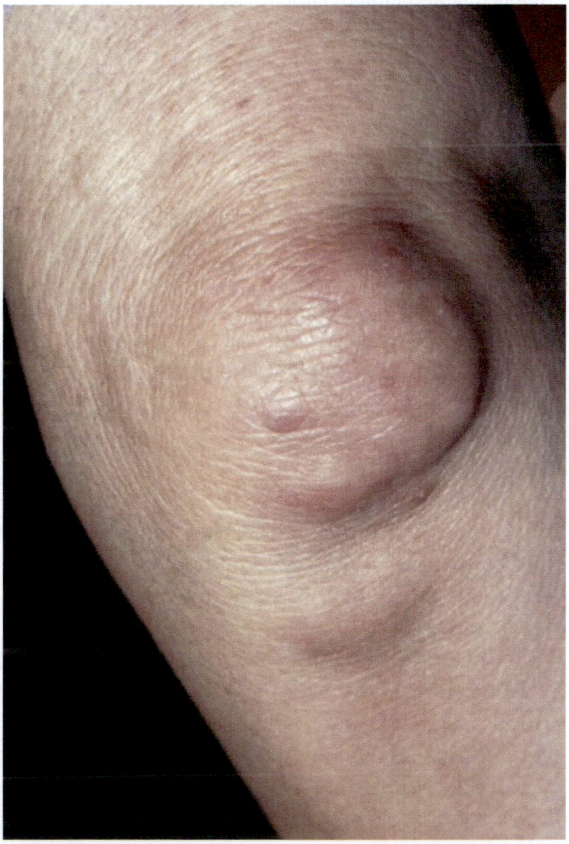

Fig. 14.22 ACA fibromatosa

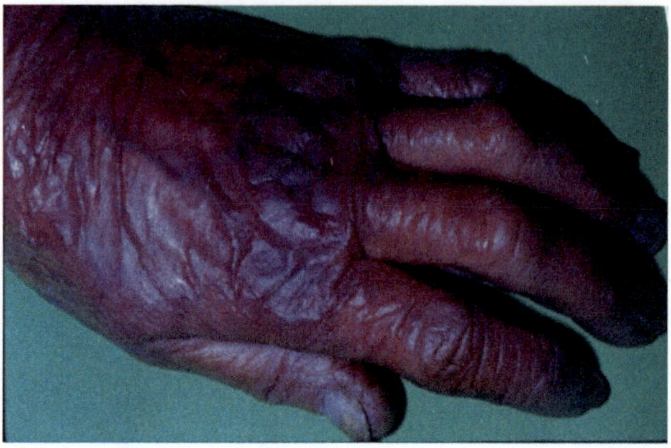

Fig. 14.23 ACA atrophicans sensu strictiori

Fibrous ACA is characterized by hard multiple nodules above elbows, small joints of the hands and ulnar part of the antebrachium. Nodules are of skin color or red, glossy, 1–3 cm in diameter.

Atrophic ACA is the true skin atrophy. Skin is thin, livid, without hairs, it could be easily injured. The inflammation leads to collagen fibres, sweat glands and subcutaneous fat atrophy [2, 5, 6, 8, 9] (Figs. 14.8, 14.9, 14.10, 14.11, 14.12, and 14.13).

Acrodermatitis chronica atrophicans		
Phase	Variants	
ACA inflammatoria	ACA maculosa	Dark red macules
	ACA oedematosa	Light red macules, oedema
ACA atrophicans	ACA teleangiectatica	Livid plaques, microvarices
	ACA fibrosa	Hard nodules by palpation
	ACA atrophicans sensu strictiori	Thin skin, hairs and sweat glands atrophy

Complications depend on the other organs ivolvement. At the early stage, the nervous system is mostly affected. ACA is mainly accompanied by arthralgias, myalgias and arthrirtis, peripheral neuropathy.

Neuroborreliosis

Acute neuroborreliosis could accompany EM. Pleocytosis in the cerebrospinal fluid with clical signs of lymphocytic meningitis are characteristic. Radiculoneuritis is presented as pain during the night, cranial paulsy or peripheral nerves palsy.

Peripheral neuropathy could be diagnosed in about one half of the ACA patients.

Rheumatic signs are typical for disseminated infection, there could be myalgias, arthralgias. Acute intermittent arthritis with oedema and arthralgias as mono- or oligoarthritis affects obviously knees (85%), small joints are speared [2, 4–6].

Cardiac symptoms are arrythmias, which can accompany or follow EM. Carditis is less common, AV-block is rarely reported.

Ophthalmologic symsptoms are follicular conjunctivitis, keratitis, virtitis and uveitis [10].

Clinical course. Untreated EM spreads centrifugally until it disappears after some months. After spontaneous healing, systemic involvement could develop. Untreated BL evolves form papule to plaque, and ACA goes from inflammatory to atrophic phases. Atrophy involves skin appendages and is irreversible.

Examination

Currently there is no laboratory test which could confirm or exclude the current Lyme borreliosis diagnosis. Lyme disease is not accompanied by increased sedimentation rate, leukocytosis, anemia, or elevated inflammatory markers.

Direct proof of *B. burgdorferi* is possible to made by using the PCR (from the skin biopsy, urin, cerebrospinal fluid, synovialis etc. Borrelial DNA could be detected by PCR even few months after therapy [26].

Other direct methods (isolation on Barbour-Stoenner-Kelly medium, electronmicroscopy, silver staining in light microscopy) are not used in daily practice [1, 6, 9, 12–14].

Serological examination. Antiborrelial antibodies are detected using the ELISA method, the confirmation should always be done by immunoblotting—there are i.e. VlsE, OspC, flagellin (p 41), antigens during the early stage and p100, p17/p18 antigens during the late phase.

The increased antiborrelial antibodies of the IgM class are found only after 3–6 weeks after the tick bite, increased levels of IgG class antibodies follow in weeks or months. The decrease of the levels of antiborrelial antibodies is very slow, it takes months and years.

The presence of increased levels on antiborrelial antibodies alone is not enough for the diagnosis of Lyme boreliosis, the diagnosis is always made based on clinical picture.

IgM antibodies are increased obviously after therapy and go down during the following months. The only increased levels of IgM antibodies in the immunocompetent patient rule out the possibility of the chronic borrelial infection—they are not specific enough.

Increased levels of IgG class immunoglobulins are regularly present during the chronic stage of borreliosis, which decrease after therapy. In the case of chronic infection prior to therapy, IgG antibodies may not reach normal levels. Another problem could be false positivity in viral diseases, autoimmune disorders, syphils, leptosirosis etc. due to cross reactions [6, 9, 15].

Diagnostics

- History of tick bite and duration of skin lesion more than one week
- Clinical picture
- Increased levels of IgG class antibodies in ACA
- Histopathology in BL, ACA
- PCR in some cases

Diferrential Diagnosis

According to *Hofmann H, Fingerle V, Hunfeld KP, Huppertz HI, Krause A, Rauer S, Ruf B; Cutaneous Lyme borreliosis: Guideline of the German Dermatology Society. Consensus group. Ger Med Sci. 2017 Sep 5;15* [6].

Erythema migrans	Persistent reaction to insect bite	Pruritus, disappears in one week
	Erysipelas/cellulitis	Fever, chills, malaise, nausea, increased CRP levels, leukocytosis
	Fixed drug exanthema	History, reccurency, pruritus
	Hypodermitis(chronic venous disease CVD)	Other symptoms of CVD-pachydermia, symmetric/ involvement
	Atrophoderma Pasini-Pierini	Erythema, atrophy, antiborrelial antibodies normal
	Morphea	Hard center by palpation, pigmentary changes
	Granuloma annulare	Nodules and plaques by palpation
	Herpes simplex (x/vesiculous EM type)	History, increased levels of the antiherpetic antibodies
	Tinea corporis	Elevated rim with scales, pruritus, dermatophyte proof
Erythemata migrantia	Urticaria	Urticarial exanthema, pruritus, course
	Multiple granulomata annularia	Nodules and plaques by palpation
	Erythema annulare centrifugum	Soft plaques by palpation, drug history
	Multiple fixed drug exanthema	Drug history, reccurence, pruritus
	Erythema infectiosum in children	Cheeks, course
Borrelial lymphocytoma	Lymphocytic infiltration	Benign pseudolymphoma
	Solitary mastocytoma	Darier sign
	Solitary B lymphoma low-grade, solitary/kožní/ cutaneuos/T cell/ lymphoma	Histopathology
Acrodermatitis chronica atrophicans—inflammatory phase	Erysipelas/cellulitis with lymphoedema	Fever, malaise, increased CRP, levels, leukocytosis
	Lupus erythematodes	Autoantibodies, histopathology
	Morphea	Different localization, histopathology
	Hypodermitis (CVD)	CDV, oedema, inflammation, ulcus
	Erytromelalgia	Dark red erythema and strong pain after warming, release of pain in cold
	Complex regional pain syndrome (before m. Sudeck)	Stp. fracturam, injury, surgery, neuritis and strong pain
	Perniones	Cold exposure history, symmetrical
	Erythema *ab igne*	Warm exposure history
ACA—atrophic phase	Skin aging	Diffuse, symmetric
	CVD	Both lower extremities, varices

Table 14.3 Lyme borreliosis therapy (*Hofmann H, Fingerle V, Hunfeld KP, Huppertz HI, Krause A, Rauer S, Ruf B; Cutaneous Lyme borreliosis: Guideline of the German Dermatology Society. Consensus group. Ger Med Sci. 2017 Sep 5;15)*

	Administration	Adults/Daily dose	Children/Daily dose	Therapy duration/ days
Erythema migrans, borrelial lymphocytoma				
Doxycycline	p.o.	200 mg	4 mg/kg (od 9 let)	14–20[a]
Amoxicillin	p.o.	3 g	50 mg/kg	14–20[a]
Cefuroxime axetil	p.o.	1 g	30 mg/kg	14–20[a]
Azithromycin	p.o.	500 mg	10 mg/kg	7–14[a]
Acrodermatitis chronica atrophicans				
Doxycycline	p.o.	200 mg	4 mg/kg	21–28
Amoxicilin	p.o.	3 g	50 mg/kg	21–28
Cefuroxime axetil	p.o.	1 g	30 mg/kg	21–28
Neuroborreliosis, AV-block, carditis				
Ceftriaxone	i.v.	2 g	50–75 mg/kg	10–28[b]
Cefotaxime	i.v.	6 g	150–200 mg/kg	10–28[b]
Penicillin G	i.v.	18–24 mil.u.	200–400 tis.u./kg	10–28[b]
Chronic arthritis				
Doxycycline	p.o.	200–400 mg	0	21–28

[a]In patients with disseminated infection (multiple EM, BL, flu-like symptoms)
[b]If parenteral therapy is shorter than 28 days, oral antibiotics are followed untill 28 days

Therapy

Therapy should be started immediatelly after the diagnosis is made. It means no serological examination is needed in typical clinical cases of skin lesions. The only exception is ACA, the increased levels of IgG class antibodies are required to confirm the diagnosis.

Antibiotic therapy (Table 14.3) includes doxycycline, event. A amoxicilin/ phenoxymethylpenicilin and in allergic patients, macrolides.

The duration of therapy should not be shorter than 2 weeks, in chronic stage 4 weeks. Prologation of therapy or repeating the antibiotics is not recommended, as well as no therapy in given only in case of the presnece of increased levels of anti-borrelial antibodies without any other clinical signs and symtpoms.

Patients with extracutaneous symptoms are treated with parenteral antibiotics (ceftriaxone) and arthritis is treated with doxycycline. Amoxicillin, penicillin G or ceftiraxone could be used during pregnancy. Tetracyclines are not used in children younger than 9 years.

Therapy can be complicated at the very beginning by Jarisch-Herxheimer reaction (darkening of skin lesions, fever), which resolves in few hours [2, 3, 5, 6].

Topical Therapy

There is no role for local therapy and anti-inflammatory topicals could cause pruritus.

Cardiac Manifestations

Cardiac manifestation may be present in 4–10% of the patients with Lyme borreliosis and can be preceded by a viral prodrome of up to 3 weeks [9, 16–18]. Medical history (including tick bite and erythema migrans), together with atrioventricular heart blocks and positive Borrelia serology are the diagnostic triad of cardiac borreliosis [17]. Cardiac symptoms usually last for 3 days to 6 weeks [4].

Clinical

Cardiac manifestation may be preceded by dermatological manifestation such as erythema migrans and could be associated with joint pain, signs and symptoms of meningoencephalitis, etc. Cardiac involvement may be asymptomatic, but also can manifest as chest pain, palpitations, syncope, dyspnea, or even sudden cardiac death [18–20]. Lyme carditis is more frequently found in men (3:1 ratio) [17]. The common cardiac manifestations are related to conduction or rhythm problems (affecting 90% of the patients with Lyme carditis) [17]. Rarely, myocarditis, pericarditis, endocarditis or fulminant pancarditis may be present [18, 21–25]. Myopericarditis may be present in 60% of the patients with Lyme carditis [17].

Conduction disturbances are reversible and self-limited in most of cases, but rarely a pacemaker may be necessary usually for with temporary use (30%) if the patients are unstable [17]. They consist of various degrees of atrioventricular block [20, 27].

Palpitations may occur as an expression of atrial fibrillation, ventricular or atrial extrasystole [28]. The attempt to control the heart rate in the absence of the etiological treatment may translate into conduction disturbance or bradycardia [29].

Myocarditis and cardiomyopathy may occur but usually the degree of severity is mild [20, 27]. There is evidence, albeit conflicting, about the role of the Borrelia infection in the development and progression of chronic congestive heart failure (CHF) [30]. Two serological tests (ELISA and Western-blot) are recommended in all patients [20].

Pericarditis may rarely appear in limited form usually associated with myocarditis [20, 27].

Endocarditis appears anecdotally in medical literature. There were only three cases of Lyme disease endocarditis of the mitral valve or aortic valve. In one case valve perforation occurred [31]. Degenerative valve disease may also manifest as a consequence of Borrelia burgdorferi infection [27].

Investigations

Investigation in borreliosis starts with usual tests including white blood count, inflammation markers. When the clinical picture is highly suggestive for borreliosis, Lyme serology IgM and IgG immunoglobulin are tested [29]. Borrelia serology at the onset of the disease may be negative [17]. The sensitivity of serology testing is about 80% in Lyme carditis [12]. Positive and indeterminate enzyme-linked immunosorbent assay (ELISA) results for Lyme disease should be followed by confirmation with immunoblots [32]. Borrelia burgdorferi immunohistochemistry and polymerase chain reaction testing using different samples from skin, urine, cerebrospinal fluid, or heart by endomyocardial biopsy should be considered [18].

Cardiac evaluation in Lyme disease is mandatory. An electrocardiogram or a 24-h Holter ECG is immediately performed for detection of conduction or rhythm problems. Signs such as a prolonged PR interval may require continuous or frequent ECG evaluation due to the risk of progressive heart block. 30% of pediatric patients with Lyme disease may show variant ECG signs. The ECG findings in Lyme carditis are ST depression or elevation, negative T waves in inferolateral leads, first, second or third-degree AV block, sinus node dysfunction, bundle blocks including alternating right and left branch bundle block, prolonged QT interval, supraventricular, junctional and ventricular tachycardia, atrial and ventricular flutter, atrial fibrillation bradycardia and asystole. Heart block may be inducible with exercise and reversible with rest [17, 33–38].

Echocardiography is essential for evaluating the heart from a structural and functional point of view. Cardiomegaly may be initially seen on a chest radiograph but echocardiography is essential for signs of myocarditis, pericarditis, endocarditis, degenerative valve disease or severe cardiomyopathy with cardiogenic shock. Information about chambers sizes, systolic and diastolic function are obtained [28].

Cardiac MRI is important to confirm the diagnosis and may demonstrate areas of myocardial wall edema (increased signal intensity on T2-weighted images), suggesting myocardial inflammation. Late gadolinium enhancement imaging will frequently reveal mid-wall or sub epicardial enhancement [17, 39].

Indium 111-monoclonal antimyosin antibody scan may be used to detecting the area of myocardial necrosis in patients suspected of having myocarditis. In some centers the confirmation of the cardiac borreliosis is given by histopathological and electronmicroscopical examination, including PCR [39].

Anatomo-pathological specimen (in a case of fatal Lyme carditis) may show diffuse pancarditis with lymphocytes infiltrates and focal interstitial fibrosis [18].

Treatment

The treatment of choice, including the cardiac borreliosis, is with antibiotics, orally for mild carditis, or intravenously for severe forms, preferably ceftriaxone [17, 20]. Orally, the treatment consists in administration for 14 weeks of doxycycline (100 mg twice daily), amoxicillin (500 mg three times daily), or cefuroxime (500 mg twice daily). Intravenous treatment includes ceftriaxone, 2 g daily or cefotaxime, 2 g every 8 h for 14 days [4].

Cardiac implications sometimes may necessitate specific treatment especially in patients with high degree AV block who may require temporary ventricular pacing. Anyhow, the patients with high degree AV block might recover in one week and with first degree AV block in six weeks [17]. Ventricular assisted devices or ECMO (extracorporeal membrane oxygenation support) may be necessary in extreme cases dominated by a fulminant myocarditis with cardiogenic shock [21].

Prognosis and Complications

If the infection is diagnosed correctly and treated accordingly, prognosis is very good including cases with heart involvement, even in extreme cases of fulminant myocarditis if correctly treated. Complete atrioventricular heart block is temporary in the majority of cases, having a good prognosis if treated. However, severe or fatal cases may occur and are reported in the literature [17, 18, 20–27].

Some authors proposed scores of risk for Lyme carditis identification in the group of patients presenting with high degree AV block. The COSTAR mnemonic was proposed (constitutional symptoms, outdoor activity, sex—male, tick bite, age < 50, rash—erythema migrans) to indicate the risk of permanent pacemaker implantation [11].

Acknowledgments All clinical pictures in this chapter are courtesy of prof. Jana Třešňák Hercogová and are part of her work Klinická dermatovenerologie, 2019, Mladá fronta, 2nd Vol—x in press already printed: Hercogová, J. Lymeská borelióza. In: Hercogová J. (ed) et al. Klinická dermatovenerologie, 2nd vol., 2019, Mladá fronta, p. 1235–1246, ISBN 987-80-204-5549-9.

References

1. Asbrink E, Hovmark A. Successful cultivation of spirochetes from skin lesions of patients with erythema chronicum migrans Afzelius and acrodermatitis chronica atrophicans. Acta Pathol Microbiol Immunol Scand B. 1985 Apr;93(2):161–3.
2. Hercogova J, Brzonova I. Lyme disease in central Europe. Curr Opin Infect Dis. 2001 Apr;14(2):133–7.
3. Hercogová J, et al. Klinická dermatovenerologie, vol. 2. Praha: Mladá fronta; 2019.
4. Alao OR, Decker CF. Lyme disease. Dis Mon. 2012;58(6):335–45.
5. Aberer E. Lyme borreliosis: an update. J Dtsch Dermatol Ges. 2007 May;5(5):406–14.
6. Hofmann H, Fingerle V, Hunfeld KP, Huppertz HI, Krause A, Rauer S, Ruf B. Cutaneous Lyme borreliosis: guideline of the German Dermatology Society. Consensus group. Ger Med Sci. 2017 Sep 5;15 https://doi.org/10.3205/000255. eCollection 2017
7. Valešová M, Hulínská D, Jirouš J. Isolation of Borrelia in the tissues of patient with Lyme borreliosis. Cas Lek Cesk. 1988;127(26):825–6.
8. Brzonova I, Wollenberg A, Prinz JC. Acrodermatitis chronica atrophicans affecting all four limbs in an 11-year-old girl. Br J Dermatol. 2002;147(2):375–8.
9. Eldin C, Raffetin A, Bouiller K, Hansmann Y, Roblot F, Raoult D, Parola P. Review of European and American guidelines for the diagnosis of Lyme borreliosis. Med Mal Infect. 2019 Mar;49(2):121–32.

10. Lesser RL. Ocular manifestations of Lyme disease. Am J Med. 1995 Apr 24;98(4A):60S–2S.
11. Besant G, Wan D, Yeung C, Blakely C, Branscombe P, Suarez-Fuster L, Redfearn D, Simpson C, Abdollah H, Glover B, Baranchuk A. Suspicious index in Lyme carditis: systematic review and proposed new risk score. Clin Cardiol. 2018;41(12):1611–6.
12. Dessau RB, van Dam AP, Fingerle V, Gray J, Hovius JW, Hunfeld KP, Jaulhac B, Kahl O, Kristoferitsch W, Lindgren PE, Markowicz M, Mavin S, Ornstein K, Rupprecht T, Stanek G, Strle F. To test or not to test? Laboratory support for the diagnosis of Lyme borreliosis: a position paper of ESGBOR, the ESCMID study group for Lyme borreliosis. Clin Microbiol Infect. 2018 Feb;24(2):118–24.
13. Hercogová J, Tománková M, Plch J, Jirouš J, Hulínská D, Frösslová D, Barták P. Borrelia burgdorferi isolates from erythema migrans. Arch Dermatol Res. 1993;285(3):171–3.
14. Hulínská D, Barták P, Hercogová J, Hancil J, Basta J, Schramlová J. Electron microscopy of Langerhans cells and Borrelia burgdorferi in Lyme disease patients. Zentralbl Bakteriol. 1994 Jan;280(3):348–59.
15. Hercogova J, Vanousova D. Syphilis and borreliosis during pregnancy. Dermatol Ther. 2008 May-Jun;21(3):205–9.
16. Kashou AH, Braiteh N, Kashou HE. Reversible atrioventricular block and the importance of close follow-up: Two cases of Lyme carditis. J Cardiol Cases. 2018 Feb 13;17(5):171–4.
17. Scheffold N, Herkommer B, Kandolf R, May AE. Lyme carditis--diagnosis, treatment and prognosis. Dtsch Arztebl Int. 2015;112(12):202–8.
18. Yoon EC, Vail E, Kleinman G, Lento PA, Li S, Wang G, Limberger R, Fallon JT. Lyme disease: a case report of a 17-year-old male with fatal Lyme carditis. Cardiovasc Pathol. 2015;24(5):317–21.
19. Kostić T, Momčilović S, Perišić ZD, Apostolović SR, Cvetković J, Jovanović A, Barać A, Šalinger-Martinović S, Tasić-Otašević S. Manifestations of Lyme carditis. Int J Cardiol. 2017 Apr 1;232:24–32.
20. Pinto DS. Cardiac manifestations of Lyme disease. Med Clin North Am. 2002 Mar;86(2):285–96.
21. Župan Ž, Mijatović D, Medved I, Kraljić S, Juranić J, Barbalić B, Oštrić M. Successful treatment of fulminant Lyme myocarditis with mechanical circulatory support in a young male adult: a case report. Croat Med J. 2017;58(2):185–93.
22. Bartůnek P, Gorican K, Mrázek V, Varejka P, Veiser T, Hercogová J, Hulínská D, Janovská D. Lyme borreliosis infection as a cause of dilated cardiomyopathy. Prague Med Rep. 2006;107(2):213–26.
23. Bartunek P, Mrázek V, Varejka P, Gorican K, Zapletalová J, Sklenár T. Borrelia burgdorferi as a cause of Morgagni-Adams-Stokes syndrome. Long time follow-up study. Wien Klin Wochenschr. 1999 Dec 10;111(22–23):964–9.
24. Bartůněk P, Mrázek V, Gorican K, Bína R, Listvanová S, Zapletalová J. Borrelia infection as a cause of carditis (a long-term study). Wien Klin Wochenschr. 2001 Jan 15;113(1–2):38–44.
25. Bartůněk P, Gorican K, Veiser T, Táborský M, Hulínská D. Significance of Borrelia infection in development of dilated cardiomypathy (a pilot study). Prague Med Rep. 2007;108(4):339–47.
26. Pícha D, Moravcová L, Vanousová D, Hercogová J, Blechová Z. DNA persistence after treatment of Lyme borreliosis. Folia Microbiol (Praha). 2014 Mar;59(2):115–25.
27. Lelovas P, Dontas I, Bassiakou E, Xanthos T. Cardiac implications of Lyme disease, diagnosis and therapeutic approach. Int J Cardiol. 2008;129(1):15–21.
28. Vujisić-Tesić B, Simin N, Petrović M, Vasiljević Z, Grujić M, Karacić A. The role of echocardiography in the evaluation of cardiac damage in Lyme disease. Glas Srp Akad Nauka Med. 1993;43:241–3.
29. Shabbir MA, Saad Shaukat MH, Arshad MH, Sacco J. Lyme carditis presenting as atrial fibrillation in a healthy young male. BMJ Case Rep. 2019;12(6):e229261.
30. Yeung C, Baranchuk A. Diagnosis and treatment of Lyme carditis: JACC review topic of the week. J Am Coll Cardiol. 2019;73(6):717–26.
31. Fatima B, Sohail MR, Schaff HV. Lyme disease: an unusual cause of a mitral valve endocarditis. Mayo Clin Proc Innov Qual Outcomes. 2018;2(4):398–401. https://doi.org/10.1016/j.mayocpiqo.2018.09.003.

32. Zwerink M, Zomer TP, van Kooten B, Blaauw G, van Bemmel T, van Hees BC, Vermeeren YM, Landman GW. Predictive value of Borrelia burgdorferi IgG antibody levels in patients referred to a tertiary Lyme centre. Ticks Tick Borne Dis. 2018;9(3):594–7.
33. Cunha BA, Elyasi M, Singh P, Jimada I. Lyme carditis with isolated left bundle branch block and myocarditis successfully treated with oral doxycycline. IDCases. 2017;11:48–50.
34. Fu Md J, Bhatta L. Lyme carditis: early occurrence and prolonged recovery. J Electrocardiol. 2018 May–Jun;51(3):516–8.
35. Kannangara DW, Sidra S, Pritiben P. First case report of inducible heart block in Lyme disease and an update of Lyme carditis. BMC Infect Dis. 2019;19(1):428.
36. Oktay AA, Dibs SR, Friedman H. Sinus pause in association with Lyme carditis. Tex Heart Inst J. 2015 Jun 1;42(3):248–50. https://doi.org/10.14503/THIJ-14-4126.
37. Rastogi U, Kumars N. Lyme Arrhythmia in an Avid Golfer: a diagnostic challenge and a therapeutic dilemma. J Atr Fibrillation. 2016;8(5):1378. https://doi.org/10.4022/jafib.1378.
38. Wan D, Blakely C, Branscombe P, Suarez-Fuster L, Glover B, Baranchuk A. Lyme carditis and high-degree atrioventricular block. Am J Cardiol. 2018;121(9):1102–4.
39. Bergler-Klein J, Sochor H, Stanek G, Globits S, Ullrich R, Glogar D. Indium 111-monoclonal antimyosin antibody and magnetic resonance imaging in the diagnosis of acute Lyme myopericarditis. Arch Intern Med. 1993;153(23):2696–700.

Syphilis

15

George-Sorin Ţiplica, Mihai Ceauşu, Cătălina Andrei, and Michel Janier

Introduction and Pathophysiology of Disease

Syphilis (syn. lues) is a systemic human disease produced by infection with the spirochete *Treponema pallidum subsp. pallidum.* Syphilis is mainly acquired by sexual contact. The infection can be transmitted during pregnancy (congenital syphilis) and, in rare situations, by blood transfusion or solid organ transplant. Acquired syphilis is divided into early and late syphilis by the duration of the infection. The World Health Organization (WHO) considers a 2 year duration of the infection as the artificial limit of the two stages [1] while other authorities (e.g. Centers for Disease Control and Prevention—Atlanta, European Center for Disease Control and Prevention) defines the limit of the two stages at 1 year. Early syphilis includes primary, secondary and early non-primary, non-secondary syphilis. Late syphilis (syphilis of unknown duration) includes cases in which the infection was produced more than 12 month ago and includes late clinical manifestations of syphilis (tertiary syphilis) [2, 3].

G.-S. Ţiplica (✉)
"Carol Davila" University of Medicine and Pharmacy, Dermatology II, Colentina Clinical Hospital, Bucharest, Romania
e-mail: george.tiplica@umfcd.ro

M. Ceauşu
"Carol Davila" University of Medicine and Pharmacy, Department of Pathology, INML "Mina Minovici", Bucharest, Romania

C. Andrei
"Carol Davila" University of Medicine and Pharmacy, Cardiology, SCU "Bagdasar-Arseni", Bucharest, Romania

M. Janier
STD Clinic, Hôpital Saint-Louis AP-HP and Hôpital Saint-Joseph, Paris, France

C. Salavastru et al. (eds.), *Skin and the Heart*,
https://doi.org/10.1007/978-3-030-54779-0_15

Treponema pallidum penetrates the cutaneous or mucosal barriers and starts local replication followed by infection in the regional lymph nodes and blood dissemination [4]. *T. pallidum* infection elicits cellular and humoral immune responses. At the infected site, an infiltrate of polymorphonuclear leukocytes will be formed and subsequently replaced by T cells (CD4+ and CD8+), monocytes, macrophages, plasma cells and dendritic cells [5]. The immune response is apparently effective in the early stages of the infection as luetic lesions disappear without treatment but, paradoxically, dissemination of *T. pallidum* is not blocked and the disease can progress in untreated patients. In secondary syphilis, *T. pallidum* bacteraemia determines multisystem involvement within the first year of infection [6–8]. *T. pallidum* spreads also to the heart, coronary ostia and aortic wall where it harbours and multiplies in the vasa vasorum of the adventitia. Small vessels are primarily affected by an infiltrate of lymphocytes and plasma cells, which leads to intimal inflammatory infiltration. The small vessel vasculitis is present from the secondary stage of syphilis and can be encountered as vasculitis of the vasa vasorum ("endarteritis obliterans") [9]. The results of the occlusion of the vasa vasorum are focal necrosis and destruction of the elastic fibers of the middle aortic layer and of the aortic valvular ring, accompanied by fibrosis and calcification. These modifications are leading to weakening of the tunica media with formation of the aneurysm and respectively to valvular aortic dysfunction with or without ostial coronaritis (due to calcification of coronary ostia). The process is mainly manifested in the aortic valve (2/3 of cases) (with valvular eversion due to fibrosis of the valvulae), the ascending aorta, the aortic arch and less frequently in the descending thoracic aorta. Histopathology is characteristic and very different from rheumatic disease and from atheromatous aortic aneurysms. Analysis of surgical material is useful to allow a retrospective diagnosis of syphilis if not made before surgery. Serological tests for syphilis should be made systemically in the case of aortic regurgitation, aortic aneurysm, stroke and myelitis.

In the late stage of infection, a cellular hypersensitivity reaction occurs to *T. pallidum*, still active in isolated sites. The reaction is demonstrated histo-pathologically by the formation of granulomas that are clinically represented by gummas [10]. Gummas develop as asymptomatic red nodules of 1–10 mm or bigger in diameter [11], on the skin or any organ, including the heart (myocarditis) [12]. The nodules have central necrotic tissue that is surrounded by epithelioid and multinucleated giant cells. As the central gumma heals, forming thickened, ridged scars, new lesions may develop from the periphery [12].

Prevalence/Population Affected

Syphilis prevalence is has had a rising trend since 2010, with an WHO estimate of 19.9 million cases worldwide (data from 2016) [13]. Most cases were reported in the WHO Western Pacific region (93.0 cases per 100,000 adult population). In Europe (EU/EEA countries) there were 33,193 cases reported in 2017 with a prevalence of 7.1 cases per 100,000 population [1]. The recent increase of syphilis incidence is related to the escalation of the infection in the population of men having sex with men (MSM) co-infected with HIV who are not using barrier protection as much as previously [14, 15]. Risk factors for syphilis are represented by multiple sex partners, unprotected sex and use of alcohol or drugs. The most vulnerable populations are represented by people living in poverty, people with poor access to health care, or those in racial, ethnic, and sexuality minority populations [16, 17].

The natural course of untreated syphilis was observed in the Oslo study [18] and in the Tuskegee study [19]. Data showed that the diagnostic of cardiovascular syphilis was made in 10% of the subjects (13% in men and 7% in women) while, during necropsy, 50–80% of cases showed various cardiovascular modifications related to the infection [19–21], aortic aneurysm being the main cardiovascular manifestation observed in 28% to 54% of patients [22]. Cardiovascular syphilis was considered the most important cause of death (11% of the subjects) [18].

Dermatological Manifestations

Cardiovascular involvement is a classical systemic manifestation of syphilis and can be encountered from the secondary stage, after the systemic spread of the bacteria. But cardiovascular syphilis is mostly seen in the late (tertiary) stage, 10–40 years after the chancre.

The dermatological manifestations of secondary syphilis are self-limited, even without treatment. All forms of elementary skin lesions can occur and are asymptomatic. A macular eruption can be observed as the first sign of this stage after 8 weeks from the inoculation. The macules are non-itchy, round, copper-reddish, 0.5–1 cm in diameter and symmetrically distributed over the trunk and extremities (roseola syphilitica). In 2–4 weeks the macular lesions disappear and another, papular, symmetrical and asymptomatic eruption will develop immediately or after a latency of 4–12 months. The lesions are round, with a diameter of 0.3–1 cm, copper-reddish, frequently with scales in the periphery (the Biett's collarette). In 4–8 weeks the lesions disappear and a new wave of syphilides will follow. Sometimes the lesions are papulo-squamous having a thick lay of scales (psoriasiform syphilides) or have a flat, shiny surface (lichenoid syphilides). The lesions can develop on the hairy regions (follicular syphilides) or evolve on the facial region with pustular aspect (acneiform syphilides) or develop on the seborrheic regions with yellowish, oily, scales (seborrheic syphilides) or can involve only the palms and soles (palmoplantar syphilides) [23]. Rarely, annular syphilides can also develop [24]. In immunocompromised patients, nodular lesions with rapid growth and central ulceration covered by crusts can develop on the face, trunk and limbs (lues maligna). It often associates with systemic manifestations [25–27].

Mucosal manifestations are the most contagious elements of secondary syphilis. On the buccal mucosa syphilides may occur as erythematous round-oval plaques, ulcerated, papulo-hypertrophic or covered by a white or gray pseudo-membrane (syphilis angina) [28]. On the genital mucosa the secondary lesions are usually papulo-erosive or papulo-hypertrophic (condyloma lata).

Hair loss can be observed in secondary syphilis with round-oval areas of alopecia of 1–3 cm in diameter (alopecia specifica). Eyebrows alopecia starting from the lateral side and non-scarring alopecia of the beard was also described [25].

The secondary syphilitic lesions appears in waves (recurrences) that clears in 4–8 weeks, sometimes leaving post-inflammatory hypo-pigmented and hyper-pigmented macules (if distributed around the neck they form "the necklace of Venus"). The recurrences are more widely spaced and most patients remain asymptomatic until tertiary syphilis starts [29].

The most common manifestations of tertiary syphilis are encountered on the skin as nodules (dermo-epidermal lesions) and gummata (hypodermal lesions) [30]. Nodular (tuberculous) syphilis is represented by isolated or grouped nodules of 0.5 cm in diameter with a copper coloured adjacent epidermis. The nodules ulcerate in time and extend from the margins. Gummatous syphilis on the skin and mucosae is represented by deep nodular lesions of 2–10 cm diameter. In time, the elastic consistence of the lesion becomes soft then fluctuant. The lesion ulcerate and necrotic tissue is eliminated on the surface through a fistula. Gummas develops with the destruction of the surrounding tissue [31]. Gumma forms usually in the areas of trauma (e.g. scalp, forehead, supraclavicular, buttock, pretibial). At the mucosal level, the gummas are frequently located in the palate, tongue, tonsils or nasally [32]. Even in the case of effective treatment, tertiary skin lesions heals with scars.

Cardiological Manifestations

In the early syphilis stage the cardiovascular disease is usually asymptomatic. However syphilitic arteritis (mainly aortitis, cerebral arteritis and medullar arteritis) can occur in the secondary period, during the first year after the chancre [33, 34] with possible meningo-vascular syphilis, stroke or myelitis [35, 36]. These events have become very rare but still represent potentially extremely severe complications with possible long term sequelae. It has been recently shown that asymptomatic aortitis documented by positron emission tomography could be more frequent that thought [37]. In early syphilis a thorough clinical examination including cardiovascular signs and symptoms must be performed but no further cardiac investigation is needed in the absence of clinical abnormalities.

During the late stage of the infection, symptoms can occur, such as: angina, heart failure, symptoms of aortic aneurysms and even sudden death. Auscultation must be performed in patients with late latent or tertiary syphilis. A chest X-ray is rarely contributory in asymptomatic patients [38].

Angina is due to coronary artery stenosis and endarteritis. Usually the patient complains of chest pain on exertion which relieves at rest. Syphilitic aortitis affects the aortic valve, producing aortic regurgitation in 10% of untreated individuals [39]. The cardiac auscultation is suggestive for aortic regurgitation with a tambour-like second heart sound and a rough diastolic murmur over the aortic area. The aortic regurgitation induces tachycardia and arrhythmia. Other clinical signs can also be observed by the clinician: the Corrigan's pulse (a pulse that is forceful and then suddenly collapses), the Quincke's pulse (nail bed pulsations), the Musset's sign (head-nodding with each cardiac pulsations). In advanced cases, aortic insufficiency and heart failure can occur. Patients complain of dyspnea on exertion, orthopnea, paroxysmal nocturnal dyspnea and reduced exercise tolerance. Clinical examination identifies peripheral edema and pulmonary rales. Syphilitic aortitis was also reported as producing the destruction of aortic valve due to vegetation [40]. Coronary artery stenosis can induce a severe reduction in the myocardial perfusion resulting in arrhythmias and sudden death [41].

Gumma can rarely develop in the heart tissue. The local infiltration and the granulomatous lesion produces symptoms [42] that are usually mis-diagnosed and a retrospective diagnosis is made post-operatory or at necropsy. There are reports of gummata that destroy the heart conduction system, inducing manifestations from arrhythmia to complete heart block [12].

Symptoms of aortic aneurysm are due to the inflammation of the aortic wall and subsequent aortitis. *T. pallidum* DNA has been detected in aortic aneurysms, demonstrating that infection of the aorta produces direct damage of the tissue [39]. The process involves all aortic layers with fibrous thickening of the adventitia, focal destruction of the media due to the cellular infiltrate and marked thickening of the intima by atherosclerotic-appearing lesions [43], grossly with a "tree bark" resemblance [44]. Syphilitic aortitis has a strong predilection toward involvement of the ascending aorta. The aneurysms are often remarkably dilated, typically sacciform or cupuliform, often with concomitant aortic regurgitation [45] but they dissect rarely [46]. Visible and palpable pulsations over the suprasternal notch can be detected in the presence of aortic aneurysm. The rupture of the aortic aneurysm is suspected by the setup of the classical triad: abdominal or back pain, hypovolemic shock and pulsatile abdominal mass. The patient also presents with a pulsatile anterior chest wall mass, palpitations, dyspnea, cough, dysphagia and chest pain. The rupture of the aortic aneurysm can produce sudden death.

There are insufficient data to determine if cardiovascular syphilis is more severe and prevalent in HIV-positive patients [47, 48].

Diagnosis/Investigations

The identification of *T. pallidum* in the lesions allows accurate diagnosis. It can be performed with polymerase chain reaction (PCR) tests from tissues (including heart or aortic samples) [49]. DNA-sequencing of *T. pallidum* is possible but used mainly for research purposes.

Pathological examination using silver staining to spot *T. pallidum* is rarely used nowadays as immunohistochemistry is more efficient and less difficult to perform [50]. The usual hematoxylin and eosin stain performed when syphilitic aortitis is suspected may present two main histological patterns (Figs. 15.1 and 15.2): (a) vasa vasorum develop endarteritis obliterans (which leads to tissue damage because of poor blood supply), which is accompanied by proliferation of intima and plasma cell infiltration; (b) development of a type IV cell-mediated immune response with the occurrence of "gummas", which consist of a central area of necrosis and activated macrophages, lymphoid and plasma cells. Obliterative changes in the vasa vasorum cause focal medial necrosis and scarring, along with disruption and disorganization of the elastic lamellae. The depressed medial scars create a roughened intimal surface, with a "tree bark" appearance. The main consequence is

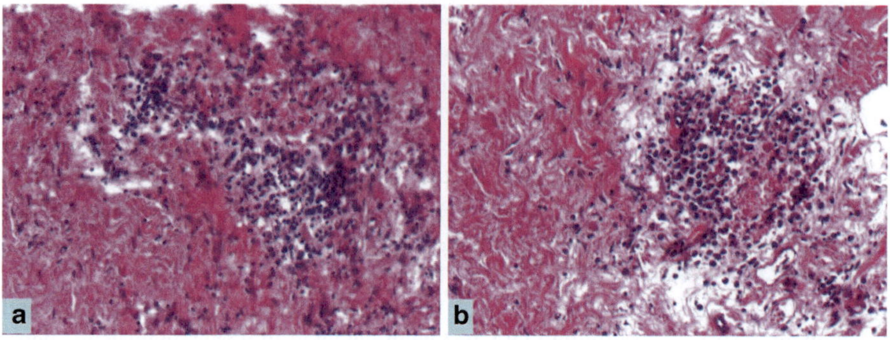

Fig. 15.1 (**a**) Nodular interstitial infiltrate with lymphocytes and plasma cells into the media of the aortic wall, HE, 100×; (**b**) nodular perivascular infiltrate (around vasa vasorum), with lymphocytes and plasma cells into the adventitia of the aortic wall, HE, 100×

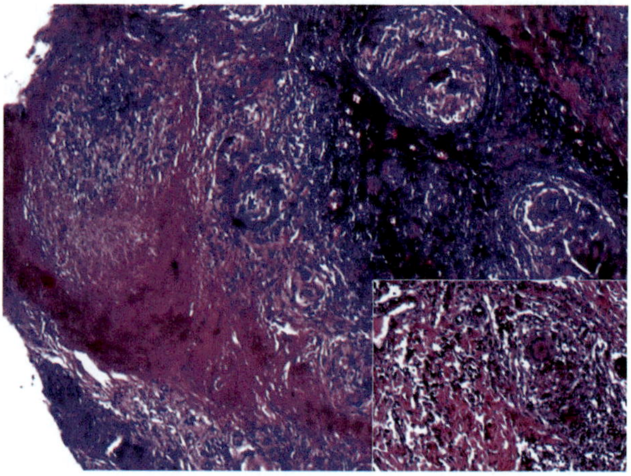

Fig. 15.2 Syphilitic granulomas with gumma necrosis, HE, 40× (inset: granuloma with multinucleated giant cell, HE, 400×)

development of thoracic aortic fusiform aneurysm and atheroma, with rupture and hemorrhage [51, 52].

Serological tests for syphilis (STS) [53, 54] contributes to the diagnosis. Non-treponemal tests (NTT)—e.g. the Venereal Diseases Research Laboratory test (VDRL), the Rapid Plasma Reagin test (RPR) and the Toluidine Red Unheated Serum Test (TRUST) are easy to perform and correlates with the activity of the disease and can be used to verify treatment efficacy. Treponemal tests (TT) are also frequently used: *T. pallidum* Haemagglutination test (TPHA), Micro-Haemagglutination Assay for *T. pallidum* (MHA-TP), *T. pallidum* Passive Particle Agglutination test (TPPA), Fluorescent Treponemal Antibody absorption test (FTA-abs test), Treponemal Enzyme Immunoassay (EIA) or Enzyme-Linked Immunosorbent Assay (ELISA), Chemiluminescence Immunoassay (CLIA), IgG or IgM immunoblot test for *T. pallidum* [55]. TT are very specific and remain positive for the whole life therefore those tests are not used to verify the treatment efficacy [55]. Other tests as the Point-of-Care tests (POCTs) have been developed [54–56] but are not used in Europe.

Investigations for the cardiovascular disease must be performed in any patient with syphilis. Chest X-ray can show the dilatation of the aorta or calcium deposits (although rare, ascending aorta calcification beginning just above the sinuses with an 'eggshell' aspect is very typical of syphilitic aneurysm) (Fig. 15.3). When heart failure is present it is possible to observe alveolar edema, Kerley B lines, pleural effusions and cardiomegaly. An aortic aneurysm can be suspected if a wide mediastinum is seen and a linear 'eggshell' configuration is present at the level of the aortic arch and descending aorta (Fig. 15.4). The electrocardiogram (ECG) can record arrhythmias, bundle branch block, atrioventricular block, ST segment elevation/

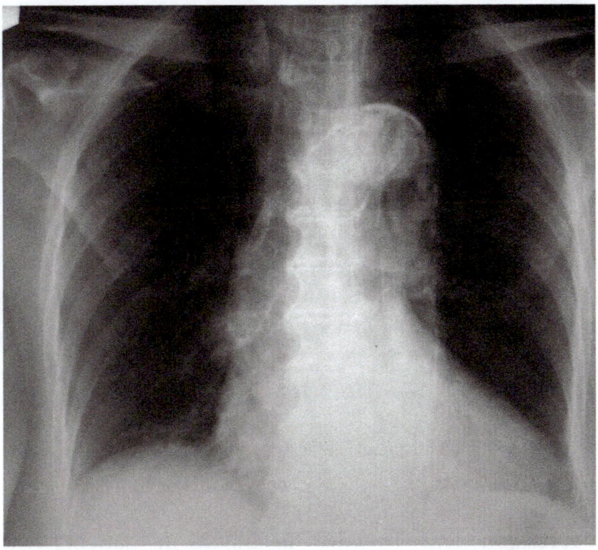

Fig. 15.3 Chest X-ray (postero-anterior view) with dilatation of the aorta and calcium deposits in a linear 'eggshell' configuration (image courtesy Dr. Sorin Paun)

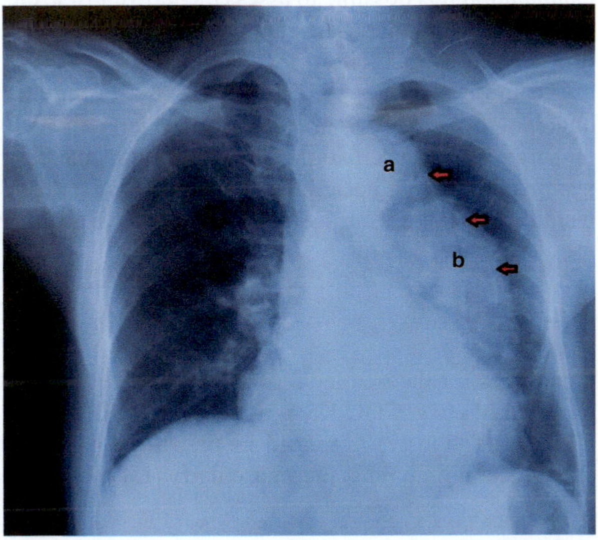

Fig. 15.4 Chest X-ray (postero-anterior view): aneurysmal dilatation at the level of the aortic arch (**a**) and descending aorta (**b**); linear "eggshell" configuration at the level of the aortic arch and descending aorta (red arrows)

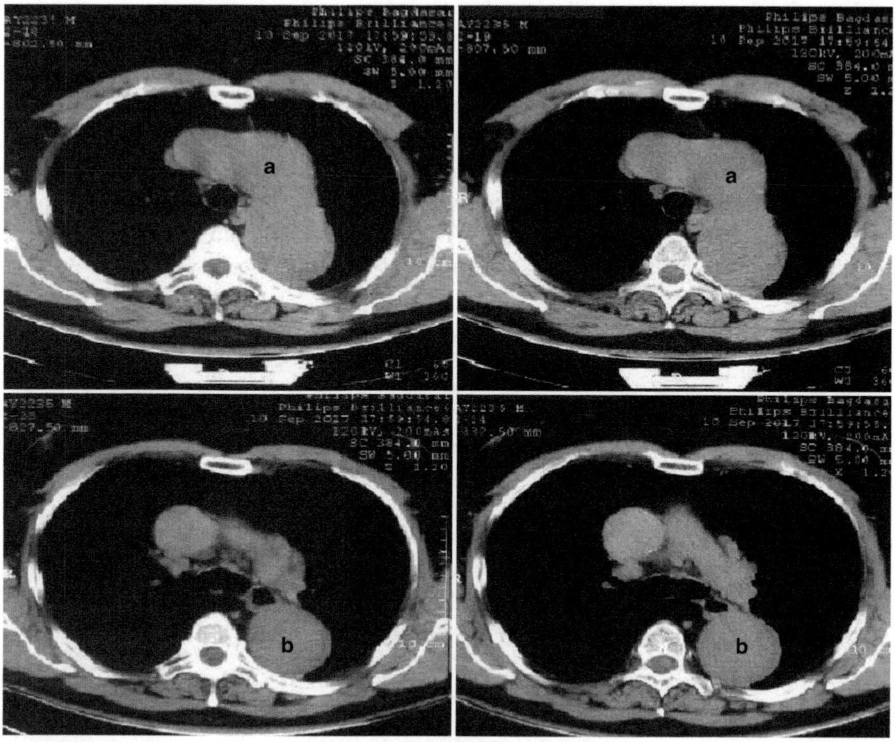

Fig. 15.5 Axial thoracic CT scans—aneurysmal dilation at the level of the aortic arch (**a**) and descending aorta (**b**)

depression and T wave inversion in patients with cardiovascular syphilis. Echocardiography shows valvular and aortic root abnormalities and in Doppler examination it is possible to assess the left ventricle ejection fraction and the degree of aortic regurgitation. The coronary angiography can detect the site and the degree of a stenosis.

An aortic aneurysm can be observed using computer tomography combined with angiography (Fig. 15.5) or in volume-rendered thoracic CT (Fig. 15.6).

Serologic cardiac biomarkers are having increasing levels in cardiovascular syphilis if acute myocarditis or heart failure occurs: CK, CK-MB, myoglobin, Cardiac troponin I, Cardiac troponin T and NT-proBNP.

Treatment

Guidelines for the treatment of syphilis are regularly up-dated by specific international bodies (e.g. CDC-USA, ECDC-EU, IUSTI) [2, 3]. Early syphilis (i.e. acquired <1 year previously) is treated as first line therapy with Benzathine penicillin G (BPG) 2.4 million units intramuscularly (IM) on day 1. Second line therapy option:

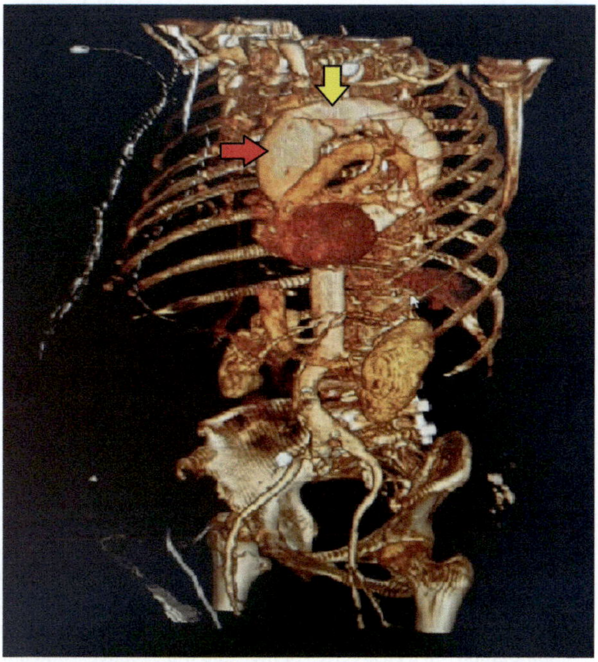

Fig. 15.6 Thoracic CT scan (coloured 3D scan—sagittal view): aneurysmal dilation at the level of the ascending aorta (red arrow) and aortic arch (yellow arrow)

Procaine penicillin 600,000 units IM daily for 10–14 days. In case of Penicillin allergy: Doxycycline 200 mg daily orally for 14 days [2].

In cases with late syphilis (i.e. acquired >1 year previously or of unknown duration)—including cardiovascular syphilis the first line therapy option is BPG 2.4 million units IM weekly on day 1, 8 and 15. Second line therapy option: Procaine penicillin 600,000 units IM daily, during 21 days. In case of Penicillin allergy: Doxycycline 200 mg orally daily, during 28 days [2]. Treatment will not cure the cardio-vascular damage (aortic valvular lesions, aneurysm) but is necessary to stop progression of the disease. Risk of severe Jarisch-Herxheimer reaction with worsening of angina pectoris, sudden death and aortic rupture are classical events in tertiary syphilis [57]. Penicillin therapy should be given with caution with in-patient management and prednisolone 20–60 mg daily for 3 days, starting syphilis treatment after 24 h of commencing prednisolone [2].

Guidelines for the management of cardiac disease are in use for the treatment of angina pectoris using nitrates, beta-blockers or calcium channel blockers [58]. For the management of coronary artery syndrome percutaneous coronary intervention (PCI) or coronary artery bypass graft can be used in selected cases followed by antiplatelet therapy [59, 60]. In the case of a patient with heart failure adequate rest, low sodium intake and reduced physical activities are recommended. Beta blockers, angiotensin converting enzyme inhibitors or diuretics will be also prescribed [61]. Cardiac transplantation or left ventricular assist devices are also taken into consideration.

In case of aortic aneurysms the patient will be closely monitored. Open surgery or endovascular stenting will be procedures used in patients with risk of aneurysmal rupture [62, 63].

References

1. European Centre for Disease Prevention and Control. Syphilis and congenital syphilis in Europe – A review of epidemiological trends (2007–2018) and options for response. Stockholm: ECDC; 2019. Stockholm, July 2019. ISBN 978-92-9498-343-5.
2. Janier M, Hegyi V, Dupin N, Unemo M, Tiplica GS, Potočnik M, French P, Patel R. 2014 European guideline on the management of syphilis. J Eur Acad Dermatol Venereol. 2014;28(12):1581–93.
3. Centers for Disease Control and Prevention. Syphilis (*Treponema pallidum*) 2018 Case Definition. Available at https://wwwn.cdc.gov/nndss/conditions/syphilis/case-definition/2018/. Last accessed on 30 November 2019.
4. French P. Syphilis. BMJ. 2007;334(7585):143–7.
5. Baker-Zander S, Sell S. A histopathologic and immunologic study of the course of syphilis in the experimentally infected rabbit. Demonstration of long-lasting cellular immunity. Am J Pathol. 1980;101(2):387.
6. Park KH, Lee MS, Hong IK, et al. Bone involvement in secondary syphilis: a case report and systematic review of the literature. Sex Transm Dis. 2014;41:532–7.
7. Davey DJ, Kojima N, Konda KA, et al. Transient aortitis documented by positron emission tomography in a case series of men and transgender women infected with syphilis. Sex Transm Infect. 2017;93:551–5.
8. Dombrowski JC, Pedersen R, Marra CM, Kerani R, Golden MR. Prevalence estimates of complicated syphilis. Sex Transm Dis. 2015;42:702–4.
9. Kennedy JL, Barnard JJ, Prahlow JA. Syphilitic coronary artery ostial stenosis resulting in acute myocardial infarction and death. Cardiology. 2006;105(1):25.
10. Wicher K, et al. Immunopathology of syphilis. In: Schell RF, et al., editors. Pathogenesis and immunology of treponemal infection. New York, NY: Marcel Dekker; 1983. p. 61.
11. Read PJ, Donovan B. Clinical aspects of adult syphilis. Intern Med J. 2012;42(6):614–20.
12. Soscia JL, Fusco JM, Grace WJ. Complete heart block due to a solitary gumma. Am J Cardiol. 1964;13(4):553–7.
13. Rowley J, Vander Hoorn S, Korenromp E, Low N, Unemo M, Abu-Raddad LJ, Chico RM, Smolak A, Newman L, Gottlieb S, Thwin SS, Broutet N, Taylor MM. Chlamydia, gonorrhoea, trichomoniasis and syphilis: global prevalence and incidence estimates, 2016. Bull World Health Organ. 2019;97(8):548.
14. Cohen SE, Klausner JD, Engelman J, Philip S. Syphilis in the modern era: an update for physicians. Infect Dis Clin N Am. 2013;27(4):705–22.
15. Centers for Disease Control and Prevention. Sexually transmitted diseases surveillance, 2017; https://www.cdc.gov/std/stats17/syphilis.htm. Last accessed November 17, 2019.
16. Centers for Disease Control and Prevention. Sexually Transmitted Disease Surveillance 2014. Atlanta: US Department of Health and Human Services, 2015.
17. Public Health England. Infection Report: Sexually Transmitted Infections. London: Public Health England, 2015.
18. Gjestland T. The Oslo study of untreated syphilis. Acta Derm Venereol (Stockh). 1955;35(Suppl. 34):3–368.
19. Talbot MD, Morton RS. The Tuskegee study of untreated syphilis. Eur J STD. 1984;1:125–32.
20. Sukthankar A. Syphilis. Medicine. 2014;42:394–8.
21. Jackman JD Jr, Radolf JD. Cardiovascular syphilis. Am J Med. 1989;87(4):425–33.
22. Heggtveit HA. Syphilitic aortitis: a clinicopathologic autopsy study of 100 cases, 1950 to 1960. Circulation. 1964;29(3):346–55.

23. Bernal Ruiz AI, Gonzalez Ruiz A, Gutierrez Rodriguez C, Garcia MM. Generalized macular rash with palmar–plantar involvement associated with lymphadenopathies. Secondary lues. Rev Clin Esp. 2001;201:101–2.
24. Dourmishev LA, Dourmishev AL. Syphilis: uncommon presentations in adults. Clin Dermatol. 2005;23(6):555–64.
25. Griffiths C, Barker J, Bleiker T, Chalmers R, Creamer D, editors. Rook's textbook of dermatology. 8th ed: Wiley Blackwell; 2016. p. 1575.
26. Baughn RE, Musher DM. Secondary syphilitic lesions. Clin Microbiol Rev. 2005;18(1):205–16.
27. Mullooly C, Higgins SP. Secondary syphilis: the classical triad of skin rash, mucosal ulceration and lymphadenopathy. Int J STD AIDS. 2010;21(8):537–45.
28. de Paulo LF, Servato JP, Oliveira MT, Durighetto AF Jr, Zanetta-Barbosa D. Oral manifestations of secondary syphilis. Int J Infect Dis. 2015;35:40–2.
29. Petzoldt D. Syphilis. In: Burgdorf WH, Plewig G, Wolff HH, Landthaler M, editors. Braun-Falco's dermatology. 3rd ed: Springer; 2009. p. 257–74.
30. Bittencourt MD, Brito AC, Nascimento BA, Carvalho AH, Drago MG. Nodular tertiary syphilis in an immunocompetent patient. An Bras Dermatol. 2016;91(4):528–30.
31. Forrestel AK, Kovarik CL, Katz KA. Sexually acquired syphilis. Part 1: Historical aspects, microbiology, epidemiology, and clinical manifestations. J Am Acad Dermatol. 2020;82(1):1–14.
32. Little JW. Syphilis: an update. Oral Surg Oral Med Oral Pathol Oral Radiol Endod. 2005;100(1):3–9.
33. Fournier A, Fournier E. Traité de la syphilis. Rueff Ed. Paris; 1904; T2 Syphilis du Coeur. p. 758.
34. Darier J. De l'artérite syphilitique. J Rueff. 1904:1–168.
35. Janier M, Pertuiset BF, Poisson M, Bleibel JM, Buge A. Early manifestations of neuromeningeal syphilis. Review of the literature apropos of 3 severe forms. In Annales de dermatologie et de venereologie 1985 (Vol. 112, No. 2, pp. 133–140).
36. Lowenstein DH, Mills C, Simon RP. Acute syphilitic transverse myelitis: unusual presentation of meningovascular syphilis. Sex Transm Infect. 1987;63(5):333–8.
37. Kösters K. Bleeker-Rovers CP, Van Crevel R, Oyen WJ, Van der Ven AJ. Aortitis Diagnosed by F–18–Fluorodeoxyglucose Positron Emission Tomography in a Patient with Syphilis and HIV Coinfection. Infection. 2005;33(5–6):387–9.
38. Dabis R, Radcliffe K. Is it useful to perform a chest X-ray in asymptomatic patients with late latent syphilis? Int J STD AIDS. 2011;22(2):105–6.
39. Katz KA. Chapter 200. Syphilis. In: Goldsmith LA, Katz SI, Gilchrest B, Paller AS, Leffell DJ, Wolff K, editors. Fitzpatrick's dermatology in general medicine. 8th ed: The McGraw-Hill Companies; 2012. p. 2471–92.
40. Hijikata S, Hongo I, Nakayama SI, Yamaguchi T, Sekikawa Y, Nozato T, Ashikaga T. Infective endocarditis due to *Treponema pallidum*: a case diagnosed using polymerase chain reaction analysis of aortic valve. Can J Cardiol. 2019;35(1):104–e9.
41. Myerburg RJ, Interian A Jr, Mitrani RM, Kessler KM, Castellanos A. Frequency of sudden cardiac death and profiles of risk. Am J Cardiol. 1997;80(5):10F–9F.
42. Hook EW III. Syphilis. Lancet. 2017;389:1550–7.
43. Roberts WC, Bose R, Ko JM, Henry AC, Hamman BL. Identifying cardiovascular syphilis at operation. Am J Cardiol. 2009;104(11):1588–94.
44. Tsokos M. Syphilitic aortic aneurysm rupture as cause of sudden death. Forensic Sci Med Pathol. 2012;8(3):325–6.
45. Maleszewski JJ. Inflammatory ascending aortic disease: perspectives from pathology. J Thorac Cardiovasc Surg. 2015;149(2):S176–83.
46. Stansal A, Mirault T, Rossi A, Dupin N, Bruneval P, Bel A, Azarine A, Minozzi C, Deman AL, Messas E. Recurrent tamponade and aortic dissection in syphilis. Ann Thorac Surg. 2013;96(5):e111–3.
47. Ro A, Mori S, Kageyama N, Chiba S, Mukai T. Ruptured syphilitic aneurysm: a cause of sudden death in a man with human immunodeficiency coinfection. J Forensic Sci. 2019;64:1555–8.

48. Maharajan M, Kumaar GS. Cardiovascular syphilis in HIV infection: a case-control study at the Institute of Sexually Transmitted Diseases, Chennai, India. Sex Transm Infect. 2005;81(4):361.
49. Marks M, Lawrence D, Kositz C, Mabey D. Diagnostic performance of PCR assays for the diagnosis of neurosyphilis: a systematic review. Sex Transm Infect. 2018;94:585–8.
50. Müller H, Eisendle K, Bräuninger W, Kutzner H, Cerroni L, Zelger B. Comparative analysis of immuno-histochemistry, polymerase chain reaction and focus-floating microscopy for the detection of *Treponema pallidum* in mucocutaneous lesions of primary, secondary and tertiary syphilis. Br J Dermatol. 2011;165:50–60.
51. Riede UN, Werner M. "Elastin Lesions: Elastin Lysis Disorders – Syphilitic aortitis", p. 58, & "Flexible Spiral Gram-Negative Bacteria", p. 262, in "Color atlas of pathology", Georg Thieme Verlag, 2004.
52. Strayer DS. Emanuel Rubin: "Blood Vessels", Chapter 16. In: Rubin's pathology – clinicopathologic foundations in medicine. 7th ed: Lippincott Williams & Wilkins; 2015. p. 613–4.
53. Larsen SA, Steiner BM, Rudolph AH. Laboratory diagnosis and interpretation of tests for syphilis. Clin Microbiol Rev. 1995;8:1–21.
54. Park IU, Fakile YF, Chow JM, et al. Performance of Treponemal Tests for the diagnosis of syphilis. Clin Infect Dis. 2019;68:913–8.
55. Ballard R, Hook III EW. Syphilis. In: Laboratory diagnosis of sexually transmitted infections, including human immunodeficiency virus. World Health Organization (WHO). 2013.
56. Gliddon HD, Peeling R, Kamb ML, Toskin I, Wi TE, Taylor MM. A systematic review and meta-analysis of studies evaluating the performance and operational characteristics of dual point-of-care tests for HIV and syphilis. Sex Transm Infect. 2017;93(S4):S3–S15.
57. Degos R, Lortat-Jacob E, Macrez P. Sero-positive syphilitic aorto-myocarditis in a woman treated during 20 years and after several years of negative serology. Bulletin de la Societe francaise de dermatologie et de syphiligraphie. 1970;77(1):32–3.
58. Zanger DR, Solomon AJ, Gersh BJ. Contemporary management of angina: part II. Medical management of chronic stable angina. Am Fam Physician. 2000;61(1):129–38.
59. Knuuti J, et al., 2019 ESC Guidelines for the diagnosis and management of chronic coronary syndromes: The Task Force for the diagnosis and management of chronic coronary syndromes of the European Society of Cardiology (ESC).
60. Nakazone MA, Machado MN, Barbosa RB, Santos MA, Maia LN. Syphilitic coronary artery ostial stenosis resulting in acute myocardial infarction treated by percutaneous coronary intervention. Case Rep Med. 2010;2010
61. Ponikowski P, Voors AA, Anker SD, Bueno H, Cleland JG, Coats AJ, Falk V, González-Juanatey JR, Harjola VP, Jankowska EA, Jessup M. 2016 ESC Guidelines for the diagnosis and treatment of acute and chronic heart failure: The Task Force for the diagnosis and treatment of acute and chronic heart failure of the European Society of Cardiology (ESC). Developed with the special contribution of the Heart Failure Association (HFA) of the ESC. Eur J Heart Fail. 2016;18(8):891–975.
62. Erbel R, Aboyans V, Boileau C, Bossone E, Di Bartolomeo R, Eggebrecht H, Evangelista A, Falk V, Frank H, Gaemperli O, Grabenwöger M. 2014 ESC guidelines on the diagnosis and treatment of aortic diseases. Rev Esp Cardiol. 2015;68(3):242.
63. Abbruzzese TA, Kwolek CJ, Brewster DC, Chung TK, Kang J, Conrad MF, LaMuraglia GM, Cambria RP. Outcomes following endovascular abdominal aortic aneurysm repair (EVAR): an anatomic and device-specific analysis. J Vasc Surg. 2008;48(1):19–28.

Viral Conditions 16

Eliza Cinteza

Varicella

Introduction and Pathophysiology of Disease

Varicella (chickenpox) is a primary infectious disease caused by varicello-zosterian virus (VZV). The varicello-zosterian virus can cause both varicella and herpes zoster (shingles) in case of reactivation. Usually, the infection is self-limiting. VZV is a DNA virus that belongs to the herpesvirus family. There are many subgroups of the herpesvirus (α, β, and γ). VZV is an α herpesvirus [1, 2].

Infection is contacted via Pflugge drops. There are two viraemic stages: the first when the virus disseminates to respiratory mucosa and ganglia where initially replicates and the second when rash onset occurs [1]. After the infection disappears, VZV remains latent in the dorsal ganglia cells [3] and reactivates in immunodeficiency conditions or in the elderly, generating herpes zoster infection involving one or more dermatomes [3]. The virus invades the cells and replicates inside the nucleus generating intranuclear inclusion bodies. Local inflammation is the factor that promotes the second viremia. The replication of the virus at the epidermal level generates focal necrosis, with immune response and infiltration with leukocytes generating vesicles and pustules. The incubation period lasts for 14–17 days. At the time of the maculopapular eruption, there are processes of vasculitis of the small vessels and fusion of the epithelial cells [3]. The "ballooning" process of the epithelial cells is responsible for the vesicular appearance. The infectivity lasts for 7 days (2 days before the onset of the rash and 5 days after) [3]. The distribution of the vesicles is centripetal. In the absence of an appropriate cellular immune response, the severity of the infection increases becoming even fatal. But with a good immune

E. Cinteza (✉)
Cardiology Department "Marie Curie" Emergency Children's Hospital, Pediatrics Department
"Carol Davila" University of Medicine and Pharmacy, Bucharest, Romania

C. Salavastru et al. (eds.), *Skin and the Heart*,
https://doi.org/10.1007/978-3-030-54779-0_16

response, the infection diminishes in intensity and stops without complete eradication of the virus. With clinical recovery, the virus remains latent into the cells, without being eliminated and this is a characteristic of the whole group of herpesviruses. Usually, there are no cutaneous scars as a consequence of the viral infection [1].

Prevalence/Population Affected

It is the most frequent disease in children associated with a pruritic vesicular rash [3]. The geographical regions where varicella is the most prevalent in children are those with a temperate climate. The incidence of varicella was approximated at 15 cases/1000 people/year [1]. 50% of the infections occur in children less than 5 years old and 85% up to the puberty. 95% of young adults have antibodies against varicella. In pregnant women in the US the incidence is rare, 0.7 per 1000 women [3, 4]. If a pregnant woman between 8 to 20 weeks gestation is affected by varicella virus, then congenital varicella syndrome may appear in a less than 2% [4].

Herpes zoster, the recurrence of the VZV infection, has an incidence of 3.4 cases/1000 persons/year in adults over 45 years old and increases to 10 cases/1000 persons/year in adults over 75 years old [3].

Dermatological Manifestations

The onset is with fever, malaise, headache and abdominal pain followed in 1 or 2 days of papules which became vesicles in a short time. These symptoms may be absent in children and well expressed in adults. Fever may be important, 40–41 °C lasting for several days. Initially, there is an erythematous pruritic rash. Shortly, the vesicles appear and they have clear content. But, in a few hours, they became pustules with turbid content and a red areola surrounding the pustules with the appearance of "dewdrop on a rose petal". They are pruriginous. The vesicles repeatedly appear, three to five times during 2–4 days being at the same time maculo-papules, vesicles, pustules, and crusts, in different stages of development (Fig. 16.1) [4]. Usually, there are 100–300 lesions, but there may be between 10 and 1500 [3]. The vesicles sometimes have different aspects, either tend to become bullous or they look umbilicated. The distribution is centripetal over the tegument of the trunk, face, scalp, limbs or at the level of the oral, genital, anal mucosa, and conjunctiva. It is more profound at the proximal part of the limbs. They can degenerate into ulcers of the mucosa [1].

In congenital varicella syndrome, there are cicatricial skin lesions, with dermatomal distribution looking pigmented and depressed associated with ocular defects (microphthalmos, nystagmus, chorioretinitis, cataracts), limb abnormalities, and intrauterine growth restriction [4].

In children, the clinical picture usually is mild to moderate, but in adults is moderate to severe [5].

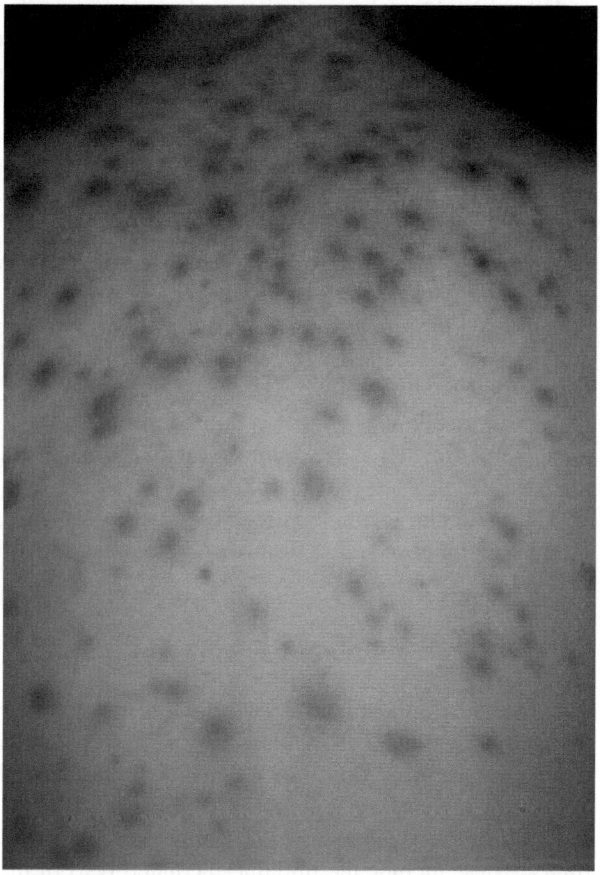

Fig. 16.1 Varicella in a 17-year-old boy

Other types of varicella may be present. In *hemorrhagic varicella,* the eruption contains hemorrhagic vesicles and it is accompanied by fever and other symptoms. Frequently is associated with malnutrition or in immunodeficiency disorders. *Varicella during pregnancy* is another serious disease for both mother and child. In these cases, the syndrome of congenital varicella may appear with neurological problems and a 30% mortality in the first year of life [1]. Secondary bacterial infection with *Streptococcus pyogenes* may lead to *varicella gangrenosa.* This is manifested as a single lesion surrounded rapidly by extended erythema.

Histological

There are many histological characteristics in varicella. The most common is "ballooning degeneration" and giant cell formation. Ballooning of the cytoplasm of the cells of the Malpighian layer is due to the intracellular edema. Multinucleated giant cells (in herpes simplex, herpes zoster, and varicella) have more than eight nuclei and they are the result of the fusion of the epithelial cells.

Other histological aspects that are found in varicella are the degenerative nuclear changes (with many forms), condensation of chromatin of the nuclear membrane, eosinophilic inclusion bodies loss of staining of the keratinocytes, and areas of focal necrosis into the liver, kidney and other organs.

Differential Diagnosis

Varicella manifestations are differentiated from other vesicular lesions that may be present in systemic viral infections such as Poxviruses, herpes simplex, varicella zoster, Coxsackie, enteroviruses, rickettsial pox, stomatitis virus, Ebola, Marburg. Also, some bacterial infections may be differentiated from varicella, most often infection with *Staphylococcus aureus*. Other situations in which the differential diagnosis of varicella is necessary may be drug reactions, contact dermatitis, or insect bites.

Also, varicella may be differentiated from diseases generating macular or maculopapular rash such as Echovirus, Rubella, Ebstein Barr, herpes virus 6 (roseola), togaviruses, measles, parvovirus.

The particular characteristics of varicella rely on centripetal distribution, rapid progression of each lesion from vesicle to crust, repetitive eruptions [1].

Cardiological Manifestations

The cardiac implication in varicella infection is very rare but it may be life-threatening. Varicella virus, like other cardiotropic viruses, may affect the heart generating myocarditis. This association is described since 1953 by Hackel as interstitial myocarditis during an epidemy of chicken pox [6]. The mechanism of myocarditis in viral infections is unknown. There are several proposed pathways of myocardial injury. These include the immune-mediated lysis of the myocardium by infiltration of immune cells targeting the infected cardiomyocytes, autoimmune-mediated destruction of cardiac cells by autoantibodies, and direct virus-induced cardiac myocyte injury. Stages of myocarditis include viral replication, acute injury of the myocytes and progression to dilated cardiomyopathy [7].

The diagnosis of pediatric myocarditis may be difficult, with a wide spectrum of clinical manifestation between asymptomatic to angina, syncope, arrhythmias, and fulminant cardiac failure or sudden death [7–11]. Another important clinical feature of the cardiac involvement in varicella infection is that skin lesions precedes myocarditis in most cases. However, diagnosis of varicella myocarditis becomes challenging when skin rash succeeds cardiac manifestations, described in a few case reports [12].

Arrhythmias may complicate the evolution with supraventricular tachycardia, ventricular tachycardia and fibrillation, and complete heart block. Other described complications are the secondary pericardial effusion and endocarditis both due to secondary bacterial infection. Cardiac tamponade or pericardial constriction may appear in the evolution of the pericardial effusion. Streptococcus and Staphylococcus are most often responsible for secondary bacterial complications [2]. Diagnosis remains largely based on clinical judgment, supported by ancillary tests. Therefore, a high index of suspicion is necessary [7].

Investigations

Of utmost importance in the diagnosis of cardiac implications are the electrocardiogram, cardiac enzymes, echocardiography (Fig. 16.2), cardiac magnetic resonance (Fig. 16.3), and endomyocardial biopsy. The electrocardiogram (Fig. 16.4) may show rhythm or conduction problems, Q wave, decreased voltage of the R waves, T waves changes, or depression of the ST interval. Echocardiography is very useful in evaluation of the heart from a structural and functional point of view. Myocarditis usually is manifesting as dilated left ventricle with poor regional and global systolic function. Both ventricles may be implicated, with increased filling pressures and dilated atria [13–16].

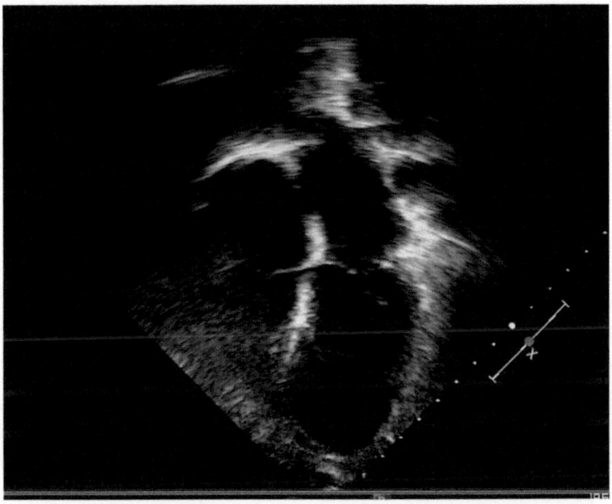

Fig. 16.2 Echocardiographic image in a 12-year-old boy with viral myocarditis. In this apical four chamber image the dilated left ventricle in the apical part can be seen

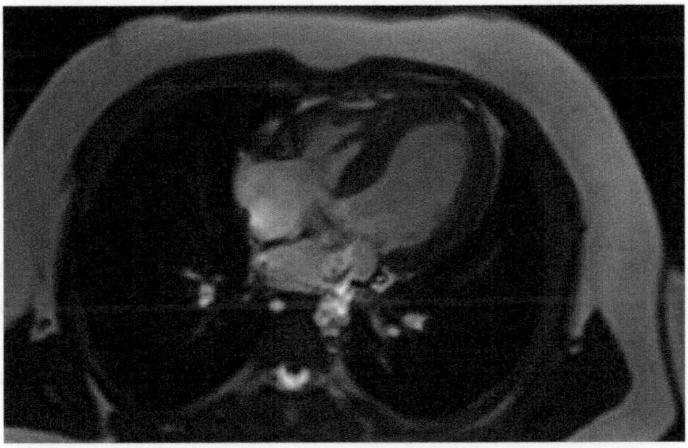

Fig. 16.3 MRI image in the same patient which confirms the echocardiographic findings

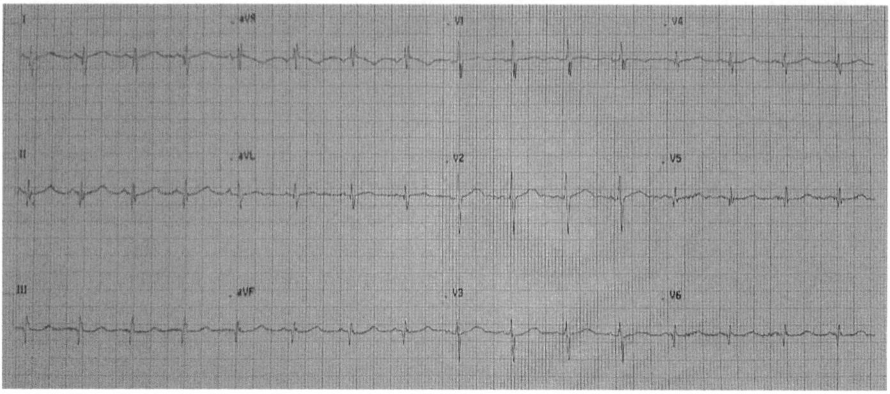

Fig. 16.4 Electrocardiographic image of the same patient which shows deep Q waves in the inferolateral leads and diminished R wave potential in D I, D II, D III, aVL, aVF, V3-V6

Cardiac magnetic resonance is very helpful in evaluating the criteria for myocarditis by showing inflammation in the myocardium as early and late myocardial gadolinium enhancement to identify edema, hyperemia, and capillary leakage and necrosis and fibrosis for late enhancement [14, 17].

The standard method for the diagnosis of myocarditis is the endomyocardial biopsy for histopathology and other techniques for identifying the viral genome. The certitude diagnosis of myocarditis is done using the Dallas criteria based on the endomyocardial biopsy.

Endomyocardial biopsy (EMB) is a widely accepted method for diagnosing myocarditis, based upon histopathology, immunohistology and molecular techniques to identify viral genomes. Rare but severe complications are associated with the biopsy such as perforation and cardiac tamponade, 0.1 to 0.5% [14, 17].

Diagnosis/Investigations

The ***usual investigations*** are needed in the first diagnostic phase. Complete blood count (CBC) may show lymphopenia and granulocytopenia. The hepatic function may be altered [3].

Helpful for the rapid diagnosis is the ***diagnostic investigations*** such as polymerase chain reaction (PCR) for detection of the DNA, Besides PCR there are other investigations that may be performed for a positive diagnosis such as virus culture, viral proteinin, examination of histological specimens, electronic microscopy for virus visualization, detection of viral antigen using direct fluorescent antibodies (DFA), and serological tests [1, 3]. The PCR is the test of choice for rapid diagnosis being used in severe or uncertain cases. It has a high sensibility and is using vesicular swabs, scabs from crusted lesions [4]. Also, the DFA may assure a rapid diagnosis but the sensibility is decreased compared with the PCR. Serological tests detect the acute and convalescent phase of varicella by evaluating IgM and IgG antibodies to VZV [3]. IgM evaluation is less specific with frequent false positive results.

There are other tests such as a fluorescent anti-membrane antibody (FAMA), enzyme-linked immunosorbent assay (ELISA), latex agglutination (LA), and complement that can be used but they are not frequently used in clinical practice [4, 14].

Treatment

There are many possibilities to intervene in varicella by actioning with pre-exposure prophylaxis, postexposure prophylaxis, etiological antiviral therapy or only with symptomatic therapy. The approach depends on the severity of the illness, of the immunological status of the patient and underlying disease [5].

Pre-exposure Prophylaxis

The first live attenuated vaccine against varicella was developed from the Oka strain, by Takahashi, during the 1970s. The vaccine has a seroconversion rate of 90% and 75% of them maintain the good level of antibodies up to 10 years [1]. Vaccination against varicella during childhood does not prevent herpes zoster in adulthood. The main indications for this vaccine are for patient's HIV positive, in patients with leukemia in remission, before immunosuppressive treatment [1]. Congenital immunodeficiencies, symptomatic HIV infection, high-dose systemic corticosteroids for longer periods, salicylates within 6 weeks, immunoglobulin within 5 months, pregnancy, exposure to varicella or zoster within 21 days are contraindications for vaccination [3]. Although mortality from VZ is rare, it is ultimately preventable through vaccination [8].

Post-exposure Prophylaxis

Within 3 days after exposure (preferably 48 h) to varicella virus, the treatment using specific zoster immunoglobulins (VariZIG, varicella zoster immune globulin) can be administered [18]. It reduces the intensity of the clinical manifestations and sometimes may even prevent it. This prophylaxis may be used also in newborns from mother exposed to varicella from 7 days before to 7 days after delivery. If the VariZIG is not available, intravenous immunoglobulin or acyclovir may be administered [4].

Antiviral Treatment

Treatment with acyclovir is recommended in varicella infection in adults, or severe varicella or zoster at any age in immunocompromised patients (malignancy, bone marrow or organ transplantation, high-dose steroid therapy, congenital T-cell immunodeficiencies, HIV infection), in neonatal varicella after maternal varicella, associated pneumonia or encephalitis) [1, 3]. In healthy children usually is necessary only symptomatic treatment with antipyretic treatment and antiseptic applications. But aspirin should be strongly avoided in varicella due to the risk of Reye syndrome [4].

For special conditions, the first line antiviral treatment in varicella is acyclovir. This should be administered within 9–10 days after exposure or in 24 h after the onset of the rash. It has to be administered for 1 week [3]. If it is not administered immediately visceral dissemination may occur, with significant morbidity and mortality in patients with immune deficiencies, or after cortico-therapy.

Acyclovir may be administered intravenously (500 mg/m^2 per dose every 8 h) or orally (20 mg/kg/dose, four times a day in children or 800 mg/dose given as five doses per day, for 5–7 days). Intravenous administration is recommended in patients with moderate to severe disease who associate pneumonia, hepatitis, thrombocytopenia, or encephalitis. Also, associated antibiotical therapy is not uncommon when secondary bacterial infection is suspected. In cases with resistance to acyclovir, Foscarnet may be used [5].

Co-administration of immunoglobulin and acyclovir it is accepted in some clinics and it may be recommended in severely immunocompromised patients [3].

The treatment of myocarditis should cover also the treatment of the heart failure, with inotropic drugs, diuretics, and angiotensin-converting-enzyme inhibitors and mechanical ventilation, mechanical cardiac support and cardiac transplantation if need it [7].

Prognosis/Complications

Mortality in high-risk patients decreased with vaccination and antiviral therapy from 10% to few [3]. But, in neonates, the mortality rate is still up to 30% [4].

Complications in varicella are rare (2%), but severe. They include pulmonary, cardiac, neurological implication, secondary bacterial infections of the skin, soft tissue or heart usually associated with *Staphylococcus aureus* or group A streptococcal infection. Cardiac and vascular complications (myocarditis, pericarditis, endocarditis, vascular thrombosis, severe arrhythmias) are rare, but life threatening [2, 19, 20]. They can appear not only in the acute phase of disease but also years after the initial infection [19]. In the case of reactivation, defined as herpes zoster, complications may still develop [21–26]. The persistence of the viral genome in myocardium generates chronic inflammation that impedes the recovery of left ventricular function. Viral persistence in the myocardium is associated with progressive cardiac dysfunction.

Varicella pneumonia—develops between 4 and 8 days in immunodeficient patients [3]. It is visible on a chest X-ray in 10% of adults.

Neurological complications include meningoencephalitis, cerebellar ataxia, transverse myelitis, ophthalmoplegia, transient hepatitis, orchitis, pancreatitis.

Secondary bacterial infection is due to *S. aureus* or *Streptococcus pyogenes*, such as pneumonia, arthritis or osteomyelitis, even fatal sepsis or necrotizing fasciitis [3].

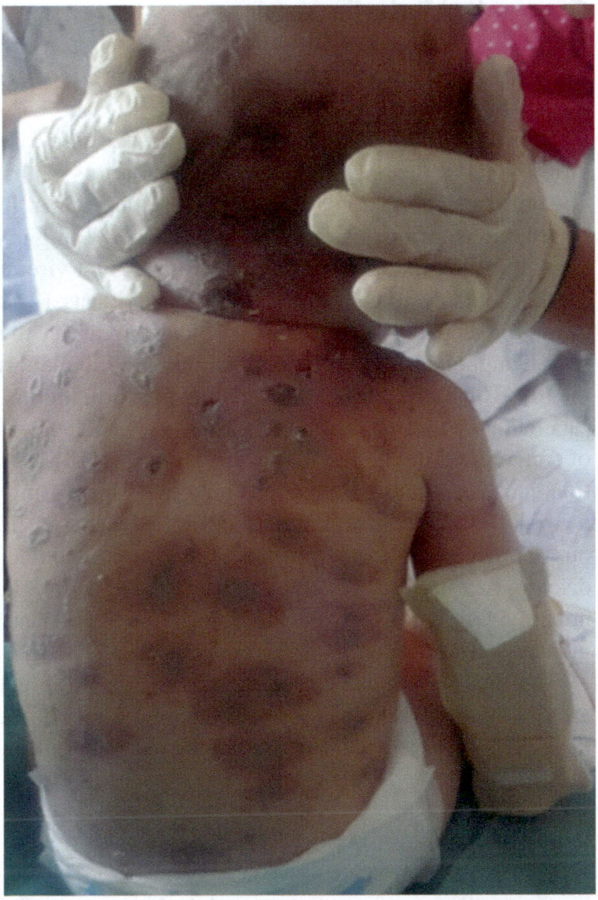

Fig. 16.5 "Varicella gangrenosa" (Archive of "Matei Bals" National Institute for Infectious Diseases, Bucharest, with permission)

Hemorrhagic complications are also described, but they are more frequently identified in adults than in children. They may be associated with thrombocytopenia—petechiae, purpura, epistaxis or with disseminated intravascular coagulopathy.

The reactivation of VZV from latency causes a localized, pruritic, vesicular rash. Although the rash is the hallmark of herpes zoster, "zoster sine herpete" is diagnosed in patients who have acute unilateral neuropathic pain but no rash [3].

Other severe complications include 'varicella gangrenosa' (Fig. 16.5) secondary to local infection, rhabdomyolysis, Reye syndrome, Stevens-Johnson syndrome, erythema multiforme.

Chronic varicella was described with persistent hyperkeratotic lesions but, usually, varicella infection confers lifelong immunity [1, 2].

Congenital Rubella

Introduction and Pathophysiology of Disease

Rubella or German measles is an infectious disease caused by an RNA virus, rubella virus, which is the only member of the Rubivirus genus and belongs to the family of Togaviridae. There are twelve genotypes, but four of them are responsible for 70% of infections. Transmission is interhuman, by Pflugge drops into the nasopharynx. After invading the respiratory epithelium, a first viremia occurs towards the reticuloendothelial system. The incubation period lasts 12–21 days. After the incubation period, a second viremia occurs which may affect the fetus by the transplacental way. Congenital rubella is the infection with rubella virus acquired during intrauterine life. The highest risk for congenital malformation is associated with acquiring of rubella in the first 10 weeks of fetal life (80–100%), with decreasing risk to the fetus of congenital infection in the second trimester (10–20%) [27]. The congenital infection causes cellular damage, has an effect on dividing cells and is associated with the risk for fetal malformations of various types such as miscarriage, stillbirth, various congenital malformation. The most common defects consist of congenital heart disease, hearing impairment, cataract or congenital glaucoma and pigmentary retinopathy. Gregg was the first to describe it in 1941 as a combination of three elements: deafness, cataract and cardiac disease [1, 28].

The precise mechanism of congenital rubella infection is not known, but there are two possibilities. One is the cytopathic effect of the virus which induces apoptosis, and the other one is related to the virus inhibition of cell division [28].

Prevalence/Population Affected

It affects all ages, from fetus to adult, being more frequent in older children and young adults [1]. Each year there are more than 100.000 new cases around the world. It is endemic mostly in an urban area during spring. America was declared free of rubella in 2015 [1, 28].

Dermatological Manifestations

Clinical manifestations are different between the classical form and congenital rubella syndrome. Classical rubella manifestations are important to be evaluated in pregnant women. It is manifested as prodromal symptoms, adenopathy, and rash which appears after the incubation period, and it is the most frequent cause of rash in older children. The onset may be with fever, not higher than 39 °C, headache, malaise. The rash has a caudal progression.

The rash is present in 60% of the infections and is represented by discrete pink macules which tend to become confluent [1] (Fig. 16.6). Any manifestation in the

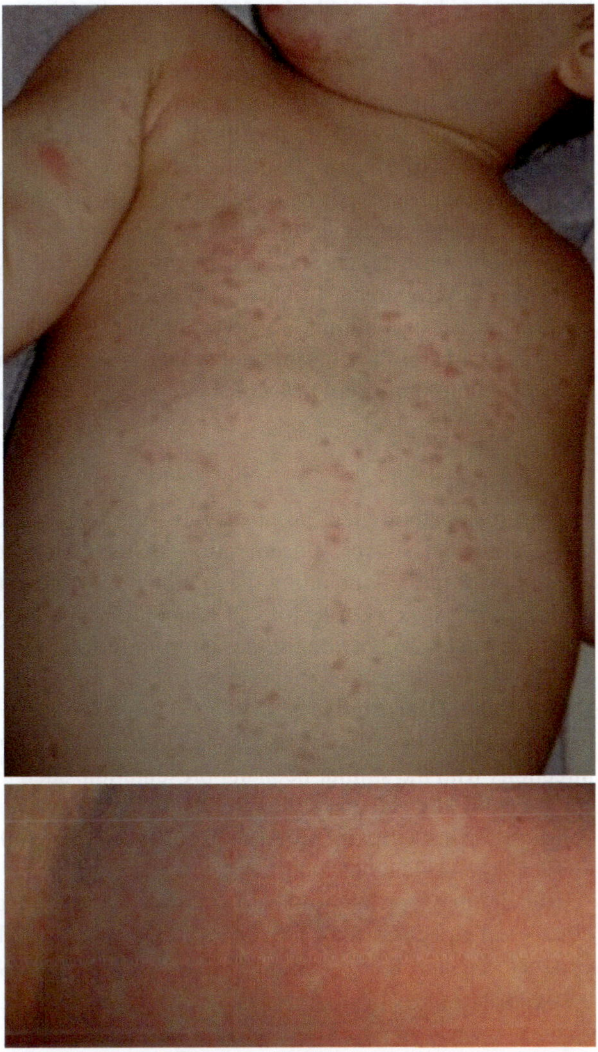

Fig. 16.6 Rubella in infant. (Courtesy of Professor Anca Chiriac, Department of Dermatology, Apollonia University, Iasi, Romania)

fetus including fetal growth restriction should be evaluated for congenital rubella syndrome [29].

As dermatological manifestation, congenital rubella syndrome may appear as "blueberry muffin lesions" with petechiae and purpura. These are occasionally found in severe cases and are usually present at birth or appear after a free interval of a few months. They represent collections of extramedullary hematopoiesis and spontaneously regress. The lesions appear as violaceous red papules and nodules 2–8 mm in diameter, in association with hyperpigmentation of the face, hyperseborrhoea and vasomotor instability with cyanosis of the extremities. Chronic erythematous exanthema is unusual, affecting preferentially the face and the four limbs.

Some reports have described cutaneous manifestations including *cutis marmorata*, seborrhea, vasculitis, recurrent urticaria and hyperpigmentation (forehead, cheeks, and umbilical area). Rarely, generalized maculopapular eruptions have been seen during the newborn period and persist for several weeks [29–31].

Together with dermatological findings, other manifestations may be part of the clinical picture in congenital rubella infection such as sensorineural deafness, cataract, glaucoma, retinopathy, hepatosplenomegaly, adenopathy, thrombocytopenia, hemolytic anemia, dysgammaglobulinemia, interstitial pneumonia, cardiac defects, meningoencephalitis, mental retardation, microcephaly, poor physical and neuromuscular development. Infants with rubella syndrome tend to have low birth weight due to a combination of prematurity and interference with intrauterine growth. Apart from the brain, the parenchymal organs rarely appear to be affected in this group of children, most of the abnormalities being in mesenchymal tissues [31, 32].

Histological

From a histopathological point of view, the features that are commonly seen are massive necrosis, severe degeneration, distortion and disorientation of the fibers. They were described including the ophthalmological pathology [33]. The histologic examination of the skin lesions in congenital rubella syndrome shows a predominantly dermal lymphocytic inflammatory infiltrate, and perivascular [29].

Differential Diagnosis

It is mandatory to differentiate congenital rubella syndrome from other congenital infections with the similar neonatal presentation, such as congenital toxoplasmosis, cytomegalovirus infection, congenital syphilis, congenital herpes simplex virus, congenital Zika virus infection or from other causes that may generate a hearing loss, cataracts, glaucoma, cardiac malformations [28].

Rubella may appear similar to smallpox, scarlet fever and drug reactions. Also, other viral infection may have a macular aspect of the rash such as echovirus, Coxsackie A and B, Ebstein-Barr virus, Human herpesvirus 6 (roseola) or human herpesvirus 7 [1].

Cardiological Manifestations: Clinical

Congenital heart disease together with ocular malformations appears if the maternal infection occurs before 18 weeks of gestational age. 80–85% of the fetuses exposed to rubella during the first trimester may have congenital malformations [28]. The most frequent congenital heart disease associated with congenital rubella syndrome are patent ductus arteriosus and pulmonary arteries stenosis. Congenital stenosis of the pulmonary branches may be single or multiple, unilateral or bilateral, peripheral or central. It may be hemodynamically benign or associated with severe right ventricular hypertrophy and dilatation.

Other rare lesions also may be associated with CRS. They are tetralogy of Fallot, ventricular septal defect, pulmonary valvular stenosis, aortic valve stenosis, aortic coarctation.

Stenosis of the coronary, cerebral, renal or peripheral vessels, by the fibromuscular proliferation of the intima and sclerosis of arteries, may appear as long-term complications in adults [28].

The patient may present with dyspnea, difficult feeding, slow weight gain, suggesting heart failure or frequent respiratory infections. Cardiovascular examination reveals a continuous systolic-diastolic murmur (for the patent ductus arteriosus) or a separate rough systolic murmur in the pulmonic area and suprasternal notch, with good transmission to the back and neck (for pulmonary artery stenosis). If there is pulmonary artery hypertension, the pulmonary component of the second sound is accentuated. The cardiac murmurs are audible in early infancy. A wide pulse pressure, an overactive right ventricular impulse or a systolic thrill may also be present [34, 35].

Investigations

Investigations should include complete blood count, evaluation of the liver function, cardiac evaluation by echocardiography and electrocardiogram, ophthalmologic exam, evaluation for hearing loss.

Electrocardiogram reveals right ventricular hypertrophy, right axis deviation or biventricular hypertrophy.

Chest X-ray shows engorged pulmonary vasculature, moderate cardiomegaly involving both ventricles and usually the left chambers [34].

Echocardiography is the investigation of choice for cardiac evaluation in CRS. Echocardiography will reveal either patent ductus arteriosus (Figs. 16.7 and 16.8), ventricular septal defect, stenosis of the pulmonary valve or branches.

Cardiac catheterization and angiocardiography may also be needed in selected cases.

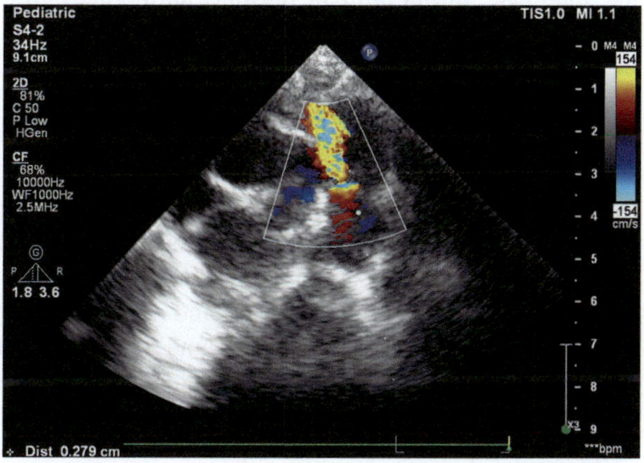

Fig. 16.7 Image of a PDA in a 4-month-old girl

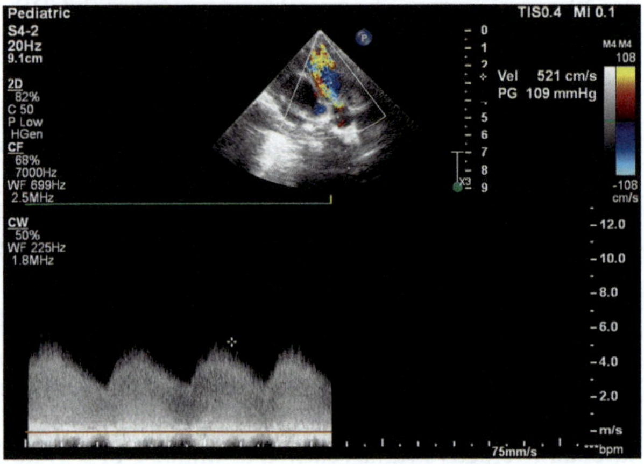

Fig. 16.8 The continuous Doppler signal registered through the PDA in the same patient

Diagnosis/Investigations

Basic investigations include the hemogram which may show leukopenia and negatives inflammatory markers [1].

Diagnosis can be confirmed by several methods: rubella virus RNA testing by polymerase chain reaction (PCR), serology evaluation (IgM and IgG), virus isolation by culture. PCR diagnosis is using samples from the amniotic or cerebrospinal liquid, respiratory secretions, throat swabs, urine samples or ocular tissue. It has good sensibility and specificity, but it is not available in all centers. Reverse transcriptase PCR (RT-PCR) amplification of viral RNA may offer a rapid diagnosis.

Serologic diagnosis evaluates the levels of specific IgM or higher levels of IgG that persists for a longer time. IgM usually is increased in the first 2 months, but in 20% of the cases, the titers will increase only at the age of 1 month. Also, there may be false positive results in infection with Parvovirus B19 [28]. Avidity test of IgG can help diagnose recent infection [27]. Also, for the mother, serology may confirm the diagnosis. In the mother, the IgM antibodies can be detected starting immediately as the rash appears. IgG antibodies appear after 2–3 weeks.

Treatment

Pre-exposure Prophylaxis

Prevention of congenital rubella is achieved by providing vaccination. The vaccine against rubella is a live attenuated rubella virus and it is given to children around 1-year-old together with the measles and mumps vaccines. Besides infants and children, also women school teachers and medical staff may require vaccination. Women who are at childbearing age should have evidence of immunity to rubella and if they are nonimmune, the recommendation is for vaccination with 1 dose of vaccine [1, 27].

Therapeutic Approach

Specific treatment of infected children is not available. All infants with confirmed CRS are considered contagious until 1 year of age, unless 2 cultures of clinical specimens obtained 1 month apart are negative for rubella virus, after 3 months of age [27].

The approach in CRS is complex and include multidisciplinarity—with medical, surgical, developmental rehabilitation involvement starting the neonatal period.

Cardiac treatment includes medical therapy with recommendations regarding improving nutrition, drug therapy of heart failure with diuretics and angiotensin-converting enzyme inhibitors. A pediatric cardiologist should decide the interventional or surgical treatment depending on the specific lesion. Closure of the defect (PDA), interventional dilatation of the pulmonary or aortic stenosis, surgery for tetralogy of Fallot has to be taken into consideration soon if the heart failure is untreatable or the oxygenation is not corresponding.

Specific treatment has to be recommended for ophthalmological problems (glaucoma, cataract, retinopathy), for hearing loss or occupational therapy for mental retardation [36].

Prognosis/Complications

The most serious complication in rubella is the congenital rubella syndrome. The mortality rate of CRS among symptomatic neonates and infants with fulminant interstitial pneumonia, severe cardiac lesions, extensive meningoencephalitis is 20% [36].

Otherwise, there are not so many complications of rubella in children. In adults, arthritis (in up to 70% of the females and 5% of the males), thrombocytopenic or non-thrombocytopenic purpura, encephalitis, hemophagocytis syndrome may complicate a rubella infection.

References

1. Sterling JC. In: Griffiths C, Barker J, Bleiker T, Chalmers R, Creamer D, editors. Viral infections in Rook's textbook of dermatology. 9th ed: Wiley; 2016.
2. Abrams D, Derrick G, Penny DJ, Shinebourne EA, Redington AN. Cardiac complications in children following infection with varicella zoster virus. Cardiol Young. 2001;11(6):647–52.
3. Arvin AM. Varicella-zoster virus. Clin Microbiol Rev. 1996;9(3):361–81.
4. Speer ME. Varicella-zoster infection in the newborn. UpToDate, Accessed Feb 2019.
5. Baljic R, Mehanic S, Imsirovic B, Ahmetspahic-Begic A, Lukovac E, Baljic I, Hasimbegovic-Ibrahimovic S, Gazibera B, Gutosic M. Therapeutic approach to chickenpox in children and adults - our experience. Med Arch. 2012;66(3 Suppl 1):21–3.
6. Hackel DB. Myocarditis in association with varicella. Am J Pathol. 1953;29:369–79.
7. May LJ, Patton DJ, Fruitman DS. The evolving approach to paediatric myocarditis: a review of the current literature. Cardiol Young. 2011;21(3):241–51.

8. O'Grady MJ, Moylett E. Cardiac-related varicella mortality in childhood: a literature review with clinical experience. Pediatr Cardiol. 2011;32(8):1241–3.
9. Thandroyen FT, Asmal AC, Armstrong TG. Varicella myocarditis producing congestive cardiomyopathy. Postgrad Med J. 1981;57(665):199–201.
10. Fiddler GI, Campbell RW, Pottage A, Godman MJ. Varicella myocarditis presenting with unusual ventricular arrhythmias. Br Heart J. 1977;39(10):1150–3.
11. Lorber A, Zonis Z, Maisuls E, Dembo L, Palant A, Iancu TC. The scale of myocardial involvement in varicella myocarditis. Int J Cardiol. 1988;20(2):257–62.
12. Sawardekar KP. Fatal varicella myocarditis in a child with down syndrome - a case report. J Trop Pediatr. 2016;62(3):250–4.
13. Pinamonti B, Alberti E, Cigalotto A, Dreas L, Salvi A, Silvestri F, Camerini F. Echocardiographic findings in myocarditis. Am J Cardiol. 1988;62:285–91.
14. Schultz JC, Hilliard AA, Cooper LT Jr, Rihal CS. Diagnosis and treatment of viral myocarditis. Mayo Clin Proc. 2009;84(11):1001–9.
15. Soongswang J, Durongpisitkul K, Nana A, Laohaprasittiporn D, Kangkagate C, Punlee K, Limpimwong N. Cardiac troponin T: A marker in the diagnosis of acute myocarditis in children. Pediatr Cardiol. 2005;26(1):45–9.
16. Lauer B, Niederau C, Kühl U, Schannwell M, Pauschinger M, Strauer BE, Schultheiss HP. J Am Coll Cardiol. 1997;30(5):1354–9.
17. Friedrich MG, Sechtem U, Schulz-Menger J, Holmvang G, Alakija P, Cooper LT, White JA, Abdel-Aty H, Gutberlet M, Prasad S, Aletras AH, Laissy JP, Paterson I, Filipchuk NG, Kumar A, Pauschinger M, Liu P. Cardiovascular magnetic resonance in myocarditis: a JACC white paper. J Am Coll Cardiol. 2009;53(17):1475–87.
18. Maranich AM, Rajnik M. Varicella-specific immunoglobulin G titers in commercial intravenous immunoglobulin preparations. Pediatrics. 2009;124:e484–8.
19. Seddon DJ. Pericarditis with pericardial effusion complicating chickenpox. Postgrad Med J. 1986;62(734):1133–4.
20. Ioannou A, Tsappa I, Metaxa S, Missouris CG. Ventricular fibrillation following varicella zoster myocarditis. Case Rep Cardiol. 2017;2017:1017686.
21. Kelly E, Cullen G, McGurk C. When an MI is not an MI: a case of varicella zoster myocarditis. Cardiology. 2008;109:193–5.
22. Dauger S, Le Goff J, Deho A, Jones P. Varicella zoster in sudden infant death. BMJ Case Rep. 2018;11(1). pii: e227034.
23. Nagel MA. Varicella zoster virus vasculopathy: clinical features and pathogenesis. J Neurovirol. 2014;20(2):157–63.
24. Kazemi V, Fernandez MC, Zide K. Herpes zoster-induced progressive heart block: a case report. Cureus. 2018;10(12):e3674.
25. Kalender E, Şensoy B, Çay S. Heart block after herpes zoster reactivation. Int J Cardiol. 2016;203:549–50.
26. Spillane JD, White PD. Herpes zoster and angina pectoris. Br Heart J. 1939;1(4):291–302.
27. Neu N, Duchon J, Zachariah P. TORCH infections. Clin Perinatol. 2015;42(1):77–103.
28. Dobson SR. Congenital rubella syndrome: clinical features and diagnosis. UpToDate. Accessed Feb 2019.
29. Lasek-Duriez A, Hubiche T, Aladjidi N, Lamireau T, Taïeb A, Léauté-Labrèze C. Chronic exanthema in a child with congenital rubella. Ann Dermatol Venereol. 2008;135(3):222–4.
30. Castrow FF II, De Beukelaer M. Congenital rubella syndrome. Unusual cutaneous manifestations. Arch Dermatol. 1968;98(3):260–2.
31. Campbell PE. Vascular abnormalities following maternal rubella. Br Heart J. 1965;27:134–8.
32. Plotkin S. Some recently recognized manifestation of the rubella syndrome. J Pediatr. 1965;67(2):182–18.
33. Zimmerman LE. Histopathologic basis for ocular manifestations of congenital rubella syndrome. Am J Ophthalmol. 1968;65(6):837–62.

34. Heiner DC, Nadas AS. Patent ductus arteriosus in association with pulmonic stenosis; a report of six cases with additional non-cardiac congenital anomalies. Circulation. 1958;17(2):232–42.
35. Franch RH, Gay BB Jr. Congenital stenosis of the pulmonary artery branches. a classification, with postmortem findings in two cases. Am J Med. 1963;35:512–29.
36. Dobson SR. Congenital rubella syndrome: management, outcome, and prevention. UpToDate, Accessed Feb 2019.

Part V

Metabolic and Endocrine Diseases

Xanthomas and Abnormalities of Lipid Metabolism and Storage

17

Efthymia Soura

Introduction

The spectrum of lipid metabolism abnormalities is wide and encompasses a variety of conditions. These include disorders that can be very common, such as xanthelasmas, disorders that are hereditary, such as primary hypercholesterolemia and disorders that can be secondary to systemic disease, such as diabetes or hypothyroidism. These conditions possess the potential to be associated with increased cardiovascular risk. Therefore, they may require systemic therapeutic interventions aimed to treat high lipid levels in addition to treatments for their cutaneous manifestations [1]. The following chapter focuses on an overview of the classification of xanthomas, dyslipidemias and their cardiovascular risk.

Overview of Lipid Metabolism

There are two main pathways of lipoprotein synthesis: the exogenous and the endogenous pathway. The initiation of the exogenous pathway requires dietary fat intake. More specifically, dietary triglycerides are catabolized in the gut to fatty acids and monoglycerides by pancreatic lipase and bile acids. These products are absorbed by intestinal epithelium, re-esterified into cholesteryl ester and triglycerides and packaged with various cholesterol esters onto apolipoprotein B-48, forming chylomicrons. Apolipoproteins can be considered as "passports" that allow access of lipoprotein particles to specific sites for delivery, storage or modification of lipids [2]. Chylomicrons gain access to systemic circulation through the thoracic duct where the core triglycerides are gradually hydrolyzed resulting to the release of free fatty acids to peripheral tissues [1]. This process is complex and requires the

E. Soura (✉)
1st University Department of Dermatology – Venereology, Andreas Syggros Hospital, National and Kapodistrian Medical School of Athens, Athens, Greece

C. Salavastru et al. (eds.), *Skin and the Heart*,
https://doi.org/10.1007/978-3-030-54779-0_17

interaction of lipoprotein lipase (LPL), which is bound to the capillary endothelium, in tissues such as adipose tissue and muscle, apolipoprotein CII (also a chylomicron component) and other lipoproteins and proteins (e.g. GPIHBP1, apo V) [2]. Chylomicrons are, therefore, progressively degraded to chylomicron remnants that contain, mainly, cholesteryl esters. These are taken up by the liver via binding to apo B-100/E receptors, re-esterified as cholesteryl esters and triglycerides and stored, while apolipoproteins such as B-48 are degraded, or exported as lipoproteins [1, 2].

The endogenous pathway follows the metabolism of fats after they are exported from the liver. More specifically, the liver produces VLDL (very low density lipoprotein) which is a very rich in triglycerides lipoprotein. Apo B100 is the major apolipoprotein of VLDL, however, the rate of transfer of triglycerides to the apo-B peptide is mediated by microsomal transfer protein (MTP) and is directly dependent to the presence of adequate amount of triglycerides [2]. After VLDL is secreted to the plasma it acquires apo E, apo CII, and apo CIII. These apoliproteins are key in the interaction of VLDL with LPL which will gradually hydrolyze the triglycerides in VLDL to fatty acids. This process, in turn, will convert VLDL to IDL, a cholesteryl ester–rich particle containing apo B and apo E. IDL can either be taken up by the liver and degraded or interact with extracellular hepatic lipases and re-enter the circulation as LDL, which consists of one molecule of apo B100 per particle and cholesteryl esters [1, 2].

HDL (high density lipoprotein) is a major component of the dynamic process of lipid metabolism. It is produced in the liver and secreted in the peripheral circulation, containing only a phospholipid disc, Apo AI and Apo AII. HDL absorbs free cholesterol and phospholipids shed from cells, surface lipids, Apo CII, Apo CIII, and Apo E (VLDL remnants), it stores cholesterol in its core after it esterifies it with the assistance of LCAT (Lecithin–Cholesterol Acyltransferase), and transports it back to the liver for excretion directly or indirectly (by interacting with VLDL) [2].

The most concise method of classifying dyslipidemias is the one proposed by Fredrickson which has been adopted by WHO [3]. A summary of the types of dyslipidemias and their cutaneous manifestations can be found in Table 17.1.

Xanthomas

Xanthomas are subcutaneous lipid deposits that, with the sole exception of familial hypercholesterolemia type II, appear during adulthood. As the term "xanthoma" (Greek: xanthos = yellow/blonde) implies, these deposits have a yellowish to orange color [4]. Although the pathogenesis of xanthomas is not well understood, it is believed that these lipid deposits originate from lipids found in the circulation. The histological picture is similar in all types of xanthomas. More specifically, all types of xanthomas contain foam cells (macrophages filled with cholesterol and cholesterol esters) and, rarely, giant touton cells. Foam cells stain positive for CD68 and adipophilin immunoperoxidase [5]. As xanthomas are slowly being degraded the appearance of clefts or connective tissue reaction around the nests of foam cells can be observed. Fibrosis can be present in older lesions [4, 6]. It must be mentioned

Table 17.1 Summary of dyslipidemias and their cutaneous and systemic manifestations

WHO classification	Serum levels	Overall symptom	Primary dyslipidaimia	Secondary causes	Cutaneous manifestations	Systemic manifestations
I (↑ CM)	↑↑ TGS ↓ HDL ↓ LDL	Hypertriglyceridaemia	• Lipoprotein lipase deficiency • ApoCII deficiency	• Alcoholism • Diabetes • Chronic renal failure	Eruptive xanthomas	• No increased risk of CV disease • Recurrent pancreatitis
IIa (↑LDL)	↑ Chol ↑ LDL	Hypercholesterolaemia	• Familial hypercholesterolaemia • Familial defective ApoB100 • Polygenic hypercholesterolaemia	• Hypothyroidism • Anorexia • Cholestatic liver disease • Nephrotic syndrome • Thiazide diuretics, corticosteroids	• Tendon xanthomas • Xanthelasmas • Interdigital planar xanthomas (homozygous FH)	Increased risk of atherosclerosis in peripheral and coronary arteries
IIb (↑LDL, ↑VLDL)	↑ Chol ↑ LDL ↑ TGS +/− ↓ HDL	Combined dyslipidaemia	Familial combined hyperlipidaemia	• Lipodystrophies • Hypothyroidism • Liver disease • Nephrotic syndrome • Chronic renal failure • Paraproteinaemias • Pregnancy • Various drugs	• Tendinous xanthomas • Tuberoeruptive xanthomas • Xanthelasmas • Interdigital planar xanthomas • Xanthomas in intertriginous areas	Increased risk of atherosclerosis in peripheral and coronary arteries
III (Broad β-VLDL)	↑ Chol ↑ LDL ↑ TGS +/− ↓ HDL	Combined dyslipidaemia	Familial dysbetalipoproteinaemia	• Diabetes • Metabolic syndrome	• Tuberous xanthomas • Palmar xanthomas	Increased risk of atherosclerosis in peripheral and coronary arteries

(continued)

Table 17.1 (continued)

WHO classification	Serum levels	Overall symptom	Primary dyslipidaimia	Secondary causes	Cutaneous manifestations	Systemic manifestations
IV (↑VLDL)	↑ Chol ↑ LDL ↑ TGS +/– ↓ HDL	Hypertriglyceridaemia and Combined dyslipidaemia	Endogenous familial hypertriglyceridemia	• Hypothyroidism • Liver disease • Nephrotic syndrome • Chronic renal failure • Paraproteinaemias • Pregnancy • Various drugs	Eruptive xanthomas	Associated with type II diabetes mellitus, obesity and alcoholism
V (↑CM,↑VLDL)	↑↑ TGS ↓ HDL ↓ LDL	Hypertriglyceridaemia	N/A	• Paraproteinaemias • Pregnancy • Various drugs (oral contraceptives, β-blockers, thiazide diuretics)	Eruptive xanthomas	type II diabetes mellitus

CM chylomicrons, *Chol* Total Cholesterol, *TGS* triglycerides, *HDL* high density lipoprotein cholesterol, *LDL* low-density lipoprotein cholesterol that although xanthomas are closely associated with increased serum lipid levels, not all patients with hyperlipidemia develop them [4]. Xanthomas are categorized as tuberous xanthomas, tendon xanthomas, eruptive xanthomas and plane xanthomas. These entities will be discussed in the sections below [6].

Tuberous Xanthomas

Tuberous xanthomas appear as pink/red-yellow nodules mainly on sites of pressure such as the elbows or knees. They usually present as small lesions that are yellowish and erythematous, and gradually increase in size ultimately attaining very large sizes that can be several centimeters in both height and diameter (can exceed 3 cm in diameter). Older lesions tend to lose their yellowish tint and become brownish and fibrotic. In some instances, tuberous xanthomas may be surrounded by smaller lesions. In this case they are called "tubero-eruptive" xanthomas. In general, tuberous and tubero-eruptive xanthomas are considered part of the same continuum [1, 4–6].

Tuberous and tubero-eruptive xanthomas have been closely associated with Type II and Type III hyperlipidemias (Table 17.1) and are considered to be linked with a high risk for cardiovascular disorders and especially coronary artery disease [6–8]. In addition, tuberous xanthomas have rarely been reported in cases of secondary dyslipoproteinemias such as nephrotic syndrome or hypothyroidism [6]. Laboratory investigations should include a complete lipid profile and, in high suspicion for primary dyslipidemias, apolipoprotein E (ApoE) genotyping and lipid electrophoresis or ultracentrifugation examinations [1]. (Tables 17.2 and 17.3).

Table17.2 Main points in the diagnosis of xanthomas [1, 6]

- The diagnosis of xanthomas is usually made clinically. If doubts exist:
  - Biopsy for histopathological assessment
- If diagnosis of xanthoma is made:
  - Personal and family history may reveal possible metabolic disorder
  - Lipid levels assessment (LDL, HDL, total cholesterol, Triglycerides, VLDL etc.)
  - Liver enzyme level assessment (AST, ALT, γ-GT, ALP, bilirubin etc.)
  - In case where abnormalities in lipid/ liver enzyme levels are observed (ultrasonography of arteries of the head and neck, intima-media thickness in the carotid arteries, ankle-brachial index) and sonography of the liver (to confirm or reject the presence of non-alcoholic fatty liver disease) should be considered especially if xanthelasmas are present
- If family hyperlipidemia is suspected:
  - Examinations specific to each type of hyperlipidemia should be performed[a]
  - Achilles tendon ultrasound could reveal thickening
- Causes of secondary hyperlipidemia should be excluded:
  - *Predominantly hypertriglyceridemia:* Obesity, Pregnancy, Diabetes mellitus, Alcoholism, Renal failure, Estrogen therapy, Steroid therapy, β-blocker therapy, Lipodystrophy, Dysglobulinemias
  - *Predominantly hypercholesterolemia*: Hypothyroidism, Nephrotic syndrome, Cholestasis, Diuretics, Cyclosporine, Hepatoma

[a]Laboratory tests are summarized in Table 17.3

Table 17.3 Specific tests used for the diagnosis of dyslipidemias [9]

- *Routine testing:*
  - Serum cholesterol
  - Serum triglycerides
  - Serum HDL cholesterol
  - Serum LDL cholesterol
  - Refrigerator test Profile to rule out secondary causes
- *Additional testing:*
  - Lipoprotein electrophoresis
  - Beta-quantification Lipoprotein lipase assay
  - Apo-E genotyping
  - Apo-C-II assay
  - Familial defective apolipoprotein B-100 screening
  - Apolipoprotein B-100 and A-1 Lp(a)
- *Special tests:*
  - Fibrinogen
  - Micronutrient antioxidants
  - LDL oxidizability
  - Homocysteine
  - Anti-phospholipid antibodies
  - LDL subclasses
  - HDL subclasses

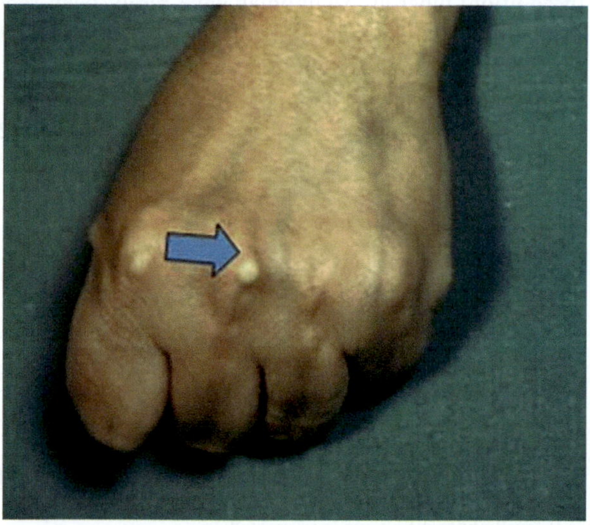

Fig. 17.1 Tendon xanthomas located on the knuckles of a patient (Courtesy of Iyengar S S, et al. Journal of Clinical lipidology, Vol. 12, no. 1, 56–109)

Tendon Xanthomas

Tendon xanthomas appear as firm, smooth papules or nodules that represent deep subcutaneous lipid deposits that affect tendons. Unlike other types of xanthomas their color is more skin colored or erythematous than yellow, since the lipid deposits are located deep within the tendons and are usually not visible. Their size ranges from 5 mm to 25 mm in diameter. Lesions are commonly located on extensor tendons of hands (knuckles), (Fig. 17.1) feet and on the Achilles tendons, (Fig. 17.2) but

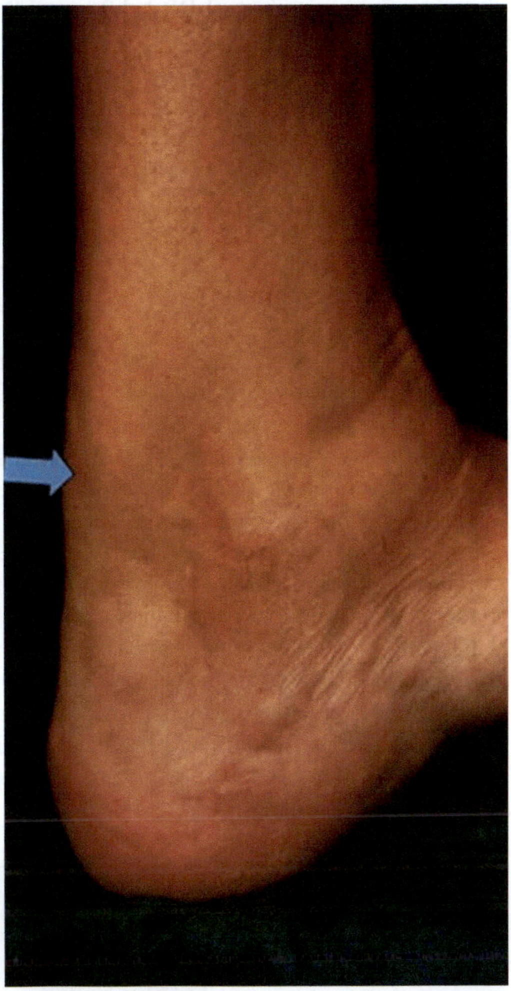

Fig. 17.2 Tendon xanthoma located on the Achilles tendon of a patient. There are very subtle changes in skin color, while the lesion is only barely visible. (Courtesy of Iyengar S. S., et al. Journal of Clinical lipidology, Vol. 12, no. 1, 56–109)

other tendons may also be affected. Tendinous xanthomas can be freely moved from side to side upon clinical examination unless they involve the periosteum, which can be the case if the patellar tendon is affected [1, 2, 4]. The lesions can be occasionally painful, especially in cases where the Achilles tendon is affected (achillodynia), and may even (rarely) be associated with spontaneous tendon rupture [10].

Tendinous xanthomas are encountered in disorders with elevated LDL cholesterol levels such as type II familial hypercholesterolemia. More specifically, 20%-50% of patients with clinically diagnosed familial hypercholesterolemia have been reported to present with tendinous xanthomas [6]. The lesions can also occur in the context of secondary hyperlipidemia associated with obstructive liver disease (cholestasis), diabetes and myxedema. In addition, special care should be taken to exclude possible diagnoses of cerebrotendinous xanthomatosis, and β-phytosterolemia [1]. Investigations assisting in the diagnosis of these lesions include imaging (e.g. Ultrasound, CT, MRI to diagnose tendon thickening), lipid assessment examinations (LDL ≥4.9 mmol/l) and liver enzyme assays [1, 9, 10]. (Table 17.2).

Tendinous xanthomas have been strongly associated with a high risk for cardiovascular disease. In a meta-analysis by Oosterveer et al. that included 22 relevant studies, it was shown that the presence of tendon xanthomas in patients with familial hypercholesterolaemia was associated with a 3.2 times higher risk of cardiovascular disease [11].

Eruptive Xanthomas

Eruptive xanthomas present as small (1 mm–5 mm) erythematous to yellow papules that arise on an erythematous base. The erythematous base is considered to be an inflammatory halo probably caused by the high triglyceride component of these lesions. They are usually located on the extensor areas of the arms and thighs, the buttocks, the inguinal and axillary folds, knees, hands and oral mucosa and their appearance is marked by a sudden eruption. (Fig. 17.3) Eruptive xanthomas can be pruritic and koebner phenomenon may be observed [1, 2, 5, 6].

The presence of eruptive xanthomas is strongly associated with severe hypertriglyceridemia (primary or secondary) and type I, IV and V hyperlipidemias. These patients may exhibit a lipaemic appearance on blood or serum levels and can present with triglyceride levels that exceed 3000 to 4000 mg/dl. Cardiovascular risk is moderately increased in these patients, mainly due to the association of eruptive xanthomas with diabetes. In addition, lipaemia retinalis is almost universaly present and is the result of the marked hypertriglyceridemia. (Fig. 17.4).

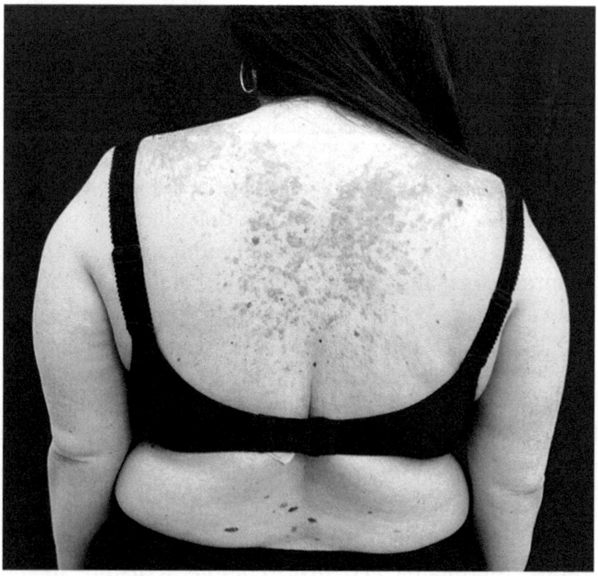

Fig.17.3 Eruptive xanthomas located on the back of a patient with type IV hyperlipidemia (Courtesy of Prof. Christina Antoniou, "Andreas Sygros Hospital of Dermatological and Venereal Diseases)

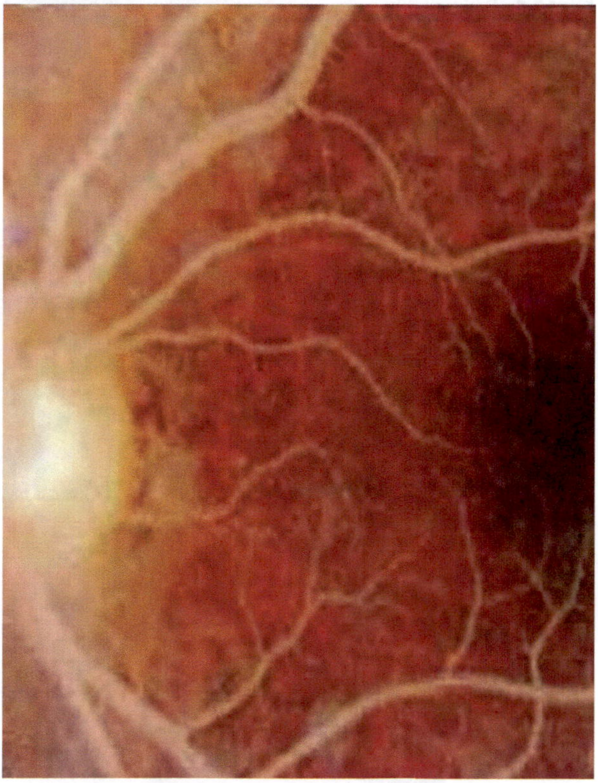

Fig.17.4 Image of a patient with lipaemia retinalis. (Courtesy of Iyengar S. S., et al. Journal of Clinical Lipidology, Vol. 12, no. 1, 56–109)

Dyslipidemic Plane (Planar) Xanthomas

Dyslipidemic plane xanthomas are divided into three categories: xanthelasmas, plane xanthomas and palmar xanthomas.

Xanthelasmas

Xanthelasmas are the most common type of xanthomas with a prevalence that has been reported to vary from 0.3% to 4.4% [6]. Females are more commonly affected than males [6]. Xanthelasmas appear as yellowish/orange plaques and affect mainly the periocular areas (upper eyelids and canthus). The lesions are usually symmetric and can be flat or nodular. In most cases they are soft when palpated but can also be solid and calcaneous [1, 12]. (Fig. 17.5) They usually appear between the fourth and sixth decades of life, however they can be observed in younger patients in the context of primary hyperlipidemias.

Although the presence of xanthelasma is indicative of hyperlipidemia, it has been reported that only half of the patients with xanthelasma actually have hyperlipidemia [5]. The clinical severity of the disorder falls under four categories: patients

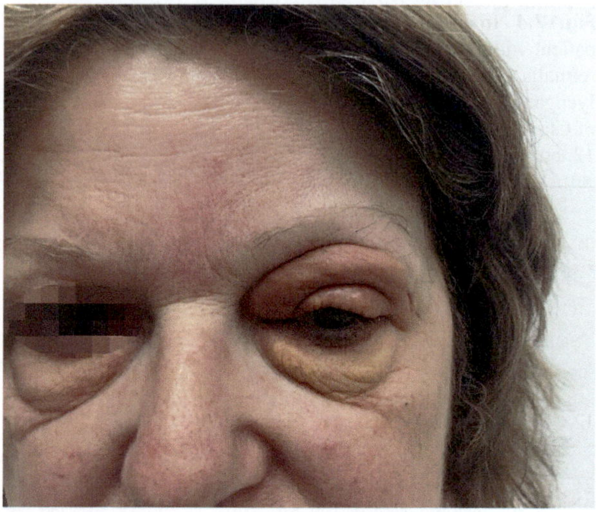

Fig. 17.5 Patient with grade IV xanthomas on the right eye. The lesion is firm upon palpation. In patients with similar lesions normal lipid lowering therapy is usually not effective in the treatment of xanthelasmas and a surgical approach may be considered. (Courtesy of Dr. Dorothea Polydorou, "Andreas Sygros Hospital of Dermatological and Venereal Diseases)

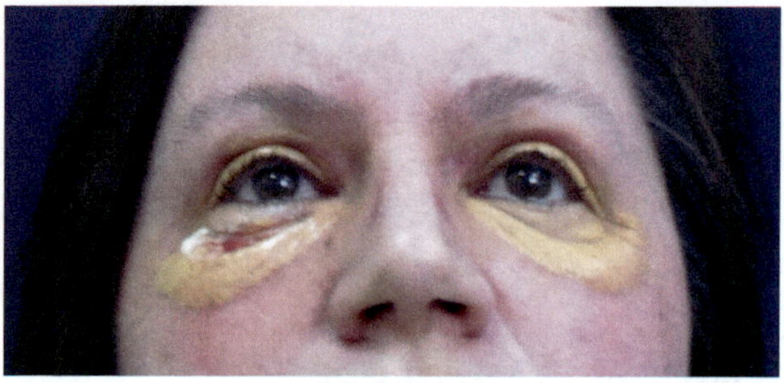

Fig. 17.6 Patient with unilateral grade IV xanthomas. The lesions possess a characteristic yellowish colour, while ulceration is present in the area under the right eye. (Courtesy of Prof. Christina Antoniou, "Andreas Sygros Hospital of Dermatological and Venereal Diseases)

with lesions on the upper eyelids are Grade I, patients with lesions extending to the medial canthal area are Grade II, patients with lesions on the medial side of both upper and lower eyelids are Grade III and patients with diffuse involvement on medial and lateral sides of the upper and lower eyelids are Grade IV. (Fig. 17.6) The height and consistency of the lesions is also noted [13].

Although the data regarding cardiovascular risk in patients with xanthelasma are inconclusive, more recent studies report a possible correlation of the disorder with coronary artery disease [14]. More specifically, in a study that included 12.745 patients, it was reported that the hazard/odds ratios for myocardial infarction, for ischaemic cerebrovascular disease and for severe atherosclerosis was 1.47, 1.56 and 2.75 respectively, for patients with xanthelasma compared to the general population [14]. It is recommended that patients with xanthelasma be evaluated with a full lipoprotein profile and a liver enzyme assay in combination to a careful history and physical examination [1, 2, 9].

Plane Xanthomas

Plane xanthomas present as yellow to orange macules, patches or plaques and can be well circumscribed or diffuse. They usually appear on the axillae, neck, shoulders or buttocks. (Fig. 17.7) Interestingly, their distribution can be unique depending on the underlying disorder [1, 2]. For instance, xanthomas located on the interdigital or intertriginous spaces may be representative for homozygous familial hypercholesterolemia [15]. Plane xanthomas can also be associated with cholestasis and may occur as a complication of diseases such as biliary atresia or primary biliary cirrhosis. It must be mentioned that plane xanthomas may also present in normolipemic patients and can be associated with paraproteinemias (multiple myeloma, monoclonal gammopathy of undetermined significance) or lymphoproliferative diseases such as cutaneous lymphomas, B cell lymphomas, chronic lymphatic leukaemia and chronic myeloid leukaemia [6, 16].

Familial hypercholesterolaemia and type III hyperlipoproteinaemia should be excluded in patients with plane xanthomas. Recommended investigations include a full lipid profile, serum electrophoresis, and autoimmune screen. In normolipemic patients examinations to exclude various blood dyscrasias should also be performed (e.g. PET/CT, flow cytometry and histological examination of lymphatic nodes) [1, 6, 9].

Palmar Xanthomas

Palmar xanthomas can affect the palms, the flexural surfaces of fingers and the creases of the palms and soles *("Xanthomata striata palmaris")*. They usually appear as yellowish nodules or plaques. In the cases that the palmar creases are affected, they can present as orange/yellow lines that follow the palmar creases and may occasionally involve the flexor creases of the wrists as well [1, 2, 5, 6].

These lesions are commonly associated with familial dysbetalipoproteinemia (Type III dyslipidemia) and are considered by some authors as pathognomonic for the condition (homozygous) [2]. Other associations include secondary dyslipidemia

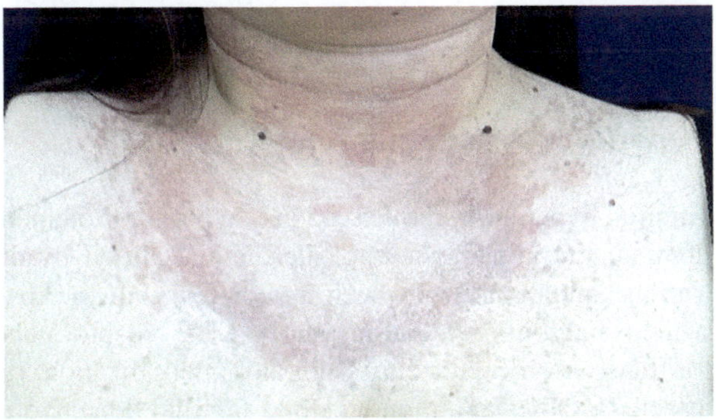

Fig. 17.7 Plane xanthomas located on the neck of a female patient. (Courtesy of Prof. Christina Antoniou, "Andreas Sygros Hospital of Dermatological and Venereal Diseases)

as a result of multiple myeloma or primary biliary cirrhosis, diabetes mellitus and hypothyreosis [17]. It has been suggested that the presence of palmar xanthomas (in the context of type III dyslipidemia) may be associated with an increased risk for coronary artery atherosclerosis [1, 6].

Investigations for patients that present with palmar xanthomas should include a complete lipid profile, fasting glucose level, liver function tests and urine and electrolytes assays. In addition, thyroid hormone levels may be useful in uncovering a possible hypothyroidism. Specific testing for primary dyslipidemia such as ApoE genotyping, lipid electrophoresis or ultracentrifugation may be suggested in specific subsets of patients [1].

Overview of Primary Dyslipidemias

Hypelipoproteinemia Type I

Type I hyperlipoproteinemia is an extremely rare condition that is caused by a deficiency of lipoprotein lipase. Several mutations affecting the function of LPL have been associated with the condition. In general, individuals that exhibit homozygous defects in the LPL gene present with lipid serum alterations during infancy. However, gene penetrance may vary. Some authors suggest that there are monogenic and polygenic forms of the disorder, with the monogenic familial forms presenting during childhood and the polygenic forms typically requiring a "trigger", such as the presence of a secondary illness, for the expression of the disease [1–3, 5].

Typical cutaneous manifestations of Type I hyperlipoproteinemia include the appearance of eruptive xanthomas. Lipemia retinalis may also be present as a result of the extremely high levels of circulating triglycerides. Blood, serum and plasma from these patients can appear milky and if the samples are centrifuged a creamy top layer may be observed. Similarly to lipemia retinalis, this observation comes as a result of the extremely prominent chylomicronemia (hypertriglyceridemia) with triglyceride levels that usually exceed >1000 mg/dL. In some patients hypercholesterolemia may also be observed. The extremely high levels of triglycerides may be associated with an increased risk of pancreatitis (which can be life-threatening). Patients may also present with hepatosplenomegaly, dyspnea, lymphadenopathy and neurologic dysfunction [1, 2, 5].

Hyperlipoproteinemia Type II

Familial hypercholesterolemia (FH, hyperlipoproteinemia type IIa) is an autosomal dominant form of hypercholesterolemia caused by defects in the LDL receptor. Various mutations have been associated with the disorder; with the majority of patients exhibiting mutations on the LDL receptor gene (receptor synthesis, receptor transport, receptor clustering and internalization, receptor recycling etc. can be affected). Other mutations include familial defective apo B (mutations that affect the ability of LDL to bind the LDL receptor) and mutations of *PCSK9* [1, 2, 5, 18, 19].

Typical cutaneous manifestations of FH include the appearance of tendon xanthomas, xanthelasmas (very rarely) and interdigital planar xanthomas (only in homozygous FH). Tendon xanthomas may first appear during childhood in patients with the homozygous type of the disease, while in patients with the heterozygous type of the disease their prevalence increases with age (e.g. 90% at age ≥ 40 years). Thickening of the Achilles tendon as well as xanthomas at the extensor tendons of the knees and hands are usually present, although it must be mentioned that clinically apparent (visible) tendon xanthomas tend to be rare and the diagnosis can be set with the use of an ultrasound examination. Other manifestations include the presence of corneal arcus (although not pathognomonic) and arthralgias. Patients usually present with high total cholesterol levels (> 300 mg/dL) and LDL cholesterol levels (> 200 mg/dL) while triglyceride levels may be normal [1, 2, 5, 20].

The condition has been closely associated with a high cardiovascular risk. Interestingly, although LDL receptor mutations are rare (1:500) it has been reported that they may be responsible for up to 5% of myocardial infarctions occurring in men younger than 55 years and women younger than 65 years. Patients that are homozygotes for the condition (1:1,000,000) present with total cholesterol levels ≥800 mg/dL and require liver transplantation to survive beyond childhood. Children and adolescents with this disease may develop aortic valve disease, although the cardiovascular risk of homozygotes may vary widely [1, 2, 7, 11].

Familial Combined Hyperlipidemia (FCH, hyperlipoproteinemia type IIb) is an autosomal dominant form of hyperlipidemia that has been reported to be present in up to 2% of the general population. Although the exact genetic defect is not yet known, it has been suggested that a secondary condition (Table 17.1) is required as a trigger for the expression of this disorder. Although the appearance of xanthomas is rare in patients with FCH, several types of xanthomas have been associated with it, including tendinous xanthomas, tuberoeruptive xanthomas, xanthelasmas, interdigital planar xanthomas and xanthomas located in intertriginous areas. Serum lipid profile includes elevated levels of triglycerides, elevated levels of LDL cholesterol or hypertriglyceridemia with low levels of HDL cholesterol [2, 5].

FCH has been associated with a high risk for cardiovascular disease and it has been suggested that it may account for up to 20% of cases of premature coronary artery disease [2].

Hyperlipoproteinemia Type III

Hyperlipoproteinemia type III is a rare condition that is associated with mutations in *ApoE*. ApoE is an apolipoprotein that mediates the binding of remnant apolipoproteins to the LDL receptor and the LDL receptor-related protein. Overall, there are three common variants of the apo E protein: E2, E3 and E4. Patients with two E2 alleles are considered to be at risk for dysbetalipoproteinemia. It must be mentioned that less than 10% of ApoE2 homozygous patients develop the condition, indicating that another key factor (environmental or genetic) may be necessary for the expression of the disease. For instance, hypothyroidism has been associated with the condition. Interestingly, patients with one or more E4 alleles have been reported to be at risk for Alzheimer's disease [1, 2, 21].

Cutaneous manifestations of hyperlipoproteinemia type III include the appearance of palmar and tuberous xanthomas. In cases where marked hypertriglyceridemia is present, lipemia retinalis and eruptive xanthomas may also be observed. Patients with dysbetalipoproteinemia present with a very characteristic serum lipid profile. More specifically, increases in the levels of VLDL and IDL are observed, while the levels of LDL may be decreased. However, since the levels of VLDL and IDL are not routinely checked, it must be mentioned that the accumulation of VLDL and chylomicron remnants is usually expressed as a marked increase in both total cholesterol (300–600 mg/dL) and triglyceride levels (300–600 mg/dL) [2, 21].

Hyperlipoproteinemia type III is considered to be highly atherogenic, and is associated with an increased risk for coronary and peripheral artery disease. More specifically, up to 50% of patients with clinical and biochemical symptoms of the disease have been reported to present with premature cardiovascular disease. Other conditions associated with hyperlipoproteinemia type III include proteinuria or nephrotic syndrome (lipoprotein glomerulopathy) [1, 2].

Hyperlipoproteinemia Type IV

Hyperlipoproteinemia type IV is a rare autosomal dominant hypertriglyceridemia disorder with heterogeneous gene penetration. It is believed that the disorder is caused by abnormalities in the metabolism of VLDL such as overproduction of VLDL in the liver or decreased VLDL catabolism (or both). The appearance of eruptive xanthomas could be a cutaneous manifestation of hyperlipoproteinemia type IV. Patients and all affected family members present with isolated elevated triglycerides that are consistently elevated on repeat analyses. In general, patients with this disorder can also present with increased plasma VLDL, while plasma cholesterol may be normal. Glucose intolerance may also be observed in these patients [1, 2, 22].

Although the association of hyperlipoproteinemia type IV and the risk for cardiovascular disease is uncertain, special care should be taken for patients that present with comorbidities (e.g. diabetes mellitus type II) that could potentially aggravate the already present hypertriglyceridemia [2].

Hyperlipoproteinemia Type V

Hyperlipoproteinemia type V is a condition that has been attributed to both genetic and environmental causes, including LPL deficiency, disorders of triglyceride production (increased) or catabolism (decreased), obesity, diabetes, alcoholism, hypothyroidism and renal failure, among others. (Table 17.1) Overall, the interplay between genetic and environmental factors has not yet been elucidated in the pathogenesis of this disorder. Patients with hyperlipoproteinemia type V may present with eruptive xanthomas. Similarly to type 1 hyperlipoproteinemia, blood serum may have a milky consistency. VLDL and chylomicron levels are elevated, while glucose intolerance and hyperuricemia may also be present. Patients with this type of hyperlipoproteinemia may present with increased cardiovascular risk, if chylomicron levels are very high. In addition, the condition may present with similar features to those of type I hyperlipoproteinemia, including high risk for pancreatitis and lipaemia retinalis [1, 23].

References

1. Flynn DP. Xanthomas and abnormalities of lipid metabolism and storage. In: Griffiths C, Barker J, Bleiker T, Chalmers RJG, Creamer D, Rook A, editors. Rook's textbook of dermatology. Hoboken, NJ: Wiley; 2016.
2. Semenkovich CF. Disorders of lipid metabolism. In: Goldman L, Schafer AI, editors. Goldman-cecil medicine. 25th ed; 2016. p. 1389–97.
3. Brahm A, Hegele RA. Hypertriglyceridemia. Nutrients. 2013;5(3):981–1001.
4. Lugo-Somolinos A, Sanchez JE. Xanthomas: a marker for hyperlipidemias. Bol Asoc Med P R. 2003;95(4):12–6.
5. James WD, Elston DM, Treat JR, Rosenbach MA, Neuhaus IM. Errors in metabolism. In: James WD, Elston DM, Treat JR, Rosenbach MA, Neuhaus IM, editors. Andrews' diseases of the skin. 13th ed. Edinburgh: Elsevier; 2020. p. 515–46.
6. Zak A, Zeman M, Slaby A, Vecka M. Xanthomas: clinical and pathophysiological relations. Biomed Pap Med Fac Univ Palacky Olomouc Czech Repub. 2014;158(2):181–8.
7. Agirbasli D, Hyatt T, Agirbasli M. Familial hypercholesterolemia with extensive coronary artery disease and tuberous and tendinous xanthomas: A case report and mutation analysis. J Clin Lipidol. 2018;12(4):863–7.
8. Maskey A, Hirachan A, Yadav D, Roka M. Large multiple tuberous xanthomas presenting with severe coronary artery disease. Eur Heart J. 2017;38(29):2313.
9. Jialal I. A practical approach to the laboratory diagnosis of dyslipidemia. Am J Clin Pathol. 1996;106(1):128–38.
10. Tsouli SG, Kiortsis DN, Argyropoulou MI, Mikhailidis DP, Elisaf MS. Pathogenesis, detection and treatment of Achilles tendon xanthomas. Eur J Clin Investig. 2005;35(4):236–44.
11. Oosterveer DM, Versmissen J, Yazdanpanah M, Hamza TH, Sijbrands EJ. Differences in characteristics and risk of cardiovascular disease in familial hypercholesterolemia patients with and without tendon xanthomas: a systematic review and meta-analysis. Atherosclerosis. 2009;207(2):311–7.
12. Nair PA, Singhal R. Xanthelasma palpebrarum - a brief review. Clin Cosmet Investig Dermatol. 2017;11:1–5.
13. Lee HY, Jin US, Minn KW, Park YO. Outcomes of surgical management of xanthelasma palpebrarum. Arch Plast Surg. 2013;40(4):380–6.
14. Christoffersen M, Frikke-Schmidt R, Schnohr P, Jensen GB, Nordestgaard BG, Tybjærg-Hansen A. Xanthelasmata, arcus corneae, and ischaemic vascular disease and death in general population: prospective cohort study. BMJ. 2011;343:d5497.
15. Sethuraman G, Thappa DM, Karthikeyan K. Intertriginous xanthomas--a marker of homozygous familial hypercholesterolemia. Indian Pediatr. 2000;37(3):338.
16. Szalat R, Arnulf B, Karlin L, Rybojad M, Asli B, Malphettes M, Galicier L, Vignon-Pennamen MD, Harel S, Cordoliani F, Fuzibet JG, Oksenhendler E, Clauvel JP, Brouet JC, Fermand JP. Pathogenesis and treatment of xanthomatosis associated with monoclonal gammopathy. Blood. 2011;118(14):3777–84.

17. Nagarajan DV, Boreham PA, Parfitt VJ. Palmar striated xanthomas. Postgrad Med J. 2003;79(938):690.
18. Timms KM, Wagner S, Samuels ME, Forbey K, Goldfine H, Jammulapati S, Skolnick MH, Hopkins PN, Hunt SC, Shattuck DM. A mutation in PCSK9 causing autosomal-dominant hypercholesterolemia in a Utah pedigree. Hum Genet. 2004;114(4):349–53.
19. Soutar AK, Naoumova RP, Traub LM. Genetics, clinical phenotype, and molecular cell biology of autosomal recessive hypercholesterolemia. Arterioscler Thromb Vasc Biol. 2003;23(11):1963–70.
20. Fellin R, Zuliani G, Arca M, Pintus P, Pacifico A, Montali A, Corsini A, Maioli M. Clinical and biochemical characterisation of patients with autosomal recessive hypercholesterolemia (ARH). Nutr Metab Cardiovasc Dis. 2003;13(5):278–86.
21. Sniderman AD, de Graaf J, Thanassoulis G, Tremblay AJ, Martin SS, Couture P. The spectrum of type III hyperlipoproteinemia. J Clin Lipidol. 2018;12(6):1383–9.
22. Schreibman PH, Wilson DE, Arky RA. Familial type IV hyperlipoproteinemia. N Engl J Med. 1969;281(18):981–5.
23. Gotoda T, Shirai K, Ohta T, Kobayashi J, Yokoyama S, Oikawa S, Bujo H, Ishibashi S, Arai H, Yamashita S, Harada-Shiba M, Eto M, Hayashi T, Sone H, Suzuki H, Yamada N. Diagnosis and management of type I and type V hyperlipoproteinemia. J Atheroscler Thromb. 2012;19(1):1–12.

The Skin and Diabetes

18

J. W. J. Lasschuit, J. R. Snaith, and J. W. Frew

Introduction

Diabetes mellitus is a condition characterised by hyperglycaemia resulting from either insulin resistance, insulin deficiency and hyperglucagonaemia (type 2 diabetes) or insulin deficiency alone (type 1 diabetes). There are numerous dermatological conditions associated with diabetes, but they do not clearly share the vascular injury mechanisms that cause the classic micro and macrovascular complications of diabetes.

This chapter will review the various cutaneous disorders associated with diabetes, their pathogenesis and management options, as well as Diabetic Foot Ulceration (DFU).

The original version of this chapter was revised. This book was inadvertently published with incorrect captions to the figures 2 and 3 in chapter 18. This has now been corrected in the book. The correction to this chapter can be found at https://doi.org/10.1007/978-3-030-54779-0_29

Authors "Lasschuit" and "Snaith" contributed equally to this chapter.

J. W. J. Lasschuit
Department of Endocrinology, St Vincent's Hospital Sydney, Darlinghurst, NSW, Australia

Clinical Diabetes, Appetite and Metabolism, Garvan Institute of Medical Research, Darlinghurst, NSW, Australia

Faculty of Medicine, University of New South Wales, Sydney, NSW, Australia
e-mail: j.lasschuit@garvan.org.au

J. R. Snaith
Department of Diabetes and Endocrinology, St Vincent's Hospital Sydney, Darlinghurst, NSW, Australia
e-mail: j.snaith@garvan.org.au

J. W. Frew (✉)
Clinical Investigation, Laboratory for Investigative Dermatology, The Rockefeller University, New York, NY, USA
e-mail: jfrew@rockefeller.edu

C. Salavastru et al. (eds.), *Skin and the Heart*,
https://doi.org/10.1007/978-3-030-54779-0_18

Diabetic Dermatological Diseases

There are numerous dermatological conditions associated with diabetes, however the degree of association varies according to the condition. These are summarised in Table 18.1.

Table 18.1 Diabetes and skin disease

Condition	Presentation	Association
Acanthosis Nigricans/ skin tags (acrochordons)	Thickened velvety plaques on posterior neck, axillary, inguinal and submammary folds	Insulin resistance
Acne vulgaris	Inflammatory papules and pustules (face, chest, upper back) in adolescents and young adults	Insulin resistance
Acquired perforating dermatosis	Highly pruritic eruption associated with dialysis and renal impairment	Longstanding diabetes
Diabetic Bullae (Bullosis Diabeticorum)	Rapidly-appearing tense bullae on lower legs and feet	Hyperglycaemia or uncontrolled disease
Diabetic Dermopathy	Violaceous atrophic macules on lower legs and forearms	Diabetes
Granuloma Annulare	Annular grouped papules, commonly on hands and feet.	Diabetes
Hidradenitis Suppurativa (acne inversa)	Chronic recurrent inflammatory nodules, abscesses and draining sinus tracts in axillae, groin and submammary folds	Insulin resistance and diabetes
Hyperhidrosis	Excessive sweating	Diabetes
Infectious conditions (Erythrasma, fungal infections, bacterial infections, mycobacterial infections,.	Various	Diabetes
Necrobiosis Lipoidica	Yellow-pink ulcerated plaques on lower legs	Diabetes (Type 1 > Type 2)
Lichen planus	Pruritic flat-topped purple papules – Commonly on wrists	Insulin resistance and diabetes
Lipodystrophy	Localised growth or destruction of subcutaneous adipose tissue	Insulin use
Pigmented purpuric dermatosis	Petechiae and pigmented macules on lower limbs	Insulin resistance and diabetes
Pruritus and Xerosis	Excoriations with no primary lesion, or itching symptoms only with minimal clinical findings. Dry, flaking skin, increased skin markings	Diabetes
Psoriasis vulgaris	*Well demarcated salmon-pink plaques with silvery scale*	Insulin resistance and diabetes
Rubeosis Facei	*Difuse facial redness and plethora*	Hyperglycaemia or uncontrolled disease
Scleredema Diabeticorum	*Hardened skin of face, shoulders, upper back with a "Woody" consistency*	Hyperglycaemia or uncontrolled disease
Vitiligo	*Areas of depigmentation- common on hands, feet, genitals, face, lips.*	Insulin resistance and diabetes
Xanthomas (eruptive)	*Yellow-pink lobulated papules on extensor surfaces of limbs, trunk.*	Type 1 and Type 2 diabetes, diabetic lipaemia

Pathogenesis of Diabetes Associated Skin Disorders

The pathological mechanisms that give rise to other diabetes-associated sequelae (diabetes nephropathy, retinopathy etc) also impact the skin [1]. The presence of hyperinsulinemia and later hyperglycaemia lead to alterations in the cutaneous innate immune response, vascular changes and neurological changes [1]. These are mediated through increased activation of protein kinase C pathways, production of superoxide radicals and advanced glycosylation end products (AGE). These metabolic disturbances result in increases in innate immune cytokines including TNF-alpha, and a reduction in the function of neutrophils leading to an increased risk of infection [1, 2]. IGF-1 is generally increased in diabetes and insulin resistance, which in turn stimulates the activation and proliferation of both keratinocytes and dermal fibroblasts. The general increase in inflammatory load with the reduction in the efficacy of anti-infectious strategies likely explains the increased propensity to chronic inflammatory skin disorders as well as infections.

Acanthosis Nigricans

Acanthosis nigricans is a condition characterised by dark velvety hyperpigmentation of the skin [2, 3]. More severe lesions develop a thickened hyperkeratotic plaque-like quality. It symmetrically affects skin fold areas and the most common sites are the folds of the neck and axillae (Fig. 18.1a). In severe cases it can affect other regions including inguinal, breast and abdominal skin folds, or mucosal surfaces. It can rarely occur in the setting of malignancy (gastrointestinal, ovarian and endometrial carcinoma) but is most commonly due to obesity and diabetes associated hyperinsulinaemia. Other endocrinological conditions [2, 3] such as polycystic ovarian syndrome (PCOS), acromegaly, mutations in the insulin receptor gene and Cushing syndrome may also be associated with IR and hence AN.

Management is targeted towards at identification and management of the underlying condition, whether malignant, endocrinological or lifestyle associated. Pharmacological treatment with metformin may assist reversal of pigmentation, but severe cases are often refractory to treatment [4].

A . Acanthosis Nigricans
B . Necrobiosis lipoidica
- i) early lesion
- ii) typical waxy atrophic plaque

C . Lipodystrophy at the site of repeated insulin injection
- i) lipoatrophy
- ii) lipohypertrophy

Fig. 18.1 Skin manifestations in diabetes. (**a**) Acanthosis Nigricans. (**b**) Necrobiosis lipoidica—(i) early lesion, (ii) typical waxy atrophic plaque. (**c**) Lipodystrophy at the site of repeated insulin injection—(i) lipoatrophy, (ii) lipohypertrophy

Acne Vulgaris

Acne vulgaris is a common condition in adolescents and young adults in modern society, but almost completely absent in non-westernized societies [5, 6]. Dietary influences in acne have been attributed to high glycaemic index foods and severity of acne has been associated with insulin resistance in multiple cohort studies. Indirect associations between insulin resistance and acne vulgaris also exist via endocrinological abnormalities including PCOS, Cushing's Syndrome and other endocrinological causes of hirsutism [5, 6].

Acquired Perforating Dermatosis

Acquired Perforating Dermatosis (APD) presents as a highly pruritic eruption, most commonly on the trunk and proximal limbs [7]. Macroscopically they appear as follicular papules and microscopically as transepidermal elimination of necrotic dermal debris. It is commonly associated with a severe underlying systemic disease, (including diabetes) and a majority of patients are on haemodialysis for nephrosclerotic renal failure. Up to 10% of all dialysis patients are estimated to suffer from various degrees of APD [7].

Diabetic Bullae

The rapid appearance of tense blisters on the legs and lower feet is the hallmark of diabetic bullae (Bullous Diabeticorum) with an estimated incidence of 0.16% of diabetic patients per year [8]. Whilst the pathogenesis is unclear, these bullae are associated with periods of hyperglycaemia or uncontrolled disease. Appropriate diagnosis involves exclusion of other autoimmune blistering diseases and infections (such as bullous impetigo). Given the risk for deterioration into chronic diabetic foot ulceration, close monitoring is mandatory [8, 9]. Although blisters are noted to heal spontaneously, some cases report the need for debridement, antibiotics and protective footwear in line with diabetic ulcer management [8, 9].

Diabetic Dermopathy

Diabetic dermopathy presents as violaceous, atrophic macules and patches on the pretibial aspect of the lower legs of diabetic patients [10]. It may also occur on the extensor surface of the forearms. It was once considered rare, however is now estimated to affect between 17–40% of diabetic patients, although some overlap with pigmented purpuric dermatosis may explain this increase in frequency. It is presumed to be microangiopathic in origin. Treatment is cosmetic only.

Granuloma Annulare

Granuloma Annulare (GA) is an inflammatory dermatosis of uncertain origin which presents as violaceous macules progressing to annular, grouped papules with an uninvolved centre [11]. They commonly occur on the hands and feet but may occur anywhere on the body. GA has been associated with diabetes, HIV, thyroid disease and internal malignancy; however good diabetic control is not definitively proven to expedite resolution of GA [11]. Differential diagnoses can include cutaneous fungal infections, eczema, psoriasis or figurate erythemas.

Hidradenitis Suppurativa

Hidradenitis Suppurativa is a chronic inflammatory condition presenting as painful nodules cysts, and purulent draining sinuses in flexural areas of the axillae, groin and submammary folds [12]. It is strongly associated with obesity and diabetes with 10.6% of HS patients suffering from diabetes. The risk of having diabetes is three times greater than the general population, even when controlled for BMI [12]. Whilst Metformin has been used as a treatment for HS, it is not efficacious as a monotherapy, but useful as an adjuvant therapy in the setting of insulin resistance and in order to aid in weight loss [13].

Hyperhidrosis

Diabetic neuropathy is known to impact the autonomic nervous system [14], and both hypohidrosis/anhidrosis and hyperhidrosis have been associated with diabetes mellitus [15]. Compensatory hyperhidrosis associated with autonomic neuropathy is more commonly seen in older patients with long standing diabetes, however undiagnosed juvenile diabetes is a potential explanation for generalised hyperhidrosis in adolescents or young adults. In the setting of hyperhidrosis, screening for undiagnosed diabetes or insulin resistance, along with thyroid function is suggested, with topical, intralesional or oral therapy options for therapy [15].

Infectious Conditions

Whilst infectious complications of diabetes mellitus are beyond the scope of this chapter. Innate immune dysfunction in diabetes mellitus does increase the risk of bacterial, fungal and mycobacterial infections secondary to ineffective neutrophil function [1, 2, 16]. Many inflammatory dermatological conditions are mimics of common infectious conditions and hence infection should always be considered and appropriately excluded in the setting of diabetic associated skin disease.

Necrobiosis Lipoidica

Necrobiosis lipioidica (NLD) presents as pink-yellow plaque most commonly on the anterior shin. Ulceration is common and can be painful [17]. 0.3% of diabetic patient s suffer from NLD, however 65% of patients with NLD reported DM (Type 1 > Type 2) and patients with DM reported a longer length of disease and poorer glycaemic control. The pathogenesis of necrobiosis lipoidica is largely unknown but is thought to involve glycoprotein deposition in small vessels leading to microangiopathic changes [8]. Other theories propose a mixture of defective collagen, impaired neutrophil migration or local hypoxia [18–20]. Histologically granulomas, inflammatory infiltrates and abnormal collagen are seen in the dermis [21]. The flat yellow appearance of chronic lesions is due to subcutaneous fat necrosis and dermal thinning.

First line treatment for non-ulcerated lesions is topical or intralesional corticosteroids and to avoid trauma to the lesion. Once ulcers form, healing is slow and difficult. Management of ulcerated lesions require emphasis on general wound care principles including appropriate dressings and avoiding malnutrition and lower limb oedema. Evidence for therapy is limited to small case series only, but there are reports of effective response with phototherapy or systemic immunomodulation including fumaric acid esters, chloroquine, hydroxychloroquine or tumour necrosis factor α (TNFα) inhibition [22]. The diagnosis and treatment of necrobiosis lipoidica requires dermatology referral and should also prompt testing for diabetes.

Lichen Planus

Lichen Planus (LP) is a chronic relapsing inflammatory dermatosis, which can also affect the genital and oral mucosa [23]. LP presents as pruritic purple flat topped papules most commonly on the wrists although it can occur on any part of the skin. Nail dystrophy can occur as well as variants associated with alopecia (Lichen Planopilaris).

Patients with DM are 2.4 times more likely to suffer from lichen planus compared with healthy controls [24], although the precise pathogenesis is poorly understood. In mucosal LP there is a risk of malignant transformation. There is no known influence of glycaemic control upon the activity of LP. Treatment consists of topical corticosteroids, oral immunomodulating agents and physical therapies including phototherapy.

Localised Lipodystrophy

Insulin therapy has the potential to cause lipodystrophy by triggering localised destruction (lipoatrophy) or stimulation (lipohypertrophy) of adipose tissue at the site of injection. (Fig. 18.1c(i)). The pathogenesis of lipoatrophy is unclear, but theories include immune reactions to either insulin or inactive substances within the insulin solution, or injury from repeated injection. There are rare reports of insulin-induced lipoatrophy distant to the site of injection likely resulting from a systemic immunological reaction [25]. Lipohypertrophy presents as soft nodules

(Fig. 18.1c(ii)) that share a consistency similar to lipomas and are found at the site of repeated insulin injection (such as periumbilical or thigh). Continued injection into lipodystrophic tissue can result in impaired absorption and erratic glucose control in diabetic patients. Rotation of injection to unaffected skin is advised.

Localised Allergic Reactions

Reactions to insulin are considered rare (estimated 2% of insulin treated patients) as modern recombinant insulin preparations have amino acid sequences more similar to human insulin [26]. There are varying degrees of reaction severity. Local injection site irritation is common and mild in severity. It can be prevented with optimisation of injection technique including avoiding injection in proximity of waistband friction, ensuring adequate depth of injection and using smaller needle tips.

Immediate hypersensitivity reactions can present as local erythema and pruritis within an hour of injection, but in severe cases cause systemic anaphylaxis. The reaction is immunoglobin E (IgE) mediated (type 1 hypersensitivity),and can begin months to years after first exposure to insulin. A change in insulin preparation and allergist referral for desensitisation may be required. Delayed reactions manifest as nodules or induration localised only to the site of injection, typically arising between 6 to 24 h after the injection. Many cases are transient and spontaneously resolving. Reactions are immune complex mediated (type III hypersensitivity), or T-cell mediated (type IV hypersensitivity). It can be managed with topical steroid creams or oral antihistamines, but if the reaction persists after several months, an allergist or dermatology referral is indicated. It is important to be aware of insulin reactions, as it can impact diabetes management and in rare cases can be life-threatening.

Pigmented Purpuric Dermatosis

Pigmented Purpuric Dermatosis (PPD) is a spectrum of disorders characterised by chronic petechiae and coalescent pigmentary macules on the lower legs with significant erythrocyte extravasation and hemosiderin deposition on histology [27]. It is associated with chronic venous hypertension and diabetes mellitus as well as drug-induced and idiopathic forms. Diabetes is estimated to be present in 10% of patients with PPD. The condition is often recalcitrant to therapy however addressing the underlying predisposing factors (including diabetes) is considered helpful.

Pruritus and Xerosis

Pruritus is a common complaint in dermatological disease and can be central to the mechanism of disease or secondary to other metabolic or systemic factors. Pruritus is estimated to affect up to half of all diabetic (49%) [28], however is largely due to secondary effects of the disease such as chronic renal impairment, autonomic neuropathy, anhidrosis, xerosis, secondary infections and diabetic neuropathy. Good glycaemic control is central to managing diabetes associated pruritus, as well as appropriate pharmacological management based upon the cause of the pruritus. General skin care with non-soap-based washes, emollients, topical corticosteroids and UV therapy are common treatments for diabetic pruritus. More recalcitrant cases may require oral neuropathic agents such as doxepin or gabapentin [28].

Psoriasis Vulgaris

Psoriasis is one of the most prevalent inflammatory skin diseases (2%–4%) with metabolic syndrome increasing the risk of disease and having psoriasis increasing the risk of metabolic disease and associated macro and microvascular complications [29]. These associations are known to be independent of BMI suggesting a common inflammatory mechanism between psoriasis and metabolic syndrome [29]. The association between diabetes and psoriasis was strongest between those individuals with severe psoriasis [30]. Vascular complications are also associated with severe psoriasis but may be confounded by the use of diuretics and methotrexate, as identified in meta-analysis of studies [30].

Rubeosis Facei

Rubeosis facei is the term given to diffuse facial redness and plethora in association with diabetes. It is considered a sign of suboptimal glycaemic control and is reported in up to half of hospitalised diabetic patients [31]. The overall prevalence is estimated as 3%–5% of diabetics, and the condition is indicative of microangiopathic complications such as retinopathy [16].

Scleredema Diabeticorum

Scleredema is a rare complication of diabetes, more common in Type 2 diabetes than Type 1. It presents with woody, non-pitting thickening and induration of the back, neck, shoulders and face [32]. Scleredema is associated with diabetes as well as post-streptococcal infection and monocloncal gammopathy. Irreversible glycosylation of dermal collagen is thought to result in accumulation of collagen and mucin [32]. In the setting of diabetes, control of the underlying disease is vital in preventing further progression of the cutaneous manifestations.

Vitiligo

Vitiligo is an autoimmune disorder which manifests as loss of pigmentation due to melanocyte apoptosis mediated by CD8+ T cells [33]. It is strongly associated with endocrinological disorders including hypothyroidism, pernicious anaemia, Addisons disease and diabetes mellitus. Vitiligo demonstrates a stronger associations with Type 1 diabetes rather than Type 2 diabetes suggesting a common CD8+ T cell autoimmune aetiology. There is no evidence to say that improved glycaemic control gives benefit to vitiligo control. Treatments for vitiligo include topical corticosteroids, topical calcineurin inhibitors, UV therapy as well as more recent trials of JAK inhibitors such as ruloxitinib.

Xanothomas (Eruptive)

Cutaneous Xanthomas are red-yellow lobulated papules which can be a cutaneous manifestation of hypertriglyceridaemia or poorly controlled diabetes mellitus [34, 35]. They have been associated with type 1 as well as type 2 diabetes and also in the setting of diabetic lipaemia [35]. Treatment involves aggressive management of hyperglycaemia as well as hypertriglyceridaemia and lipaemia.

Diabetic Foot Ulceration

The Association Between Diabetic Foot Ulceration and Cardiovascular Disease

Diabetic foot ulceration (DFU) affects approximately 15% of people during the course of diabetes mellitus [36], and has important implications for cardiovascular health. Five-year mortality is independently predicted by DFU in multivariate analyses that include other prevalent diabetes complications, with a hazard ratio of 2.48 (95% confidence interval 2.43–2.54) compared to people with diabetes without DFU [37]. In fact, the mortality rate is comparable to many common types of cancer [38].

Mortality in people with DFU is attributable to ischaemic heart disease in up to two-thirds of cases [39]. Ulcer aetiology should be considered in cardiovascular risk assessment, as the presence of ischaemia denotes higher mortality than neuropathy alone [39]. Significant peripheral vascular disease likely indicates atherosclerotic disease burden in the coronary and cerebral vasculature [40]. However, the presence of microvascular disease is also of relevance. Increased mortality is observed in people with diabetes mellitus and cardiovascular autonomic neuropathy with a relative risk of 2.14 (95% confidence interval 2.66–4.47), with asymptomatic ischaemia and arrhythmias a probable precipitant for sudden death [41].

People with DFU are more likely to have dyslipidaemia, microalbuminuria or proteinuria, higher glycosylated haemoglobin (HbA1c), and greater prevalence of macro- and microvascular diabetes complications [42]. Intensive cardiovascular risk management has been shown to improve mortality [39]. Of note, those with neuropathic ulceration also benefit with such strategies, albeit to a lesser degree [39]. Therefore, the presence of peripheral neuropathy may in itself suggest significant macrovascular disease in some individuals with diabetes.

General Assessment and Management of Diabetic Foot Ulceration

Given the high morbidity and mortality associated with the condition [43], and the deleterious consequences on quality of life [44], the personal and society costs of DFU are significant. Management of lower-limb complications in diabetes mellitus constitutes up to one third of healthcare expenditure in diabetes care [38]. Therefore, the need for concerted efforts to systematically prevent and manage DFU is well recognised.

Foot assessment forms part of the routine diabetes complication screen performed at least annually, and incorporates patient education and review of footwear. Beyond identifying active ulceration, a brief history and neurovascular foot examination allows for risk stratification. The 'high-risk foot' is defined by the presence of two or more risk factors, including peripheral neuropathy, peripheral arterial disease and foot deformity, or by the presence of previous foot ulceration or amputation [45, 46]. Following ulcer healing, the risk of recurrence within one year is approximately 40% [38].

Standard evaluation of DFU should cover the mechanism of injury, duration, site, depth, neurovascular status and signs of infection. Ill-fitting footwear is the most common precipitant of ulceration [47]. Chronic and deep ulceration increases the likelihood of underlying osteomyelitis, which can be further investigated using a probe and imaging. The site and appearance of the ulcer may suggest a particular aetiology (see Fig. 18.2). Bedside assessment provides valuable outcome stratification by use of validated grading systems, such as The Society for Vascular Surgery Lower Extremity Threatened Limb Classification System (Wound extent, Ischemia, and foot Infection [WIfI]) [43].

Key elements to consider in DFU management include [36, 45, 47, 48]:

- Pressure offloading and non-weight bearing
- Revascularisation
- Treatment of infection, which may involve debridement or amputation
- Regular dressings and advanced wound management (e.g. negative pressure therapy, bioengineered tissues)
- Glycaemic control and diabetes education, noting that hyperglycaemia (especially blood glucose levels greater than 12 mmol/L) impairs wound healing [44]
- Treatment of other cardiovascular risk factors, including hypertension and dyslipidaemia
- Smoking cessation strategies
- Social and psychological support
- Preventative education regarding regular foot checks, first aid and footwear

Wholistic management of DFU is resource intensive and complex. People with DFU should be managed by specialised multidisciplinary teams, especially when ulceration is deep, ischaemic, infected or non-healing. Specialised services have been shown to reduce amputation risk [47], emergency department admissions, inpatient cost and length of hospitalisation (Fig. 18.3) [49].

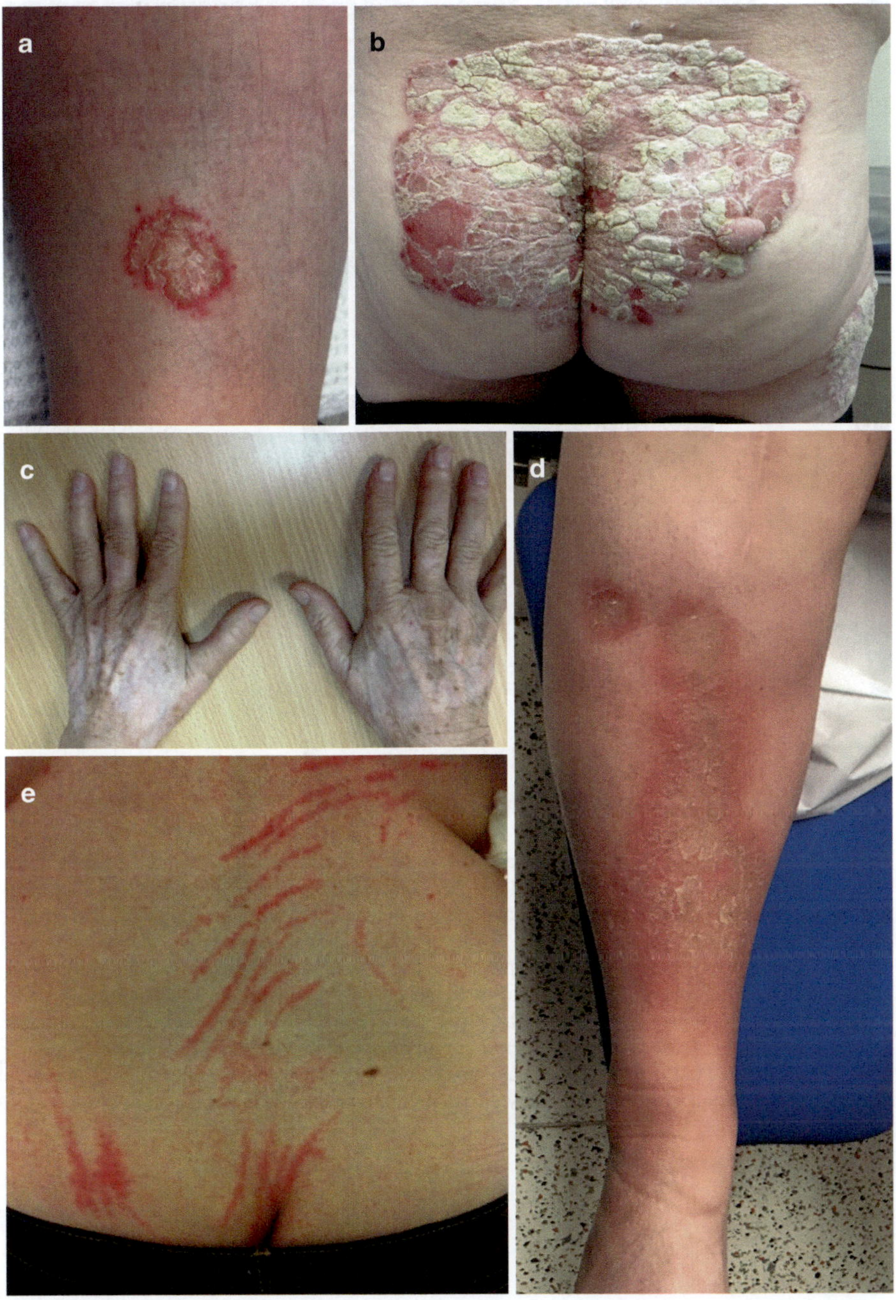

Fig. 18.2 Assorted Clinical Conditions Associated with Diabetes Mellitus including (**a**) Infections including Tinea Corporis, (**b**) Chronic Plaque Psoriasis, (**c**) Vitiligo of the dorsum of the hands, (**d**) Necorbiosis Lipoidica of the pretibial aspect of the lower leg, (**e**) Excoriations in the absence of primary skin disease (Endogenous Pruritus)

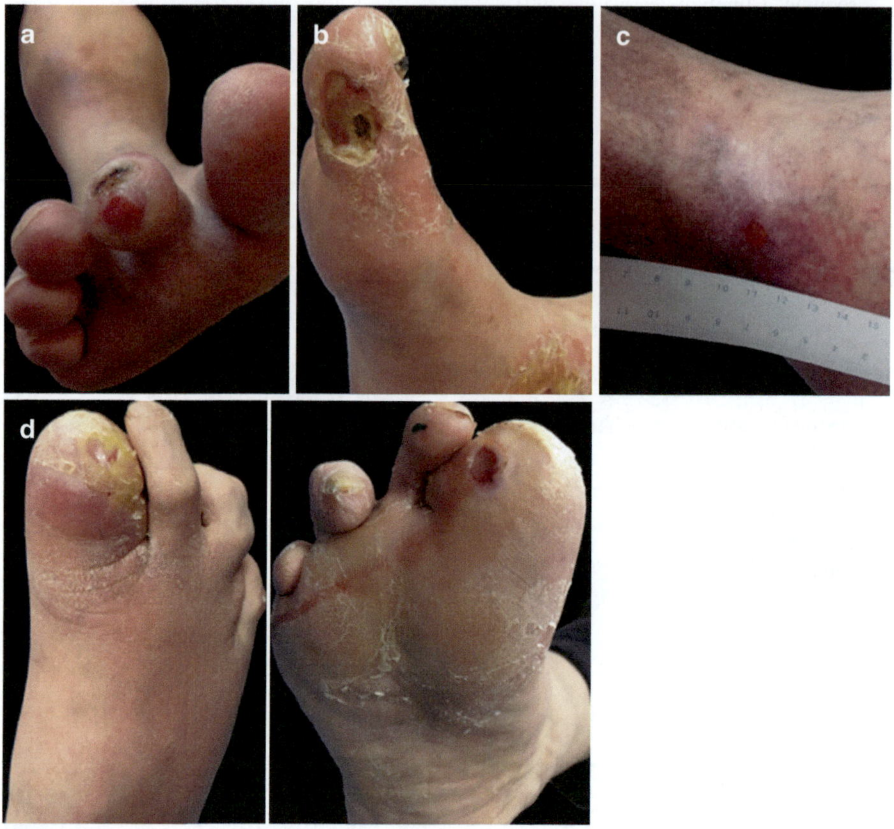

Fig. 18.3 The clinical presentation of diabetic foot ulceration is varied, and clinical features are often suggestive of the underlying aetiology. (**a**) Neuropathic ulceration: Mallet toe deformity leading to ulceration in an area of abnormal pressure, evidenced by surrounding callus and onychauxis. There is also xerosis and erythema. (**b**) Arterial ulceration: Irregular deep ulceration with a necrotic base in a location vulnerable to pressure. The skin is characteristically anhidrotic, cool, shiny and thin, with reduced hair. Pedal pulses are absent. (**c**) Venous ulceration: Shallow irregular ulceration, which is typically located in the gaiter area. There is accompanying oedema, lipodermatosclerosis and varicose veins. (**d**) Ulceration probing-to-bone: Plantar hallux ulceration, which on probing extended to the promixal phalanx and to the dorsal surface through a sinus. The dactylitic appearance is concerning for osteomyelitis and cellulitis extends to the dorsal midfoot

Investigation of Cardiovascular Disease in Diabetic Foot Ulceration

While the high prevalence of cardiovascular disease in people with DFU is irrefutable, the optimal approach to screen such individuals for subclinical disease is uncertain. In people with diabetes, those with DFU are more likely to have major electrocardiogram abnormalities, left ventricular hypertrophy, abnormal regional wall motion, abnormal carotid intima-media thickness and carotid plaque on Doppler ultrasound [42].

An annual electrocardiogram is a feasible investigation to identify subclinical conduction abnormalities, as it may direct avoidance of medications with the potential to cause hypoglycaemia or QTc prolongation. In people with DFU and HbA1c below 7.5% (58 mmol/mol), the presence of QTc prolongation has been associated with high mortality (92% compared to 49% at 8 years) [50]. QTc prolongation is a feature of cardiac autonomic neuropathy, and when compounded by hypoglycaemic unawareness due to loss of typical adrenergic warning symptoms, it predisposes the individual to cardiac arrhythmia [50]. Cardiac autonomic neuropathy as defined by an abnormal R-R ratio or orthostatic hypotension is more common in people with diabetic peripheral neuropathy, especially in those with DFU [51].

Screening for subclinical myocardial ischaemia should also be considered in people with DFU, particularly if major procedures are planned. In people with diabetes and no symptoms or history of ischaemic heart disease, those with peripheral neuropathy more likely had myocardial ischaemia as identified on electrocardiographically gated Technetium-99 m (Tc-99 m) sestamibi single-photon emission computed tomographic (SPECT) [51]. In individuals requiring peripheral revascularisation for DFU, targeted stress echocardiography identified the need for concomitant coronary revascularisation in approximately half of cases [52].

People hospitalised for DFU appear to be at particularly high risk of major cardiovascular events. Non-ST elevation myocardial infarction and sudden cardiac arrest comprise almost half of inpatient complications, and a minority have typical chest pain [53]. Major cardiovascular events generally occur within 10 days of admission or major procedure (for example amputation), and most have non-specific ST-T wave changes or new left bundle branch block on electrocardiogram [53]. Where stress echocardiography identifies myocardial ischaemia, coronary revascularisation at the time of peripheral revascularisation for DFU appears to result in favourable limb salvage and survival outcomes [52].

Conclusion

Although largely benign and a cosmetic nuisance for patients, it is important that physicians recognise the range of skin manifestations of diabetes mellitus and insulin treatment. The presence of acanthosis nigricans and necrobiosis lipoidica should alert the physician to investigate for a diagnosis of diabetes, and lipodystrophy may signal inappropriate insulin injection technique, potentially compromising treatment efficacy. Further studies are required to better understand their pathogenesis and treatment options.

Diabetic foot ulceration is associated with high cardiovascular morbidity and mortality. Assessment of DFU is not only of importance in directing ulceration management; moreover, identifying the aetiology of ulceration has important implications for cardiovascular risk factor modification and screening. Recognition of subclinical conduction abnormalities and myocardial ischaemia, and early intervention is likely to improve clinical outcomes for people with DFU.

References

1. Graves DT, Kayal RA. Diabetic complications and dysregulated innate immunity. Front Biosci. 2008;13:1227–39.
2. Torley D, Bellus GA, Munro CS. Genes, growth factors and acanthosis nigricans. Br J Dermatol. 2002 Dec;147(6):1096–101.
3. Ahmad S, Mahmoudi H, Naeem M, Betz RC. Autosomal recessive isolated familial acanthosis nigricans in a Pakistani family due to a homozygous mutation in the insulin receptor gene. Br J Dermatol. 2013 Aug;169(2):476–8.
4. Romo A, Benavides S. Treatment options in insulin resistance obesity-related acanthosis nigricans. Ann Pharmacother. 2008 Jul;42(7):1090–4.
5. Emiroglu N, Cengiz FP, Kemeriz F. Insulin resistance in severe acne vulgaris. Postepy Dermatol Alergol. 2015;32(4):281–5.
6. Cerman AA, Aktas E, Altunay IK, Arici JE, Tulunay A, Ozturk FY. Dietary glycaemic factors, insulin resistance and adiponectin levels in acen vulgaris. J Am Acad Dermatol. 2016;75(1):155–62.
7. Lynde CB, Pratt MD. Acquired perforating dermatosis; association with diabetes and renal failure. CMAJ. 2009;181(9):615.
8. Shahi N, Bradley S, Vowden K, Vowden P. Diabetic bullae: a case series and a new model of surgical management. J Wound Care. 2014;23(6):326.
9. Larsen K, Jensen T, Karlsmark T, Holstein PR. Incidence of bullosis diabeticorum - a contraversial ause of chronic foot ulceration. Int Wound J. 2008;5(4):591–6.
10. Iversen L, Bygum A. Diabetic dermopathy. BMJ. 2018;363:k4882.
11. Wang J, Khachemoune A. Granuloma Annulare: a focused review of therapeutic options. Am J Clin Dermatol. 2018;19(3):333–4.
12. Bui TL, Silva-Hirschberg C, Torres J, Armstrong AW. Hidradenitis Suppurativa and diabetes mellitus: a systematic review and meta-analysis. J Am Acad Dermatol. 2018;78(2):395–402.
13. Frew JW, Hawkes JE, Krueger JG. Topical, systemic and biologic therapies in hidradenitis suppurativa: pathogenic insights by examining therapeutic mechanisms. Ther Adv Chron Dis. 2019;10 https://doi.org/10.1177/2040622319830646.
14. Scheinberg N, Salbu RL, Goswami G, Cohen K. Treatment of diabetic autonomic neuropathy in older adults with diabetes melitus. Consult Pharm. 2016;31(11):633–45.

15. Amano M, Namiki T, Munetsugu T, et al. Dyshidrosis associated with diabetes mellitus: hypohidrosis associated with diabetic neuropathy and compensated hyperhidrosis. J Deramtol. 2019;46:e292–3. https://doi.org/10.1111/1346-8138.14840.
16. Duff M, Demidova O, Blackburn S, Shubrook J. Cutaneous manifestations of diabetes mellitus. Clin Diabetes. 2015;33(1):40–8.
17. Erfurt-Berge C, Dissemond J, Schwede K, Seitz A-T, Al Ghazal P, Wollina U, et al. Updated results of 100 patients on clinical features and therapeutic options in necrobiosis lipoidica in a retrospective multicentre study. Eur J Dermatol. 2015 Dec;25(6):595–601.
18. Reid SD, Ladizinski B, Lee K, Baibergenova A, Alavi A. Update on necrobiosis lipoidica: a review of etiology, diagnosis, and treatment options. J Am Acad Dermatol. 2013 Nov;69(5):783–91.
19. Evans CD, Pereira RS, Yuen CT, Holden CA. Anti-collagen antibodies in granuloma annulare and necrobiosis lipoidica. Clin Exp Dermatol. 1988 Jul;13(4):252–4.
20. Gange RW, Black MM, Carrington P. Defective neutrophil migration in granuloma annulare, necrobiosis lipoidica, and sarcoidosis. Arch Dermatol. 1979 Jan;115(1):32–5.
21. Alegre VA, Winkelmann RK. A new histopathologic feature of necrobiosis lipoidica diabeticorum: lymphoid nodules. J Cutan Pathol. 1988 Apr;15(2):75–7.
22. Peckruhn M, Tittelbach J, Elsner P. Update: treatment of necrobiosis lipoidica. J Dtsch Dermatol Ges. 2017;15(2):151–7.
23. Atzmony L, Reiter O, Hodak E, Gdalevich M, Mimouni D. Treatments for cutaneous lichen planus: a systematic review and meta analysis. Am J Clin Dermatol. 2016;17(1):11–22.
24. Otero Rey EM, Yanez-Busto A, Rosa-Henriquez IF, Lopez-Lopez J, Blanco-Carrion A. Lichen planus and diabetes mellitus: systematic review and meta-analysis. Oral Dis. 2018;25(5):1253–64. https://doi.org/10.1111/odi.12977.
25. Kondo A, Nakamura A, Takeuchi J, Miyoshi H, Atsumi T. Insulin-induced distant site lipoatrophy. Diabetes Care. 2017 Jun 1;40(6):e67–8.
26. Ghazavi MK, Johnston GA. Insulin allergy. Clin Dermatol. 2011 May 1;29(3):300–5.
27. Kim DH, Seo SH, Ahn HH, Kye YC, CHoi JE. Characteristics and clinical manifestations of pigmented purpuric dermatoses. Ann Dermatol. 2015;27(4):404–10.
28. Babakinejad P, Walton S. Diabetes and pruritus. Br J Diabetes. 2016;16:154–5.
29. Wan MT, Shin DB, Hubbard RA, Ne MH, Mehat NN, Gelfand JM. Psoriasis and the risk of diabetes: a prospective population-based cohort study. J Am Acad Dermatol. 2018;78(2):315–22.
30. Armstrong AW, Harskamp CT, Armstrong EJ. Psoraisis and the risk of diabetes mellitus: a systematic review and meta analysis. JAMA Dermatol. 2013;149(1):84–91.
31. Namazi MR, Jorizzo JL, Fallahzadeh MK. Rubeosis faciei diabeticorum: a common, but often unnoticed, clinical manifestation of diabetes mellitus. Sci World J. 2010;10:70–1.
32. Namas R, Ashrat A. Scleredema of Buschke. Eur J Rheumatol. 2016;3(4):191–2.
33. Frisoli ML, Harris JE. Vitiligo: mechanistic insights lead to novel treatments. J Allergy Clin Immunol. 2017;140(3):654–62.
34. Mendes AL, Miot HA, Junior VH. Diabetes mellitus and the skin. An Bras Dermatol. 2017;92(1):8–20.
35. Tsuchiya S, Sawada S, Takeda K, et al. Erupive xanthomas in a patient with soft ftink diabetic ketoacdiosis and apolipoprotein E4/2. Endocr J. 2019;66(1):107–14.
36. Frykberg RG, Zgonis T, Armstrong DG, et al. Diabetic foot disorders. A clinical practice guideline (2006 revision). J Foot Ankle Surg. 2006;45:S1–66.
37. Walsh JW, Hoffstad OJ, Sullivan MO, Margolis DJ. Association of diabetic foot ulcer and death in a population-based cohort from the United Kingdom. Diabet Med. 2016;33:1493–8.
38. Armstrong DG, Wrobel J, Robbins JM. Guest editorial: are diabetes-related wounds and amputations worse than cancer? Int Wound J. 2007;4:286–7.
39. Young MJ, McCardle JE, Randall LE, Barclay JI. Improved survival of diabetic foot ulcer patients 1995-2008: possible impact of aggressive cardiovascular risk management. Diabetes Care. 2008;31:2143–7.
40. Moulik PK, Mtonga R, Gill GV. Amputation and mortality in new-onset diabetic foot ulcers stratified by etiology. Diabetes Care. 2003;26:491–4.

41. Vinik AI, Ziegler D. Diabetic cardiovascular autonomic neuropathy. Circulation. 2007;115:387–97.
42. Pinto A, Tuttolomondo A, Di Raimondo D, et al. Cardiovascular risk profile and morbidity in subjects affected by type 2 diabetes mellitus with and without diabetic foot. Metabolism. 2008;57:676–82.
43. Causey MW, Ahmed A, Wu B, et al. Society for vascular surgery limb stage and patient risk correlate with outcomes in an amputation prevention program. J Vasc Surg. 2016;63:1563–73. e2
44. Jeffcoate WJ, Harding KG. Diabetic foot ulcers. Lancet. 2003;361:1545–51.
45. National Health and Medical Research Council. National evidence-based guideline on prevention, identification and management of foot complications in diabetes (Part of the guidelines on management of Type 2 diabetes). Melbourne, Australia 2011.
46. McCabe CJ, Stevenson RC, Dolan AM. Evaluation of a diabetic foot screening and protection programme. Diabet Med. 1998;15:80–4.
47. Apelqvist J, Bakker K, van Houtum WH, Schaper NC, International Working Group on the Diabetic Foot Editorial B. Practical guidelines on the management and prevention of the diabetic foot: based upon the International Consensus on the Diabetic Foot (2007) Prepared by the International Working Group on the Diabetic Foot. Diabetes Metab Res Rev. 2008;24(Suppl 1):S181–7.
48. Armstrong DG, Boulton AJM, Bus SA. Diabetic foot ulcers and their recurrence. N Engl J Med. 2017;376:2367–75.
49. Lasschuit JWJ, Greenfield JR, Tonks KT. High risk foot service reduces number of emergency department presentations and length of stay. Diabetes Metab. 2018;46(3):252–5.
50. Fagher K, Londahl M. The impact of metabolic control and QTc prolongation on all-cause mortality in patients with type 2 diabetes and foot ulcers. Diabetologia. 2013;56:1140–7.
51. Tesfaye S, Chaturvedi N, Eaton SE, et al. Vascular risk factors and diabetic neuropathy. N Engl J Med. 2005;352:341–50.
52. Rigatelli G, Cardaioli P, Dell'avvocata F, Giordan M, Lisato G, Mollo F. Endovascular management of patients with coronary artery disease and diabetic foot syndrome: a long-term follow-up. J Geriatr Cardiol. 2011;8:78–81.
53. Hung SY, Huang YY, Hsu LA, et al. Treatment for diabetic foot ulcers complicated by major cardiac events. Can J Diabetes. 2015;39:183–7.

19 Lysosomal Storage Disorders: Fabry Disease

P. Geenty, M. Tchan, and L. Thomas

Introduction

The lysosomal storage disorders (LSD) are a heterogeneous group of more than 50 rare, inherited deficiencies in specific proteins involved in lysosomal biology, that result in abnormal accumulation of the relevant substrate. Further discussion will be largely limited to Anderson Fabry disease (Fabry disease), an example of a LSD affecting both the heart and the skin, amongst various other organ systems. In addition to Fabry disease, other lysosomal storage disorders are known to affect the heart causing a hypertrophic cardiomyopathic phenotype, including glycogen storage diseases (Pompe and Danon diseases), as well as the sphingolipidoses which include Fabry, Gaucher and Niemann-Pick diseases. [1, 2] Gaucher disease is the most well-known of the lysosomal storage diseases, however cardiac manifestations are rare, and Fabry disease is unique amongst LSD as there is no infantile form that is lethal in childhood. [3]

Fabry disease, an X-linked lysosomal disorder, is characterised by the absence or deficiency of α-galactosidase, which is responsible for the breakdown of glycosphingolipids. Consequent accumulation, primarily of globotriaosylceramide (Gb3), occurs in various tissues leading to the major clinical manifestations of childhood neuropathic pain, and renal failure, hypertrophic cardiac disease and cerebrovascular disease (CVD) in adulthood. Intracellular accumulation of Gb3 begins in utero [4] and continues throughout life, with Gb3 accumulating in most cell types, particularly vascular endothelium throughout the body. Fabry disease can thus be considered primarily a systemic vasculopathy, although the downstream

P. Geenty · L. Thomas (✉)
Cardiology Department, Westmead Hospital, Westmead, NSW, Australia
e-mail: paul.geenty@health.nsw.gov.au; liza.thomas@sydney.edu.au

M. Tchan
Genetic Medicine Department, Westmead Hospital, Westmead, NSW, Australia
e-mail: michel.tchan@health.nsw.gov.au

C. Salavastru et al. (eds.), *Skin and the Heart*,
https://doi.org/10.1007/978-3-030-54779-0_19

pathophysiological consequences of Gb3 deposition are complex and remain poorly understood.

In addition to Gb3, one of its degradation products Lyso-Gb3 (globotriaosylsphingosine), also accumulates in Fabry disease, and is worthy of particular mention due to its increasingly recognised role both in the pathophysiology of the disease, as well as its use in diagnosis and monitoring response to therapy [5]. Lyso-Gb3 has been implicated in contributing to endothelial and myocyte hypertrophy [6], and its role as a biomarker has been demonstrated, with it correlating with mutation type and predicting phenotype severity, as well as discriminating between classic and delayed onset phenotypes [7, 8]. Importantly it was shown to identify disease in females with normal enzyme activity [9].

Prevalence/Population Affected

Unlike the majority of Lysosomal Storage Disorders, which show autosomal recessive inheritance, Fabry disease is inherited in an X-linked pattern, as are Danon disease and Hunter syndrome [2]. Whilst it was initially believed that females were asymptomatic carriers, it is now known that female patients eventually exhibit some or all the manifestations of the disease. Indeed, female patients may develop severe manifestations, albeit at a later age with a slower rate of disease progression [10].

The *GLA* gene encoding alpha galactosidase is 7 exons long, and located on the X-chromosome (Xq22.1). More than 900 mutations have been identified. Single base changes and small deletions or insertions account for over 90% of mutations in the *GLA* gene [11], with most families having "private" mutations. There is significant heterogeneity between families with regard to enzyme activity and severity of clinical phenotypes (discussed in more detail below) [1]. Significant variability may also be seen within members of the same family, suggesting contributions from epigenetic, environmental or comorbid processes determining natural history [12].

Classical Fabry disease is rare, with a reported incidence ranging from 1:40,000 to 117,000 of live male births [1, 13]. More recently, centres performing newborn screening have reported rates of 1:1368 to 1:8882 of live births. [8] It is thus apparent that there are many more patients with non-classical phenotypes (generally presenting with isolated late-onset cardiac disease), than classically affected males. These non-classical phenotypes largely result from mutations that allow for residual enzyme activity, and can additionally be distinguished on clinical grounds as well as lower Lyso-Gb3 levels.

Due to its multisystem and variable manifestations as well as its rarity, interest has been applied to screening within those with end stage renal failure, LVH/HCM, as well as early or cryptogenic stroke. Fabry disease should be considered in patients undergoing workup for possible HCM, in particular those that lack a known HCM sarcomeric mutation. This is of particular importance since the advent of targeted therapeutic options for Fabry disease. Prevalence of Fabry disease within HCM cohorts range from 0 to 12%, depending on the populations studied [14, 15]. Most studies report rates of 0.5 to 1% amongst HCM patients, [5, 16] rising to 5% when limited to patients lacking sarcomeric mutations [17]. Amongst a cohort of females with presumed late onset HCM, 12% were subsequently found to have Fabry disease. Similarly, cohort studies of male patients with unexplained LVH have provided variable rates of 3–10% [18, 19]. Rates amongst patients with early or cryptogenic stroke also vary from 1–5% [20–22], and amongst patients receiving haemodialysis, up to 1% [23].

Clinical Manifestations

The accumulated substrates in Fabry disease, of which Gb3 is the hallmark, can be found in various tissues, the most clinically relevant including cardiac, skin, renal, neural and vascular. The disease carries significant morbidity and mortality, due to adult onset cardiac hypertrophy, renal impairment, and stroke.

By comparison, childhood symptoms, typically with onset between the ages of 5–10 in males, are distinct from the above and include neuropathic pain/acroparasthesia, gastrointestinal symptoms, heat/cold or exercise intolerance, and the angiokeratoma characteristic of the disease. [1] The non-dermatological early manifestations are likely due to involvement of the peripheral and autonomic nervous systems [24]. Proteinuria can be detected from the second decade of life onwards, whilst neurological and cardiac manifestations typically follow from the third decade. (Fig. 19.1).

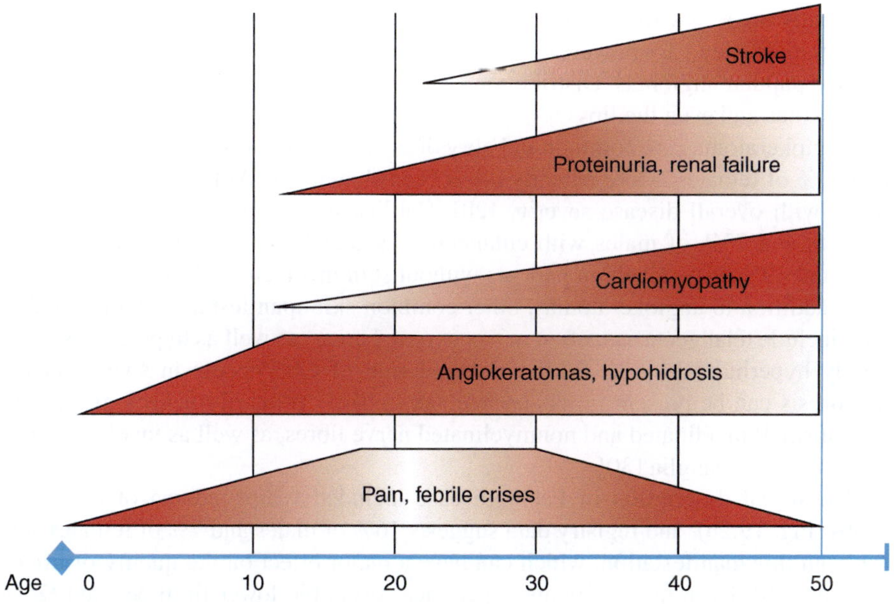

Fig. 19.1 Diagrammatic representation of the age distribution related to the various multisystem manifestations of Anderson Fabry disease. From " *Natural History and typical clinical manifestations of Fabry Disease" (Linhart et al; Heart 2007;93:528–535)*. Pending permission from Publisher

The above clinical manifestations describe classical Fabry disease in males, with the additional biochemical marker of greatly elevated Lyso-Gb3. Non-classical presentations of Fabry disease are, as previously mentioned, usually associated with isolated cardiac findings and much lower levels of Lyso-Gb3. Specific mutations, such as p.N215S and IVS4 + 919G > A, are known to be associated with non-classical disease [25].

Dermatological Manifestation

Fabry disease was initially identified as a dermatological condition, first described in 1898, independently by dermatologist Johanes Fabry and surgeon William Anderson, and given the term Angiokeratoma Corporis Diffusum [14]. However, when autopsy studies revealed its systemic involvement, it was considered more than an isolated dermatological condition. Among the various non-cardiac manifestations now recognised, the most common remain dermatological. Dermatological symptoms contribute to the early morbidity seen in Fabry disease, with hypohidrosis and associated heat intolerance, the commonest symptoms [26].

Angiokeratomas usually emerge between the age of 5 and 13 years. They are telangiectatic lesions of the capillaries in the upper dermis, covered by a hyperkeratotic epidermis and surround by epidermal "collars" (Fig. 19.2a) [27]. They classically present initially as small, maculopapular, non-blanching angiectasias, purplish-red in colour, which subsequently increase in size and number with age, classically in a "swimming trunk" distribution and around the umbilicus [12]. Appearances may vary however, including macular angiomas lacking hyperkeratosis, and papular angiomas. Distribution can also vary, involving the proximal limbs, palms/soles and even the lips.

Angiokeratomas are common in Fabry disease, and are present in 70% of males, and 39% of females. More recently it has been shown that skin manifestations correlate with overall disease severity [28]. Cardiac involvement is seen in 80% of females and 73% of males with cutaneous vascular lesions, compared with only 38% and 49% respectively in patients without skin involvement [29].

In addition to angiokeratomas, other common skin manifestations in Fabry disease include telangectasias, often in sun exposed areas, as well as hypo or less commonly hyperhidrosis [13]. Whilst accumulation of Gb3 occurs in sweat glands, anhidrosis can be present in its absence and is likely primarily neurological, with loss of small myelinated and nonmyelinated nerve fibres, as well as involvement of the dorsal root ganglia [30].

The initial description of Fabry disease included lymphoedema of the lower limbs (Fig. 19.2b), and registry data suggests 16% of males and 7% of females suffer from this manifestation, which can have a major effect on the quality of life of patients [28]. Even more patients experience reversible lower limb oedema (25% and 17% in males and females respectively). Exact mechanisms are unknown, and it is unclear if accumulation of Gb3 damages lymphatic networks, however fluorescence microangiography has shown fragmentation of the microlymphatic network

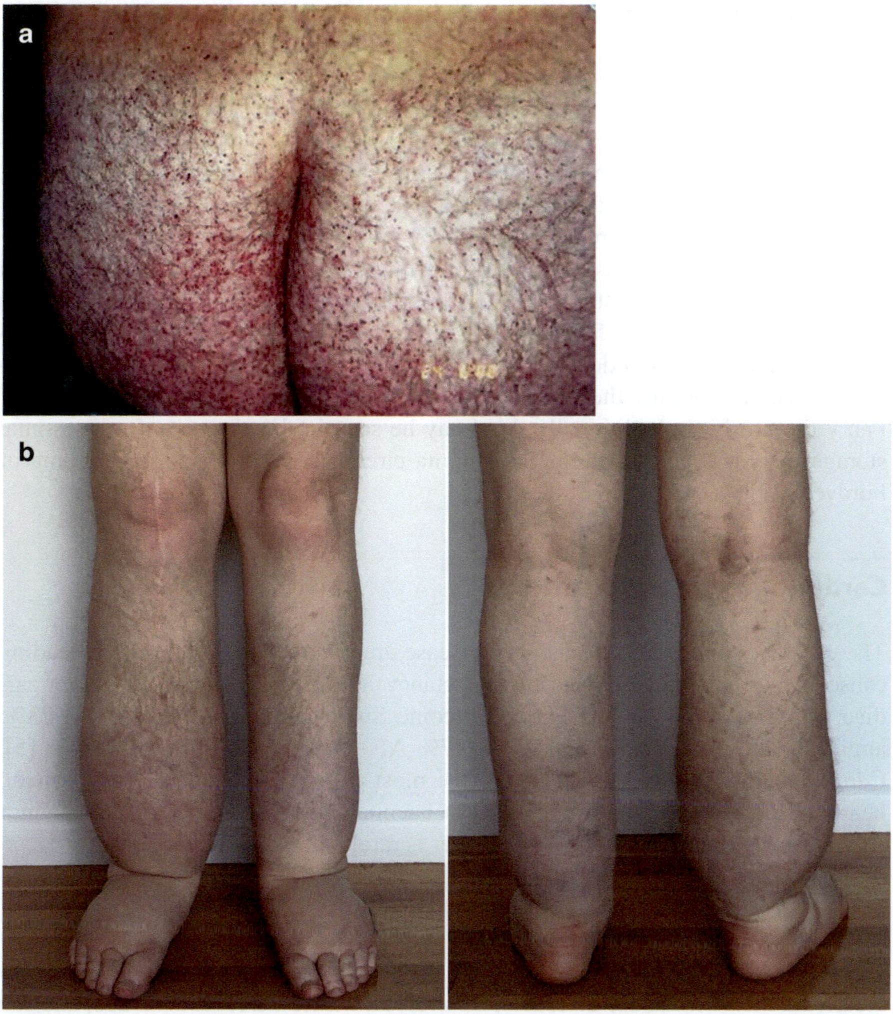

Fig. 19.2 (**a**) Typical appearance of angiokeratoma in the "swimming trunk" distribution. (**b**) Bilateral lower limb lymphoedema in a patient with Anderson Fabry disease is a common manifestation

[31]. Concomitant cardiac and renal failure associated with Fabry disease can further exacerbate oedema; however their presence does not correlate with the presence of lymphoedema.

Although not a strictly dermatological manifestation, males with classical Fabry disease often have characteristic facies; with features including periorbital fullness, prominent lobules of the ears, bushy eyebrows, recessed forehead, pronounced nasal angle, generous nose/bulbous nasal tip, prominent supraorbital ridges, shallow midface, full lips, prominent nasal bridge, broad alar base, coarse features, posteriorly rotated ears, and prognathism [32].

Histological Findings

Accumulation of Gb3 can be demonstrated in vascular endothelial cells, smooth muscle cells, fibroblasts and eccrine sweat glands [12]. Histology typically shows dilated, ectatic papillary dermal capillaries, epidermal acanthosis, and focal orthohyperkeratosis [33]. Histological evidence of Fabry disease is not limited to areas of skin lesions, with dermal cells obtained from unaffected skin also showing accumulation of glycosphingolipids. Gb3 can be readily detected by immunohistochemistry.

Whilst angiokeratoma is considered a hallmark of Fabry disease, they are seen in several other lysosomal storage disorders, including oligosaccharidoses such as fucosidosis (seen in over 50%), alpha-N-galactosaminidase deficiency, beta mannosidosis and galactosialidosis. [34–37] As is the case with cardiac and ocular manifestations, chloroquine therapy may mimic the dermatological manifestations of Fabry disease [38]. Additionally they may be seen in the absence of a lysosomal storage disorder, such as in angiokeratoma circumscriptum, or angiokeratoma of Fordyce [39].

Cardiological Manifestations

The cardiac manifestations of Fabry disease are diverse, and are now the leading cause of mortality and reduced life expectancy. The majority of patients suffer cardiac symptoms (60% in the Fabry Outcome Survey), namely dyspnoea in 23%, angina in 23%, palpitations in 27% (17% AF, 8% NSVT), syncope in 4% [5]. Cardiac manifestations include LVH (the most common), left atrial enlargement, heart failure, arrhythmias, small vessel ischaemia and sudden cardiac death. Minor valvular involvement is common, however is rarely clinically significant.

Left Ventricular Hypertrophy

Nearly all men with Fabry disease develop LVH, which increases with age, and can be severe. This is typically concentric (Fig. 19.3a), however asymmetric hypertrophy which mimics sarcomeric HCM is also seen. In rare cases, LV outflow tract obstruction is seen [40]. Another feature is prominent and hypertrophied papillary muscles (Fig. 19.3b). Heart failure is a leading cause of morbidity in Fabry disease, with average age of onset of 32 and 40 years in males and females respectively [41].

Most patients have preserved systolic function, with progressive diastolic dysfunction, worsening hypertrophy, and eventually fibrosis and scar formation predisposing to ventricular arrhythmia and sudden cardiac death. Thus, the Fabry cardiomyopathy is progressive, and is the most common cause of death in Fabry disease [42].

Transthoracic echocardiography has been the mainstay for screening, though MRI may be complimentary. More recently, echocardiographic strain imaging has detected subclinical and regional impairment early on in the disease course,

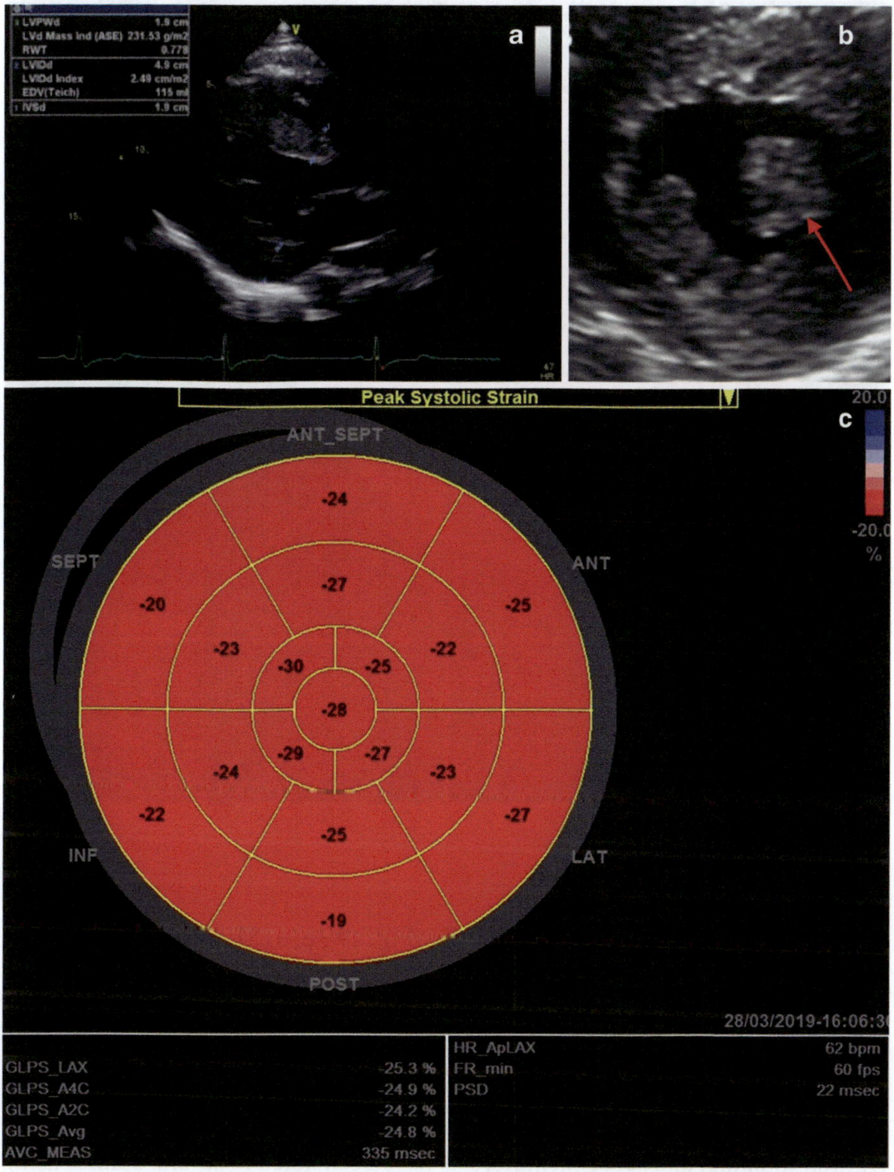

Fig. 19.3 (**a**) Transthoracic echocardiogram showing typical left ventricular hypertrophy, seen on parasternal long axis view. (**b**) Prominent papillary muscles (arrow) seen on short axis view. C: "Bullseye" plot showing LV longitudinal strain in a healthy control. D: Typical distribution of LV peak systolic strain, with impairment primarily in inferoposterior segments (arrow)

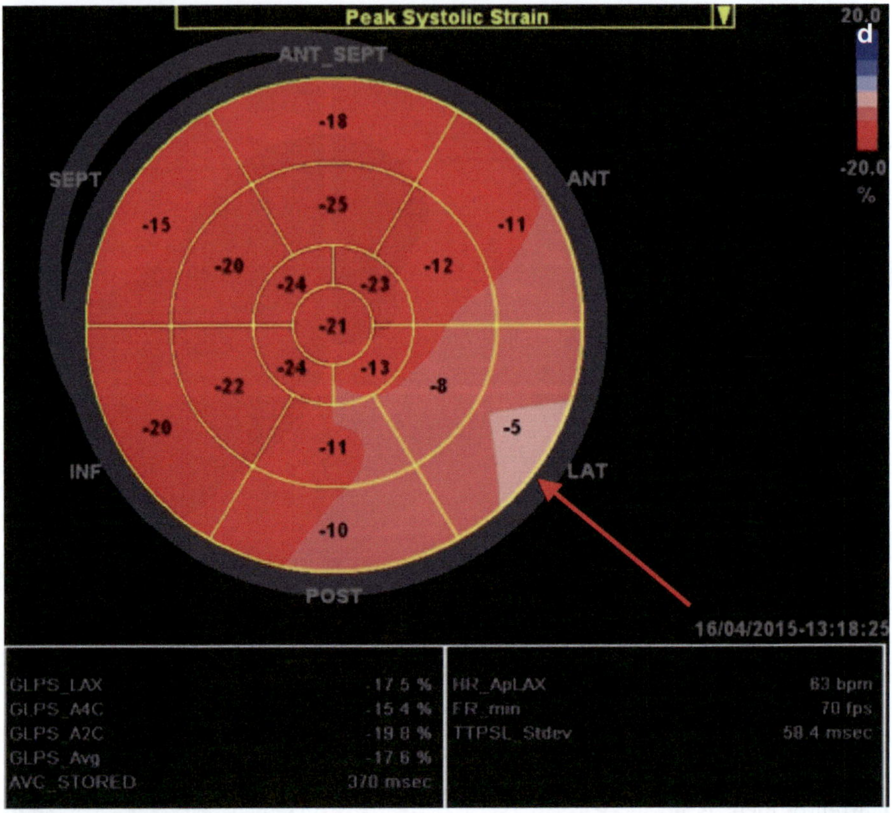

Fig. 19.3 (continued)

independent of the presence of LVH. [42] (Fig. 19.3c, d) Strain imaging has also shown promise in differentiating Fabry cardiomyopathy from other forms of hypertrophic cardiomyopathy. Whilst the focus has been on left ventricular function, recent studies have shown reduced strain in the right ventricle and both atria, which reflects that accumulation of Gb3 is not limited to the left ventricle [43].

Despite the classical concentric pattern of hypertrophy, regional variations in LV wall thinning, and subsequent fibrosis have been noted in several studies using cardiac magnetic resonance (CMR) imaging with gadolinium contrast enhancement. Intramural fibrosis progresses to transmural, and usually involves the basal posterolateral segments of the LV [1]. It is thought that the predilection for both wall thinning and fibrosis to occur in the posterior wall may be due to increased wall stress [26]. Interestingly, CMR studies with late gadolinium enhancement have shown that unlike male patients in whom hypertrophy always precedes fibrosis, female patients can develop fibrosis in the absence of LVH [44]. MRI has also demonstrated consistently low T1 signal, even prior to the development of hypertrophy or scarring [45].

Angina/Ischaemia

Exertional symptoms of angina are common (13–23%) [1], reflecting microvascular ischaemia, as significant epicardial coronary artery lesions are uncommon, and myocardial infarction is rare (2%). In addition to small vessel disease, increased oxygen demand due to hypertrophy, and endothelial dysfunction may contribute to exertional chest pain [46]. Assessment of myocardial blood flow using Positron Emission Tomography (PET) imaging has shown severe impairment in coronary microvascular function, in the absence of coronary artery disease [47].

Arrhythmia

Arrhythmias are common in Fabry disease, the most common being sinus bradycardia followed by atrial arrhythmias (atrial fibrillation (AF), atrial flutter and supraventricular tachycardias) [13]. Holter monitoring demonstrated AF in 17%, with non sustained ventricular tachycardia (VT) in 15–38% [5, 48]. Disturbances are largely due to direct involvement of the conducting system, with Gb3 demonstrated throughout the conduction system, including the sinoatrial and atrio-ventricular nodes, the His bundle and its branches [49]. In the case of ventricular arrhythmias, fibrosis and scar formation is causative. Loss of heart rate variability and chronotropic incompetence, one of the earliest cardiac manifestations, are likely due to autonomic nervous system involvement [13].

Common ECG findings include a shortened PR interval without a delta wave, evidence of LV hypertrophy, sinus bradycardia and AV conduction disturbances including bundle branch block. With age, conduction abnormalities become more common, with resting bradycardia and chronotropic incompetence. 3% eventually require permanent pacing due to progressive sinus node dysfunction, AV block, or as treatment for difficult to manage atrial arrhythmias [26]. Another study reported a 8% cumulative incidence of PPM insertion over 5-years [5].

Valvular

As mentioned previously, valvular involvement is common. Thickening of mitral and aortic valve leaflets, or mitral valve prolapse, resulting in mild regurgitation is reported [13].

Aortic/Arterial Involvement

Dilatation of the ascending aorta is seen in 30–56% in male patients, with one study reporting aneurysms in 9.6% and 1.9% in males and females respectively [50]. Aneurysms were asymptomatic and limited to the ascending aorta. Vascular remodelling has also been demonstrated in small and medium sized arteries, with significant increases in the intima-media thickness of radial and common carotid arteries [51]. Aortic dissection remains rare.

Cardiac Pathophysiology

Gb3 is known to accumulate throughout the heart, including cardiac myocytes, vascular endothelial cells, smooth muscle cells, valvular fibroblasts, as well as the conducting system. This widespread involvement accounts for the range of cardiac manifestations of Fabry disease, though the actual pathophysiology remains poorly understood.

Marked left ventricular hypertrophy, often mimicking HCM is a hallmark of cardiac involvement in Fabry disease, however the accumulation of Gb3 itself only accounts for 1–3% of LV mass [10]. Rather it likely triggers a cascade of factors leading to LVH, including trophic factors such as lyso-Gb3, and vascular endothelial dysfunction due to oxidative stress. There is also evidence that Gb3 may disrupt mitochondrial metabolism, leading to a compensatory LVH [52].

The development of Fabry cardiomyopathy likely shares common histopathological processes with other organs. Secondary tissue defects occur, including apoptosis, activation of inflammatory cascades, deposition of extracellular matrix, hypertrophy and finally replacement fibrosis [4]. As in other organ systems, it is likely that microvascular damage due to involvement of the vascular endothelium plays a significant role in organ dysfunction [24]. Conversion of endothelial cells to storage cells has been shown to lead to induction of oxidative stress, endothelial dysfunction, and a predisposition to thrombosis with upregulation of adhesion molecules [53–55]. Advanced Fabry cardiomyopathy classically results in myocardial replacement fibrosis, which likely acts as the substrate for the ventricular arrhythmias [56].

Impaired mitochondrial function and therefore energy metabolism has been proposed as a mechanism for Fabry cardiomyopathy, as is the case in other metabolic and sarcomeric cardiomyopathies. Accumulation of lysosomal material may affect the function of the inner mitochondrial membrane, thereby decreasing ATP synthase activity. Myocytes become unable to maintain energy levels required for contraction leading to increased hypertrophy signalling. In a study of 23 patients, MR spectroscopy showed decreased levels of high energy phosphate molecules, and that his correlated with increased cardiac mass [57]. Improvements in energy metabolism were detected after enzyme replacement therapy.

Histologically, endomyocardial biopsy typically shows empty myocytes on light microscopy, with electron microscopy showing dense osmiophilic bodies ('zebra bodies') containing Gb3. Interestingly, the histopathological findings resemble changes seen with chloroquine and amiodarone toxicity, both of which affect lysosomal function.[13]Myocardial accumulation of Gb3 begins early in life, followed by a significant lag of several decades before LVH can be clinically detected [48].

Other Manifestations

Neurological

Neurological symptoms are typically acroparasthaesia and hypohidrosis/heat intolerance. Neuropathic pain can be chronic or occur as pain crises, triggered by pain or heat, lasting from a few minutes to several weeks, and can be accompanied by low grade fevers, fatigue and arthralgias [12, 26]. Small fibre peripheral neuropathy occurs, manifesting as loss of distal hot/cold temperature sensitivity.

Up to 25% of patients experience transient ischaemic attacks or stroke in vertebrobasilar and posterior circulations. Vestibular dysfunction and sensorineural hearing loss are also common. In a study of 33 Fabry patients, 24% had suffered a stroke, with a mean age for first stroke of 29 [26].

Neurological involvement is likely primarily due to ischaemic injury and metabolic failure, due to accumulation in neurovascular endothelial cells, vasa vasorum, and neurons within the central and peripheral nervous systems, including dorsal root and autonomic ganglia. This leads to loss of both small myelinated and unmyelinated fibres, and even an ischaemic small vessel multifocal leukoencephalopathy [12]. Epidermal nerve fibre density is reduced in Fabry disease which mirrors other neuropathic pathologies such as diabetic neuropathy, familial dysautonomia and HIV-associated neuropathy [58, 59]. Axons terminating in the epidermis arise entirely within the dorsal root ganglia, and post mortem studies of Fabry disease patients have shown severe changes in these ganglia.

GI

Gastrointestinal symptoms are common early in life, are generally non-specific, including cramping pain, bloating, diarrhoea and constipation. A combination of microvascular, and autonomic dysfunction may be responsible [12]. GI issues may impact significantly on quality of life. These symptoms respond modestly to ERT.

Renal

Most patients develop a progressive nephropathy with proteinuria detected as early as childhood. Focal and global glomerulosclerosis can be seen in the second decade of life in males, with early tubular dysfunction in the form of impaired urine concentrating ability. Classical male patients typically progress to renal failure by the age of 40 [60].

Gb3 accumulates in all renal cells, including podocytes, mesangium, glomerular endothelium, and tubular and interstitial cells. This produces a variety of pathologies including glomerular sclerosis, tubular atrophy and interstitial fibrosis [17]. Progression occurs at a rate comparable to diabetic nephropathy.

Cornea

Corneal involvement is seen in 90% of patients, and include one of the hallmark signs of Fabry disease, namely cornea verticillata, a pattern of pale, spiral streaks in the corneal epithelium. Vision is rarely affected, however sudden vision loss has been described due to central retinal artery occlusion and ischaemic optic neuropathy [12]. These findings are also seen with long term amiodarone or chloroquine use.

Diagnosis/Investigations

Fabry disease is diagnosed by detecting either an absence or deficiency of α-galactosidase, genetic mutation analysis, or increased levels of accumulated substrates. Whilst levels of Gb3 and lyso-Gb3 in serum and urine have been investigated as screening tools, diagnosis of Fabry disease is largely limited to the first two methods. Due to its nonspecific and variable presentation, a degree of suspicion is required to consider the diagnosis when reviewing the patient with hypertrophic cardiomyopathy, renal impairment or early/cryptogenic stroke.

Diagnosis

α-galactosidase activity can be measured in plasma, dried blood spots, and leukocytes, the last of which is generally preferred, due to a lower level of false negatives [41]. In males, this is commonly the first test performed, and if suggestive of Fabry disease (absent or low enzyme activity), is confirmed by genetic testing. Mutation analysis should be performed in all patients at diagnosis, as it allows confirmation of diagnosis, occasionally genotype-phenotype prediction, as well as guiding amenability to oral chaperone therapy. Importantly, genetic testing is crucial for the screening and genetic counselling of family members.

In females, the diagnostic paradigm is different, as enzymatic testing will miss a large proportion of female patients due to residual, and even normal α-galactosidase activity. Likewise, Lyso-Gb3 is not reliably elevated in women. For this reason, testing should proceed directly to genetic mutation analysis in female patients. Combined genetic testing panels targeted at the patient with unexplained LVH are now widely available [1].

Investigations

Fabry cardiomyopathy is most commonly monitored using echocardiography; however cardiac involvement is present for several decades before LVH is apparent. Myocardial strain imaging can detect subclinical systolic and diastolic dysfunction, even in the absence of LVH [42], and detects response to ERT. In addition to LVH, prominence of papillary muscles is typical [14]. Regional strain abnormalities correlate with fibrosis which would otherwise require CMR for detection.

Cardiac MRI is a valuable addition to echocardiography. It allows accurate assessment of LVH and mass with hypertrophied papillary muscles (Fig. 19.4a). Additionally, the presence of late gadolinium enhancement enables detection of fibrosis or scar formation, with implications for both prognosis and response to ERT. Inferolateral wall involvement is typical for Fabry disease (Fig. 19.4b), [61] with fibrosis and thinning of the posterior wall associated with an increased risk of adverse cardiac events including death [62]. Non-contrast T1 shortening, attributed directly to accumulation of Gb3 and related products within the myocardium, is

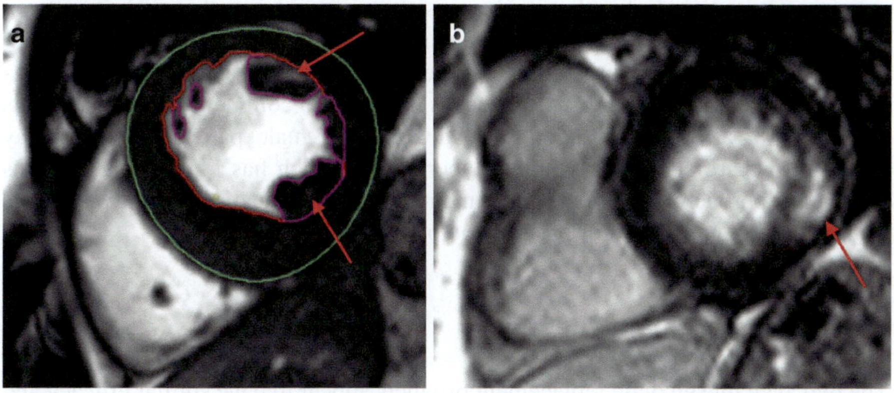

Fig. 19.4 (**a**) Cardiac Magnetic Resonance Imaging showing concentric Left ventricular hypertrophy with prominence of papillary muscles (arrows). (**b**) Gadolinium enhancement demonstrating scar tissue typically in the inferolateral segments (arrow). (Images courtesy of Dr. R Kozor)

specific to Fabry disease, discriminating from normal controls as well as hypertensive, HCM and AL-amyloidosis patients [63]. T1 analysis may also show 'pseudo-normalisation" in regions of late gadolinium enhancement. This method also avoids gadolinium contrast in patients with renal impairment.

Lyso-Gb3 appears to be a superior biomarker to the primary substrate itself, both in monitoring response to treatment, and in differentiating classical from cardiac variant disease. High sensitivity troponin T (HsTnT) and NT-proBNP have also both been investigated and shown to correlate with late gadolinium enhancement on MRI, suggesting they may have a role in monitoring for cardiac involvement in Fabry disease [64, 65].

Proteinuria can be detected from childhood, therefore monitoring for renal involvement should begin early, and continue throughout life. Accurate monitoring of creatinine clearance, rather than estimates of the glomerular filtration rate, should be performed periodically. Typically there is a period of hyperfiltration prior to gradual loss of renal function.

Treatment

Treatment in Fabry disease is divided into directed therapy targeted at the primary disease process, and non specific therapy for various organ systems affected. All directed therapy shares the principle of lowering amount of stored substrate, either by enhanced degradation, or reduced production [6]. Treatment of Fabry disease was revolutionised in 2001 with the introduction of a disease-specific, enzyme replacement therapy (ERT), with two commercially available products, agalsidase alpha and beta. More recently, an oral chaperone therapy (migalastat) has become available.

International treatment guidelines for ERT in Fabry disease vary; however it is common practise to initiate treatment at the time of diagnosis in classical male patients. The rationale for this is clear, as there is evidence that early treatment improves outcomes, particularly commencing treatment prior to the development of myocardial fibrosis. The situation is less clear for female patients or those with cardiac variant disease. A common consensus has been to commence ERT in patients with LVH or arrhythmia [14, 44]. However unlike male patients, females may develop myocardial fibrosis without hypertrophy, which has implications for this treatment approach. Initiation of treatment for renal indications usually includes significant proteinuria and/or progression of chronic kidney disease.

Enzyme Replacement Therapy

The two available enzyme replacement products appear to have similar efficacy and safety, are administered as fortnightly intravenous infusions, and are effective in reducing levels of Gb3 in serum, urine and on tissue biopsy [41]. ERT additionally reduces neuropathic pain, improves gastrointestinal symptoms, as well as stabilising renal function or slowing its decline, and delays progression to cardiac events. Evidence for the benefit of ERT on stroke risk is lacking.

Overall, longer term results of ERT have been mixed. Numerous studies have shown improvements in LV mass and improved diastolic function, which is limited to those patients without fibrosis. Other studies have failed to show any lasting clinical benefit [14, 66]. In a meta-analysis of six studies [67], LV mass remained stable or increased at a slower rate on ERT compared to placebo, with little effect on renal function. Whilst a Cochrane meta-analysis showed unclear benefits on long term outcome, this was limited to randomised control trials which are of limited duration and few in number. Subsequent pooled analysis of cohort studies suggested significantly lower renal, cardiovascular and cerebrovascular events compared to placebo [68].

The development of neutralising antibodies to ERT is common, and may contribute to the mixed results described above. This is less common in females, likely due to their residual enzyme levels, but occur in up to 70% of male patients. Their significance is unclear, and resistance may be overcome with increased dose; however numerous studies show that the presence of antibodies is associated with increased LV mass, higher levels of lyso-Gb3, and worse severity scores [8].

Oral Chaperone Therapy

Any oral therapy presents a significant improvement to patient quality of life to the fortnightly ERT infusions. In the past few years, migalastat, an oral chaperone therapy which is given second daily, has been approved for Fabry disease. The term chaperone refers to its action in reversibly binding to the active site of mutant enzymes, thereby facilitating their trafficking to lysosomes and increasing enzymatic activity [5, 69]. Comparison with ERT in several trials has shown similar improvements in renal, cardiac and composite outcomes, including reversal of LVH even in the presence of fibrosis. A trial of combined chaperone + ERT therapy showed a 1.2–5.1 fold increase in enzyme levels over ERT alone [8]. In addition, a further possible advantage is a larger volume of distribution than ERT, which may allow wider treatment benefit. The main disadvantage of migalastat is that is effective only in patients with amenable, mainly missense, mutations (comprising 35–50% of all Fabry disease).

Future Directed Therapies

Substrate reduction therapies include oral treatments which reduce the amount of accumulated substance. Lucerastat directly inhibits glucosulceramide synthase, thereby reducing Gb3. Unlike current chaperone therapy, these treatments act across all genotypes.

Preliminary work on gene therapy for Fabry disease has been published. Studies in mice have shown increased enzyme levels at 6 months [8].

Ancillary/Supportive Therapies

Standard advice around cardiovascular risk remains important in Fabry disease. Smoking cessation, control of blood pressure, treatment of hypercholesterolemia and weight management improve long term outcomes [70].

Despite clearing Gb3 from the skin, ERT has little effect on angiokeratoma, for which treatment has primarily been with laser therapy. Results of this are mixed but overall appear effective [71]. Laser therapy does not provide a long term solution, as angiokeratoma recur.

Aggressive treatment of proteinuria with ACEI/ARB is standard of care. Patients often require renal replacement therapy; Gb3 does not appear to accumulate in transplanted kidneys.

AF and flutter are common, and pharmacological options can be limited. Beta-blockers must be used with caution due to the risk of exacerbating bradycardia and AV block, both of which are common in Fabry disease [41]. Amiodarone is generally avoided due to its potential to further interfere with lysosomal metabolism and function [26]. If rhythm/rate control prove difficult, electrophysiological ablation and insertion of pacemaker is required [5]. Ventricular arrhythmias, likely due to myocardial fibrosis, are a significant cause of death. Patients are closely monitored for NSVT, and if clinical concern is high, implantable cardiac defibrillator is indicated.

Additional treatments include targeting neuropathic pain, motility agents for GI symptoms, and moisturisers and compression stockings for lymphoedema. Heart transplantation has been used in end stage disease, with case reports showing favourable outcomes, with no disease recurrence out to 14 years post transplant [72, 73]. Importantly, treatment should be individualised, and multi-disciplinary.

Prognosis/Complications

Despite the significant advances in treatment options in the past two decades, patients with Fabry disease continue to have a significantly reduced life expectancy, with review of the Fabry registry in 2009 showing 58.2 years in males, and 75.4 years in females [74]. Cardiovascular causes are the most common cause of death, followed by cerebrovascular and renal disease in men. The majority of patients who died had received renal replacement therapy. Hypertension and the presence of LVH appear to be the most strongly associated with major cardiovascular events [75]. Patients with Fabry disease commonly die due to heart failure, and ventricular arrhythmias. Heart failure is common and seen in 60% of patients. In a systematic review of 4185 patients 75% of deaths were due to cardiovascular events, 62% of which were sudden cardiac death [5], with 15.3% suffering VT.

References

1. Yousef Z. Left ventricular hypertrophy in Fabry disease: a practical approach to diagnosis. Eur Heart J. 2013;34:802–8.
2. Nair V, Belanger EC, Veinot JP. Lysosomal storage disorders affecting the heart: a review. Cardiovasc Pathol. 2019;39:12–24.
3. Elstein D. Summary: Fabry disease, a uniquely different lysosomal storage disorder. In: Elstein D, Altarescu G, editors. Fabry disease. Dordrecht: Springer; 2010. p. 499–504.
4. Weidemann F, et al. The Fabry cardiomyopathy: models for the cardiologist. Annu Rev Med. 2011;62:59–67.
5. Hagège A, et al. Fabry disease in cardiology practice: literature review and expert point of view. Arch Cardiovasc Dis. 2019;112:278–87.
6. Aerts J, et al. Biomarkers in the diagnosis of lysosomal storage disorders: proteins, lipids and inhibodies. J Inherit Metab Dis. 2011;34:605–19.
7. Nowak A, et al. Genotype, phenotype and disease severity reflected by serum LysoGb3 levels in patients with Fabry disease. Mol Genet Metab. 2018;123(2):148–53.
8. Cairns T, et al. Hot topics in Fabry disease. Postgrad Med J. 2018;94:709–13.
9. Nowak A, Mechtler TP, Desnick RJ, et al. Plasma LysoGb3: a useful biomarker for the diagnosis and treatment of Fabry disease heterozygotes. Mol Genet Metab. 2017;120:57–61.
10. Echevarria L, et al. X-chromosome inactivation in female patients with Fabry disease. Clin Genet. 2016;89:44–54.
11. Winchester B, Young E. Laboratory diagnosis of Fabry disease. In: Elstein D, Altarescu G, editors. Fabry disease. Dordrecht: Springer; 2010. p. 111–32.
12. Eng C, et al. Fabry disease: guidelines for the evaluation and management of multi-organ system involvement. Genet Med. 2006;8(9):539–48.
13. Gambarin F, et al. When should cardiologists suspect Anderson-Fabry disease? Am J Cardiol. 2010;106:1492–9.
14. Yeung D, et al. Echocardiographic assessment of patients with Fabry disease. J Am Soc Echocardiogr. 2018;31(6):639–649.e2.
15. Elliott P, et al. Prevalence of Anderson-Fabry disease in patients with hypertrophic cardiomyopathy: the European Anderson-Fabry disease survey. Heart. 2011;97:1957–60.
16. Tsujiuchi M, et al. Long-term effects of enzyme replacement therapy for Anderson-Fabry disease: differences in three siblings with the same genotype. Int Heart J. 2019;60:208–14.
17. Havndrup, et al. Fabry Disease mimicking hypertrophic cardiomyopathy; genetic screening needed for establishing the diagnosis in women. Eur J Heart Fail. 2010;12:535–40.

18. Nakao S, et al. An atypical variant of Fabry's disease in men with left ventricular hypertrophy. N Engl J Med. 1995;333:288–93.
19. Sachdev B, et al. Prevalence of Anderson-Fabry disease in male patients with late onset hypertrophic cardiomyopathy. Circulation. 2002;105:1407–11.
20. Brouns R, et al. Belgian Fabry study: prevalence of Fabry disease in a cohort of 1000 young patient with cerebrovascular disease. Stroke. 2010;41:863–8.
21. Baptista M, et al. Mutations of the GLA gene in young patients with stroke: the PORTYSTROKE Study – screening genetic conditions in Portuguese young stroke patients. Stroke. 2010;41:431–6.
22. Rolfs A, et al. Prevalence of Fabry disease in patients with cryptogenic stroke: a prospective study. Lancet. 2005;366:1794–6.
23. Kotanko P, Kramer R, Devrnja D, et al. Results of a nationwide screening for Anderson- Fabry disease among dialysis patients. J Am Soc Nephrol. 2004;15(5):1323–9.
24. Wanner C. Fabry disease model: a rational approach to the management of Fabry disease. Clin Ther. 2007;29(Suppl A):S2–5.
25. Alharbi FJ, et al. Globotriasoylsphingosine (Lyso-Gb3) as a biomarker for cardiac variant (N215S) Fabry disease. J Inherit Metab Dis. 2018;41(2):239–47.
26. O'Mahony C, Elliott P. Anderson-Fabry disease and the heart. Prog Cardiovasc Dis. 2010;52(4):326–35.
27. Elleder M. Subcellular, cellular and organ pathology of Fabry disease. In: Elstein D, Altarescu G, editors. Fabry disease. Dordrecht: Springer; 2010. p. 39–79.
28. Orteu C, Janssen T, Lidove O, et al. Fabry disease and the skin: data from the Fabry outcome survey. Br J Dermatol. 2007;157:331–7.
29. Dhoat S, Orteu CH, Navarro C, Lidove O, Jansen T, Clarke J. Patients with Fabry disease with cutaneous vascular lesions have higher disease severity scores and more multi- system involvement: data from 1354 patients registered on FOS, the Fabry outcome survey. Br J Dermatol. 2009;161(Suppl 1):45.
30. Gadoth N, Sandbank U. Involvement of dorsal root ganglia in Fabry's disease. J Med Genet. 1983;20(4):309–12.
31. Amann-Vesti BR, Gitzelmann G, Widmer U, Bosshard NU, Steinmann B, Koppensteiner R. Severe lymphatic micrangiopathy in Fabry disease. Lymphat Res Biol. 2003;1(3):185–9.
32. Ries M, Moore DF, Robinson CJ, Tifft CJ, Rosenbaum KN, Brady RO, Schiffmann R, Krasnewich D. Quantitative dysmorphology assessment in Fabry disease. Genet Med. 2006 Feb;8(2):96–101.
33. Navarro C, Teijeira S, Dominguez C, et al. Fabry disease: an ultrastructural comparative study of skin in hemizygous and heterozygous patients. Acta Neuropathol (Berl). 2006;7:1–8.
34. Fleming C, Rennie A, Fallowfield M, McHenry PM. Cutaneous manifestations of fucosidosis. Br J Dermatol. 1997;136(4):594–7.
35. Kanzaki T, Yokota M, Irie F, et al. Aniokeratoma corporis diffusum with gly- copeptiduria due to deficient lysosomal alpha-N-acetylgalactosaminidase activity. Clincal, morphologic and biochemical studies. Arch Dermatol. 1993;129:460–5.
36. Rodriguez-Serna M, Botella-Estrada R, Chabas A, et al. Angiokeratoma cor- poris diffusum associated with beta-mannosidase deficiency. Arch Dermatol. 1996;132(10):1219–22.
37. Paller SA. Metabolic disorders characterized by angiokeratomas and neurologic dysfunction. Neurol Clin. 1987;5(3):441–6.
38. Albay D, Adler SG, Philipose J, Calescibetta CC, Romansky SG, Cohen AH. Chloroquine-induced lipidosis mimicking Fabry disease. Mod Pathol. 2005;18(5):733–8.
39. Schiller PI, Itin PH. Angiokeratomas: an update. Dermatology. 1996;193(4):275–82.
40. Gruner C, et al. Systolic myocardial mechanics in patients with Anderson-Fabry disease with and without left ventricular hypertrophy and in comparison to nonobstructive hypertrophic cardiomyopathy. Dent Echo. 2012;29:810–7.
41. Weidemann F, Linhart A, Monserrat L, Strotmann J. Cardiac challenges in patients with Fabry disease. Int J Cardiol. 2010;141:3–10.

42. Shanks M. Systolic and diastolic function assessment in Fabry disease patients using speckle-tracking imaging and comparison with conventional echocardiographic measurements. J Am Soc Echocardiogr. 2013;23:1407–14.
43. Morris D, et al. Global cardiac alterations detected by speckle-tracking echocardiography in Fabry disease: left ventricular, right ventricular, and left atrial dysfunction are common and linked to worse symptomatic status. Int J Card Imaging. 2015;31:301–13.
44. Niemann M, et al. Differences in Fabry cardiomyopathy between female and male patients – consequences for diagnostic assessment. J Am Coll Cardiol Img. 2011;4:592–601.
45. Vijapurapu R, et al. Global longitudinal strain, myocardial storage and hypertrophy in Fabry disease. Heart. 2019 Mar;105(6):470–6. https://doi.org/10.1136/heartjnl-2018-313699.
46. Linhart A, et al. Cardiac manifestations of Anderson-Fabry disease: results from the international Fabry ouytcome survey. Eur Heart J. 2007;28:1228–35.
47. Tomberli B, et al. Coronary microvascular dysfunction is an early feature of cardiac involvement in patients with Anderson-Fabry disease. Eur J Heart Fail. 2013 Dec;15(12):1363–73.
48. Namdar M, et al. Electrocardiographic changes in early recognition of Fabry disease. Heart. 2011;97:485–90.
49. Becker AE, Schoorl R, Balk AG, van der Heide RM. Cardiac manifestations of Fabry's disease. Report of a case with mitral insufficiency and electrocardiographic evidence of myocardial infarction. Am J Cardiol. 1975;36(6):829–35.
50. Barbey F. Aortic remodeling in Fabry disease. Eur Heart J. 2010;31:347–53.
51. Collin C, et al. Long-term changes in arterial structure and function and left ventricular geometry after enzyme replacement therapy in patients affected with Fabry disease. Eur J Cardiovasc Prev Rehabil. 2012;19(1):43–54.
52. Elleder M, Bradova V, Smid F, Budesinsky M, Harzer K, Kustermann-Kuhn B, et al. Cardiocyte storage and hypertrophy as a sole manifestation of Fabry's disease. Report on a case simulating hypertrophic non-obstructive cardiomyopathy. Virchows Arch A Pathol Anat Histopathol. 1990;417(5):449–55.
53. Utsumi K, Yamamoto N, Kase R, et al. High incidence of thrombosis in Fabry's disease. Intern Med. 1997;36(5):327–9.
54. Heare T, Alp NJ, Priestman DA, et al. Severe endothelial dysfunction in the aorta of a mouse model of Fabry disease; partial prevention by N-butyldeoxynojirimycin treatment. J Inherit Metab Dis. 2007;30(1):79–87.
55. Park JL, Whitesall SE, D'Alecy LG, Shu L, Shayman JA. Vascular dysfunction in the alpha-galactosidase A-knockout mouse is an endothelial cell-, plasma membrane-based defect. Clin Exp Pharmacol Physiol. 2008;35(10):1156–63.
56. Kramer J, et al. Two-dimensional speckle tracking as a non-invasive tool for identification of myocardial fibrosis in Fabry disease. Eur Heart J. 2013;34:1587–96.
57. Machann W, et al. Cardiac energy metabolism is disturbed in Fabry disease and improves with enzyme replacement therapy using recombinant human galactosidase A. Eur J Heart Fail. 2011;13:3.
58. Lauria G, McArthur JC, Hauer PE, Griffin JW, Cornblath DR. Neuropathological alterations in diabetic truncal neuropathy: evaluation by skin biopsy. J Neurol Neurosurg Psychiatry. 1998;65:762–6.
59. Polydefkis M, Yiannoutsos CT, Cohen BA, et al. Reduced intraepidermal nerve fiber density in HIV-associated sensory neuropathy. Neurology. 2002;58:115–9.
60. Schiffmann R, et al. Fabry disease: progression of nephropathy, and prevalence of cardiac and cerebrovascular events before enzyme replacement therapy. Nephrol Dial Transplant. 2009;24:2102–11.
61. Weidemann F. The variation of morphological and functional cardiac manifestation in Fabry disease: potential implications for the time course of the disease. Eur Heart J. 2005;26:1221–7.
62. Yeung D, et al. Echocardiographic assessment of patients with Fabry disease. J Am Soc Echocardiogr. 2018 Jun;31(6):639–49.

63. Sado D, et al. Identification and assessment of Anderson-Fabry disease by cardiovascular magnetic resonance noncontrast myocardial T1 mapping. Circ Cardiovasc Imaging. 2013;6:39.2–398.
64. Seydelmann N, Liu D, Kramer J, et al. High-sensitivity troponin: a clinical blood biomarker for staging cardiomyopathy in Fabry disease. J Am Heart Assoc. 2016;5:e002839.
65. Coats CJ, Parisi V, Ramos M, et al. Role of serum N-terminal pro-brain natriuretic peptide measurement in diagnosis of cardiac involvement in patients with Anderson-Fabry disease. Am J Cardiol. 2013;111:111–7.
66. Motwani M, et al. Enzyme replacement therapy improves cardiac features and severity of Fabry disease. Mol Genet Metab. 2012;107:197–202.
67. Rombach S, et al. Natural course of Fabry disease and the effectiveness of enzyme replacement therapy: a systematic review and meta-analysis. J Inh Metab Disease. 2014;37:341–52.
68. El Dib R, et al. Enzyme replacement for Anderson-Fabry disease: A complementary overview of a Cochrane publication through a linear regression and a pooled analysis of proportions from cohort studies. PLoS One. 2017;12(3):e0173358.
69. Hughes DA, et al. Oral pharmacological chaperone migalastat compared with enzyme replacement therapy in Fabry disease: 18-month results from the randomised phase III ATTRACT study. J Med Genet. 2017;54:288–96.
70. Sirrs SM, et al. Outcomes of patients treated through the Canadian Fabry disease initiative. Mol Genet Metab. 2014 Apr;111(4):499–506. https://doi.org/10.1016/j.ymgme.2014.01.014.
71. Orteu CH. Dermatological manifestations of Fabry disease. In: Elstein D, Altarescu G, editors. Fabry disease. Dordrecht: Springer; 2010. p. 259–74.
72. Verocai F, Clarke JT, Iwanochko RM. Case report: long-term outcome post-heart transplantation in a woman with Fabry's disease. J Inherit Metab Dis. 2010;33(Suppl 3):S385–7.
73. Roman-Monserrat IS, et al. Comprehensive clinical evaluation of a large Spanish family with Anderson-Fabry disease, novel GLA mutation and severe cardiac phenotype. Med Clin (Barc). 2014;142(11):497–504.
74. Waldeck S, et al. Life expectancy and cause of death in males and females with Fabry disease: findings from the Fabry registry. Genet Med. 2009;11(11):790–6.
75. Patel M, et al. Cardiovascular events in patients with Fabry disease- natural history data from the Fabry registry. J Am Coll Cardiol. 2011;57:1093–9.

Mastocytosis

20

Cristina Bulai Livideanu, Olivier Lairez, and Carle Paul

Dermatological Manifestations

Summary

1. Mastocytosis: introduction and mast cell activation symptoms
2. Diagnosis criteria of mastocytosis
3. Prognosis of mastocytosis patient
4. Diagnosis approach
5. Treatment of mastocytosis

Mastocytosis: Introduction and Mast Cell Activation Symptoms

Introduction

Mastocytosis are a heterogeneous group of pathologies first described in 1872 by Nettleship and Tay [1].

It corresponds to the accumulation or proliferation of abnormal mast cells in one or more organs.

C. B. Livideanu (✉) · C. Paul
Excellence Centre for Mastocytosis (CEREMAST), Toulouse, France

Department of Dermatology, Toulouse University Hospital, Paul Sabatier University, Toulouse, France
e-mail: livideanu.c@chu-toulouse.fr

O. Lairez
Excellence Centre for Mastocytosis (CEREMAST), Toulouse, France

Department of Cardiology, Toulouse University Hospital, Paul Sabatier University, Toulouse, France

C. Salavastru et al. (eds.), *Skin and the Heart*,
https://doi.org/10.1007/978-3-030-54779-0_20

It is named an isolated cutaneous mastocytosis (CM) when the skin is the only organ affected or a systemic mastocytosis (SM) if at least one internal organ is involved.

The most commonly affected organs are skin and bone marrow: more than 80% of patients with mastocytosis have a compatible skin eruption [2]. This is a rare disease, whose prevalence is estimated at 1 to 5/10,000 [3].

There are two peaks of incidence with very different clinical manifestations:

- In childhood between 6 months and 2 years
- In adult patient >40 years

Clinical manifestations are related, on the one hand, to mast cell activation, and, on the other hand, to tissue infiltration with abnormal mast cells [4].

Since 2016, mastocytosis have been divided into isolated cutaneous mastocytosis, systemic mastocytosis - indolent, smoldering, systemic mastocytosis with an associated hematological neoplasm, aggressive SM, mast cell leukemia and mast cell sarcoma according to WHO classification [5–8].

Regarding the cutaneous mastocytosis, it is divided in:

- maculopapular cutaneous mastocytosis:
- pigmented maculopapular mastocytosis in more than 80% of cases (formerly urticaria pigmentosa) (Fig. 20.1)

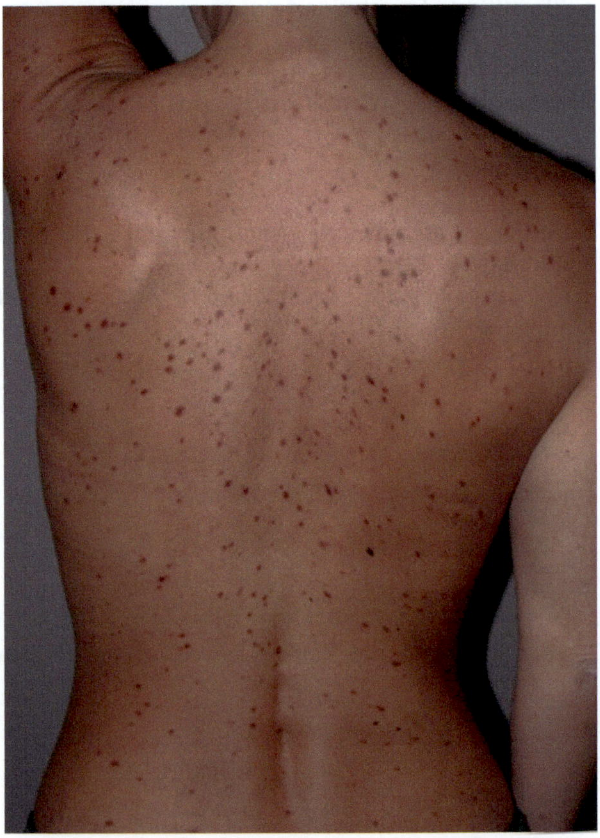

Fig. 20.1 Pigmented maculopapular cutaneous mastocytosis

- not pigmented maculopapular mastocytosis in 14% of cases of cutaneous mastocytosis in adulthood (previous named telangiectasia macularis eruptiva perstans) (Fig. 20.2) [9]
- diffuse cutaneous mastocytosis (1%) (Fig. 20.3)
- mastocytoma described mainly during childhood (Fig. 20.4), is very rarely in adulthood.

Some other forms of cutaneous mastocytosis more rarely in adulthood can be diagnosed in clinical practice as such tumoral cutaneous mastocytosis (Fig. 20.5), cutaneous mast cell sarcoma (Fig. 20.6) or genital mucosal involvement (Fig. 20.7) [10].

Unlike systemic involvement, cutaneous mastocytosis is usually diagnosed in children. Its prognosis in childhood is favorable: the evolution is frequently marked by a spontaneous disappearance during puberty [11].

Systemic mastocytosis is usually seen in adults. Mast cell infiltration can involve many organs including bone marrow. According to the same WHO classification of 2016, systemic mastocytosis is divided into subtypes: indolent SM (46-68%), smoldering SM (1.8%) (data from unpublished our cohort), SM associated with another neoplastic hemopathy (8.6-40%), aggressive SM (20-21%) and very rare forms: mast cell leukemia (1%) and mast cell sarcoma (0.4%) (data from unpublished our cohort) [12].

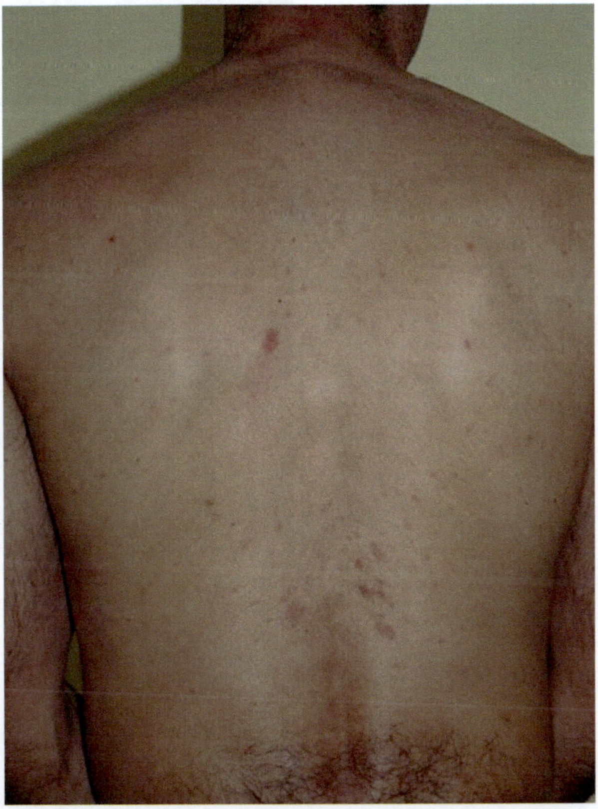

Fig. 20.2 Not pigmented maculopapular cutaneous mastocytosis

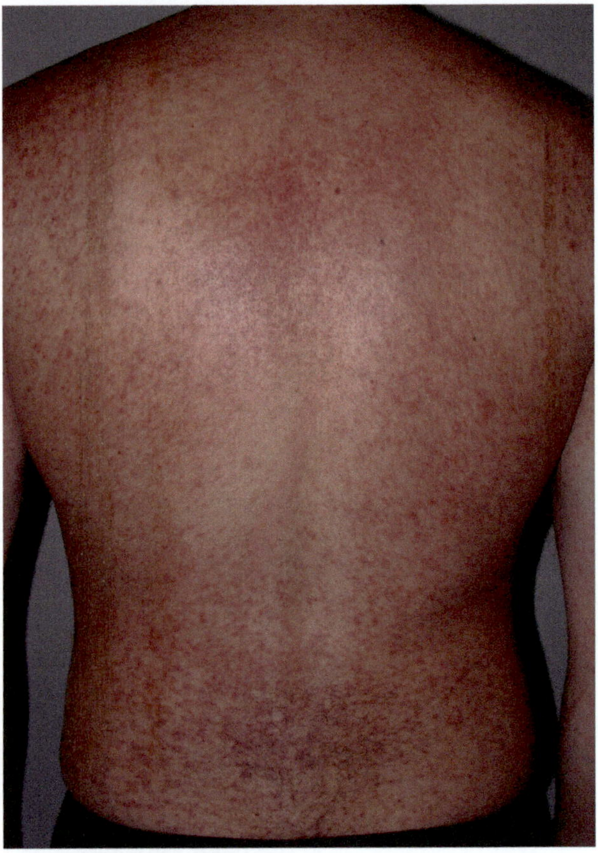

Fig. 20.3 Diffuse cutaneous mastocytosis

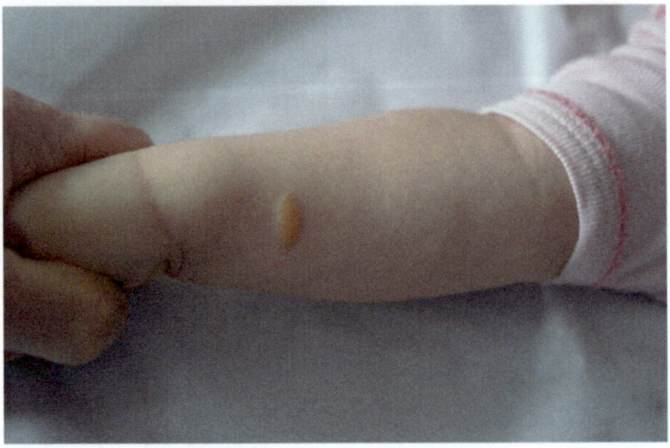

Fig. 20.4 Mastocytoma on the arm in a child

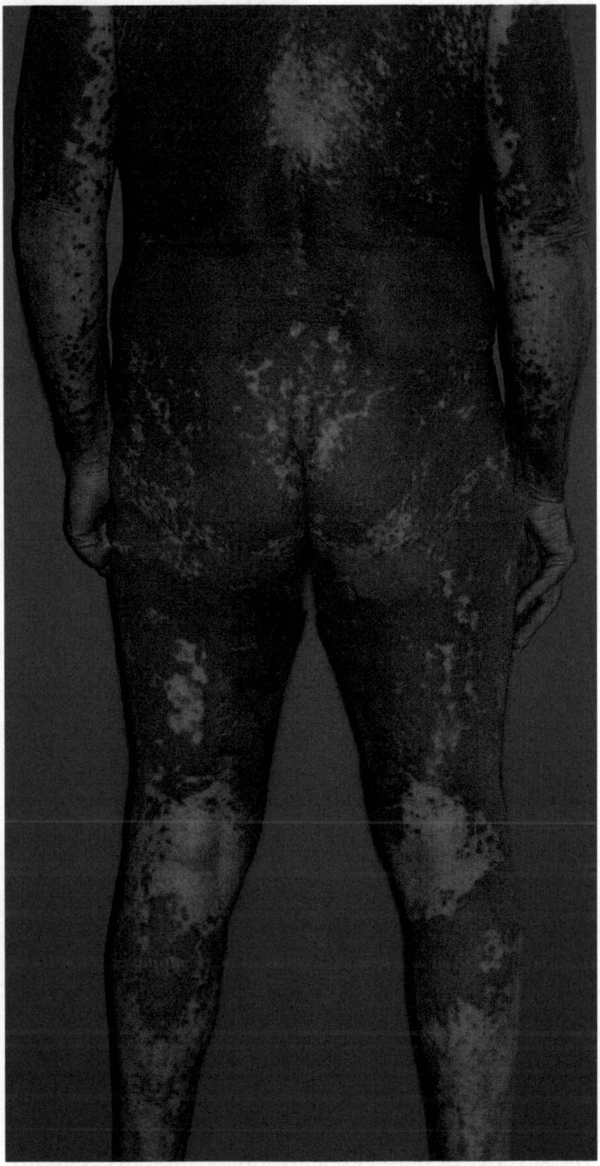

Fig. 20.5 Diffuse and tumoral cutaneous mastocytosis

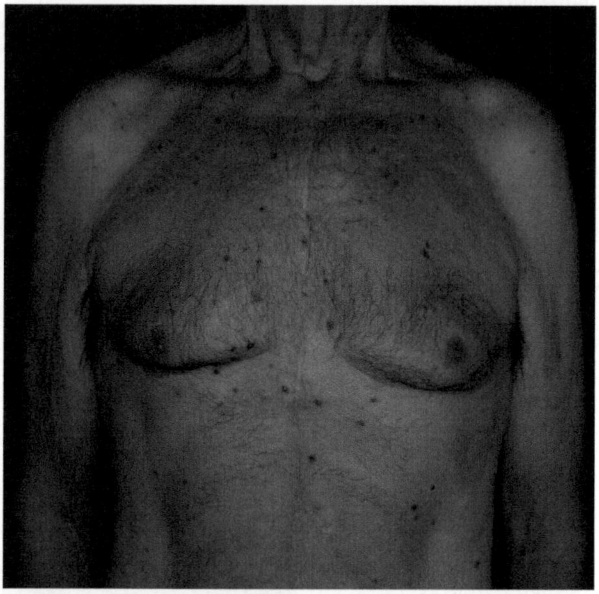

Fig. 20.6 Mast cell sarcoma with cutaneous involvement

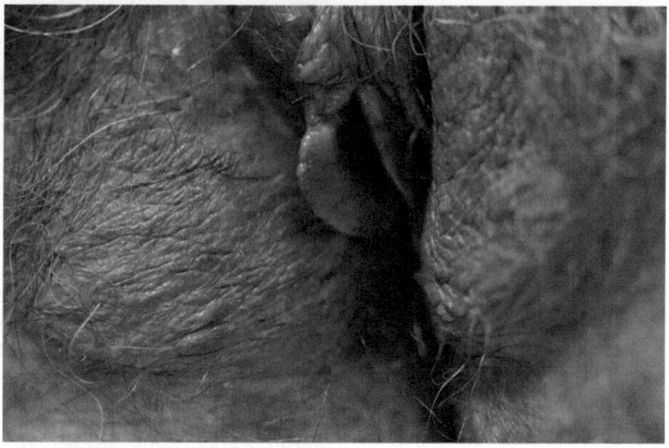

Fig. 20.7 Genital mucosal mastocytosis

Mast Cell Activation Symptoms

The severity of mast cell activation symptoms is highly variable, regardless of mast cell infiltration. The symptoms are nonspecific and multiple. These may be:

- Flushing or paroxysmal flushes corresponding to a rash erythema and heat strokes limited or generalized
- Localized or generalized pruritus
- Chronic spontaneous urticaria and dermographism
- Paroxysmal digestive symptoms such as diarrhoea, abdominal pain, nausea, vomiting or bloating

- Neuropsychic manifestations such as depression, attention deficit or memory disorders, anxiety
- Urological symptoms with pollakiuria type, bladder instability
- ORL or respiratory manifestations such as rhinitis, cough, dyspnoea
- Idiopathic anaphylactic reactions up to anaphylactic shock
- General symptoms as fever and asthenia

Diagnosis Criteria of Mastocytosis

Systemic Mastocytosis

Systemic mastocytosis requires extensive exploration and is based on major and minor criteria that were redefined in 2008 and 2016 by the WHO classification [6–8] (Table 20.1). These criteria are searched on blood and bone marrow. The SM diagnostic is made when the major criterion and one minor criterion or three minor criteria are present.

SM is associated with CM (see below) in more of 80% of cases. It is divided in indolent systemic mastocytosis, smouldering systemic mastocytosis (the presence of ≥2 B-findings including high mast cell burden, organomegaly, and evidence for multilineage involvement) [13], aggressive SM (the presence of ≥1 C-findings including any organopathy), systemic mastocytosis associated with associated haematological neoplasm, mast cell leukaemia (≥ 20% mast cells on bone marrow aspirate smears or ≥ 10% circulating mast cells) (12.) and mast cell sarcoma (histological criterion) [14].

Often SM associated with another neoplastic haematology and sometime aggressive SM are not associated with CM.

The Tables 20.2 and 20.3 shown the B-findings and C-findings need to make the diagnosis of smouldering and aggressive systemic mastocytosis respectively.

It is important to note that the patients with SM without CM can present cutaneous mast cell activation symptoms as such: flush (Fig. 20.8), prurit us, chronic spontaneous urticaria and symptomatic dermographism.

Table 20.1 The diagnosis of SM requires the major criterion and one minor criterion or at least three minor criteria

Major criterion	Multifocal, dense infiltrates of mast cells (≥15 mast cells in aggregates) detected in sections of bone marrow and/or other extracutaneous organs
Minor criteria	(a). In biopsy sections of bone marrow or other extracutaneous organs, >25% of the mast cells in the infiltrate are spindle-shaped or have atypical morphology or, of all mast cells in bone marrow aspirate smears, >25% are immature or atypical
	(b). Detection of an activating point mutation at codon 816 of *KIT* in bone marrow, blood or other extracutaneous organ
	(c). Mast cells in bone marrow, blood or other extracutaneous organ express CD25 with/without CD2 in addition to normal mast cell markers
	(d). Serum total tryptase persistently exceeds 20 μg/L (unless there is an associated myeloid neoplasm, in which case this parameter is not valid)

Table 20.2 B-findings: need 2/3 criteria for diagnosis of smouldering SM

B-findings	Clinical events
1. High mast cell burden	Bone marrow biopsy: >30% infiltration of cellularity by mast cells (focal, dense aggregates) and/or serum total tryptase level > 200 ng/mL
2. Dysplasia	Signs of dysplasia or myeloproliferation, in non-mast cell lineage(s), but insufficient criteria for definitive diagnosis of an associated hematological neoplasm (AHN), with normal or only slightly abnormal blood counts
3. Organomegaly	Hepatomegaly without impairment of liver function, palpable splenomegaly without hypersplenism, and/or lymphadenopathy on palpation or imaging

Table 20.3 C-findings: need 1/4 criterion for the diagnosis of aggressive SM

C-findings	Clinical events
1. Bone marrow dysfunction caused by neoplastic mast cell infiltration	≥1 cytopenia(s) defined by absolute neutrophil count; <1.0 × 109/L, hemoglobin <10 g/dL, and/or platelet count <100 × 109/L
2. Palpable hepatomegaly with impairment of liver function	Ascites and/or portal hypertension
3. Skeletal involvement	Large osteolytic lesions with/without pathological fractures
4. Palpable splenomegaly	Hypersplenism
5. Malabsorption with weight loss	Gastrointestinal mast cell infiltrates identified

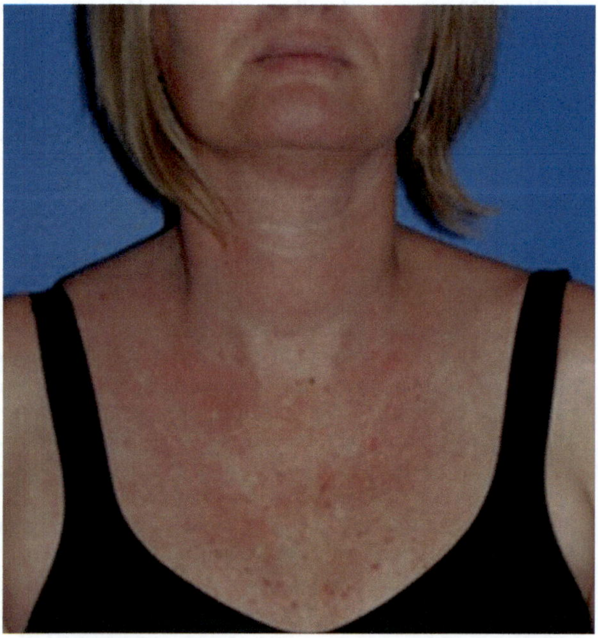

Fig. 20.8 Cutaneous mast cell activation symptoms: flush

Cutaneous Mastocytosis

Diagnosis of CM is carried out if there is a typical mastocytosis eruption associated with a significant histological mast cell infiltration and/or the detection of the *D816V* mutation in the cutaneous lesion [15]. This last diagnostic criteria of cutaneous mastocytosis seems to be better than the previous criteria, which require the presence of a cut-off of mast cells in the dermis on the 40X magnfication field [16]. In fact, the number of mast cell in the dermis is variable according to the histological sections analysed by pathologist [17].

Often the skin lesions of mastocytosis are bilateral and symmetrical. However, sometimes the CM lesions are only unilateral (Fig. 20.9).

It is helpful if the Darier sign is present as this is, specific to CM. It corresponds to the rapid onset of erythema, localized oedema and sometimes pruritus, a few minutes after the rubbing of a skin lesion of mastocytosis (Fig. 20.10). It is the result of mechanically induced histamine release. However, this sign is not always present in CM patients.

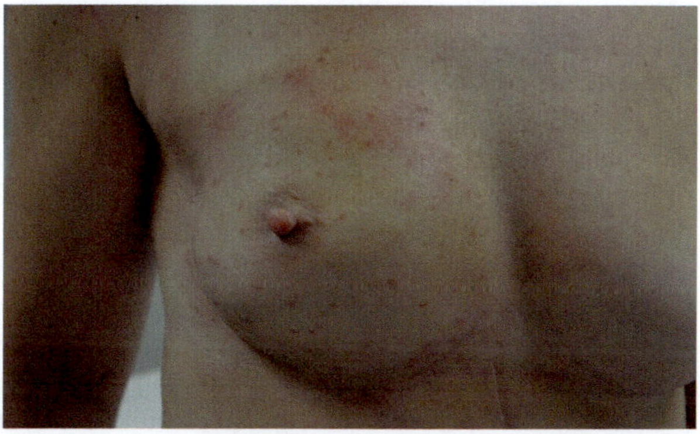

Fig. 20.9 Unilateral lesions of cutaneous mastocytosis

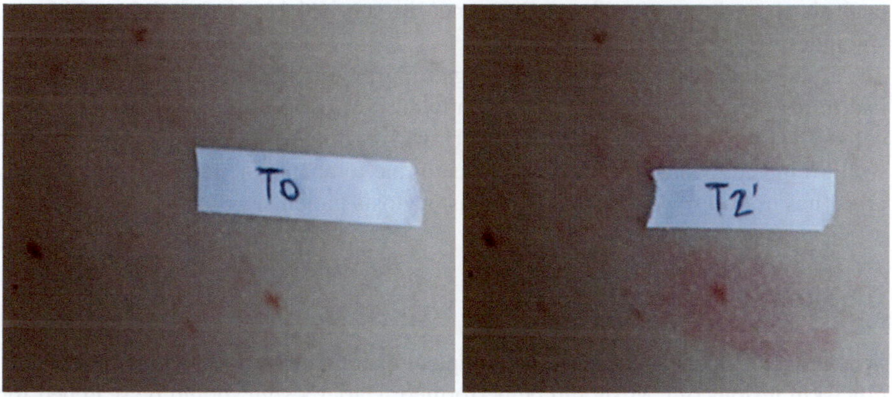

Fig. 20.10 Darier's sign: Erythema and oedema appearing 2 min after rubbing a skin lesion

Isolated Cutaneous Mastocytosis

The diagnosis of isolated CM is made according to international criteria (see upper table) provided all SM criteria are absent [18]. Its frequency is low in adulthood: 15 to 17% [18–20].

A level of serum tryptase <20 μg/L does not differentiate isolated CM from SM. In fact, in our unpublished cohort, the frequency of patients with serum tryptase <20 μg/L and cutaneous lesions of mastocytosis was associated with systemic involvement (SM) in 21% (23/108) patients.

Undetermined Mastocytosis

Patients with CM and only one or two minor criteria of SM, currently, can be classified as undetermined mastocytosis. Because almost 20% of patients with CM are diagnosed with an undetermined mastocytosis [18], the new criteria diagnose of SM are required. Two new tools for SM diagnosis were published: *KIT* mutation in blood [21] and a level of bone marrow tryptase ≥50 μg/L [22].

Prognosis of the Mastocytosis Patient

Patients with isolated CM or indolent SM have a survival prognosis identical to that of the general population of the same age group [23]. On the contrary, the survival prognosis is worst for aggressive systemic mastocytosis and the SM associated with an associated haematological neoplasm. Currently, these two last entities are included with mast cell leukaemia in the new group named advanced SM [24]. The factors predicting the worst prognosis regarding the survival in mastocytosis patient are: advanced SM, age > 60 years, thrombocytopenia, anaemia, alkaline phosphatase, and/or the presence of other molecular abnormalities [25, 26]. Regarding smouldering SM the survival prognosis was recently evaluated and in multivariable analysis there is no significant difference in survival between indolent SM and smouldering SM [27].

On the other hand, the prognosis regarding the quality of life is probably very bad in patients with isolated CM and indolent SM, who present with several mast cell activation symptoms [12, 28–30]. However, this aspect of prognosis was not well evaluated. Moreover, the risk of death due to anaphylactic shock and cardiac arrest has not been well evaluated in mastocytosis patients.

Diagnostic Approach

When mastocytosis is suspected, a complete examination of the tegument for specific skin lesions of CM should be performed. Darier's sign should be searched for in skin lesions of mastocytosis. The exception is for mastocytoma in childhood, when the important mass of mast cell, can lead to the severe mast cell activation symptoms.

At adulthood, a skin biopsy must be performed secondarily, confirming the abnormal mast cell infiltration and/or the presence of KIT mutation in skin.

Then, it is necessary to search for an extra-cutaneous systemic involvement, currently, performing:

- an osteo-medullary biopsy (major diagnostic criterion and cytological minor criterion),
- a myelogram for cytological minor criteria
- an immunophenotype of bone marrow mast cells to search an abnormal expression of CD2 and/or CD25
- a genetic search for the mutation of the KIT in bone marrow cells
- a blood test with serum tryptase assay

If the diagnosis of SM is performed, other exams depending on the symptoms of patient can be necessary. The realization of a bone densitometry is also recommended seen the risk of osteoporosis and bone fracture in SM patient [18, 31].

It is important to note that an isolated CM diagnosis seems can be performed just using the result of KIT cutaneous mutation and a level of bone marrow tryptase ≥50 μg/L, without having to perform a bone marrow biopsy (Fig. 20.11) [18].

When a SM is suspected in a patient without CM, because he/she present recurrent unexplained anaphylactic symptoms, the score of REMA can be calculated in order to decide whether the check-up looking for SM is necessary or not (Table 20.4) [32].

On the contrary, when a SM is suspected in a patient without CM, because he/she presents with only unexplained osteoporosis and/or bone fractures there is no score in order to decide whether the check-up looking for SM is necessary or not. In this

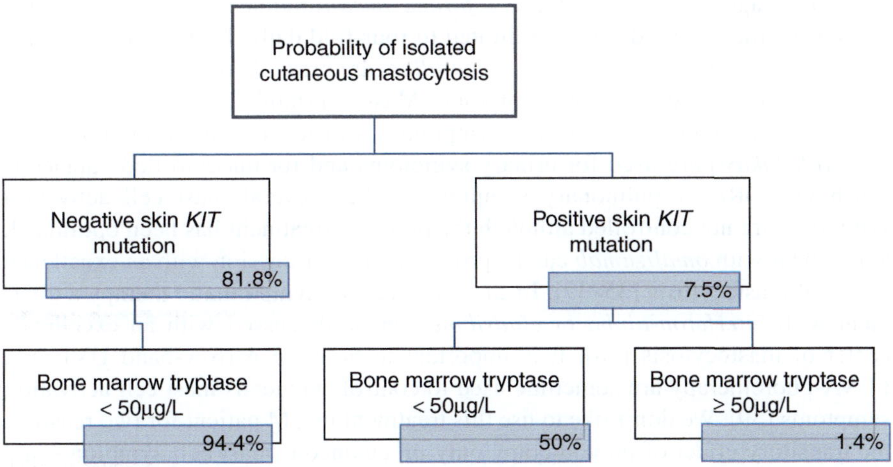

Fig. 20.11 Diagnostic algorithm: probability of isolated CM according to skin KIT mutation and bone marrow tryptase level ≥ 50 μg/L

Table 20.4 REMA score ≥ 2 is required achieving a complete diagnostic work-up of systemic mastocytosis

Variable		Score
1. **Gender**		
	Male	+1
	Female	–1
2. **Clinical symptoms**		
	Absence of urticaria, pruritus and angioedema	+1
	Urticaria, pruritus and/or angioedema	–2
	Presyncope and/or syncope	+3
3. **Tryptase**		
	<15 μg/l	–1
	<15 μg/l and > 25 μg/l	0
	>25 μg/l	+2

last case a close collaboration between rheumatologist and the mastocytosis expert is necessary.

Treatment of the Mastocytosis Patient

Currently, very few treatments have marketing authorization for mastocytosis. *imatinib* is used for KIT-negative systemic mastocytosis and *midostaurin* in advanced systemic mastocytosis. Regarding these drugs only an evaluation on CM was performed [33]. Some drugs are in development for indolent SM and advanced SM, as such: *masitinib, avapritinib* [34].

All treatments use for control of mast cell activation symptoms have not received marketing authorisation for mastocytosis. Often, we use histamine 1 receptor antagonists (*levocetirizine*, *ketotifen, desloratadine*) for cutaneous symptoms, sometimes with dosage up-titrated to four-fold daily. Histamine 2 receptor antagonists (*ranitidine, cimetidine, famotidine*) are prescribed for digestive symptoms or uncontrolled cutaneous symptoms. Mast cell stabilizer (*cromolyn sodium*) is used for uncontrolled digestive symptoms. Anti-leukotriene drugs (*montelukast, zafirlukast*) are used for urinary symptoms and for uncontrolled cutaneous (flushing), ORL or pulmonary symptoms. When several mast cell activation symptoms are not controlled although the previous treatment has been optimized, a treatment with *omalizumab* can be proposed after discussion with an excellence center of mastocytosis [35–37]. In case of failure of symptomatic therapy a treatment with *interferon-alpha* or *cladribine* can be discussed with an excellence center of mastocytosis [38]. It is important to note the narrow-band UVB and PUVA-phototherapy are sometime used to control cutaneous mast cell activation symptoms [39]. We don't like to use this treatment in CM patient for two reasons: the transitory effect of phototherapy only on cutaneous mast cell symptoms and for theoretical risk of melanoma in mastocytosis patient [40].

Cardiological Manifestations

Summary

1. Cardiac events in mastocytosis patients
2. Cardiac surgery in patient with mastocytosis
3. Mast cell mediators and the heart

1. Cardiac events in mastocytosis patients

The most frequent cardiac events described in patients with mastocytosis are Kounis syndrome, unexplained recurrent syncope, arrythmia, and unexplained cardiac arrest. Sometimes these events can be associated in the same patient.

The Kounis syndrome is defined as coronary artery spasm occurring in the setting of an anaphylactic reaction [41]. Kounis syndrome (also described as 'allergic angina') is an increasingly appreciated pathogenic entity which may overlap with systemic mastocytosis [41]. Three types of Kounis syndrome have been defined in the literature, categorized according to coronary findings at angiography [42]. Types 1 and 2 of Kounis syndrome are defined respectively as spontaneous release of inflammatory mediators in the setting of normal coronary arteries with isolated vasospasm (type 1) or atheromatous coronary arteries with acute plaque rupture (type 2). Type 3 of Kounis syndrome is associated with intracoronary thrombosis, including stent thrombosis [42].

A recent literature review of systemic mastocytosis and cardiac events identified 24 cases of systemic mastocytosis presenting with cardiac symptoms [43]. The short-term mortality was reported in 5/24 (20.8%) cases. Twenty of 24 patients (83.3%) with cardiac presentations of mastocytosis were male and age ranged from 33–85 years (mean age 53-year-old). Twenty-one patients (91%) had a history of recurrent unexplained syncope. Eleven patients (45.8%) presented with a Kounis syndrome of type 1 or 2. Seven patients (29%) had a cardiac arrest as their first manifestation of systemic mastocytosis. Pulseless electrical activity was the most common mechanism of cardiac arrest, but asystolic arrest and ventricular fibrillation were also reported [44]. Apart from their cardiovascular presentations, few patients had any additional clinical features of mastocytosis. Eight patients (33%) had no additional identified symptoms, six patients (25%) had a rash, seven patients (29%) had gastrointestinal symptoms of occasional diarrhoea or reflux, two patients (9%) had an associated haematological disorder, one patient had splenomegaly, and one patient had osteoporosis [43].

We recently took care of a 43-year-old patient had a recent history of an anaphylactic reaction with unconscious for 12 h and two concomitant cardiac arrests. His ECG exams show initially some anomalies of ST segment in the anterolateral /lateral derivations (Fig. 20.12) and one hour later diffuse ST segment anomalies (Fig. 20.13). His ECG exam performed remotely from event was normal without any anomalies (Fig. 20.14). A dermatological exam allowed diagnosing cutaneous

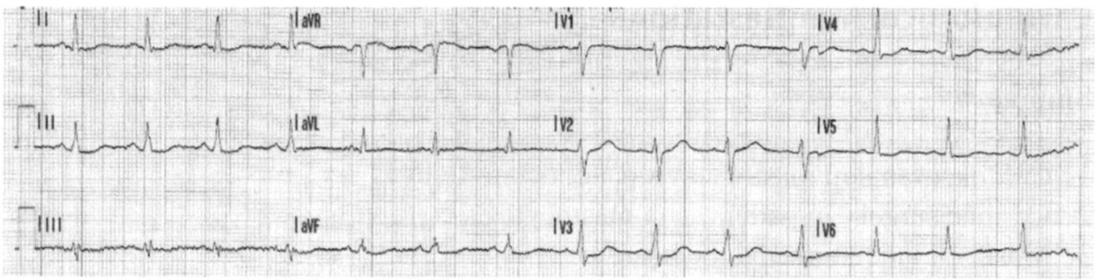

Fig. 20.12 Initial ECG tracing showing elevation of ST in the anterolateral/lateral derivations

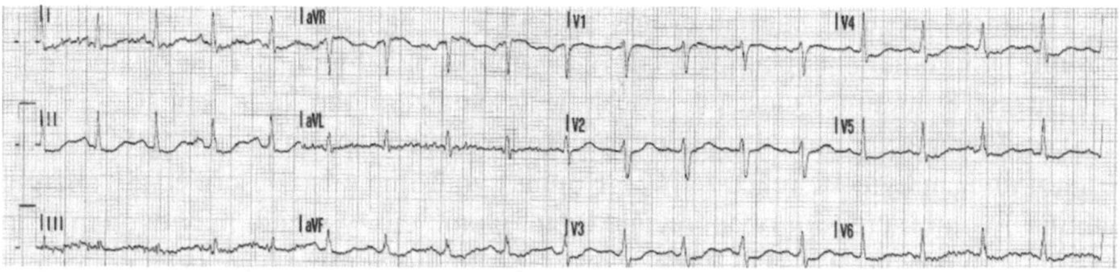

Fig. 20.13 ECG tracing performed 1 h later showing diffuse elevation of ST segment

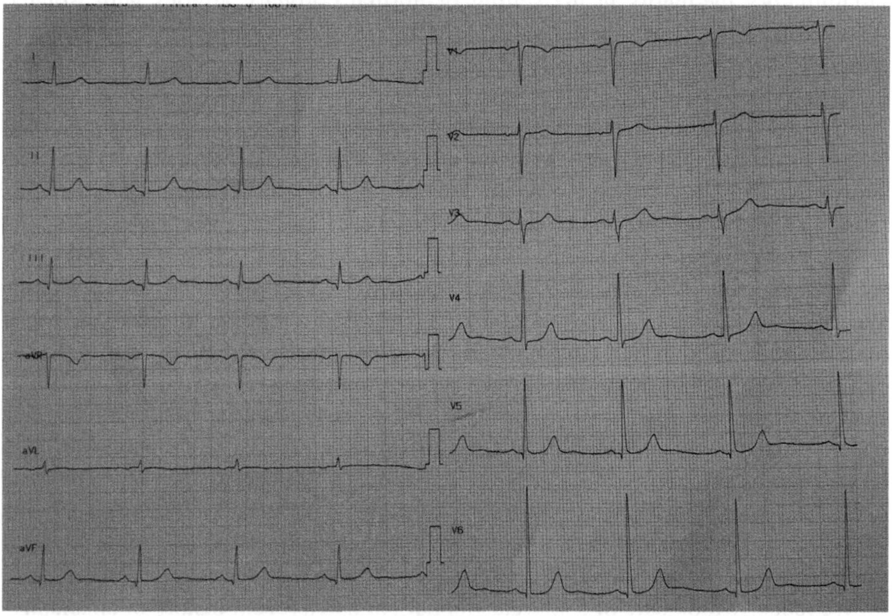

Fig. 20.14 Normal ECG tracing in the same patient performed remotely from event

mastocytosis (Fig. 20.15). The final diagnostic (after complete evaluation) was systemic mastocytosis with cutaneous involvement.

Patients with a history of recurrent unexplained syncope, an episode of Kounis syndrome or unexplained cardiac arrest should be considered for diagnostic workup of possible systemic mastocytosis. A guideline for approaching the diagnosis of mastocytosis in patient with unexplained cardiac events is summarized in Fig. 20.16.

Ulrich W. Kolck et al., reported the cardiovascular symptoms in patients with mastocytosis and the mainly symptoms are dysrhythmias, palpitations, pericarditis, syncope, hypotension and cardiac arrest. Many other symptoms were reported as possible cardiovascular symptoms of mast cell disease [45].

In 2016, Sigurd Broesby-Olsen et al., reported the results of a nationwide population-based study using Danish medical registries. For venous thromboembolism they found a hazard ration of 1.9 (95% CI 1.2-3.0), with a 10-year absolute risk

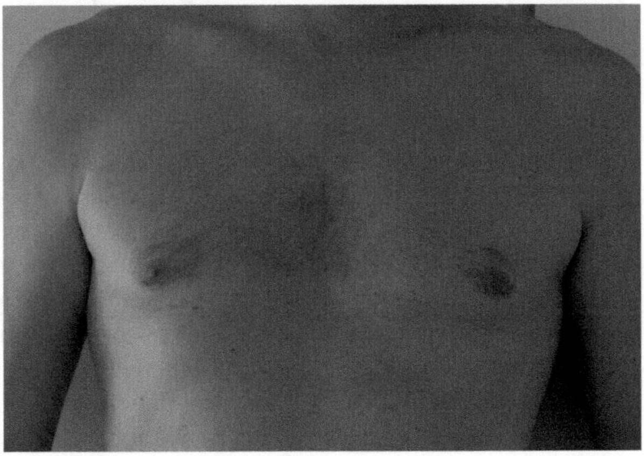

Fig. 20.15 Pigmented maculopapular cutaneous mastocytosis

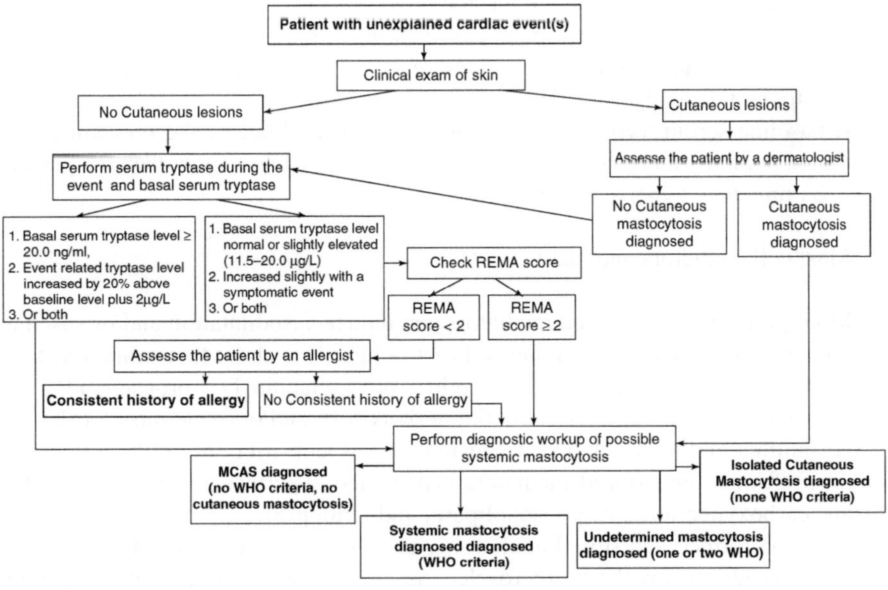

Fig. 20.16 Diagnostic algorithm of mastocytosis in patient with unexplained cardiac events

of 3.9% (95% CI 2.3-6.1) and for stroke a hazard risk of 1.6 (95% CI 1.1-2.3) with 10-year absolute risk of 4.6% (95% CI 2.8-6.9) [40].

In a recent study, Indhirajanti et al., reported a prevalence of cardiovascular disease higher in patients with SM compared to healthy controls (20% vs. 6%, $p = 0.04$) [46].

Patients with a diagnosis of mastocytosis require a varying amount of therapy. Avoidance of any known triggers is important, as well as symptomatic management. Histamine receptor antagonists are considered first-line therapy for treatment of symptomatic mastocytosis, and leukotriene antagonists are typically then added in as second-line therapy. For refractory cases, a treatment with *omalizumab* or cytoreductive therapies such as *interferon-alpha, cladribine* or tyrosine kinase inhibitors may have an emerging role.

2. Cardiac surgery in patient with mastocytosis

There is a high theoretical possibility of cardiac surgery to act as a trigger for degranulation of mast cells in patients with mastocytosis [47, 48]. Currently, there are limited data about the management of patients with mastocytosis undergoing cardiac surgery [49]. On the other hand, the risk due to cardiac surgery to act as a trigger for degranulation of mast cells is not more than it due to other surgery. So, the management of mastocytosis patient's needing cardiac surgery must be identical to the mastocytosis patient's need for other surgery.

The perioperative management of a patient with mastocytosis includes: avoidance of the triggers of mast cell degranulation, such as stress, temperature changes, mechanical factors and pharmacological factors. *Atracurium*, *Mivacurium* and *Nefopam* are not recommended in mastocytosis patients [50]. It is important to note that pain by itself may induce mast cell degranulation. So, the use of analgesics, specifically avoiding opioids which trigger mast cells, is indicated for intraoperative and postoperative analgesia [51].

A baseline serum tryptase level should be measured before the procedure as a reference point. It can be compared with serum tryptase levels after eventual perioperative immediate hypersensitivity [50].

3. Mast cell mediators and heart

More preformed and stored mediators can induce vasodilatation and/or vascular permeability with hypotension and/or heart failure. It is about histamine, tryptase, chymase, vasoactive intestinal polypeptide, prostaglandin D2, prostaglandin E2, platelet activating factor, interleukin 6, interleukin 10 and/or oxide nitric [45].

Histamine, endothelin 1 and 3 can induce vasoconstriction and hypertension. Other preformed and stored mediators can induce hypertension by other mechanisms: carboxypeptidase A, phospholipase, and renin [45].

Some preformed and stored mediators can induce a strong vasoconstriction and coronary syndromes without atherosclerosis, as like serotonin, leukotriene, endothelin 1 and 3.

On the contrary, other mediators can induce atherosclerosis and coronary syndromes by attraction of leukocytes to the atherosclerotic lesion and activation of immune cells. It is about of interleukin 8, chemokine ligand 5, 4, 3, and 2. Moreover, other mediators can promote the induction of plaque angiogenesis and so atherosclerosis: vascular endothelial growth factor and fibroblast growth factor-2 and -7 [45].

Some mediators can induce a fibroblast proliferation and/or activation and so fibrosis: histamine, tryptase, interleukin 4, fibroblast growth factor-2 and -7, and transforming growth factor beta [45, 52].

In conclusion, the set of mediators secreted by activated mast cells can lead to multiple cardiac effects and, hence, several clinical cardiac manifestations.

References

1. Group BMJP. Reports of medical and surgical practice in the hospitals of Great Britain. Br Med J. 1869;2:323–5.
2. Akin C, Metcalfe DD. Systemic Mastocytosis. Annu Rev Med. 2004;55:419–32.
3. https://www.orpha.net/consor/cgibin/OC_Exp.php?lng=FR& Expert=98292. Accessed on 18th August 2019.
4. Damaj G, Hermine O. Systemic mastocytosis in adults: pathophysiology and clinical manifestations. Correspondances en Onco-Hématologie. 2015;X:6.
5. Valent P, Akin C, Metcalfe DD. Mastocytosis: 2016 updated WHO classification and novel emerging treatment concepts. Blood. 2017;129:1420–7.
6. Arber DA, Orazi A, Hasserjian R, et al. The 2016 revision to the World Health Organization classification of myeloid neoplasms and acute leukemia. Blood. 2016;127:2391–405.
7. Valent P, Horny HP, Li CY, et al. In: Jaffe ES, Harris NL, Stein H, Vardiman JW, editors. World Health Organization (WHO) classification of tumours pathology and genetics of tumours of the haematopoietic and lymphoid tissues. Lyon: International Agency for Research on Cancer; 2001. p. 291–302.
8. Horny HP, Akin C, Metcalfe DD, et al. In: Swerdlow SH, Campo PE, Harris NL, Jaffe ES, Pileri SA, Stein H, editors. World Health Organization (WHO) classification of tumours pathology and genetics of tumours of the haematopoietic and lymphoid tissues. Lyon: International Agency for Research on Cancer; 2008. p. 54–63.
9. Severino M, Chandesris MO, Barete S, et al. Telangiectasia macularis eruptiva perstans (TMEP): a form of cutaneous mastocytosis with potential systemic involvement. J Am Acad Dermatol. 2016;74:885–91.
10. Bulai Livideanu C, Severino-Freire M, Jendoubi, et al. Image gallery: the vulva: an atypical localization of mastocytosis in adulthood. Br J Dermatol. 2019;181:e33. https://doi.org/10.1111/bjd.17897.
11. Méni C, Bruneau J, Georgin-Lavialle S, et al. Paediatric mastocytosis: a systematic review of 1747 cases. Br J Dermatol. 2015;172:642–51.
12. Pardanani A. Systemic mastocytosis in adults: 2017 update on diagnosis, risk stratification and management. Am J Hematol. 2016;91:1147–59.
13. Valent P, Akin C, Sperr WR, Horny HP, Metcalfe DD. Smouldering mastocytosis: a novel subtype of systemic mastocytosis with slow progression. Int Arch Allergy Immunol. 2002;127:137–9.
14. Monnier J, Georgin-Lavialle S, Canioni D, et al. Mast cell sarcoma: new cases and literature review. Oncotarget. 2016;7:66299–309.
15. Hartmann K, Escribano L, Grattan C, et al. Cutaneous manifestations in patients with mastocytosis: consensus report of the European Competence Network on Mastocytosis; the American

Academy of Allergy, Asthma & Immunology; and the European Academy of Allergology and Clinical Immunology. J Allergy Clin Immunol. 2016;137:35–45.
16. Valent P, Akin C, Escribano L, et al. Standards and standardization in mastocytosis: consensus statements on diagnostics, treatment recommendations and response criteria. Eur J Clin Investig. 2007;37:435–53.
17. Kirsten N, Tournier E, Lepage B, et al. Immunohistochemical staining for diagnosis of cutaneous mastocytosis. J Eur Acad Dermatol Venereol. 2016; https://doi.org/10.1111/jdv.13946.
18. Fradet M, Negretto M, Tournier E, et al. Frequency of isolated cutaneous involvement in adult mastocytosis: a cohort study. J Eur Acad Dermatol Venereol. 2019; https://doi.org/10.1111/jdv.15638.
19. Merante S, Ferretti V, Elena C, et al. The Italian Mastocytosis registry: 6-year experience from a hospital-based registry. Future Oncol. 2018;14:2713–23.
20. Valent P, Arock M, Bischoff SC, et al. The European Competence Network on Mastocytosis (ECNM). Wien Klin Wochenschr. 2004;116:647–51.
21. Kristensen T, Vestergaard H, Bindslev-Jensen C, Møller MB, Broesby-Olsen S, Mastocytosis Centre, Odense University Hospital (MastOUH). Sensitive KIT D816V mutation analysis of blood as a diagnostic test in mastocytosis. Am J Hematol. 2014;89:493–8.
22. Bulai Livideanu C, Apoil PA, Lepage B, et al. Bone marrow tryptase as a possible diagnostic criterion for adult systemic mastocytosis. Clin Exp Allergy. 2016;46:133–41.
23. Lim KH, Tefferi A, Lasho TL, et al. Systemic mastocytosis in 342 consecutive adults: survival studies and prognostic factors. Blood. 2009;113:5727–36.
24. Ustun C, Arock M, Kluin-Nelemans HC, et al. Advanced systemic mastocytosis: from molecular and genetic progress to clinical practice. Haematologica. 2016;101:1133–43.
25. Pardanani A, Shah S, Mannelli F, et al. Mayo alliance prognostic system for mastocytosis: clinical and hybrid clinical-molecular models. Blood Adv. 2018;13:2964–72.
26. Mannelli F, Gesullo F, Rotunno G, et al. Validation of the Mayo alliance prognostic system for mastocytosis. Blood Cancer J. 2019;18:4–8.
27. Tefferi A, Shah S, Reichard K, Hanson AC, Pardanani A. Smoldering mastocytosis: survival comparisons with indolent and aggressive mastocytosis. Am J Hematol. 2019;94:E1–2.
28. Siebenhaar F, Förtsch A, Krause K, et al. Rupatadine improves quality of life in mastocytosis: a randomized, double-blind, placebo-controlled trial. Allergy. 2013;68:949–52.
29. Hermine O, Lortholary O, Leventha P, et al. Case-control cohort study of patients' perceptions of disability in mastocytosis. PLoS One. 2008;3:e2266. https://doi.org/10.1371/journal.pone.0002266.
30. Jennings S, Slee V, Zack R, et al. Patient perceptions in mast cell disorders. Immunol Allergy. 2018;38:505–25.
31. Degboé Y, Eischen M, Apoil PA, et al. Higher prevalence of vertebral fractures in systemic mastocytosis, but not in cutaneous mastocytosis and idiopathic mast cell activation syndrome. Osteoporos Int. 2019;30:1235–41.
32. Alvarez-Twose, González-de-Olano D, Sánchez-Muñoz L, et al. Validation of the REMA score for predicting mast cell clonality and systemic mastocytosis in patients with systemic mast cell activation symptoms. Int Arch Allergy Immunol. 2012;157:275–80.
33. Bulai Livideanu C, Casassa E, Tournier E et al. Mastocytosis treated with midostaurine: evaluation of response to treatment. Poster No. 376, JDP 2016, Paris.
34. https://clinicaltrials.gov Accessed on 18 August 2019.
35. Fatma Jendoubi, Maella Severino-Freire, Carle Paul, Cristina Bulai Livideanu. Omalizumab in the treatment of mast cell disorders: a systematic review of the literature. Poster N°330, JDP 2018, Paris.
36. Lemal R, Fouquet G, Terriou L, et al. Omalizumab therapy for mast cell-mediator symptoms in patients with ISM, CM, MMAS, and MCAS. J Allergy Clin Immunol Pract. 2019;19:30322–8.
37. González-de-Olano D, Padial-Vilchez MA, Núñez-Acevedo B, et al. Usefulness of omalizumab and sting challenge test in hymenoptera venom allergy and mastocytosis. J Investig Allergol Clin Immunol. 2019; https://doi.org/10.18176/jiaci.0395.

38. Barete S, Lortholary O, Damaj G, et al. Long-term efficacy and safety of cladribine (2-CdA) in adult patients with mastocytosis. Blood. 2015;126:1009–16.
39. Brazzelli V, Grassi S, Merante S, et al. Narrow-band UVB phototherapy and psoralen-ultraviolet a photochemotherapy in the treatment of cutaneous mastocytosis: a study in 20 patients. Photodermatol Photoimmunol Photomed. 2016;32:238–46.
40. Broesby-Olsen S, Farkas DK, Vestergaard H, et al. Risk of solid cancer, cardiovascular disease, anaphylaxis, osteoporosis and fractures in patients with systemic mastocytosis: a nationwide population-based study. Am J Hematol. 2016;91:1069–75.
41. Kounis NG, Zavras GM. Histamine-induced coronary artery spasm: the concept of allergic angina. Br J Clin Pract. 1991;45:121–8.
42. Fassio F, Losappio L, Antolin-Amerigo D, et al. Kounis syndrome: a concise review with focus on management. Eur J Intern Med. 2016;30:7–10.
43. Paratz DE, Khav N, Burns TA. Systemic mastocytosis, kounis syndrome and coronary intervention: case report and systematic review. Heart Lung Circ. 2017;26:772–8.
44. Ridolo E, Triggiani M, Montagni M, et al. Mastocytosis presenting as cardiac emergency. Intern Emerg Med 2013; 8: 749–52; Rohr SM, Rich MW, Silver KH. Shortness of breath, syncope and cardiacarrest caused by systemic mastocytosis. Ann Emerg Med 2 005; 45: 592–4.
45. Kolck WU, Haenisch B, Molderings JG. Cardiovascular symptoms in patients with systemic mast cell activation disease. Transl Res. 2016;174:23–32.
46. Indhirajanti S, Van Daele LA, Bos P, et al. Systemic mastocytosis associates with cardiovascular events despite lower plasma lipid levels. Atherosclerosis. 2018;268:152–6.
47. Magovern GJ, Moraca RJ. Aortic valve replacement in patients with systemic mastocytosis. J Card Surg. 2012;27:189–91.
48. Brockow K, Bonadonna P. Drug allergy in mast cell disease. Curr Opin Allergy Clin Immunol. 2012;12:354–60.
49. Giraldo-Grueso M, Montes RF, Echeverri D, Umana P, Mitral J. Valve replacement in a patient with systemic mastocytosis. J Cardiothorac Vasc Anesth. 2019;33:877–86.
50. Dewachter P, Castells CM, Hepner LD, Mouton-Faivre C. Perioperative management of patients with mastocytosis. Anesthesiology. 2014;120:753–9.
51. Dewachter P, Mouton-Faivre C, Cazalaà JB, Carli P, Lortholary O, Hermine O. Mastocytosis and anaesthesia. Ann Fr Anesth Reanim. 2009;28:61–73.
52. Hermans A, Roeters WM, van Lennep JE, LAP VD, Bot I. Mast cells in cardiovascular disease: from bench to bedside. Int J Mol Sci. 2019;20(14):3395. https://doi.org/10.3390/ijms20143395.

Part VI

Infectious Diseases

Medication Induced Cardiotoxicity and Skin Reactions

21

Carmen Salavastru, Stefana Cretu, Adelina Sendrea, and George Sorin Tiplica

Introduction

A drug, or medication is a substance or compound offered for the investigation, prevention or treatment of symptoms or clinical conditions [1]. According to the definition provided by the World Health Organization, an adverse drug reaction (ADR) is the undesirable, unpleasant or harmful clinical manifestation that results from the administration of a drug at usual doses in humans. An adverse drug event is defined as the occurrence of clinical manifestation temporally associated to the use of a medicinal product, without necessary being causally related [2, 3].

Negative outcomes related to drug therapy are an important cause of patient morbidity, can sometimes be lethal, they generate high economic costs and may lead to negative changes in the doctor-patient relationship, as patients are tempted to lose trust in their caring physician [1, 4]. It is estimated that hospitals in many countries spend around 15–20% of their budgets to care for patients suffering from drug related complications [5].

C. Salavastru (✉)
Paediatric Dermatology Department, "Carol Davila" University of Medicine and Pharmacy, Bucharest, Romania

S. Cretu
"Carol Davila" University of Medicine and Pharmacy, Bucharest, Romania

A. Sendrea
"Carol Davila" University of Medicine and Pharmacy, Bucharest, Romania

Dermato-Oncology Research Unit, "Colentina" Clinical Hospital, Bucharest, Romania

G. S. Tiplica
"Carol Davila" University of Medicine and Pharmacy, Dermatology II, Colentina Clinical Hospital, Bucharest, Romania
e-mail: george.tiplica@umfcd.ro

C. Salavastru et al. (eds.), *Skin and the Heart*,
https://doi.org/10.1007/978-3-030-54779-0_21

Therefore, it is very important to obtain a detailed medication history for all patients. Over-the-counter, herbal or other alternative medicine remedies should be noted, as well as other substances consumed by the patient, such as alcohol, nicotine, illegal drugs, topical cosmetic products [1, 4].

Pathophysiology

The pathogenesis of most adverse-drug reactions is not fully understood. They can be caused by either of the following compounds, collectively or individually: drugs in their original form, metabolites of drugs or altered self [4].

Adverse drug reactions may be predictable or unpredictable. The former are usually dose related and non-immunologic in nature, as opposed to the latter, which can occur via both immunologic and non-immunologic mechanisms and are not dose related [1, 6] (Table 21.1).

Prevalence/Population Affected

It is difficult to estimate the true prevalence of adverse drug reactions. Data vary greatly amongst different studies, mainly due to study design. Also, many are performed in emergency departments, intensive care units or hospital wards, few investigate outpatient settings and almost none, primary care [8, 9].

Apart from the above mentioned limitations, a lack of standardized coding for adverse drug reactions is an important issue an leads to difficulties in comparing results from different studies [3, 9, 10]. Moreover, a great challenge is also underreporting [11].

Sometimes adverse drug reactions result from human error and in some cases, due to the fear of litigation, they are not reported. Others, occur independent of human intervention.

Rare adverse reactions reported in anecdotal studies published in the medical literature are subsequently validated by the monitoring agencies after thorough investigation. Promulgated criteria for the assessment of a potential drug reaction include:

- Presence of a pharmacologic basis for the reaction
- Immunologic anomalies
- Recurrence upon challenge
- The occurrence of:

  Immediate acute or local reactions at the time of administration

  Previously known reactions with a new route of administration

  Repeated rare reactions [1]

In Europe, for example, depending on the study, between 3.3 and 6.5% of all hospital admissions are caused by an adverse drug reaction, and between 10% and 20% develop an adverse drug reaction during their hospital stay [12, 13].

Table 21.1 Predictable and unpredictable drug reactions

Predictable adverse drug reactions (ADRs) [1,6]		• ADRs resulting from overdose occurring at doses considered therapeutic, due to patient related characteristic or to drug interactions • Side effects • Unwanted or toxic events linked to the pharmacologic action of the drug • Cumulative toxicity occurring after prolonged exposure • Delayed toxicity • Drug interactions • Teratogenicity • Drug induced chromosomal damage • Exacerbation of disease • Metabolic alterations • Non-immunologic activation of effector pathways. e.g.: binding of the drug to receptors on basophils and mast cells, leading to their degranulation via non-immunologic mechanisms
Unpredictable adverse drug reactions [1, 4, 6, 7]	**Immunologic** (according to the Gell-Coombs classification system)	• Type I: IgE-mediated drug reactions, leading to urticarial, angioedema and anaphylaxis • Type II: involving the interaction between an antibody and a fixed antigen (the drug or its metabolites), resulting in cytotoxic drug induced reactions • Type III: involving immune complex mediated cytotoxicity, without the presence of a fixed antigen, leading to vasculitis, serum sickness and certain forms of urticarial • Type IV: cell mediated, delayed type hypersensitivity reactions, resulting in a plethora of clinical manifestations ranging from exanthematous eruptions to Stevens-Johnson syndrome and toxic epidermal necrolysis
	Non-Immunologic	• Intolerance - unusually small amounts of the drug cause an exaggeration of its characteristic effects • Idiosyncrasy - effect not characteristic to the drug, occurring without the involvement of immunologic mechanisms, resulting from inter-individual variations of drug metabolism

Risk factors for the development of adverse drug reactions include: female gender, old age, chronic renal disease, prolonged hospital stays and the concomitant use of multiple drugs [11, 13, 14].

Also, in children, adverse drug reactions are a great concern. One reason is that in this age group the physiology is different from that of adults. However, there is a very limited number of studies focusing on or including children and many drugs are prescribed *off-label*. Toxicity in children is different compared to that observed in adults, due to different drug pharmacodynamics and pharmacokinetics, with some effects only becoming apparent many years later. Additionally, in neonates, due to particular features, characteristic to this age group, drug toxicity seems to be relatively frequent [14, 15].

Although in many cases, adverse drug reactions can be prevented, only a minority of the severe ones can be avoided through increased risk awareness [1, 9, 11].

The skin is commonly involved in adverse drug reactions. Some authors observed that up to 6.7% of hospitalized patients suffer from some form of adverse cutaneous drug reaction and that between 0.33% and 3% are severe [16].

Cancer patients are amongst the population most affected by adverse drug reactions. One reason is that their treatment sometimes involves the presence of multiple drugs. Another reason is that some of the targets of antineoplastic medication are also found in healthy tissues [1, 17].

Dermatological Manifestation

Cases of adverse cutaneous reactions requiring or prolonging hospital stay, resulting in persistent or significant disability or threatening survival may classify as severe. This category includes: anaphylaxis, exfoliative dermatitis, fixed drug eruptions, acute generalized exanthematous pustulosis (AGEP)—5% mortality, drug induced hypersensitivity syndrome (DISH)/ drug rash with eosinophilia and systemic symptoms (DRESS)-10% mortality, Stevens-Johnson syndrome, toxic epidermal necrolysis-mortality ranging between 25–30% [1, 16].

With regard to adverse events involving antineoplastic drugs, the National Cancer Institute-Common Terminology Criteria for Adverse Events v5.0, classifies their severity into five major forms: grade 1 (mild), grade 2 (moderate), grade 3 (severe), grade 4 (life-threatening) and grade 5 (death). In case of grade 1 severity, symptoms are absent or mild in intensity, only clinical or diagnostic observations are present and no intervention is needed. Grade 2 severity involves the same clinical characteristics as in the previous, having in addition the indication for minimal, local or non-invasive intervention and the limitation of age-appropriate activities of daily living. In grade 3 severity clinical findings although significant, are not immediately life-threatening, however they do indicate hospitalization or prolongation of hospitalization, associating disability, limiting self-care. Despite these features, the patient is not bedridden. Grade 4 severity adverse drug events have life-threatening consequences leading to urgent need for intervention [18].

Clinical Findings

Adverse drug reactions can affect the skin at any level (epidermis, dermis, subcutis), its appendages (hair, nails, apocrine, eccrine and sebaceous glands) and mucous membranes. Because the skin has a limited way to respond to different aggressions, in many cases causality is difficult to assess. Although not necessarily present simultaneously, all types of elementary lesions can be found in adverse drug reactions.

In patients where adverse drug reactions are suspected, appropriate management begins with clinical evaluation of the eruption and morphological approach can prove very useful [6].

Cardiologic Adverse Drug Reactions

Introduction and Pathophysiology of Disease

Drug induced cardiotoxicity remains one of the most common side effects of many drug classes (including over the counter prescriptions and illicit substances), despite of significant advances in medical and pharmacological research, becoming a global concern of healthcare, especially in the field of oncology.

It represents one of the most serious adverse drug reactions associated with development of novel molecules, being associated with almost all drug classes, not only oncological treatments. The major concern of drug induced cardiotoxicity is determined by drugs that are administered in a chronic manner, for long-lasting diseases, such as chemotherapeutics and neuro-psychiatric molecules, because the cardiac toxic effects may become clinically evident only after a prolonged systemic accumulation of the drug itself or its metabolites [19]. Cardiotoxicity is defined, in very general terms, by The National Cancer Institute, as "toxicity that affects the heart" [20] which comprises a very broad spectrum of manifestations and doesn't define very well this term, leading to a lack of clear understanding of what it means. It is a very well-known fact that the most cardiotoxic drug class is represented by various chemotherapeutics. This is why one of the most accurate definitions of drug induced cardiotoxiciy has been formulated by the cardiac review and evaluation committee that supervised clinical trials with trastuzumab (monoclonal antibiody used in breast cancer treatment), as one of the following:

- Cardiomyopathy (left ventricular/ septal ejection fraction reduction)
- Symptoms associated with heart failure
- Signs associated with heart failure (S3 gallop, tachycardia)
- Reduction of left ventricular ejection fraction from baseline ($\leq 5\% - \leq 55\%$) associated with signs or symptoms of heart failure OR reduction of left ventricular ejection fraction ($\geq 10\% - < 55\%$), without any associated signs or symptoms [20].

The limits of the above mentioned definition are represented by the fact that it doesn't rely to the early, subclinical cardiovascular damage induced by certain drugs. Therefore, currently an ideal, comprehensive definition is lacking.

Currently, according to International Conference of Harmonization Expert Working Group for all drugs in development, assessing the risk of drug-induced cardiotoxicity is mandatory for all new chemical molecules, being a part of their standard preclinical evaluation. However, despite significant efforts made to determine the cardiotoxic potential of therapeutic agents in their preclinical phase of development, drug induced cardiotoxicity is still a significant safety concern [19].

Drug associated cardiotoxic effects can be classified into two types, based on structural anomalies and potential of reversibility: type I cardiotoxicity (characterized by myocardial injury, which usually is permanent and irreversible) and type II cardiotoxicity (which is reversible, being characterized by a higher probability of cardiac function restoration after disruption of offending drug) [21, 22].

Additionally, drug induced cardiotoxicity, can be divided into acute, subacute or chronic, according to the onset time in relation to treatment time span, as it is summarized in Table 21.2.

Various drugs can determine cardiotoxicity either through a direct effect on the cardiovascular system, or through an indirect effect, by increasing certain pre-existing cardiovascular risk factors, as is highlighted in Table 21.3.

Other classification system of drug-induced cardiotoxicity is based on the effect of the drugs either on the heart, on the vascular system or on both of them. Cardiac and respectively, vascular effects of drugs are listed in Table 21.4.

The common pathophysiological mechanism of all drug related cardiotoxic manifestations is represented by the oxidative stress, associated with free radicals

Table 21.2 Clasification of drug induced cardiotoxicity. Types of drug-induced cardiotoxicity related to treatment time span [20]

	Acute cardiotoxicity	Subacute cardiotoxicity	Chronic cardiotoxicity
Onset	During/immediately after the treatment (up to 2 weeks after treatment discontinuation)		**Type I** = early (within the first year after treatment discontinuation) **Type II** = late (> 1 year after treatment discontinuation)
Manifestations	Transient Ventricular repolarization anomalies ECG QT-interval changes Supraventricular and ventricular arrhythmias Acute coronary syndromes Myocarditis-like syndromes		Asymptomatic systolic / diastolic left ventricular dysfunction → severe congestive cardiomyopathy → death

Table 21.3 Types of drug-induced cardiotoxic effects [23]

	Direct cardiotoxic effects	Indirect cardiotoxic effects (increase of cardiovascular risk factors)
Manifestations	Acute coronary syndromes Vascular hypertension Arrhythmias Left ventricle dysfunction → heart failure	Impaired endothelial function Atherosclerosis Arterial thrombosis Arterial hypertension
Common involved drugs	Anthracyclines	Anti-hormonal preparations used in breast/prostate cancers • GnRH antagonists • Aromatase inhibitors • Anti-androgens • Anti-estrogens

Table 21.4 Cardiac and vascular—drug induced toxicities [24]

Cardiac-drug induced toxicity	Vascular drug-induced toxicity
Dysrhythmias (Brady/tachydysrhythmias) Myocardial ischemia Left ventricular dysfunction / heart failure Myocarditis Cardiac valves impairment Pericardial disease induction	Arterial blood pressure effects: • Systemic hypertension • Systemic hypotension • Pulmonary hypertension Thromboembolic events • Arterial • Venous

Table 21.5 Mechanisms of anthracyclines-induced cardiotoxicity

Multiple mechanisms theory [26]	**Multiple hit theory** [22, 26]
Iron-anthracyclines metabolites development Reactive oxygen species development Topoisomerase B inhibition *Associated with* Genetic predisposition → enhancement of the damage induced by each agent at the myocyte level	Sequential injuries determined by a single pharmacological agent on the myocytes *Associated with* Genetic predisposition Cardiac risk factors (arterial hypertension, diabetes mellitus, dyslipidemia)

production and hypoxia. The chronic, prolonged exposure to drugs that have cardiotoxic potential induces apoptosis and myocontractility disorders. Therefore, the cardiotoxic effect of drugs is induced through two main mechanisms: affecting the performance of cardiac muscles and alteration of the ion-channels (voltage gated Na-K ion channel) and pumps (Na-K ATPase pump). Furthermore, drugs with cardiotoxic potential can determine both prolonged cardiac repolarization (prolonged QT interval on the ECG) and arrhythmia (for example torsades de pointes) [25]. But, in specific terms, the pathophysiology of cardiotoxic effects is much more complex at a molecular level, varying according to which drug class is involved and, much more, with the dosage that has been used.

On a more specific level, the mechanisms behind drug induced cardiotoxicity can vary significantly among different drug classes. The most widely known drug class that causes toxic cardiac effects are the chemotherapeutics. Regarding the specific term of "chemotherapy-induced cardiotoxicity", there are two hypotheses proposed as potential mechanisms, summarized in Table 21.5.

The tyrosine kinase inhibitors associated cardiac toxicity can be induced by several mechanisms, according to each drug's target, which are listed in Table 21.6.

On the other hand, the anthracycline-induced cardiotoxicity, is based on the oxidative stress mechanism, which generates reactive oxygen species during the metabolism of these drugs, by a rapidly transfer of the unpaired electrons to an oxygen molecule. The resulting superoxide anions can determine various degrees of cellular injury, through sarcomere degradation, mitochondrial dysfunction and DNA damage. Moreover, the reduction of the carbonyl group of these drugs generates toxic metabolites in the myocardium, which, once accumulated, determine an

Table 21.6 Mechanisms of tyrosine kinase inhibitors-induced cardiotoxicity [27]

Drug target	Cardiac effect
c-Jun N-terminal kinase Pyruvate dehydrogenase kinase Protein kinase A	Disruption of the normal function of cardiomyocytic mitochondria → interruption in the oxidative phosphorylation → mitochondrial morphological anomalies and cardiomyocite hypertrophy & caspase-mediated mitochondrial apoptosis
PDGFR (platelet-derived growth factor receptor) ErbB Raf-1 Shp2	Cardiomyopathy and reduced contractility Alterations in ion channel activation (e.g.: reduced phosphorylation of the hERG K^+ channel → blockade of this channel → clinical = QT interval prolongation)
VEGFR (vascular endothelial growth factor receptor)	Hypertension

inhibition of the Ca^{2+} and Na^+ pumps located in the mitochondrial membrane, leading subsequently to certain mycocardial energetics disturbances and finally to systolic dysfunction. Additionally, anthracyclines determine release of pro-inflammatory cytokines (like IL-1β, IL-6) by macrophage stimulation, cytokines that can modulate apoptosis. Other mediators with important, but incompletely understood role in anthracycline-induced cardiotoxicity are topoisomerase 2β (Top 2β) and anthracycline-sensitive cardiac ankyrin repeat protein (CARP). It has been shown that deletion of Top 2β protected a mouse model myocardium from anthracycline-induced cardiotoxicity and hypertension upregulates CARP expression. All the mechanisms mentioned above, can determine eventually cardiomyocytic death [28].

In the case of antiretroviral nucleoside reverse transcriptase inhibitors-induced cardiotoxicity, the mechanism is mainly based on the induction of cardiac mitochondrial dysfunction determined by an inhibition of the DNA polymerase-gamma which, in turn, leads to mitochondrial DNA mutations and eventually to cardiomyopathy [19].

Prevalence/Population Affected

The exact prevalence of cardiotoxic events determined by drugs is unknown.

In the past four decades, almost 10% of the drugs have been withdrawn from the market worldwide due to concerns regarding their cardiovascular safety profile, drugs like rofecoxib, tegasterod and sibutramine [19].

The most well-known and studied drugs with cardiotoxic effects are the ones used in the oncological field, among which the greatest risk is associated with anthracyclines. In cancer survivors, the most common cause of death is cardiovascular disease, which results either from the treatment or from certain associated cardiovascular risk factors that also increase the likelihood of developing cardiac toxicity. These cardiac drug-induced toxic effects affect all age groups, including children [29].

The incidence of cancer therapy induced cardiotoxicity varies significantly, according to which therapeutic agent is being used, in which dosage and for how long, depending also on patient's associated cardiovascular comorbidities. It has been shown that cardiac dysfunctions represent the leading cause of mortality in breast cancer patients with an age over 50 years old and in elderly patients it seems to contribute more to the mortality rates compared to younger ones [30].

In the pediatric population of long-term cancer survivors, the cardiovascular disorders are the leading non-cancer related cause of both morbidity and mortality, with almost 75% of children developing a chronic cardiac disease within 30 years after the initial diagnosis [29] and 33% of long-time survivals of pediatric cancers die of cardiovascular cause [19]. More specifically, it has been shown that children who have survived cancer have an 8.2-fold higher rate of cardiac death, a 15-fold increased rate of congestive heart failure and a 9-fold higher rates of stroke compared to age and sex-matched controls [30].

Certain risk factors are associated with development of drug induced cardiotoxic manifestations, such as extreme age at time of drug exposure (<4 years old and elderly patients), associated cardiovascular comorbidities or risk factors (personal history of cardiac disease or left ventricular dysfunction, preexisting hypertension, obesity, dyslipidemia, diabetes, sedentariness, smoking), therapeutic regimen dosage and treatment duration, concomitant radiotherapy or cardiac irradiation, female gender, black ethnicity and genetic predisposition [19]. For example, patients who are either overweight or obese have a higher risk of developing anthracycline- and trastuzumab-induced cardiotoxicity [31]. Another important susceptibility factor for development of anthracycline-induced cardiotoxicity is represented by the number of myocardial cells that is established during the embryonic development, which is controlled by a protein with a key-role in progression of mitosis in general and in cardiomyocyte replication in particular—called survivin [28].

According to the Galician consensus statement (a joint oncologist/cardiologist initiative focused on prevention and management of cardiotoxicity in breast cancer patients), an overall risk score of developing cardiotoxicity in cancer patients can be determined prior to treatment initiation. In order to be able to determine the risk, it's needed to assess which drugs are being used and patient-related data (socio-demographic data and associated cardiovascular comorbidities), as it can be seen in Table 21.7 [33, 34].

The maximum cardiotoxicity risk score that can be obtained is 14 and it can be interpreted as it follows:

- Score > 6: very high risk
- Score = 5–6: high risk
- Score = 3–4: intermediate risk
- Score = 1–2: low risk
- Score = 0: very low risk [32]

Risk assessment in patients that undergo certain treatments with well-known cardiotoxic potential is essential prior treatment initiation in order to be able to make the proper therapeutic decisions for each patient and to organize early preventive measures. However, drug-induced cardiotoxicity may be determined also in an idiosyncratic manner, without any associated risk factors [19].

Table 21.7 Risk assessment of drug-induced cardiotoxicity in oncological patient [32].

Drug-Related Risk
High risk (4 points): Anthracyclines (cytotoxic antibiotics), cyclophosphamide, ifosfamide, trastuzumab, clofarabine **Intermediate risk (2 points):** Docetaxel, pertuzumab, sunitinib, sorafenib **Low risk (1 point):** Bevacizumab, dasatinib, imatinib, lapatinib, etoposide, rituximab, thalidomide
Patient-Related Risk (1 point each)
Female gender **Extreme ages (< 15 years old or > 65 years old)** **Personal history of:** • Cardiomyopathy/heart failure • Ischemic heart disease • Arrhythmias under treatment • QTc > 500 ms (ECG) **Hypertension** **Diabetes mellitus** **Previous use of anthracyclines** **Radiotherapy of the mediastinal area**

Cardiovascular Manifestation

The adverse events are graded, according to U.S. Department of health and human services into five severity grades, ranging from mild adverse events to death, as it follows:

- Grade 1 (mild)—asymptomatic or mild symptoms
- Grade 2 (moderate)—moderate symptoms
- Grade 3 (severe)—severe or medically significant, but not immediately life-threatening
- Grade 4 (life threatening)—symptoms that are immediately life-threatening
- Grade 5—death related to adverse event [18].

Treatment

- Grade 1 (mild)—clinical observation; intervention not indicated
- Grade 2 (moderate)—minimal, local or noninvasive intervention indicated
- Grade 3 (severe)—hospitalization or prolongation of hospitalization; limiting self-care and activities of daily living
- Grade 4 (life threatening)—urgent intervention indicated [18].

Table 21.8 summarizes the most common skin and cardiotoxic reactions of the most commonly used medication.

Table 21.8 Summary of the most common skin and cardiotoxic reactions of the most commonly used medication

DRUG CLASS		DERMATOLOGICAL ADVERSE EVENT [1,6,35-42]						CARDIOLOGIC ADVERSE EVENT [1,35-111]		PREDISPOSING FACTORS OF ADVERSE EVENTS [1,5]
		Type of eruption	Morphology	Mucous membrane involvement	Time of onset	Differential diagnosis	Frequency (Percentage of patients treated)	Manifestation	Frequency	
Beta-lactams	Penicillins	Urticaria	Pruritus Wheals	Absent	Min-1h	Idiopathic Other possible etiologies for urticaria Insect bites	10%	Pericarditis Arrythmias Sudden cardiac death Vasovagal hypotension Tachycardia Bradycardia Miocarditis	3.2%(% of total adverse drug reactions in cases of betalactamine administration)[5]	Renal impairment Young to middle aged patients are more at risk Pre-existing cardiac disease,especially: -aortic insufficiency -mitral stenosis -mitral regurgitation
		Angioedema	Swollen deep dermis and subcutaneous tissue	Present/ Absent		Idiopathic Other possible etiologies Dermatomyositis Insect bites				
		Exanthematous	Erythematous No blistering	Absent	>72 h	Viral exanthems Toxins Syphilis	2%			
		Palpable purpura (serum sickness)	Palpable purpura	Absent	>72 h	Infectious Autoimmune Hemopathies Paraneoplastic	Rare			
		Erythema multiforme	Typical targetoid lesions	Present	Variable	Fixed drug eruption Stevens-Johnson syndrome Toxic epidermal necrolysis	Rare			
		Bullous pemphigoid	Erythema Tense bullae	Infrequent	Variable	Fixed drug eruption Stevens-Johnson syndrome Toxic epidermal necrolysis Pemphigus Epidermolysis bullosa aquisita Erythema multiforme	Rare			

(continued)

Table 21.8 (continued)

Beta-lactams (continued)		Pemphigus	Flaccid bullae Erosions	Present	Weeks-months	Fixed drug eruption Stevens-Johnson syndrome Toxic epidermal necrolysis Bullous pemphigoid	Rare			
		Pustular psoriasis	Non-follicular, sterile pustules arising on background of edematous erythema	Absent	Variable	Acute generalized exanthematous pustulosis	Rare			
		Drug-induced hypersensitivity syndrome	Severe exanthematous rash	Infrequent	1–6 weeks	Viral diseases Hemopathies	Rare			
	Ampicillin	Exanthematous	Erythematous No blistering	Absent	7-12 days	See above	5-10%	Myocarditis QT prolongation	Rare	Mononucleosis Cytomegalo virus infection Chronic lymphatic leukemia Renal impairment Concomitant administration of Allopurinol
		Urticaria	Pruritus Wheals	Absent	Min-1h	See above	1.5%			
		Palpable purpura (serum sickness)	Palpable purpura	Absent	>72 h	See above	Rare			
		Erythema multiforme	Typical targetoid lesions	Present	Variable	See above	Rare			
		Bullous pemphigoid	Erythema Tense bullae	Infrequent	Variable	See above	Rare			
		Pemphigus	Flaccid bullae Painful erosions	Present	Weeks-months	See above	Rare			
		Fixed drug eruption	One or more round well-circumscribed erythematous plaques Sometimes central bullae	Absent	First exposure: 1–2 weeks Re-exposure: > 48 h, usually within 24 h	Erythema multiforme	Rare			
		Stevens-Johnson syndrome	Atypical targetoid leasions; 10 % body surface area	Present	4–28 days	SSSS Erythema multiforme	Rare			
		Toxic epidermal necrolysis	Confluent and extensive epidermal detachment	Present	4–28 days	SSSS Erythema multiforme Pemphigus	Rare			

			>30 % body surface area								
Beta-lactams (continued)	**Amoxicillin**	Exanthematous	Erythematous No blistering	Absent	7-12 days	See above	1-2%		Acute myocardial infarction Atrial fibrillation/Atrial flutter(AFI/AFL) Ventricular arrhythmia Non-AFI/AFL arrhythmia		
		Urticaria	Pruritus Wheals	Absent	Min-1h	See above					
		Fixed drug eruption	One or more round well-circumscribed erythematous plaques Sometimes central bullae	Absent	First exposure: 1–2 weeks Re-exposure: > 48 h, usually within 24 h	See above	Rare				
		Palpable purpura (serum sickness)	Palpable purpura	Absent	>72 h	See above	Rare				
		Acute generalized exanthematous pustulosis	Non-follicular, sterile pustules arising on background of edematous erythema	Present/ Absent	<4 days	Pustular psoriasis	Rare				
Beta-lactams (continued)	**Cephalosporins**	Exanthematous	Erythematous No blistering	Absent	7-12 days	See above	Variable	1-10%	Pericarditis Coronary spasm Myocardial infarction Atrioventricuar node block		
		Urticaria	Pruritus Wheals	Absent	Min-1h	See above	1-3%				
		Angioedema	Swollen deep dermis and subcutaneous tissue	Present/ Absent							
		Palpable purpura (serum sickness)	Palpable purpura	Absent	>72 h	See above	Rare				
		Fixed drug eruption	One or more round well-circumscribed erythematous plaques Sometimes central bullae	Absent	First exposure: 1–2 weeks Re-exposure: > 48 h, usually within 24 h	See above	Rare				
		Erythema multiforme	Typical targetoid lesions	Present	>72 h	See above	Rare				
		Toxic epidermal necrolysis	Confluent and extensive	Present	4–28 days	See above	Rare				

(continued)

Table 21.8 (continued)

			epidermal detachment >30 % body surface area								
Tetracyclines E.g. Doxicycline, Tetracycline, Minocycline		Photosensitivity	Erythema ± Blistering after sun exposure	Absent	Variable	Eczema Lichen planus	Variable		Supraventricular arrythmia Sporadic Wenckebach heart block	Rare	Long term treatment
		Pseudoporphyria	Erythema, skin fragility, blistering and scarring of photo-exposed areas	Absent	Variable	Porphyria cutanea tarda Bullous pemphigoid	Variable				
		Exanthematous	Erythematous No blistering	Absent	23-35 days	See above	Variable				
		Urticaria	Pruritus Wheals	Absent	Min-1h	See above	Variable				
		Erythema multiforme	Typical targetoid lesions	Present	>72 h	See above	Variable				
		Stevens-Johnson syndrome	Atypical targetoid leasions, 10 % body surface area	Present	4–28 days	See above	Rare				
		Toxic epidermal necrolysis	Confluent and extensive epidermal detachment >30 % body surface area	Present	4–28 days	See above	Rare				
		Fixed drug eruption	One or more round well-circumscribed erythematous plaques Sometimes central bullae	Absent	First exposure: 1–2 weeks Re-exposure: > 48 h, usually within 24 h	See above	Rare				
		Bullous pemphigoid	Erythema Tense bullae	Infrequent	Variable	See above	Rare				
		Pemphigus	Flaccid bullae Painful erosions	Present	Weeks-months	See above	Rare				
		Psoriasiform	Mostly scalp, palmoplantar	Absent	Variable	Psoriasis vulgaris	Rare				

		(vulgar and pustular), and diaper area			Acropustulosis Eczema				
Minocycline	Pigmentation	Blue-black macules in areas of previous inflammation or scarring/ Brown-grey macules in sunexposed areas	Present/ Absent	>5 months		1-4%	Pigmentation of endocardium Systemic Vasculitis		Co-treatment with: -cyproterone acetate+ethinylestradiol -amitriptyline -phenothiazines -13-cis-retinoic acid
	Palpable purpura (serum sickness)	Palpable purpura	Absent	15 days	See above	Rare			
	Drug-induced systemic inflammatory response syndrome (fever >38.5 °C; tachypnea: >20 breaths/min; tachycardia: >90 beats/min; leukocytosis: >12.000 cells/mm³ or >10 % immature forms)	Generalized erythematous rash (may be absent)	Absent	Hours–weeks	Infection Septic shock	Rare			
Sulphonamides, E.g. Sulfasalazine, Sulfametoxypyridazine, Sulfadoxine	Urticaria	Pruritus Wheals	Absent	Min-1h	See above	Rare	Tachycardia Toxic myocarditis Myocardial infarction Pericarditis Bradycardia	Rare	AIDS patients
	Exanthematous	Erythematous No blistering	Absent	Variable	See above	1-5%			
	Erythema multiforme	Typical targetoid lesions	Present	>72 h	See above	Rare			
	Stevens-Johnson syndrome	Atypical targetoid leasions, 10 % body surface area	Present	4–28 days	See above				
	Toxic epidermal necrolysis	Confluent and extensive epidermal detachment >30 % body surface area	Present	4–28 days	See above				

(continued)

Table 21.8 (continued)

	Fixed drug eruption	One or more round well-circumscribed erythematous plaques Sometimes central bullae	Absent	First exposure: 1–2 weeks Re-exposure: > 48 h, usually within 24 h	See above		1-5%			
	Drug-induced lupus	Similar to idiopathic subacute cutaneous LE (SCLE): scaly papules and plaques, some with annular configuration	Absent/ present	Variable	Idiopathic SCLE Polymorphous light eruption					
	Palpable purpura (serum sickness)	Palpable purpura	Absent	15 days	See above					
	Drug-induced hypersensitivity syndrome	Severe exanthematous rash	Infrequent	1–6 weeks	See above					
Trimtethoprim-sulfamethoxazole(co-trimoxazole)	Erythema multiforme	Typical targetoid lesions	Present	11 days	See above		3%	QT prolongation Torsade de pointes Pericardial tamponade Cardiac arrest Arrythmias due to hyperkaliemia Ventricular tachycardia		
	Stevens-Johnson syndrome	Atypical targetoid leasions 10 % body surface area	Present		See above					
	Toxic epidermal necrolysis	Confluent and extensive epidermal detachment >30 % body surface area	Present		See above					
	Fixed drug eruption	One or more round well-circumscribed erythematous plaques Sometimes central bullae	Absent		See above					

	Bullous pemphigoid	Erythema Tense bullae	Infrequent	Variable	See above	Rare				
	Pemphigus	Flaccid bullae Painful erosions	Present	Weeks-months	See above	Rare				
Trimethoprim	Fixed drug eruption	One or more round well-circumscribed erythematous plaques Sometimes central bullae	Absent	Variable	See above	Rare		Hypotension Arrythmias	Rare	
	Urticaria	Pruritus Wheals	Absent	Min-1h	See above	Rare				
Aminoglycosides E.g: Gentamicin, Tobramycin Streptomycin Kanamycin	Exanthematous	Erythematous No blistering	Absent	Variable	See above	5%		Myocardial toxicity* *occurring at very high concentrations	Rare	
	Urticaria	Pruritus Wheals	Absent	Min-1h	See above					
Macrolides E.g. : Azithromicyn Clarithromycin Erythromicyn Spiramycin	Exanthematous	Erythematous No blistering	Absent	Variable	See above	1%	10-15%	Systemic vasculitis		Older adults Preexisting heart disease
	Erythema multiforme	Typical targetoid lesions	Present		See above	Rare		QT-interval prolongation	9.8% (of patients treated)	
	Stevens-Johnson syndrome	Atypical targetoid leasions, 10 % body surface area	Present		See above			Cardiac arrhythmias	0.91%	
	Fixed drug eruption	One or more round well-circumscribed erythematous plaques Sometimes central bullae	Absent		See above			Cardiac arrest Torsade de pointes	Variable	

(continued)

Table 21.8 (continued)

	Palpable purpura (serum sickness)	Palpable purpura	Absent		See above	<1%		Ventricular tachycardia	0.08%	
Clindamycin	Exanthematous	Erythematous No blistering	Absent	7-12 days	See above	10%		QT interval prolongation Torsade de pointes	Rare	
	Erythema multiforme	Typical targetoid lesions	Present	Variable	See above	Rare				
Chloramphenicol	Exanthematous	Erythematous No blistering	Absent	Variable	See above	Rare		Cardiomyopathy Cardiovascular collapse	Variable	Extreme ages Preexisting heart conditions
	Urticaria	Pruritus Wheals	Absent	Min-1h	See above	Rare				
	Angioedema	Swollen deep dermis and subcutaneous tissue	Present/ Absent							
	Acute generalized exanthematous pustulosis	Non-follicular, sterile pustules arising on background of edematous erythema	Present/ Absent	<4 days	See above	Rare				
	Erythema multiforme	Typical targetoid lesions	Present	Variable	See above	Rare				
	Toxic epidermal necrolysis	Confluent and extensive epidermal detachment >30 % body surface area	Present	Variable	See above	Rare				
Metronidazole and tinidazole	Exanthematous	Erythematous No blistering	Absent	Variable	See above	Rare		QT interval prolongation	Rare	Old age Preexisting cardiac conditions
	Erythema multiforme	Typical targetoid lesions	Present		See above					

Nitrofurantoin	Exanthematous	Erythematous No blistering	Absent	Variable	See above	Rare	Left bundle branch block Tachycardia	Rare	Old age Preexisting heart conditions
	Erythema multiforme	Typical targetoid lesions	Present	Variable	See above				
	Drug-induced lupus	Similar to idiopathic SCLE	Absent/ present	Variable	See above				
Quinolones E.g. Ciprofloxacin Norfloxacin Levofloxacin	Photosensitivity	Erythema ± Blistering after sun exposure	Absent	Variable	See above	Variable	Ventricular arrhythmia QT-prolongation Torsade de pointes	Variable	Old age Preexisting heart conditions
	Exanthematous	Erythematous No blistering	Absent	Variable	See above	0.5-2%			
	Urticaria	Pruritus Wheals	Absent	Min-1h	See above	Rare			
	Angioedema	Swollen deep dermis and subcutaneous tissue	Present/ Absent						
	Acute generalized exanthematous pustulosis	Non-follicular, sterile pustules arising on background of edematous erythema	Present/ Absent	<4 days	See above	Rare			
	Palpable purpura (serum sickness)	Palpable purpura	Absent	7-21 days	See above	Rare			
	Radiation recall reaction	Erythema +/- blisters at sites of previous radiotherapy	Absent	Variable	Photosensitivity	Variable			
	Stevens-Johnson syndrome	Atypical targetoid leasions, 10 % body surface area	Present	4-28 days	See above	Rare			
	Toxic epidermal necrolysis	Confluent and extensive epidermal detachment	Present	4-28 days					

(continued)

Table 21.8 (continued)

		>30 % body surface Area							
Vancomycin	Exanthematous	Erythematous No blistering	Absent	Variable	See above	5%	Cardiac arrest	Rare	
Isoniazid	Exanthematous	Erythematous No blistering	Absent	Variable	See above	1%	Systemic vasculitis	Rare	Slow inactivators of the drug Co-administraton of multiple drugs
	Acneiform eruptions	Inflammatory lesions No comedones Atypical sites	Absent	Variable	Acne Rosacea Tuberculids	Rare	Pericarditis	30%	
	Urticaria	Pruritus Wheals	Absent	Min-1h	See above	Rare	Acute eosynophilic myocarditis Tachycardia Hypotension	Rare	
	Palpable purpura (serum sickness)	Palpable purpura	Absent	7-21 days	See above	Rare			
	Drug-induced lupus	Similar to idiopathic SCLE	Absent/ present	Variable	See above	Rare			
	Drug-induced hypersensitivity syndrome	Severe exanthematous rash	Infrequent	1–6 weeks	See above	Rare			
	Stevens-Johnson syndrome	Atypical targetoid leasions, 10 % body surface area	Present	4-28 days	See above	Rare			
Pyrazinamide	Exanthematous	Erythematous No blistering	Absent	Variable	See above	Rare	Tachycardia Myocarditis* *animal studies	Variable	HIV/AIDS patients
	Photosensitivity	Erythema ± Blistering after sun exposure	Absent	Variable	See above	Rare			
	Urticaria	Pruritus Wheals	Absent	Min-1h	See above	Rare			
	Drug-induced hypersensitivity syndrome	Severe exanthematous rash	Infrequent	1–6 weeks	See above	Uncommon			

Rifampicin	Exanthematous	Erythematous No blistering	Absent	Variable	See above	Uncommon	Ventricular tachycardia	Rare	MDRD-TB Co-administration of other drugs Multiple comorbities
	Drug-induced lupus	Similar to idiopathic SCLE	Absent/ present	Variable	See above	Rare			
	Toxic epidermal necrolysis	Confluent and extensive epidermal detachment >30 % body surface area	Present	4-28 days	See above	Rare			
	Pemphigus	Flaccid bullae Painful erosions	Present	Weeks-months	See above	Rare			
	Photosensitivity	Erythema ± Blistering after sun exposure	Absent	Variable	See above	Rare			
	Drug-induced hypersensitivity syndrome	Severe exanthematous rash	Infrequent	1–6 weeks	See above	Uncommon			
Clofazimine	Pigmentation	Brown-orange pigmentation of the skin Reddish-blue pigmentation of scarred areas	Present/Absent	Variable	See above	Rare	« Torsade de pointes » Ventricular tachycardia	Rare	Multiple comorbities Co-administration of other drugs
	Exanthematous	Erythematous No blistering	Absent	Variable	See above	Rare			
	Acneiform eruptions	Inflammatory lesions No comedones Atypical sites	Absent	Variable	See above	Rare			
	Photosensitivity	Erythema ± Blistering after sun exposure	Absent	Variable	See above	Rare			
Dapsone	Fixed drug eruption	One or more round well-circumscribed	Absent	Variable	See above	3%	Myocardial injury Venticular arrhythmia Cardiac arrest	Variable	

(continued)

Table 21.8 (continued)

		erythematous plaques Sometimes central bullae					Shock		West-African patients High starting dose of dapsone Co-treatment with clofazimine Melanesian population (genetic susceptibility) Slow acetylators Glucose-6-phosphate dehydrogenase deficiency Old age
	Exanthematous	Erythematous No blistering	Absent	Variable	See above	Uncommon	Complete atrioventricular block Hypersensitivity myocarditis Pericarditis Pericardial effusion Congestive heart failure	Rare	
	Erythema multiforme	Typical targetoid lesions	Present	>72 h	See above				
	Drug induced hypersnsitivity syndrome (dapsone or sulphone syndrome)	Fever Erythematous eruption+pustules Exfoliative dermatitis Hepatitis+lymphadenopaty+anemia	Present/absent	2-7 weeks(29 days)	Viral diseases Hemopathies Infection Septic shock Psoriasis vulgaris Acropustulosis Pustular psoriasis				
	Stevens-Johnson syndrome	Atypical targetoid leasions, 10 % body surface area	Present	4-28 days	See above	Rare			
Thalidomide	Exanthematous	Erythematous No blistering	Absent	Variable	See above	46%	Deep vein trombosis	Variable	HIV patients Multiple comorbidities
	Erythema multiforme	Typical targetoid lesions	Present	>72 h	See above				
	Drug-induced hypersensitivity syndrome	Severe exanthematous rash	Infrequent	1–6 weeks	See above		Coronary artery spasm	Rare	
	Toxic epidermal necrolysis	Confluent and extensive epidermal detachment >30 % body surface area	Present	4-28 days	See above		Bradycardia Ventricular tachycardia Ventricular fibrilation Atrioventricula block	Variable	
	Exanthematous	Erythematous No blistering	Absent	Variable	See above	1.1%	Heart failure Cardiomegaly Arrhythmias	Variable	Old age

Itraconazole	Fixed drug eruption	One or more round well-circumscribed erythematous plaques Sometimes central bullae	Absent	First exposure: 1–2 weeks Re-exposure: > 48 h, usually within 24 h	See above	Rare	Hypertension Cardiac arrest	Rare	Multiple comorbities Co-administration of other drugs
	Palpable purpura (serum sickness)	Palpable purpura	Absent	>72 h	See above	Rare			
	Acute generalized exanthematous pustulosis	Non-follicular, sterile pustules arising on background of edematous erythema	Present/ Absent	<4 days	See above	Rare			
Fluconazole	Exanthematous	Erythematous No blistering	Absent	Variable	See above	1.8%	Heart failure QT prolongation Torsade de pointes	Variable	Old age Multiple comorbities Co-administration of other drugs AIDS patients
	Fixed drug eruption	One or more round well-circumscribed erythematous plaques Sometimes central bullae	Absent	First exposure: 1–2 weeks Re-exposure: > 48 h, usually within 24 h	See above	Rare			
	Angioedema	Swollen deep dermis and subcutaneous tissue	Present/ Absent	Min-1h	See above	Rare	Ventricular fibrilation Cardiac arrest	Rare	
	Stevens-Johnson syndrome	Atypica targetoid leasions, 10 % body surface area	Present	4-28 days	See above	Rare			
Ketoconazole	Urticaria	Pruritus Wheals	Absent	Min-1h	See above	Uncommon	Heart failure QT prolongation « Torsade de pointes »	Variable	Old age Multiple comorbities Co-administration of other drugs
	Angioedema	Swollen deep dermis and subcutaneous tissue	Present Absent	Min-1h	See above				

(continued)

Table 21.8 (continued)

	Exanthematous	Erythematous No blistering	Absent	Variable	See above	Rare			
Terbinafine	Exanthematous	Erythematous No blistering	Absent	Variable	See above	2.7-3%	Tachycardia Bradycardia	Rare	Co-administration of other drugs
	Urticaria	Pruritus Wheals	Absent	Min-1h	See above				
	Stevens-Johnson syndrome	Atypical targetoid leasions, 10 % body surface area	Present	4-28 days	See above				
	Toxic epidermal necrolysis	Confluent and extensive epidermal detachment >30 % body surface area	Present	4-28 days	See above				
	Erythema multiforme	Typical targetoid lesions	Present	>72 h	See above				
	Palpable purpura (serum sickness)	Palpable purpura	Absent	>72 h	See above				
	Acute generalized exanthematous pustulosis	Non-follicular, sterile pustules arising on background of edematous erythema	Present/ Absent	<4 days	See above				
	Drug-induced lupus	Similar to idiopathic SCLE	Absent/ present	Variable	See above				
	Bullous pemphigoid	Erythema Tense bullae	Infrequent	Variable	See above				
	Fixed drug eruption	One or more round well-circumscribed erythematous plaques Sometimes central bullae	Absent	First exposure: 1–2 weeks Re-exposure: > 48 h, usually within 24 h	See above				

Amphotericin	Grey syndrome	Ashed colour Acral cyanosis Prostration	Absent	Immediate reaction to infusion	Pigmentation disorders Peripheral ischemia	Rare	Heart failure Cardiac arrest	Variable	Old age Multiple comorbities Co-administration of other drugs
	Exanthematous	Erythematous No blistering	Absent	Variable	See above				
Griseofulvin	Exanthematous	Erythematous No blistering	Absent	Variable	See above	Uncommon	Tachycardia Hypotension	Rare	Alcohol consumption
	Photosensitivity	Erythema ± Blistering after sun exposure	Absent	Variable	See above				
	Urticaria	Pruritus Wheals	Absent	Min-1h	See above				
	Angioedema	Swollen deep dermis and subcutaneous tissue	Present/ Absent	Min-1h	See above				
	Fixed drug eruption	One or more round well-circumscribed erythematous plaques Sometimes central bullae	Absent	First exposure: 1–2 weeks Re-exposure: > 48 h, usually within 24 h	See above				
	Palpable purpura (serum sickness)	Palpable purpura	Absent	>72 h	See above				
	Toxic epidermal necrolysis	Confluent and extensive epidermal detachment >30 % body surface area	Present	4-28 days	See above				
	Exanthematous	Erythematous No blistering	Absent	Variable	See above	Rare	QT interval prolongation	Variable	Old age Multiple comorbities

(continued)

Table 21.8 (continued)

Voriconazole	Pseudoporphyria	Erythema, skin fragility, blistering and scarring of photo-exposed areas	Absent	Variable	See above		Ventricular tachycardia	Rare	Co-administration of other drugs HIV paties
	Photosensitivity	Erythema ± Blistering after sun exposure	Absent	Variable	See above		Bradycardia	Variable	
	Drug-induced lupus	Similar to idiopathic SCLE	Absent/ present	Variable	See above		Torsade de pointes	Variable	
	Erythema multiforme	Typical targetoid lesions	Present	Variable	See above				
	Stevens-Johnson syndrome	Atypical targetoid leasions, 10 % body surface area	Present	4-28 days	See above				
	Toxic epidermal necrolysis	Confluent and extensive epidermal detachment >30 % body surface area	Present	4-28 days	See above				
α-2 mimetics E.g.: Metyldopa Clonidine	Exanthematous	Erythematous No blistering	Absent	4-21 days	Viral exanthems Toxins Syphilis	Variable	Bradycardia Hypotension	Variable	Old age Preexisting cardiac conditions Co-administration of other drugs
	Palpable purpura	Palpable purpura	Absent	7-21 days	Infectious Autoimmune Hemopathies Paraneoplastic				
	Lichenoid	Purple flat-topped papules Pruritus	Absent	Variable	Lichen planus Eczema				
	Psoriasiform / exacerbation of preexisting psoriasis	Mostly scalp, palmo-plantar (vulgar and pustular types), diaper area	Absent	Variable	Psoriasis vulgaris Acropustulosis Eczema				
	Drug-induced lupus	SCLE-like	Absent/present	Variable	Idiopatic subacute cutaneous lupus erythematosus				

	Drug-induced hypersensitivity syndrome	Severe exanthematous eruption	Infrequent	1-6 weeks	Viral infections Hemopathies				
β -1 mimetics (Dobutamine)	Exanthematous	Erythematous No blistering	Absent	4-21 days	See above	Variable	Tachycardia Direct toxic effect on cardiomyocytes	Variable	
β -2 mimetics (Salbutamol, Clenbuterol, Albuterol)	Urticaria	Wheals Pruritus	Absent	Minutes-hours	Idiopathic urticaria Other etiologies Insect bites	Variable	Tachycardia Ischemia Hypotension (higher doses)	Variable	Old age Preexisting cardiac conditions Co-administration of other drugs
	Exanthematous (hands, 3 pregnant women)	Erythematous No blistering	Absent	4-21 days	See above	Variable			
β –blockers (Metoprolol, Acebutolol, Atenolol)	Exanthematous	Erythematous No blistering	Absent	4-21 days	See above	Variable	Tachycardia Bradycardia Ischemia Hypotension Hypertension Reversible effect on contractility	Variable	Old age Preexisting cardiac conditions Co-administration of other drugs
	Lichenoid	Purple flat-topped papules Pruritus	Absent	Variable	See above	Variable			
	Psoriasiform / exacerbation of preexisting psoriasis	Mostly scalp, palmo-plantar (vulgar and pustular types), diaper area	Absent	Variable	Psoriasiform / exacerbation of preexisting psoriasis	Variable			
	Drug-induced lupus	Subacute cutaneous lupus erythematosus-like	Absent/present	Variable	See above	Variable			
	Palpable purpura	Palpable purpura	Absent	7-21 days	See above	Rare			
	Pemphigus	Flaccid bullae Painful erosions	Present	Weeks-months	See above	Rare			
	Erythema multiforme	Typical target-like lesions – regular round-	Present/ absent	Variable	SJS/TEN Fixed drug eruption	Variable			Old age

(continued)

Table 21.8 (continued)

Calcium channel blockers (Verapamil Diltiazem, Amlodipine)		oval shape, sharp margins					Bradycardia Reversible effect on contractility Hypotension	Variable	Preexisting cardiac conditions Co-administration of other drugs
	Palpable purpura	Palpable purpura	Absent	7-21 days	See above	Rare			
	Urticaria	Pruritus Wheals	Absent	Min-1h	See above	Variable			
	Psoriasiform	Mostly scalp, palmoplantar (vulgar and pustular), and diaper area	Absent	Variable	See above	Rare			
	Exanthematous	Erythematous No blistering	Absent	7-12 days	See above	Rare			
	Acute generalized exanthematous pustulosis (AGEP)	Non-follicular sterile pustules on an erythematous background	Present/ Absent	<4days	Pustular psoriasis	Rare			
	Drug-induced lupus	Subacute cutaneous lupus erythematosus-like	Absent/prese nt	Variable	*See above*	*Variable*			
	Lichenoid	Purple flat-topped papules Pruritus	Absent	Variable	See above	*Variable*			
	Angioedema (facial)	Deep edema of dermis and subcutaneous tissue	Present/ Absent	Minutes-hours	Idiopatic angioedema	Variable			
Phosphodiesterase inhibitors E.g. Sildenafil Vardenafil Tadalafil	Fixed drug eruption	One or more round well-circumscribed erythematous plaques Sometimes central bullae	Absent	First exposure: 1–2 weeks Re-exposure: > 48 h, usually within 24 h	See above	Rare	Hypotension	Variable	Old age Preexisting cardiac conditions Co-administration of other drugs
	Lichenoid	Purple flat-topped papules Pruritus	Absent	Variable	See above	Variable			

Sodium channel blockers E.g. Lidocaine Mepivacaine Bupivacaine Prilocaine Ropivacaine Articaine Procaine	Exanthematous	Erythematous No blistering	Absent	4-21 days	See above	Variable	Cardiovascular manifestations of LAST (local anesthetic systemic toxicity): -tachycardia -bradycardia -hypotension -chest pain -dyspnea -hypertension -ventricular ectopy -ventricular tachycardia -ventricular fibrillation -asystole Cardiac arrest	Variable	Old age Preexisting cardiac conditions Co-administration of other drugs
	Angioedema	Deep edema of dermis and subcutaneous tissue	Present/ Absent	Minutes-hours	See above	Variable			
	Urticaria	Wheals Pruritus	Absent	Minutes-hours	See above	Variable			
Non-steroidal antiinflammatory drugs (Rofecoxib, Ibuprofen, Aspirin, Piroxicam, Diclofenac)	Urticaria	Pruritus Wheals	Absent	Min-1h	See above	Variable	Ischemia Hypertension Strokes (ischemic stroke, transient ischemic attack) Thrombotic cardiovascular events Cardiovascular death Nonfatal recurrent myocardial infarction Systemic arterial emboli	Variable	Old age Multiple comorbities Co-administration of other drugs
	Angioedema	Deep edema of dermis and subcutaneous tissue	Present/ Absent	Minutes-hours	See above	Variable			
	Palpable purpura	Palpable purpura	Absent	7-21 days	See above	Rare			
	Exanthematous	Erythematous No blistering	Absent	7-12 days	See above	Rare			
	Erythema multiforme	Typical targetoid lesions	Present	Variable	See above	Rare			
	Fixed drug eruption	Single/multiple round, well-circumscribed erythematous plaques with central bullae (sometimes)	Absent	First exposure: 1-2 weeks Reexposure > 48 h, usually 24 h	See above	Variable			
	Psoriasiform	Mostly scalp, palmoplantar (vulgar and pustular), and diaper area	Absent	Variable	See above	Rare			
	Stevens-Johnson syndrome	Atypical targetoid lesions that affect < 10% BSA	Present	4-28 days	See above	Variable			

(continued)

Table 21.8 (continued)

	Palpable purpura	Palpable purpura	Absent	7-21 days	See above	Rare			
	Bullous pemphigoid	Erythema Tense bullae	Infrequent	Variable	See above	Rare			
	Exanthematous	Erythematous No blistering	Absent	7-12 days	See above	Variable			
	Lichenoid	Purple flat-topped papules Pruritus	Absent	Variable	See above	Variable			
Estrogen + progestin (combined oral contraceptives)	Acneiform	Just inflammatory lesions, without comedones, +/- hyperseborrhoea on atypical sites	Absent	Variable	Acne Rosacea Tuberculids	Variable	Ischemia Hypertension Venous thromboembolism Strokes	Variable	Multiple comorbities Co-administration of other drugs
	Pigmentation	Blue-black macules in areas of previous inflammation and in sunexposed areas	Present/ Absent	Variable	See above	Variable			
Corticosteroids (prednisone, prednisolone, methylprednisolone)	Acneiform	Just inflammatory lesions, without comedones, +/- hyperseborrhoea on atypical sites	Absent	Variable	Acne Rosacea Tuberculids	Variable	Hypertension Coronary heart disease Ischemic heart disease Heart failure Sudden death	Variable	Old age Multiple comorbities Co-administration of other drugs
	Dermatoporosis	Atrophy, teleangiectasia and hematoma	Absent	Variable	Poikiloderma Trauma	5%			
Antihistamines (antiH1 and antiH2)	Fixed drug eruption	One or more round well-circumscribed erythematous plaques Sometimes central	Absent	First exposure: 1–2 weeks Re-exposure: > 48 h, usually within 24 h	See above	Rare	Palpitations QT interval prolongation Torsade de pointes	Variable	Old age Multiple comorbities

		bullae							Co-administration of other drugs
	Exanthematous	Erythematous No blistering	Absent	7-12 days	See above	Variable			
	Drug-induced lupus	Similar to idiopathic SCLE	Absent/ present	Variable	See above	Rare			
	Urticaria	Pruritus Wheals	Absent	Min-1h	See above	Variable			
	Psoriasiform (exacerbation of preexisting psoriasis)	Mostly scalp, palmoplantar (vulgar and pustular), and diaper area	Absent	Variable	See above	Rare			
	Lichenoid	Purple flat-topped papules Pruritus	Absent	Variable	See above	Variable			
Interferon + ribavirin	Drug-induced lupus	Similar to idiopathic SCLE	Absent/ present	Variable	See above	Rare	Dilated cardiomyopathy Myocarditis Hypertension (reversible) Arrhythmia Ischemic heart disease	Uncommon	Women Old age
	Exanthematous	Erythematous No blistering	Absent	7-12 days	See above	Variable			
	Pigmentation	Blue-black macules in areas of previous inflammation and in sunexposed areas	Present/ Absent	Variable	See above	Variable			
	Sarcoidosis	Erythema Nodules	Present/ Absent	15 days-30 months	Infections Autoimmune conditioins	60%			
	Vasculitis	Palpable purpura, usually located on the lower extremities	Absent	Variable	See above	Rare			
	Lichenoid	Purple flat-topped papules Pruritus	Absent	Variable	See above	*Variable*			
	Stevens-Johnson syndrome	Atypical target lesions that affect < 10% BSA	Present	4-28 days	See above	Rare	Bradycardia		Old age

(continued)

Table 21.8 (continued)

	Telaprevir Boceprevir	Drug-induced hypersensitivity syndrome	Severe exanthematous rash	Infrequent	1–6 weeks	See above	Uncommon	Heart block Asymptomatic heart failure	3.6% (small series)	Multiple comorbities Co-administration of other drugs
		Acute generalized exanthematous pustulosis	Non-follicular, sterile pustules arising on background of edematous erythema	Present/ Absent	<4 days	See above	Rare			
Alkinating Agents	**Alkyl sulphonates e.g.Busulfan**	Urticaria	Pruritus Wheals	Absent	Min-1h	See above	Uncommon	Endomyocardial fibrosis Pericarditis Tamponade Cardiac ischemia Hypertension Myocarditis Heart failure Arrhythmias	Variable	High doses Old age Multiple comorbities Co-administration of other drugs
		Erythema multiforme	Typical targetoid lesions	Present	>72 h	See above	Rare			
		Pseudoporphyria	Erythema, skin fragility, blistering and scarring of photo-exposed areas	Absent	Variable	See above	Variable			
		Palpable purpura	Palpable purpura	Absent	7-21 days	See above	Rare			
	Nitrogen mustard derivates e.g. Chlorambucil	Urticaria	Pruritus Wheals	Absent	Min-1h	See above	Uncommon	Endomyocardial fibrosis Pericarditis Tamponade Cardiac ischemia Hypertension Myocarditis Heart failure Arrhythmias	Variable	High dose therapy Co-administration of other drugs
		Exanthematous	Erythematous No blistering	Absent	7-12 days	See above	Variable			
		Toxic epidermal necrolysis	Confluent and extensive epidermal detachment >30 % body surface area	Present	4-28 days	See above	Rare			
		Alopecia	Loss of hair	Absent	Variable	Alopecia areata Fungal infections	Common	Endomyocardial fibrosis Pericarditis		

	Cyclophosphamide and Mesna					Factitial alopecia		Tamponade Cardiac ischemia Hypertension Myocarditis Heart failure Arrhythmias	Variable	High dose therapy Co-administration of other drugs
		Allergic Exanthems	Erythematous No blistering	Absent	Variable	See above	Rare			
		Urticaria	Pruritus Wheals	Absent	Min-1h	See above	Uncommon			
		Angioedema	Swollen deep dermis and subcutaneous tissue	Absent/ Present	Min 1h	See above	Uncommon			
		Fixed drug eruption	One or more round well-circumscribed erythematous plaques Sometimes central bullae	Absent	First exposure: 1–2 weeks Re-exposure: > 48 h, usually within 24 h	See above	Rare			
		Erythema multiforme	Typical targetoid lesions	Present	>72 h	See above	Rare			
	Melphalan	Angioedema	Swollen deep dermis and subcutaneous tissue	Absent/ Present	Min-1h	See above	Uncommon	Supraventricular tachycardia Atrial fibrillation	Common	High dose therapy Co-administration of other drugs Old age
	Nitrosoureas **e.g. Carmustine .Dacarbazine,Procarbzine**	Fixed drug eruption	One or more round well-circumscribed erythematous plaques Sometimes central bullae	Absent	First exposure: 1–2 weeks Re-exposure: > 48 h, usually within 24 h	See above	Rare	Ischemia Chest pain Miocardial infaction, Heart failure Arrhythmias Pericardial effusions Pericarditis	Variable	Co-administration of other drugs, especially chemotherapeutic agents

(continued)

Table 21.8 (continued)

		Angioedema	Swollen deep dermis and subcutaneous tissue	Absent/ Present	Min-1h	See above	Rare	Hemodynamic abnormalities		
		Photosensitivity	Erythema ± Blistering after sun exposure	Absent	Variable	See above	Variable			
		Exanthematous	Erythematous No blistering	Absent	7-12 days	See above	Variable			
Cytotoxic antibiotics	Bleomycin	Alopecia	Loss of hair	Absent	Variable	See above	Common	Arterial hypertension Heart failure Thromboembolic events	Variable	Co-administration of other drugs, especially chemotherapeutic agents
		Exanthematous	Erythematous No blistering	Present/Abse nt	7-12 days	See above	Variable			
		Neutrophilic eccrine hidradenitis	Erythematous and edematous patches, papules and plaques with acral distribution	NA	8–10 days	Infectious Palmoplantar hidradenitis	Variable			
		Pigmentation	Blue-black macules	Present/ Absent	Variable	See above	Variable			
	Dactinomycine (Actinomycine)	Acneiform	Just inflammatory lesions, without comedones, +/- hyperseborrhoea on atypical sites	Absent	Variable	See above	Variable	Heart failure	Variable	Co-administration of other drugs, especially chemotherapeutic agents
	Daunorubicin	Angioedema	Deep edema of dermis and subcutaneous tissue	Present/ Absent	Minutes-hours	See above	Variable	Cardiomyopathy Direct toxic effect on cardiomyocytes	Variable	Long term therapy High doses Co-administration of other drugs
		Urticaria	Wheals Pruritus	Absent	Minutes-hours	See above	Variable			
		Pigmentation	Blue-black macules on skin and nails	Present/ Absent	Variable	See above	Variable			

	Doxorubicyne (Adriamycine)	Urticaria	Wheals Pruritus	Absent	Minutes-hours	See above	3%	Phlebitis Tachycardia Cardiomyopathy Direct toxic effect on cardiomyocytes	Variable	Long term therapy High doses Co-administration of other drugs
		Pigmentation	Blue-black macules on skin and nails	Present/Absent	Variable	See above	Variable			
		Exanthematous	Erythematous No blistering	Present/Absent	4-21 days	See above	Variable			
Antimetabolites	Azathioprine	Exanthematous	Erythematous No blistering	Absent	4-21 days	See above	Variable	Hypotension	Well recognized	Homozygotes for the low activity allele for thyomethil transferase
		Urticaria	Wheals Pruritus	Absent	Minutes-hours	See above	Variable			
		Vasculitis	Palpable purpura, usually located on the lower extremities	Absent	Variable	See above	Rare			
		Erythema multiforme	Typical target-like lesions – regular round-oval shape, sharp margins	Present/absent	Variable	See above	Variable			
	Cytarabine	Acral erythema	Symmetric, painful erythema of palms and soles Blisters	NA	1–3 weeks	History of the patients—highly suggestive	53%	Ischemia Pericarditis Heart failure Cardiogenic shock	Variable	Long term therapy High doses Co-administration of other drugs
		Neutrophilic eccrine hidradenitis	Erythematous and edematous patches, papules and plaques with acral distribution	NA	8–10 days	Infectious Palmoplantar hidradenitis				
		Exanthematous	Erythematous No blistering	Absent	4-21 days	See above				

(continued)

Table 21.8 (continued)

	Urticaria	Wheals Pruritus	Absent	Minutes-hours	See above				
Fluorouracil	Alopecia	Loss of hair	Absent	Variable	See above	Variable	Angina-like chest pain Coronary artery thrombosis Myocardial infarction Arteritis Arrhythmias Vasospasm Ventricular tachycardia QT prolongation with torsades de pointes	Variable	Long term therapy High doses Co-administration of other drugs
	Pigmentation	Black-brown macules in sun exposed areas	Present/ Absent	Variable	See above	Variable			
	Photosensitivity	Erythema ± Blistering after sun exposure	Absent	Variable	See above	Variable			
	Acral erythema	Symmetric, painful erythema of palms and soles Blisters	NA	1–3 weeks	History of the patients—highly suggestive	Variable			
	Erythema multiforme	Typical target-like lesions – regular round-oval shape, sharp margins	Present/ absent	Variable	See above	Variable			
Capecitabine	Acral erythema	Symmetric, painful erythema of palms and soles Blisters	NA	1–3 weeks	History of the patients - highly suggestive	50%	Ischemia Pericarditis Heart failure Cardiogenic shock	Variable	Long term therapy High doses Co-administration of other drugs
	Sarcoidosis	Erythema Nodules	Present/absent	15 days-30 months	See above	Rare			
Gemcitabine	Radiation recall reaction	Erythema +/- blisters at sites of previous radiotherapy	Absent	Variable	Photosensitivity	Variable	Atrial fibrillation	Variable	Old age Long term therapy High doses Co-administration of other drugs
	Alopecia	Loss of hair	Absent	Variable	See above	6% (low dose therapy) 8%(high dose therapy)			

		Urticaria	Wheals Pruritus	Absent	Minutes-hours	See above	4% (for low dose therapy)	Cardiac ischemia Chest pain Myocardial infarction Heart failure Arrhythmias Pericardial effusions Pericarditis Hemodynamic abnormalities	Variable	Long term therapy High doses Co-administration of other drugs
	Methotrexate	Photosensitivity	Erythema ± Blistering after sun exposure	Absent	Variable	See above	5%			
		Exanthematous	Erythematous No blistering	Absent	4-21 days	See above	15%			
		Vasculitis	Palpable purpura, usually located on the lower extremities	Absent	Variable	See above	Rare			
		Toxic epidermal necrolysis	Confluent and extensive epidermal detachment >30 % body surface area	Present	4–28 days	See above	Rare			
Vinca alkaloids and etoposide	**Etoposide**	Alopecia	Loss of hair	Absent	Variable		Variable	Atrial fibrillation	Variable	Newly diagnosed Hodgkin disease Old age Long term therapy High doses Co-administration of other drugs
		Stevens-Johnson syndrome	Atypical targetoid lesions that affect < 10% BSA	Present	4-28 days	See above	Variable			
		Radiation recall reaction	Erythema +/- blisters at sites of previous radiotherapy	Absent	Variable	Photosensitivity	Variable			
		Exanthematous	Erythematous No blistering	Absent	5-9 days after initiation of therapy	See above	Variable			
		Photosensitivity	Erythema ± Blistering after sun exposure	Absent	Variable	See above	Common	Hypotension or hypertension Cardiac ischemia		Old age
		Alopecia	Loss of hair	Absent	Variable	See above	Variable			

(continued)

Table 21.8 (continued)

Vinblastine	Erythema multiforme	Typical target-like lesions – regular round-oval shape, sharp margins	Present/ absent	Variable	See above	Variable	Angina Myocardial infarction Bradycardia Arrhythmias Conduction abnormalities Heart failure	Variable	Long term therapy High doses Co-administration of other drugs
Anti-EGFR E.g. Cetuximab, Erlotinib, Imatinib, Sorafenib	Acneiform	Just inflammatory lesions, without comedones, +/- hyperseborrhoea on atypical sites	Absent	Variable	See above	Common	Heart failure Edema Pericardial effusion Pericarditis Hypertension Arrhythmias Prolonged QT interval Cardiac ischemia Chest pain	Variable	Old age Long term therapy High doses Co-administration of other drugs
	Pigmentation	Black-brown macules	Present/ Absent	Variable	See above	Variable			
	Exanthematous	Erythematous No blistering	Absent	4-21 days	See above	Variable			
	Neutrophilic eccrine hidradenitis	Erythematous and edematous patches, papules, and plaques with acral distribution	NA	8–10 days	See above	Variable			
	Vasculitis	Palpable purpura, usually located on the lower extremities	Absent	Variable	See above	Rare			
Platinum agents e.g. Carboplatin and cisplatin	Exanthematous	Erythematous No blistering	Absent	4-21 days	See above	1-30%	Cardiomyopathy Congestive heart failure Acute myocardial infarction Hypertension and hypotension Arrythmias Myocarditis Angina		Co-adminstration of other chemotherapeutic agent Atopic subjects
	Urticaria	Wheals Pruritus	Absent	Minutes-hours	See above	5-20%			
Hydroxycarbamide (hydroxyureea)	Alopecia	Loss of hair	Absent	Variable	See above	Variable			
	Pigmentatio-generalized or	Black-brown macules	Present/Absent	6 weeks	See above	5%			

	limited to pressure areas n								
	Fixed drug eruption	One or more round well-circumscribed erythematous plaques Sometimes central bullae	Absent	First exposure: 1–2 weeks Re-exposure: > 48 h, usually within 24 h	See above	Rare	Vaso-oclusive effcts Acute chest syndrome Vasculo-endothelial disfunction	Variable	High hematocrit Older age
	Acral erythema	Symmetric, painful erythema of palms and soles Blisters	NA	1–3 weeks	History of the patients—highly suggestive	Variable			
	Photosensitivity	Erythema ± Blistering after sun exposure	Absent	Variable	See above	Rare			
	Vasculitis	Palpable purpura, usually located on the lower extremities	Absent	Variable	See above	Rare			
	Radiation recall reaction	Erythema +/- blisters at sites of previous radiotherapy	Absent	Variable	Photosensitivity	Variable			
	Lichenoid	Purple flat-topped papules Pruritus	Absent	Variable	See above	Variable			
Taxanes e.g. Docetaxel, Paclitaxel	Exanthematous	Erythematous No blistering	Absent	4-21 days	See above	81 %	Bradycardia	Variable	Co-adminstration of other drugs
	Alopecia	Loss of hair	Absent	Variable	See above	Variable			
	Fixed drug eruption	Single/multiple round, well-circumscribed erythematous plaques with central bullae (sometimes)	Absent	First exposure: 1-2 weeks Reexposure > 48 h, usually 24 h	See above	Variable			

(continued)

Table 21.8 (continued)

Ciclosporine	Reversible hypertrichosis	Presence of excess hair on face, eyebrows, upper back, upper arms	NA	Variable	Endocrine conditions Other causes of hypertrichosis	Common	Hypertension Arteriolar vasoconstriction	Variable	Long term use High doses Co-administration of other drugs
	Vasculitis	Palpable purpura, usually located on the lower extremities	Absent	Variable	See above	Rare			
	Alopecia	Loss of hair	Absent	Variable	See above	Variable			
Erythropoietin	Exanthematous	Erythematous No blistering	Absent	4-21 days	See above	Variable	Hypertension Venous thromboembolism Strokes	Variable	Old age Multiple comorbities Co-administration of other drugs
Anti VEGF e.g. Bevacizumab Sorafenib	Exanthematous	Erythematous No blistering	Absent	4-21 days	See above	Variable	Ischemia Reversible effect on contractility Hypertension Strokes Direct toxic effect on cardiomyocytes Venous thromboembolism	Variable	Multiple comorbities Co-administration of other drugs
HER2i and others e.g.Transtuzumab	Angioedema	Deep edema of dermis and subcutaneous tissue	Present/ Absent	Minutes-hours	See above	Variable	Direct toxic effect on cardiomyocytes Reversible effect on contractility	Variable	Co-treatment with paclitaxel
	Photosensitivity	Erythema ± Blistering after sun exposure	Absent	Variable	See above	Rare			
	Urticaria	Wheals Pruritus	Absent	Minutes-hours	See above	Variable			
Tricyclic antidepressants e.g. Nortryptiline Amineptine	Acneiform	Inflammatory lesions, without comedones, +/- hyperseborrhoea on atypical sites	Absent	Variable	See above	Variable			

Amitriptyline Clomipramine Imipramine Maprotiline		Alopecia	Loss of hair	Absent	Variable	See above	Variable	Tachycardia Cardiac ischemia Hypotension Hypertension	Variable	Old age Multiple comorbities Co-administration of other drugs
		Photosensitivity	Erythema ± Blistering after sun exposure	Absent	Variable	See above	Rare			
		Urticaria	Wheals Pruritus	Absent	Minutes-hours	See above	Variable			
		Vasculitis	Palpable purpura, usually located on the lower extremities	Absent	Variable	See above	Rare			
Selective serotonin reuptake inhibitors e.g. Fluoxetine, Paroxetine, Sertraline		Alopecia	Loss of hair	Absent	Variable	See above	Rare	Bradycardia Prolongation of QT intervals Dysrhythmia syncope Orthostatic hypotension	Variable	Low enzyme activity (CYP2B6 and CYP2C19)
		Palpable purpura	Palpable purpura	Absent	7-21 days	See above	Variable			
		Urticaria	Wheals Pruritus	Absent	Minutes-hours	See above	Variable			
		Vasculitis	Palpable purpura, usually located on the lower extremities	Absent	Variable	See above	Rare			
Hypnotics, sedatives and anxiolytics	**Barbiturates E.g.Pheno barbital**	Coma blisters	Seen in patients with impaired consciousness Pressure/no pressure area	NA	Variable	Eccrine necrosis	8%	Hypotension	34.1%	Status epilepticus Co-administration of other drugs
		Erythema multiforme	Typical target-like lesions – regular round-oval shape, sharp margins	Present/ absent	Variable	See above	Rare	Cardiac rhythm disturbances	3.3%	
		Exanthematous	Erythematous No blistering	Absent	4-21 days	See above	Rare			
		Palpable purpura (serum sickness)	Palpable purpura	Absent	7-21 days	See above	Rare			
		Fixed drug eruption	One or more round well-circumscribed	Absent	First exposure: 1–2 weeks	See above	Well known			

(continued)

Table 21.8 (continued)

			erythematous plaques Sometimes central bullae		Re-exposure: > 48 h, usually within 24 h					
		Photosensitivity	Erythema ± Blistering after sun exposure	Absent	Variable	See above	Rare			
		Toxic epidermal necrolysis	Confluent and extensive epidermal detachment >30 % body surface area	Present	4–28 days	See above	Rare			
	Benzodia-zepines e.g. Alprazolam Diazepam and nitrazepam Lormetazepam	Photosensitivity	Erythema ± Blistering after sun exposure	Absent	Variable	See above	Rare	Trombophlebitis at injection sites	Variable	Status epilepticus Co-administration of other drugs
		Exanthematous	Erythematous No blistering	Absent	4-21 days	See above	Variable	Hypotension	31.6%	
		Urticaria	Wheals Pruritus	Absent	Minutes-hours	See above	Variable	Cardiac rhythm disturbances	2.1%	
		Toxic epidermal necrolysis	Confluent and extensive epidermal detachment >30 % body surface area	Present	4–28 days	See above	Rare			
		Erythema multiforme	Typical target-like lesions – regular round-oval shape, sharp margins	Present/ absent	Variable	See above	Rare			
		Fixed drug eruption	Single/multiple round, well-circumscribed erythematous plaques with central bullae (sometimes)	Absent	First exposure: 1-2 weeks Reexposure > 48 h, usually 24 h	See above	Rare			
		Vasculitis	Palpable purpura, usually located on the lower extremities	Absent	Variable	See above	Rare			

Anti-psychotics	**Phenothiazines e.g. Chlorpromazine, Levomepromazin**	Lichenoid	Purple flat-topped papules Pruritus	Absent	Variable	See above	Variable	Cardiac arrhythmias Sudden death	Variable	Diabetes Insulin resistance Administration of other drugs
		Exanthematous	Erythematous No blistering	Absent	4-21 days	See above	Variable			
		Erythema multiforme	Typical target-like lesions – regular round-oval shape, sharp margins	Present/ absent	Variable	See above	Variable			
		Photosensitivity	Erythema ± Blistering after sun exposure	Absent	Variable	See above	Well known			
	Risperidone	Erythema multiforme	Typical target-like lesions – regular round-oval shape, sharp margins	Present/ absent	Variable	See above	Variable	Ventricular arrhythmias	Rarely	Alcohol dependence
Anti-convulsivants	**Carbamazepine**	Exanthematous	Erythematous No blistering	Absent	8-60 days	See above	3-12%	Tachycardia Hypotension Electrocardiographic ventricular extrasystoles and repolarization disorders	Variable	Females History of reaction to another antiepileptic drug
		Urticaria	Wheals Pruritus	Absent	Minutes-hours	See above				
		Toxic epidermal necrolysis	Confluent and extensive epidermal detachment >30 % body surface area	Present	8-60 days	See above				
		Erythema multiforme	Typical target-like lesions – regular round-oval shape, sharp margins	Present/ Absent		See above				
		Drug-induced lupus	SCLE-like	Absent/ Present		See above				
		Photosensitivity	Erythema ± Blistering after sun exposure	Absent		See above				

(continued)

Table 21.8 (continued)

	Lamotrigine	Stevens-Johnson syndrome	Atypical target lesions that affect < 10% BSA	Present	8 weeks	See above	5-10%	Heart failure	Variable	Co-administration of other drugs
		Toxic epidermal necrolysis	Confluent and extensive epidermal detachment >30 % body surface area	Present		See above				
		Exanthematous	Erythematous No blistering	Absent		See above				

References

1. Breathnach SM. Chapter 75: Drug reactions. In: Burns T, Breathnach S, Cox N, Griffiths C, editors. Rook's textbook of dermatology, vol. 4. 8th ed. Hoboken, NJ: Wiley; 2010.
2. https://www.who.int/medicines/areas/quality_safety/safety_efficacy/trainingcourses/definitions.pdf- Accessed 20.02.2019
3. Seger D, Barker K, McNaughton C. Misuse of the Naranjo adverse drug reaction probability scale in toxicology. Clin Toxicol. 2013 Jul 1;51(6):461–6.
4. Shear NH, Knowles SR, Shapiro L.(2008).Chapter 40:Cutanous reactions to drugs. In: Fitzpatrick's dermatology in general medicine, 7th edn, vol. 1 (K. Wolff, L.A. Goldsmith, S.I. Katz, et al.). McGraw-Hill: New York
5. Qing-ping S, Xiao-dong J, Feng D, Yan L, Mei-ling Y, Jin-xiu Z, Shu-qiang Z. Consequences, measurement, and evaluation of the costs associated with adverse drug reactions among hospitalized patients in China. BMC Health Serv Res. 2014 Dec;14(1):73.
6. Revuz J, Valeyrie-Allanore L. Chapter 21: Drug reactions. In: Bolognia JL, Jorizzo JL, Schaffer JV, editors. Dermatology, vol. 1. 3rd ed. Philadelphia, PA: Elsevier Saunders; 2012.
7. Riedl MA, Casillas AM. Adverse drug reactions: types and treatment options. Am Fam Physician. 2003 Nov 1;68(9):1781–94.
8. Alhawassi TM, Krass I, Bajorek BV, Pont LG. A systematic review of the prevalence and risk factors for adverse drug reactions in the elderly in the acute care setting. Clin Interv Aging. 2014;9:2079.
9. Hakkarainen KM, Hedna K, Petzold M, Hägg S. Percentage of patients with preventable adverse drug reactions and preventability of adverse drug reactions–a meta-analysis. PLoS One. 2012 Mar 15;7(3):e33236.
10. Belhekar MN, Taur SR, Munshi RP. A study of agreement between the Naranjo algorithm and WHO-UMC criteria for causality assessment of adverse drug reactions. Indian J Pharm. 2014 Jan;46(1):117–20.
11. Rydberg DM, Holm L, Engqvist I, Fryckstedt J, Lindh JD, Stiller CO, Asker-Hagelberg C. Adverse drug reactions in a tertiary care emergency medicine ward-prevalence, preventability and reporting. PLoS One. 2016 Sep 13;11(9):e0162948.
12. Bouvy JC, De Bruin ML, Koopmanschap MA. Epidemiology of adverse drug reactions in Europe: a review of recent observational studies. Drug Saf. 2015 May 1;38(5):437–53.
13. Ribeiro MR, Motta AA, Marcondes-Fonseca LA, Kalil-Filho J, Giavina-Bianchi P. Increase of 10% in the rate of adverse drug reactions for each drug administered in hospitalized patients. Clinics. 2018;73:1–6.
14. Langerová P, Vrtal J, Urbánek K. Adverse drug reactions causing hospital admissions in childhood: a prospective, observational, single-centre study. Basic Clin Pharmacol Toxicol. 2014 Dec;115(6):560–4.
15. Thiesen S, Conroy EJ, Bellis JR, Bracken LE, Mannix HL, Bird KA, Duncan JC, Cresswell L, Kirkham JJ, Peak M, Williamson PR. Incidence, characteristics and risk factors of adverse drug reactions in hospitalized children–a prospective observational cohort study of 6,601 admissions. BMC Med. 2013 Dec;11(1):237.
16. Deng Q, Fang X, Zeng Q, Lu J, Jing C, Huang J. Severe cutaneous adverse drug reactions of Chinese inpatients: a meta-analysis. An Bras Dermatol. 2017 Jun;92(3):345–9.
17. Fabbrocini G, Cameli N, Romano MC, Mariano M, Panariello L, Bianca D, Monfrecola G. Chemotherapy and skin reactions. J Exp Clin Cancer Res. 2012 Dec;31(1):50.
18. https://ctep.cancer.gov/protocoldevelopment/electronic_applications/docs/CTCAE_v5_Quick_Reference_5x7.pdf. Accessed 01.08.2019.
19. Kelleni MT, Abdelbasset M. Drug induced cardiotoxicity: mechanism, prevention and management. In: InCardiotoxicity. London: IntechOpen; 2018 Nov 14.
20. Albini A, Pennesi G, Donatelli F, Cammarota R, De Flora S, Noonan DM. Cardiotoxicity of anticancer drugs: the need for cardio-oncology and cardio-oncological prevention. J Natl Cancer Inst. 2010 Jan 6;102(1):14–25.

21. Madeddu C, Deidda M, Piras A, Cadeddu C, Demurtas L, Puzzoni M, Piscopo G, Scartozzi M, Mercuro G. Pathophysiology of cardiotoxicity induced by nonanthracycline chemotherapy. J Cardiovasc Med. 2016 May 1;17(1):S12–8.
22. Wickramasinghe CD, Nguyen KL, Watson KE, Vorobiof G, Yang EH. Concepts in cardio-oncology: definitions, mechanisms, diagnosis and treatment strategies of cancer therapy-induced cardiotoxicity. Future Oncol. 2016 Mar;12(6):855–70.
23. Faithfull S, Burton C, Clarke S, Kirby M, Lyon A, Levitt G, Poole K, Walter F. Mitigating risk of cardiovascular disease in people living with and beyond cancer. Cancer Nurs Pract. 2017 Feb 8;16(1):18–23.
24. Mladěnka P, Applová L, Patočka J, Costa VM, Remiao F, Pourová J, Mladěnka A, Karlíčková J, Jahodář L, Vopršalová M, Varner KJ. Comprehensive review of cardiovascular toxicity of drugs and related agents. Med Res Rev. 2018 Jan 5, 38, 4, https://doi.org/10.1002/med.21476
25. Iqubal A, Haque SE, Sharma S, Ansari MA, Khan V, Iqubal MK. Clinical updates on drug-induced cardiotoxicity. Int J Pharm Sci Res. 2018 Jan 1;9(1):16–26.
26. Loar RW, Noel CV, Tunuguntla H, Colquitt JL, Pignatelli RH. State of the art review: chemotherapy-induced cardiotoxicity in children. Congenit Heart Dis. 2018 Jan;13(1):5–15.
27. Chaar M, Kamta J, Ait-Oudhia S. Mechanisms, monitoring, and management of tyrosine kinase inhibitors–associated cardiovascular toxicities. Onco Targets Ther. 2018;11:6227–37.
28. Chung WB, Youn HJ. Pathophysiology and preventive strategies of anthracycline-induced cardiotoxicity. Korean J Intern Med. 2016 Jul;31(4):625–33.
29. Manolis AA, Manolis TA, Mikhailidis DP, Manolis AS. Cardiovascular safety of oncologic agents: a double-edged sword even in the era of targeted therapies–part 1. Expert Opin Drug Saf. 2018 Sep 2;17(9):875–92.
30. Curigliano G, Cardinale D, Dent S, Criscitiello C, Aseyev O, Lenihan D, Cipolla CM. Cardiotoxicity of anticancer treatments: epidemiology, detection, and management. CA Cancer J Clin. 2016 Jul;66(4):309–25.
31. Guenancia C, Lefebvre A, Cardinale D, Yu AF, Ladoire S, Ghiringhelli F, Zeller M, Rochette L, Cottin Y, Vergely C. Obesity as a risk factor for anthracyclines and trastuzumab cardiotoxicity in breast cancer: a systematic review and meta-analysis. J Clin Oncol. 2016 Sep 10;34(26):3157–65.
32. Larsen CM, Mulvagh SL. Cardio-oncology: what you need to know now for clinical practice and echocardiography. Echo Res Pract. 2017 Mar 1;4(1):R33–41.
33. Cueva JF, Antolín S, Calvo L, Fernández I, Ramos M, de Paz L, Mata JG, Lopez R, Constenla M, Perez E, González A. Galician consensus on management of cardiotoxicity in breast cancer: risk factors, prevention, and early intervention. Clin Transl Oncol. 2017 Sep 1;19(9):1067–78.
34. Barros-Gomes S, Herrmann J, Mulvagh SL, Lerman A, Lin G, Villarraga HR. Rationale for setting up a cardio-oncology unit: our experience at Mayo Clinic. Cardio-Oncology. 2016 Dec;2(1):5.
35. Salavastru CM. Approach to the evaluation and management of drug eruptions. Curr Dermatol Rep. 2016 Mar 1;5(1):49–57.
36. Kokado R, Hagiya H, Koyama T, Matsui E, Okuno H, Morii D, Hamaguchi S, Yoshida H, Miwa Y, Tomono K. Antibiotic-associated adverse drug events at a Japanese academic hospital. J Infect Chemother. 2019 May 1;25(5):392–5.
37. Deharo C, Berbis P, Privat Y. Dermatological complications caused by oral contraceptives. Fertil Contracept Sex. 1988 Apr 1;16(4):299–304.
38. Oray M, Abu Samra K, Ebrahimiadib N, Meese H, Foster CS. Long-term side effects of glucocorticoids. Expert Opin Drug Saf. 2016 Apr 2;15(4):457–65.
39. Mistry N, Shapero J, Crawford RI. A review of adverse cutaneous drug reactions resulting from the use of interferon and ribavirin. Can J Gastroenterol Hepatol. 2009;23(10):677–83.
40. Shuster M, Do D, Nambudiri V. Severe cutaneous adverse reaction to telaprevir. Dermatol Online J. 2015;21(1):13030.
41. Stalling SS, Vu JR, English JC. Telaprevir-induced pityriasis rubra pilaris–like drug eruption. Arch Dermatol. 2012 Oct 1;148(10):1215–7.

42. Biesbroeck LK, Scott JD, Taraska C, Moore E, Falsey RR, Shinohara MM. Direct-acting antiviral-associated dermatitis during chronic hepatitis C virus treatment. Am J Clin Dermatol. 2013 Dec 1;14(6):497–502.
43. Saleh AA. Kounis syndrome: acute inferior myocardial infarction with atroventricular node block due to ceftriaxone: a first reported case. Ann Saudi Med. 2014 May;34(3):250–3.
44. Polgreen LA, Riedle BN, Cavanaugh JE, Girotra S, London B, Schroeder MC, Polgreen PM. Estimated cardiac risk associated with macrolides and fluoroquinolones decreases substantially when adjusting for patient characteristics and comorbidities. J Am Heart Assoc. 2018 Apr 21;7(9):e008074.
45. Youssef MS. Sudden ventricular dysrhythmias after unintentional mediastinal washout with tetracycline containing solution. Anaesthesia. 1988 Nov;43(11):992–3.
46. Waite RA, Malinowski JM. Possible mesalamine-induced pericarditis: case report and literature review. Pharmacotherapy. 2002 Mar;22(3):391–4.
47. Asirvatham S, Sebastian C, Thadani U. Severe symptomatic sinus bradycardia associated with mesalamine use. Am J Gastroenterol. 1998 Mar;93(3):470–1.
48. Jose A, Cramer AK, Davar K, Gutierrez G. A case of drug-induced lupus erythematosus secondary to trimethoprim/sulfamethoxazole presenting with pleural effusions and pericardial tamponade. Lupus. 2017 Mar;26(3):316–9.
49. Bienias P, Ciurzyński M, Paczyńska M, Pruszczyk P. Cardiac arrest and electrical storm due to recurrent torsades de pointes caused by concomitant clarithromycin, cotrimoxazole and amiodarone treatment. Polski merkuriusz lekarski: organ Polskiego Towarzystwa Lekarskiego. 2014 Nov;37(221):285–8.
50. Sharma AK, Heist K, Russell G, Krahn T, Ferrell M. A true MI? Am J Med. 2011 Jul 1;124(7):608–10.
51. Lopez JA, Harold JG, Rosenthal MC, Oseran DS, Schapira JN, Peter T. QT prolongation and torsades de pointes after administration of trimethoprim-sulfamethoxazole. Am J Cardiol. 1987 Feb 1;59(4):376–7.
52. Aviado DM, Singh G, Berkley R. Pharmacology of new antimalarial drugs sulfonamides and trimethoprim. Chemotherapy. 1969;14(1):37–53.
53. Hendry PJ, Taichman GC, Taichman SJ, Keon WJ. Human myocardial responses to antibiotics: gentamicin, tobramycin and cephalothin. Can J Cardiol. 1988;4(5):219–22.
54. Valdés SO, Kim JJ, Niu MC, Caridad M, Miyake CY, Moffett BS. Cardiac arrest in pediatric patients receiving azithromycin. J Pediatr. 2017 Mar 1;182:311–4.
55. Maduranga PB, Chathurangani KC, Dharmaratne CJ, De Silva UD, Amarasinghe S. Long QT interval induced by clindamycin. Ceylon Med J. 2018 Mar 1;63:29–30.
56. Viskin S, Justo D, Halkin A, Zeltser D. Long QT syndrome caused by noncardiac drugs. Prog Cardiovasc Dis. 2003 Apr 1;45(5):415–27.
57. Mehta DA, Warwick GL, Goldberg MJ. QT prolongation after ampicillin anaphylaxis. Heart. 1986 Mar 1;55(3):308–10.
58. Suarez CR, Ow EP. Chloramphenicol toxicity associated with severe cardiac dysfunction. Pediatr Cardiol. 1992 Jan 1;13(1):48–51.
59. Altin C, Kanyilmaz S, Baysal S, Özin B. QT interval prolongation due to metronidazole administration/metronidazol uygulamasina bagli QT uzamasi. Anadulu Kardiyoloji Dergisi. 2011 Aug 1;11(5):468.
60. Gandotra SD, Smotrys MA, Patel DB, Chadha A. Systemic inflammatory response syndrome (SIRS) and a left bundle branch block (LBBB) due to nitrofurantoin. BMJ Case Rep. 2017 May 22;2017. bcr-2016
61. Westermann GW, Böhm M, Bonsmann G, Rahn KH, Kisters K. Chronic intoxication by doxycycline use for more than 12 years. J Intern Med. 1999 Dec;246(6):591–2.
62. Zhang SN, He QX, Yang NB, Ni SL, Lu MQ. Isoniazid-induced drug rash with eosinophilia and systemic symptoms (DRESS) syndrome presenting as acute eosinophilic myocarditis. J Intern Med. 54, 3511
63. Siddiqui MA, Khan IA. Isoniazid-induced lupus erythematosus presenting with cardiac tamponade. Am J Ther. 2002 Mar 1;9(2):163–5.

64. Jung HY, Park S, Shin B, Lee JH, Lee SJ, Lee MK, Lee WY, Yong SJ, Kim SH. Prevalence and clinical features of drug reactions with eosinophilia and systemic symptoms syndrome caused by antituberculosis drugs: a retrospective cohort study. Allergy Asthma Immunol Res. 2019 Jan;11(1):90–103.
65. National Toxicology Program. Bioassay of pyrazinamide for possible carcinogenicity. National Cancer Institute carcinogenesis Technical Report Series. 1978;48:1.
66. Li H, Li R, Qu J, Yu X, Cao Z, Liu Y, Cao B. Ventricular tachycardia in a disseminated MDR-TB patient: a case report and brief review of literature. Front Med. 2014 Jun 1;8(2):259–63.
67. Choudhri SH, Harris L, Butany JW, Keystone JS. Clofazimine induced cardiotoxicity--a case report. Lepr Rev. 1995 Mar;66(1):63–8.
68. Kang KS, Kim HI, Kim OH, Cha KC, Kim H, Lee KH, Hwang SO, Cha YS. Clinical outcomes of adverse cardiovascular events in patients with acute dapsone poisoning. Clin Exp Emerg Med. 2016 Mar;3(1):41–5.
69. Zhu KJ, He FT, Jin N, Lou JX, Cheng H. Complete atrioventricular block associated with dapsone therapy: a rare complication of dapsone-induced hypersensitivity syndrome. J Clin Pharm Ther. 2009 Aug;34(4):489–92.
70. Ali A, Hothi SS, Thompson A, Malik N. Negative chronotropic effects and coronary ischaemic abnormalities following thalidomide therapy. Cardiology. 2013;125(1):34–7.
71. Denolle T, Azizi M, Massart C, Zennaro MC. Itraconazole: a new drug-related cause of hypertension. InAnnales de cardiologie et d'angeiologie. 2014 Jun;63(3):213–5.
72. Hauben M, Hung EY. A quantitative analysis of the spontaneous reporting of congestive heart failure-related adverse events with systemic anti-fungal drugs. J Clin Pharmacol. 2013 Jul;53(7):762–72.
73. Tsimogianni AM, Andrianakis I, Betrosian A, Douzinas E. Cardiac arrest provoked by itraconazole and amiodarone interaction: a case report. J Med Case Reports. 2011 Dec;5(1):33.
74. Okamoto J, Fukunami M, Kioka H. Frequent premature ventricular contractions induced by itraconazole. Circ J. 2007;71(8):1323–5.
75. Tholakanahalli VN, Potti A, Hanley JF, Merliss AD. Fluconazole-induced torsade de pointes. Ann Pharmacother. 2001 Apr;35(4):432–4.
76. Pham CP, de Feiter PW, van der Kuy PH, van Mook WN. Long QTc interval and torsade de pointes caused by fluconazole. Ann Pharmacother. 2006 Jul;40(7–8):1456–61.
77. Chakravarty C, Singh PM, Trikha A, Arora MK. Fluconazole-induced recurrent ventricular fibrillation leading to multiple cardiac arrests. Anaesth Intensive Care. 2009 May;37(3):477–80.
78. Boyce MJ, Baisley KJ, Warrington SJ. Pharmacokinetic interaction between domperidone and ketoconazole leads to QT prolongation in healthy volunteers: a randomized, placebo-controlled, double-blind, crossover study. Br J Clin Pharmacol. 2012 Mar;73(3):411–21.
79. MOK NS, Lo YK, Tsui PT, Lam CW. Ketoconazole induced torsades de pointes without concomitant use of QT interval-prolonging drug. J Cardiovasc Electrophysiol. 2005 Dec;16(12):1375–7.
80. Vena GA, Micali G, Santoianni P, Cassano N, Peruzzi E. Oral terbinafine in the treatment of multi-site seborrheic dermatitis: a multicenter, double-blind placebo-controlled study. Int J Immunopathol Pharmacol. 2005 Oct;18(4):745–53.
81. Bebawi E, Jouni SS, Tessier AA, Frenette AJ, Brindamour D, Doré M. A metoprolol–terbinafine combination induced bradycardia. Eur J Drug Metab Pharmacokinet. 2015 Sep 1;40(3):295–9.
82. Fett DL, Vukov LF. An unusual case of severe griseofulvin-alcohol interaction. Ann Emerg Med. 1994 Jul 1;24(1):95–7.
83. Philips JA, Marty FM, Stone RM, Koplan BA, Katz JT, Baden LR. Torsades de pointes associated with voriconazole use. Transpl Infect Dis. 2007 Mar;9(1):33–6.
84. Dewan P, Gomber S, Arora V. Ventricular tachycardia: a rare side effect of Voriconazole. Indian J Pediatr. 2017 Feb 1;84(2):152–3.

85. Uludağ D, Özdemir N, Tüysüz G, Eroğlu AG, Celkan T. Voriconazole induced bradycardia. Pediatr Hematol Oncol. 2013 Oct 1;30(7):674–6.
86. Alkan Y, Haefeli WE, Burhenne J, Stein J, Yaniv I, Shalit I. Voriconazole-induced QT interval prolongation and ventricular tachycardia: a non—concentration-dependent adverse effect. Clin Infect Dis. 2004 Sep 15;39(6):e49–52.
87. Prosser JM, Mills A, Rhim ES, Perrone J. Torsade de pointes caused by polypharmacy and substance abuse in a patient with human immunodeficiency virus. Int J Emerg Med. 2008 Sep;1(3):217–20.
88. Singh BK, Haque SE, Pillai KK. Assessment of nonsteroidal anti-inflammatory drug-induced cardiotoxicity. Expert Opin Drug Metab Toxicol. 2014 Feb 1;10(2):143–56.
89. Marsico F, Paolillo S, Filardi PP. NSAIDs and cardiovascular risk. J Cardiovasc Med. 2017 Jan 1;18:e40–3.
90. Zhao W, Ji F, Yu S, Li Z, Deng H. Dilated cardiomyopathy and hypothyroidism associated with pegylated interferon and ribavirin treatment for chronic hepatitis C: case report and literature review. Braz J Infect Dis. 2014 Jan;18(1):110–3.
91. Teragawa H, Hondo T, Amano H, Hino F, Ohbayashi M. Adverse effects of interferon on the cardiovascular system in patients with chronic hepatitis C. Jpn Heart J. 1996;37(6):905–15.
92. Ucciferri C, Occhionero A, Vecchiet J, Falasca K. Cardiac toxicity associated with HCV direct antiviral agents. Mediterr J Hematol Infect Dis. 2018;10(1):e2018069.
93. Yanamandra U, Gupta S, Khadwal A, Malhotra P. Melphalan-induced cardiotoxicity: ventricular arrhythmias. BMJ Case Rep. 2016 Dec 15;2016:bcr2016218652.
94. Feliz V, Saiyad S, Ramarao SM, Khan H, Leonelli F, Guglin M. Melphalan-induced supraventricular tachycardia: incidence and risk factors. Clin Cardiol. 2011 Jun;34(6):356–9.
95. Doyle MK, Berggren R, Magnus JH. Interferon-induced sarcoidosis. J Clin Rheumatol. 2006 Oct 1;12(5):241–8.
96. Kang SM, Baek JY, Hwangbo B, Kim HY, Lee GK, Lee HS. A case of capecitabine-induced sarcoidosis. Tuberc Respir Dis. 2012 Mar 1;72(3):318–22.
97. Kushner JP, Hansen VL, Hammar SP. Cardiomyopathy after widely separated courses of adriamycin exacerbated by actinomycin-D and mithramycin. Cancer. 1975 Nov;36(5):1577–84.
98. Dorr RT, Bozak KA, Shipp NG, Hendrix M, Alberts DS, Ahmann F. In vitro rat myocyte cardiotoxicity model for antitumor antibiotics using adenosine triphosphate/protein ratios. Cancer Res. 1988 Sep 15;48(18):5222–7.
99. Wang WC, Ware RE, Miller ST, Iyer RV, Casella JF, Minniti CP, Rana S, Thornburg CD, Rogers ZR, Kalpatthi RV, Barredo JC. A multicenter randomised controlled trial of hydroxyurea (hydroxycarbamide) in very young children with sickle cell anaemia. Lancet. 2011 May 14;377(9778):1663–72.
100. Tshilolo L, Tomlinson G, Williams TN, Santos B, Olupot-Olupot P, Lane A, Aygun B, Stuber SE, Latham TS, McGann PT, Ware RE. Hydroxyurea for children with sickle cell anemia in sub-Saharan Africa. N Engl J Med. 2019 Jan 10;380(2):121–31.
101. Platt OS, Thorington BD, Brambilla DJ, Milner PF, Rosse WF, Vichinsky E, Kinney TR. Pain in sickle cell disease: rates and risk factors. N Engl J Med. 1991 Jul 4;325(1):11–6.
102. Ilgin S, Kilic V, Baysal M, Aydogan-Kilic G, Ucarcan S, Dermenci B, Atli O. Evidence for cardiotoxicity associated with sertraline in rats. Toxicology Research. 2018;7(5):817–25.
103. Glauser T, Shinnar S, Gloss D, Alldredge B, Arya R, Bainbridge J, Bare M, Bleck T, Dodson WE, Garrity L, Jagoda A. Evidence-based guideline: treatment of convulsive status epilepticus in children and adults: report of the Guideline Committee of the American Epilepsy Society. Epilepsy Currents. 2016 Jan;16(1):48–61.
104. Abosi O, Lopes S, Schmitz S, Fiedorowicz JG. Cardiometabolic effects of psychotropic medications. Horm Mol Biol Clin Invest. 2018 Jan10;36(1) https://doi.org/10.1515/hmbci-2017-0065.
105. Jolly DT, Stiell IG. Cardiotoxicity associated with an intentional overdose of maprotiline and perphenazine: a case report. Can Fam Physician. 1987 Nov;33:2627.

106. Grubisha MJ, Brennan JL, Douaihy A. Isolated sinus tachycardia following reinitiation of risperidone in a patient with suspected autonomic hypersensitivity. J Pharmacol Pharmacother. 2015 Jan;6(1):42–4.
107. Todorović V, Randelović S, Joksović D, Jović-Stosić J, Vucinić S, Glisović L. Carbamazepine cardiotoxicity in acute poisoning. Vojnosanit Pregl. 1993;50(2):143–6.
108. Qureshi WS, Memon S, Latif ML, Garle MJ, Parker TL, Pratten MK. Carbamazepine toxic effects in chick cardiomyocyte micromass culture and embryonic stem cell derived cardiomyocyte systems–possible protective role of antioxidants. Reprod Toxicol. 2014 Dec 1;50:49–59.
109. Biton V, Shneker BF, Naritoku D, Hammer AE, Vuong A, Caldwell PT, Messenheimer JA. Long-term tolerability and safety of lamotrigine extended-release: pooled analysis of three clinical trials. Clin Drug Investig. 2013 May 1;33(5):359–64.
110. Li WH, Liu HN, Lee DD. Myocarditis in dapsone-induced drug reaction with eosinophilia and systemic symptoms—a case report and review of the literature. Dermatol Sin. 2011 Jun 1;29(2):63–6.
111. Shiohara T, Mizukawa Y. Drug-induced hypersensitivity syndrome (DiHS)/drug reaction with eosinophilia and systemic symptoms (DRESS): an update in 2019. Allergol Int. 2019 Apr 16;68(3):301–8.

22 Cardiovascular Side Effects of Medications for Skin Diseases

Carmen Salavastru, Alina Suru, Monica Popescu, and George Sorin Tiplica

The cytochrome P450s (CYPs) are members of a superfamily of oxidative enzymes, which represent the major system for the oxidative metabolism of therapeutic substances. Sequencing of the human genome has revealed 58 different human CYP genes, which encode various CYP isoenzymes. The most important enzyme for most dermatological drugs is CYP3A.

Inducers are drugs that increase the levels of CYP3A, leading to increased metabolism and decrease of effectiveness of other drugs; Rifampin is one example of drugs used in dermatology that are inducers.

Inhibitors block CYP3A and lead to decreased metabolism and increased effectiveness; examples of systemic dermatological medication include antifungals (Itraconazole, Ketoconazole) and antibiotics (Erythromycin, Clarithromycin).

The substrate drugs are primarily metabolized by CYP3A and are the most influenced; examples: immunosuppressive agents (Cyclosporine, Tacrolimus), macrolides (Erythromycin, Clarithromycin); some drugs are both inhibitors and substrates [1].

The cardiovascular toxicity of the medication used in current practice is important to be considered by any prescribing physician. Mladěnka *et al.* identified in their 2017 review of the cardiovascular toxicity of drugs and related agents several types of cardiovascular insults: disturbances in cardiac rhythm, functional and

C. Salavastru (✉) · A. Suru
Paediatric Dermatology Department, "Carol Davila" University of Medicine and Pharmacy, Bucharest, Romania

M. Popescu
"Carol Davila" University of Medicine and Pharmacy, Bucharest, Romania

Dermato-oncology Research Unit, "Colentina" Clinical Hospital, Bucharest, Romania

G. S. Tiplica
"Carol Davila" University of Medicine and Pharmacy, Dermatology II, Colentina Clinical Hospital, Bucharest, Romania

C. Salavastru et al. (eds.), *Skin and the Heart*,
https://doi.org/10.1007/978-3-030-54779-0_22

structural heart impairment, arterial and venous thrombo-embolism, effects on blood pressure [2].

In the last decades more and more systemic agents are being used alone, or combined with topical therapy.

Some of the most frequently used classes of systemic drugs that are in the daily armamentarium of dermatologists, together with information on the mechanism of action, cardiovascular effects and interactions with cardiovascular drugs are shown in Annex (Table 22.1).

Dapsone

Dapsone is an aniline derivative; it combines both antimicrobial/antiprotozoal properties and anti-inflammatory effects resembling those of non-steroidal anti-inflammatory drugs. As an antimicrobial agent, dapsone is bacteriostatic in action [17]. Dapsone is a competitive antagonist of Para-AminoBenzoic Acid (PABA) interfering with normal synthesis of folic acid by bacteria.

Dapsone is effective in dermatoses with abnormal neutrophil accumulation, through many potential mechanisms. Dapsone interferes with neutrophil chemotactic migration and β2 integrin (CD11b/ CD18)—mediated adherence of human neutrophils in vitro. Dapsone interferes with the activation or function of the G-protein that initiates the signal transduction cascade common to chemotactic stimuli. This inhibition suppresses neutrophil recruitment and local production of toxic respiratory and secretory products of neutrophils [18].

The well-established indications are leprosy and dermatitis herpetiformis. It is also indicated for linear IgA dermatosis, bullous lupus, erythema elevatum et diutinum as well as other autoimmune bullous dermatoses, vasculitis, neutrophilic dermatoses (Sweet syndrome, pyoderma gangrenosum, Behçet syndrome) and other dermatoses [133].

Cardiovascular side effects: hypersensitivity myocarditis has been associated with Dapsone at therapeutic doses [19] [20]. Dapsone-induced DRESS, with fever, maculo-papular eruptions that progresses to exfoliative dermatitis, cervical lymphadenopathy, transaminitis, and cardiac involvement has been described in just a few cases [20]. The cardiac involvement in DRESS syndrome is represented by hypersensitivity myocarditis that can occur in two forms: hypersensitivity myocarditis (also known as acute eosinophilic myocarditis) and acute necrotizing eosinophilic myocarditis. Hypersensitivity myocarditis is usually self-limited, with a good prognosis once the offending agent is discontinued and the hypersensitivity reaction is suppressed by immunotherapy. ECG evaluation often shows nonspecific ST segment or T-wave abnormalities, conduction delay, or sinus tachycardia. Acute necrotizing eosinophilic myocarditis is a much more severe form of hypersensitivity myocarditis that presents with chest pain, ST segment elevation, elevated cardiac enzymes, and normal coronary arteries. The prognosis is poor and the mortality rate associated with this type of myocarditis is greater than 50% [21].

Antimalarial Agents

Chloroquine (CQ) and hydroxy-chloroquine (HCQ) have immunomodulatory, anti-inflammatory, and antiproliferative properties; they alleviate UV-induced inflammation, inhibit thrombocyte aggregation, enhance glucose tolerance, and cause increased porphyrin excretion [40]. They act by inhibition of antigen processing and presentation, inhibition of cytokine release, inhibition of stimulation of toll-like receptors that participate in immune response. Antimalarials decrease the activity of natural killer cells, inhibit the activity of cytotoxic T lymphocytes, regulate apoptosis; they competitively inhibit anti-DNA antibodies and decrease prostaglandin and leukotriene levels and they block superoxide radicals [40].

Antimalarials are effective for the treatment of the specific skin lesions of cutaneous lupus erythematosus whether acute, subacute, or chronic. Off-label indications include photosensitivity dermatoses (porphyria cutanea tarda, polymorphous light eruption, solar urticaria, dermatomyositis), granulomatous dermatoses (sarcoidosis, granuloma annulare), lymphocytic infiltrates, panniculitis and other dermatoses [41].

Cardiovascular side effects: At normal dosages, CQ/HCQ have no negative effects on the heart. There are case reports, however, on conduction disorders, cardiomyopathy, and even death [40].

At the time of writing, several potential treatments for treating Coronavirus disease 2019 (COVID-19), caused by SARS-CoV-2 were under investigation. Some candidate drugs may cause PR prolongation (e.g. lopinavir/ritonavir) and/or QT prolongation (chloroquine, hydroxychloroquine, azithromycin, lopinavir/ritonavir, and others). The expectedly short treatment duration for COVID-19 (5–10 days) mitigates the drugs' cardiac risks to an extent [134].

Antimalarials induced cardiomyopathy is a rare, probably under-recognized, complication of prolonged treatment with antimalarials. It presents as hypertrophic, restrictive cardiomyopathy with or without conduction abnormalities [42].

Retinoids

Retinoids are small-molecule hormones that exert their effects on target cells by binding and activating nuclear retinoid receptors [43–45]. For several decades, systemic retinoids have been used to treat psoriasis and disorders of keratinization [135]. FDA approved systemic retinoid use in three dermatoses: Acitretin is indicated for psoriasis, Isotretinoin for acne vulgaris and Bexarotene for selected cases of mycosis fungoides. Other indications for dermatologic disorders include: follicular disorders (acne-related conditions, hidradenitis suppurativa, dissecting cellulitis of the scalp), disorders of keratinization (Darier's disease, pityriasis rubra pilaris, ichthyosis, keratodermas), rosacea, chemoprevention of malignancies (syndromes with increased risk of cutaneous malignancy, xeroderma pigmentosum, Kaposi's sarcoma) and other inflammatory dermatoses [43].

Cardiovascular side effects: There are limited reports on the adverse cardiac effects of isotretinoin in literature. According to case reports, systemic isotretinoin therapy can cause cardiac side effects, like atrial tachycardia, congenital heart disease, cardiac remodeling and sinus tachycardia [46, 47]. Premature ventricular contractions were also reported to be associated with isotretinoin use [47, 48].

Regarding isotretinoin it is stipulated that a major mechanism of teratogenesis is a deleterious effect on cephalic neural-crest cell activity that results in craniofacial, cardiac, thymic malformations. The cardiac malformations included conotruncal heart defects and aortic-arch abnormalities [136].

The most common laboratory abnormality observed in patients taking systemic retinoids is elevation in serum lipids. Patients with obesity, diabetes or excessive alcohol intake are at increased risk. Triglycerides levels are affected to a greater degree than cholesterol levels. The magnitude of this effect, in terms of both percentage of patients affected and severity of elevation, is much greater with bexarotene than with other systemic retinoids [43].

Corticosteroids

Glucocorticoids are primary stress hormones that regulate a variety of physiological processes and are essential for life. Systemic glucocorticoids are one of the most important dermatological medication due to their anti-inflammatory, immunosuppressive and antiproliferative role.

The actions of glucocorticoids are predominantly mediated through the classic glucocorticoid receptor.

Oral administration of steroids is particularly useful in acute hypersensitivity diseases, connective tissue diseases, immunological blistering diseases, and the commoner dermatoses when they are very severe and widespread [49].

Dermatological indications include: severe dermatitis, erythrodermas, bullous dermatoses, vasculitis (cutaneous and systemic), collagen vascular diseases, neutrophilic dermatoses and others (sarcoidosis, panniculitis, urticaria) [50].

Cardiovascular side effects: the cardiovascular effects of systemic corticosteroids are vasoconstriction, sodium retention and increases renin levels. These factors will lead to hypertension; the fluid retention can determine or exacerbate heart failure [51].

Another major adverse effect of glucocorticoids on the cardiovascular system is dyslipidemia. Glucocorticoids may predispose treated patients to coronary artery disease if high doses and prolonged courses are used. Accordingly, they should be employed carefully in patients with other risk factors for cardiovascular disease [52].

Atrial fibrillation and cardiac sudden death have been reported as risks of pulse iv corticosteroids. To date there has been no study prospectively monitoring for cardiac effects in dermatologic patients. White et al. recommend that monitoring of dermatologic patients during pulse iv corticosteroids should be titrated according to the individual patient's active and past medical problems, concomitant drug therapy, and any previous reactions to pulse iv corticosteroids. Continuous cardiac monitoring is clearly indicated for patients with cardiac or renal disease who receive systemic corticosteroids [53].

Immunosuppressive Agents

Azathioprine is an immunosuppressive agent that acts as an antagonist of purine metabolism, resulting in the inhibition of DNA, RNA, and protein synthesis. It is an approved agent for the prevention of organ transplant rejection and severe rheumatoid arthritis. In dermatology it is indicated for autoimmune bullous disorders, lupus erythematosus, dermatomyositis and polymyositis and other inflammatory skin diseases such as eczema, psoriasis and vasculitis [54].

Interactions with cardiovascular drugs The use of angiotensin-converting enzyme inhibitors to control hypertension in patients on azathioprine has been reported to induce anemia and severe leukopenia; azathioprine may inhibit the anticoagulant effect of warfarin [54–56].

Cyclophosphamide is a precursor of an alkylating nitrogen mustard antineoplastic and immunosuppressive agent that is metabolized primarly in the liver to aldophosphamide that will be converted to active metabolites.

Its specific mechanism used in treating autoimmune diseases is not well understood, but has been postulated to include apoptosis, decreased immunoglobulin G production due to B-cell suppression and decreased production of adhesion molecules and cytokines [57]. Dermatologic indications: mycosis fungoides, systemic vasculitis, bullous dermatoses, neutrophilic dermatoses, autoimmune connective tissue disease, neoplasms.

Cardiovascular side effects: Cardiotoxicity is an uncommon complication in high-dose chemotherapy regimens. The cardiovascular side effects can present as a syndrome of congestive heart failure, myocarditis or both, and can be fatal [57].

The precise mechanism of cyclophosphamide cardiotoxicity is not known, but it is thought that it may cause endothelial injury with outpouring of toxic metabolites that result in damage to the cardiomyocytes [58].

Clinical manifestations of cardiotoxicity range from asymptomatic pericardial effusions to heart failure and myopericarditis. The risk of cardiotoxicity appears to be dose related and occurs within 1 to 10 days after the administration of the first dose of cyclophosphamide [59, 60].

Cyclosporine is a potent immunomodulatory agent that blocks the transcription of cytokine genes in activated T cells; in particular, cyclosporine inhibits the transcription of interleukin 2. Although cyclosporine's major actions are on T cells, there is some evidence that it produces direct effects on other cell types [137, 138]. While indicated only for the treatment of moderate to severe psoriasis, cyclosporine has also been used as an off-label drug for the treatment of various inflammatory skin conditions, including atopic dermatitis, blistering disorders, connective tissue diseases, neutrophilic dermatosis, neoplastic disorders, alopecia and granulomatous dermatoses [62, 139, 140, 141].

Cardiovascular side effects: hypertension is the most important cardiovascular side effect. The risk of developing hypertension increases with the dose and duration of therapy. Potential mechanisms for cyclosporine-induced hypertension are: activation of neurohormonal vasoconstrictors, alterations in vascular reactivity, renal tubular reabsorption of sodium in association with volume expansion, alterations in regulation of intracellular calcium ions, excess production of vasoconstrictors (prostaglandins, thromboxane, endothelin), decreased production of vasodilatory prostaglandins, stimulation of the renin-angiotensin system [61].

Methotrexate competitively and reversibly binds to dihydrofolate reductase preventing the conversion of dihydrofolate to tetrahydrofolate. Methotrexate is indicated in proliferative dermatoses, immuno-bullous dermatoses, autoimmune connective tissue diseases, vasculitis and neutrophilic dermatoses [67].

Cardiovascular side effect: Methotrexate may have a cardio-protective effect for patients with early onset rheumatoid arthritis [142], as well as for patients with psoriasis. Meta-analysis data from studies that involved patients with psoriasis showed that patients treated with methotrexate had fewer cardiovascular incidents compared to patients not treated with methotrexate [63, 64].

There is some in vitro and in vivo proof that methotrexate might have a combination of anti-inflammatory, blood pressure lowering, and vasculoprotective effects. Some mechanisms were proposed for the potential antiatherosclerotic, blood pressure lowering, and vasculoprotective effects of methotrexate, particularly cytokine modulation, adenosine accumulation, and activation of 5′ adenosine monophosphate-activated protein kinase [65]. However, Ridker et al. concluded in a recent publication that among patients with stable atherosclerosis, low-dose methotrexate (at a target dose of 15 to 20 mg weekly) did not reduce levels of interleukin-1β, interleukin-6, or C-reactive protein and did not result in fewer cardiovascular events than placebo [66].

Interactions with cardiovascular drugs: Methotrexate may decrease serum levels of inotropic cardiac drugs and of digoxin [67].

Mycophenolate mofetil (MMF) is a lymphocyte selective immunosuppressive agent that inhibits de novo purine synthesis via its active metabolite, mycophenolic acid. Mycophenolic acid depletes guanosine nucleotides by noncompetitively, selectively, and reversibly inhibiting inosine monophosphate dehydrogenase. Off-label dermatological indications of MMF include inflammatory skin conditions, psoriasis, autoimmune blistering disorders, connective tissue disorders and neutrophilic dermatosis (e.g. refractory pyoderma gangrenosum) [143, 144].

Cardiovascular side effects: MMF is very well tolerated. The most common side effects are gastrointestinal but there are reports about MMF improving hypertension [68, 69].

Antiandrogens

Spironolactone is an aldosterone antagonist with weak antiandrogen effect; by blocking the androgen receptor spironolactone inhibits the effects of androgens in the body. Of label dermatological indications are: hirsutism, acne, androgenetic alopecia and hidradenitis suppurativa. The main cardiovascular side effect is venous thrombosis [70].

Cyproterone acetate is available in European countries and is used off label for hirsutism. Cyproterone acetate, as one of the components of the combined oral contraceptive (COC) use has been associated with venous thrombosis (VT) (i.e., deep venous thrombosis and pulmonary embolism). Risk of venous thrombosis for combined oral contraceptives with 30-35μg ethinylestradiol and gestodene, desogestrel, cyproterone acetate and drospirenone were similar [70].

A case of cerebral vascular accident associated with cyproterone acetate–ethinyl estradiol has been reported [71], as well as cases of increased plasma apolipoprotein A-I and HDL-phospholipid levels in women with polycystic ovary syndrome treated with cyproterone acetate [72].

Biologic Therapeutics

Biologic therapeutics are used in several chronic dermatoses (e.g. psoriasis, atopic dermatitis) and other skin conditions (e.g hydradenitis suppurativa). Various cardiovascular adverse events have been associated with biological therapies. Heart failure is one of the most important adverse reactions reported in the medical literature. Arrhythmias were also reported in patients receiving infliximab. Data regarding the effect of biological therapies on the vascular system is contradictory. Some authors considered that TNF blockers etanercept and adalimumab might have a favorable effect on the lipid profile and reduce the rate of cardiovascular events while others consider that long-time treatment with infliximab could be pro-therogenic [145].

Psoriasis, Crohn's colitis, rheumatoid arthritis, and a variety of spondyloarthropathies benefit from using the biological agents [78, 79].

Monoclonal antibodies (e.g. Adalimumab, Avelumab, Brodalumab, Dupilumab, Ixekizumab, Nivolumab) are molecules that alter the normal cellular immune response, pathways of cell signaling, activation and cytokine production [78–80].

Anti-TNFα agents (e.g. *Infliximab, Adalimumab*) reduce inflammation and can stop inflammatory disease progression.

Cardiovascular side effects: Although TNF has been shown to have negative inotropic effects on the myocardium and may further contribute to left ventricular dysfunction and cardiomyopathy, the anti TNFα agents etanercept and infliximab did not show anticipated protective cardiovascular effect in clinical trials. While no benefit was seen, several patients did experience adverse cardiac outcomes and worsening of congestive cardiac failure with TNFα blockers are reported to occur [78–81, 54].

Rituximab is an anti-CD20 monoclonal antibody with considerable potential in dermatology due to an increase in off-label indications [146].

Cardiovascular side effects Fatal infusion reactions include myocardial infarction, ventricular fibrillation, and cardiogenic shock [83]. In patients with a history of cardiorespiratory disease can cause exacerbations of angina, arrhythmias and heart failure [84].

Cardiovascular toxicity in the form of cardiac dysrhythmias has been reported in 8% of patients treated with rituximab. These include monomorphic ventricular tachycardia, supraventricular tachycardia, trigeminy and irregular pulse, and an isolated case of a fatal infusion secondary to myocardial infarction [84].

Ustekinumab is a human monoclonal antibody that binds to the p40 subunit common to both interleukin (IL)-12 and IL-23 [147].

Cardiovascular side effects: the totality of the available clinical data suggests neither a detrimental nor a beneficial effect of ustekinumab on serious CV events [86]. Other reports accuse exacerbation or new onset of congestive heart failure [87].

Omalizumab is a recombinant humanized monoclonal antibody targeting the high-affinity Fc receptor of IgE, registered for the treatment of chronic spontaneous urticaria and severe allergic asthma [148]; off label it has been used in atopic dermatitis [149].

Cardiovascular side effects: Omalizumab has been linked to higher incidence rate of cardiovascular or cerebrovascular events such as transient ischemic attack, myocardial infarction, pulmonary hypertension, pulmonary embolism or venous thrombosis and unstable angina [89].

Dupilumab is an interleukin 4 (IL-4) receptor α-antagonist that inhibits IL-4 and IL-13 signaling through blockade of the shared IL-4α subunit used in atopic dermatitis [150].

Cardiovascular side effects: Cardiovascular thromboembolic events (cardiovascular deaths, non-fatal myocardial infarctions and non-fatal strokes) were reported in clinical trials as associated with a small percentage of patients receiving dupilumab [92].

Chronic inflammatory diseases are characterized by an increased cardiovascular risk. IL-17A has a defined role in both aspects [151].

Secukinumab is a fully human anti-IL-17A monoclonal antibody, ixekizumab is a humanized IgG4 monoclonal antibody that neutralizes IL-17 and brodalumab is a human, anti-IL17RA monoclonal antibody which blocks the activity of IL17RA, 17A/F and 17E.

Several pre-clinical data indicate that IL-17 inhibitors may be effective in multiple mucocutaneous disorders beyond psoriasis. The possible targets for IL-17 inhibitors include oral lichen planus, alopecia areata, pyoderma gangrenosum, palmo-plantar pustulosis, systemic lupus erythematosus, systemic sclerosis, mixed connective tissue disease, pemphigus vulgaris, pemphigoid, dermatitis herpetiformis, atopic dermatitis and chronic periodontitis [96].

Cardiovascular side effects: It is too early to conclude if IL-17 targeting will show protective CV effects in patients with chronic inflammatory diseases with Ixekizumab having a neutral impact on cardiovascular-related parameters in patients with psoriasis [95].

Still, from the clinical trials come reports of cardiac death due to cardiac arrest and cardiomyopathy linked to brodalumab [96].

Fusion Antibody Proteins

Fusion antibody proteins (e.g. Etanercept, Alefacept, Abatacept, Onercept), also known as chimeric proteins, are proteins which are created by the fusion of the receptor domain of a human protein with the constant region of human IgG

Cardiovascular side effects: etanercept can cause congestive heart failure [98] as well as silent ischaemic heart disease and diastolic dysfunction.

Less data exists on the association of anakinra, abatacept with cardiovascular adverse effects [80].

Recombinant Human Cytokines and Growth Factors

Recombinant Human Cytokines and Growth Factors can be grouped as follows:

(a) Interferons: Interferon α (IFNα), Interferon γ (IFNγ)

Interferon therapy for HCV infection is cardiac safe in patients who have structurally normal heart. Female patients have a propensity of adverse events like severe diastolic dysfunction and mild pericardial effusion [105].

(b) Granulocyte macrophage colony stimulating factor (GM- CSF)

GM-CSF may have multiple direct and indirect beneficial cardiovascular effects including neovascularization of ischemic myocardium and reducing the extent of myocardial damage after infarction [106].

(c) Platelet derived growth factor (PDGF)

PDGFs drive pathological mesenchymal responses in vascular disorders such as atherosclerosis, restenosis, pulmonary hypertension and cardiac fibrosis [107].

Intravenous Immunoglobulin

Immunoglobulin infusion adverse reactions include arrhythmia occurring during or after (supraventricular tachycardia and bradycardia), stroke, myocardial infarction, and pulmonary embolism [112].

Immune Checkpoint Inhibitors: Anti PD-1

The development of immune checkpoint inhibitors has revolutionized the treatment of melanoma. However, immunotherapy is not without side effects. Cardiotoxicity is an under-recognized and potentially life-threatening complication of targeted immune checkpoint therapy [152].

(a) Ipilimumab. The first case of cardiotoxicity induced by ipilimumab was reported in 2013, which presented as myocardial fibrosis within a retrospective study among 752 ipilimumab-treated patients for melanoma [117]. Other cardiac reported side effects induced by ipilimumab: cardiac arrest [118], myocarditis, myocardial fibrosis [117] congestive heart failure [119], left ventricular dysfunction, reduction in ejection fraction, paroxysmal atrial fibrillation, ischemia [120], pericarditis, pericardial effusion [121] and biventricular failure [122].

The overall incidence of cardiac adverse events in the published literature was rare, occurring in approximately 1% of treated cases. However, the cardiovascular-specific mortality rate was 42% in patients who developed cardiotoxicity while on the drug [118, 153].

(b) Nivolumab and Ipilimumab. Myocarditis occurred with greater severity in patients who received combination therapy of ipilimumab and nivolumab [153]. They can determine as well immune-induced myocarditis and cardiomyopathy [119] or lymphocytic myocarditis [125].

(c) Pembrolizumab. In the published pembrolizumab monotherapy cohorts, the rates of adverse cardiac events were higher, occurring in approximately 1.2% of treated patients.

The published articles revealed during the treatment with pembrolizumab autoimmune cardiomyopathy (grade 3 CTCAE) and myocarditis [128], ventricular arrhythmia, left ventricular systolic dysfunction, myocarditis with cardiomyopathy, cardiac atrial flutter, hypertension, sinus tachycardia, stable angina pectoris [129], congestive cardiac failure [127], myocardial infarction [130, 131].

Annex

Table 22.1 Cardiovascular interactions and side effects with dermatologic drug therapy

Class	Drug	Mechanism of action	Cardiovascular contraindications/side effects	Interactions with cardiovascular drugs
Antiviral Agents				
	Acyclovir	Blocks viral DNA polymerase [3,4]	N/A	Antiviral agents may increase the serum levels and potential toxicity of inotropic agents (digoxin) [4]
	Valacyclovir	Prodrug of acyclovir; converted in first pass through the gastrointestinal tract and liver to acyclovir [4]		
	Famciclovir	The oral prodrug of penciclovir [3,4]		
	Brivudine	Blocks viral DNA synthesis by interacting with deoxythymidine kinase and DNA polymerase [5,6]		
Antibacterial Agents				
ß-lactam antibacterial agents	Penicillins	The ß-lactam antibacterial agents bind to penicillin - binding-proteins in the bacterial cell membrane and	Vasospasm seen with parenteral or intramuscular formulations	Penicillins may elevate serum levels or potentiate the therapeutic effects of anticoagulants and may prolong prothrombin times [15]

	Cephalosporins	bacterial cell wall peptidoglycan synthesis.		Cefotetan and cefoperazone (containing N-methylthiotetrazole ring) may determine hypoprothrombinemia [16]
Macrolides	Erythromycin Azithromycin Clarithromycin	Bind reversibly to the bacterial ribosome, inhibiting RNA - dependent protein synthesis; they also possess anti inflammatory effect [7]	Cardiac conduction abnormalities; in utero exposure to erythromycin was linked by some authors to cardiovascular malformation [11], while others dispute this association [12]	Erythromycin inhibits CYP leading to decreased metabolic clearance of digoxin and warfarin Erythromycin and clarithromycin may alter the metabolism of drugs known to influence cardiac conduction ex terfenadine and their combination is contraindicated [7]
Fluoroquinolones	Ciprofloxacin Gatifloxacin Gemifloxacin Levofloxacin Lomefloxacin Moxifloxacin Norfloxacin Ofloxacin	Interfere with bacterial DNA replication by inhibition of DNA gyrase and topoisomerase IV [8]	Gatifloxacin and moxifloxacin are associatedwith QTc interval prolongation [8] Gatifloxacin, moxifloxacin, and levofloxacin had a higher risk of serious arrythmias [13]	Fluoroquinolones increase serum levels for antiarrhythmic agents (ex. mexiletine); in combination with warfarin may increase the risk of hemorrhage [8] Gatifloxacin and moxifloxacin may increase the risk of QT interval prolongation in combination with antiarrhythmic agents (ex amiodarone, bepridil, disopyramide, dofetilide, ibutilide, procainamide, quinidine) and beta blockers (especially sotalol) [8]
Tetracyclines	Tetracycline Doxycycline Minocycline	Are bacteriostatic and inhibit bacterial protein synthesis by binding to the 30S subunit of the bacterial ribosome. Tetracyclines also have anti-inflammatory and anti-collagenolytic effects [9]	Protective effect on the murine myocardium [14]	Tetracyclines may increase the serum levels of oral anticoagulants [9]

(continued)

Table 22.1 (continued)

Rifamycins	Rifampin Rifabutin	Rifamycins inhibit RNA synthesis by inhibiting DNA - dependent RNA polymerase [10]		Rifamycins decrease the drug level of cardiovascular drugs as: digoxin, mexiletine, propafenone, quinidine, warfarin (risk of thrombosis), carvedilol, all calcium channel blo ckers [10]
Dapsone		Competitive antagonist of PABA interfering with normal synthesis of folic acid by bacteria; antineutrophil action [17, 18]	Contraindications: severe cardiovascular disease Side effects: may determine hypersensitivity myocarditis [19,20] Dapsone-induced DRESS [20,21]	
Antifungal Agents		Oral antifungals interfere with the enzymes involved in producing ergosterol, a key component of fungal cell walls [22]		
	Griseofulvin	Is incorporated into keratin; it interferes with microtubule formation [23]		Impairs action of coumarin antiarrhythmic drugs and calcium channel blockers [22]
Allylamines	Terbinafine	Inhibits sterol biosynthesis by blocking squalene peroxidase causing accumulation of squalene and cell death [24, 25]		Impairs action of coumarin; enhances the effect of antiarrhythmic drugs and beta blockers [22]
Azoles	Ketoconazol		Ketokonazol use has been limited due to serious liver damage and harmful interactions [28, 29]	

Triazoles	Itraconazole Fluconazole	Triazoles impair synthesis of ergosterol by inhibiting C14 -a sterol demethylase [26, 27]	Itraconazol, fluconazol: QT interval prolongation torsades de pointes risk of sudden death [30] Itraconazol: cardiac contractility reduction, dilated cardiomyopathy in animal models [31]; hypertension premature ventricular contractions, ventricular fibrillation, heart failure [32, 33]	As inhibitors of CYP450 enzymes, triazoles can impair metabolism of coadministered drugs, increasing the risk of toxicity [26] Itraconazole and fluconazole can enhance coumarin effect and the risk of hemorrhagic complications Enhance the effect of antiarrhythmic drugs and calcium channel blockers. Coadministration of azole drugs with cisapride, pimozide, quinidine, dofetilide, or levacet ylmethadol is contraindicated. These combinations may cause severe cardiac events including ventricular tachycardia, torsades de pointes, cardiac arrest and/or sudden death[22]
Antihistamins		Block the action of histamine by competing for receptor sites [34]		
Sedating H1 Ethanolamine Ethylenediamine Piperazine Alkylamine Phenothiazine Piperidine	Diphenhydramine Clemastine Tripelennamine Hydroxyzine Chlorpheniramine Promethazine Cyproheptadine		Dose-related sinus tachycardia, reflex tachycardia supraventricular arrhythmias, dose related prolongation of the QT interval, ventricular arrhythmias [35]	H1 antihistamins may enhance CYP 2D6 substrates as antiarrhythmic agents and beta blockers[36]
Non Sedating H1	Azelastine Cetirizine Levocetirizine Ebastine Fexofenadine Loratadine Desloratadine	Poorly lipophilic; do not cross the blood-brain barrier; highly selective action; little or no anticholinergic activity [36]	Terfenadine: life threatening cardiac arrhythmias (no longer available) [36] Fexofenadine- no effect on QTc interval [37] Loratadine: no clinical effect upon the potassium	

(continued)

Table 22.1 (continued)

	Mizolastine		channels without QT modification [38]	
Tricyclic antidepressant	Doxepin	Doxepin is a psychotropic agent with tricyclic antidepressantand anxiolytic properties	Dose-related CV adverse effects: hypotension, hypertension, tachycardia, palpitations [39]	Metabolized by CYP2D6; quinidine may increase risk of QTc prolongation Antiarrhythmic agents (CYP 2C9 inhibition) and antiplatelet drugs (CYP 2C19) may increase serum levels and potential toxicity of doxepin [39]
Other antiallergic agents	Cromolyn Ketotifen Rupatadine	Mast cell stabilizer H1 receptor antagonist and mast cell stabilizer Dual histamine H1 receptor and platelet activating factor receptor antagonist [34]	Flushing, tachycardia, premature ventricular contractions, palpitations, chest pain No cardiovascular side effect	Precaution is recommendedin the case of rupatadine use in combination with isoenzyme CYP3A4 inhibitors, in patients with prolonged QT interval, ongoing hypokalemia or in other cases that might result in arrhythmia such as clinically significant bradycardia or acute myocardial ischemia [34]
Antimalarials	Chloroquine Hydroxychloroquine Quinacrine	Antimalarials s tabilize membranes; downregulate expression of MHC molecules; interact with the complement system, inhibit prostaglandin synthesis [40, 41]	EKG abnormalities: depression of T wave hypotension, cardiomyopathy [40 -42]	Increase levels of digoxin and antiarrhythmic agents as propafenone [41]
Retinoids	Tretinoin Isotretinoin Etretinate Acitretin Bexarotene	Modulate the differentiation and keratinization of keratinocytes, alter fibroblast activity and modulate T-cell response [43-45]	Atrial tachycardia, congenital heart disease, cardiac remodeling, sinus tachycardia [46, 47], premature ventricular contractions [47, 48], incresed lipid blood levels [43]	

Corticosteroids	Hydrocortisone Prednisolone Prednisone Methylprednisolone Triamcinolone Dexamethasone	Immunosuppressive and anti-inflammatory effects	Hypertension Heart failure Coronary artery disease [49-52] For pulse iv: Cardiac dysrhythmias Risk of sudden death [53]	Increase renal clearance of aspirin Hypokalemia may lead to digitalis toxicity Enhances/impaires warfarin With other QT „prolongers" (antiarrhythmic agents, macrolides, fluoroquinolones) may increase the risk of QT prolongation and torsades de pointes [49, 52]
Immunosuppressive agents	Azathioprine	Purine antagonist that interferes with NK,T and B cells [54]		Angiotensin-converting enzyme inhibitors may increase the risk of leukopenia and anemia [54, 55] Azathioprine may decrease the anticoagulant effect of warfarin [56]
	Cyclophosphamide	Alkylating agent, blocks DNA and RNA	Cardiotoxicity congestive heart failure, myocarditis [57-59]	Reduces absorption of digoxin Increases the anticoagulanteffect of warfarin; may decrease the GI absorbtion of digoxin [60]
	Cyclosporine	Inhibits helper T-cell function by blocking IL-2 function; also blocks the release of other lymphokines	Hypertension [61]	Amiodarone increases cyclosporine levels Diltiazem and verapamil increase cyclosporine levels Cyclosporine increases the levels of digitalis [62]
	Methotrexate	Folic acid antagonist	Protective effect (antiatherosclerotic, lowers blood pressure, vasculoprotective effect) [63-65]. Did not reduce levels of interleukin-1β, interleukin-6, or C-reactive protein and did not result in fewer cardiovascular events than placebo[66]	May decrease serum levels of inotropic cardiac drugs and of digoxin [67]
	Mycophenolate mofetil	Inhibits lymphocytic inosine monophosphate dehydrogenase; influences mast cell	Improves hypertension [68, 69]	

(continued)

Table 22.1 (continued)

		degranulation and lipoxygenase activity		
Antiandrogens	Spironolactone	Aldosterone antagonist		Spironolactone together with angiotensin-converting enzyme inhibitors may decrease aldosterone and increase the risk of hyperkalemia. May give falsely elevated serum digoxin levels; enhances digoxin [73, 74]
	Cyproterone acetate	Progestin with antiandrogenic properties	Venous thrombosis [70] Cerebral vascular accident [71] Increased plasma apolipoprotein A -I and HDL -phospholipid levels in women wit h polycystic ovary syndrome [72]	Inhibitors and inducers of the cytochrome P450 enzyme CYP3A4 (ex: Amlodipine, Clopidogrel, Disopyramide, Lovastatin, Quinidine) may interact with Cyproterone acetate [74]
Colchicine		Inhibits microtubular system, interfering with cell division, migration, other neutrophil functions, collagen synthesis and deposition of amyloid [75]	May have cardiovascular benefits [76]	Colchicine is a substrate of Cytochrome P450 3A4 (CYP3A4) and concentrations may be increased by drugs that are inhibitors such as diltiazem, verapamil [77]
Biologic therapeutics				
Monoclonal antibodies	· Anti-TNΦα: Infliximab, Adalimumab, Certolizumab, Golimumab	Molecules that alter the normal cellular immune response, pathways of cell signaling, activation	Negative inotropic effects worsening of congestive cardiac failure [78-81]	It is worth stressing that TNF inhibitors very ra rely cause drug interactions [82]

		and cytokine production [78,79,80]		
	· Anti-CD20: Rituximab	The antibody labels B lymphocytes, which have the CD20 cell marker. These cells are then killed by 1 of 3 mechanisms: antibody-dependent cytotoxicity, complement-dependent cytotoxicity, or stimulation of apoptosis [83]	Fatal infusion reactions include myocardial infarction, ventricular fibrillation, and cardiogenic shock [83]. In patients with a history of cardiorespiratory disease can cause exacerbations of angina, arrhythmias and heart failure [84].	Clinically important, potentially hazardous interaction with Benazepril, Captopril, Clevidipine, Enalapril, Fosinopril, Irbesartan, Lisinopril, O lmesartan, Quinapril, Ramipril [85]
	· Anti-IL-12 and anti-IL-23 monoclonal antibody: Ustekinumab	Binds with specificity to the p40 protein subunit used by both the interleukin (IL)-12 and IL-23 cytokines	Neither a detrimental nor a beneficial effect [86] Exacerbation or new onset of congestive heart failure [87]	The risks of atrial fibrillation and major adverse cardiovascular events associated with the use of ustekinumab vs TNF inhibitors were not different in patients with psoriasis or psoriatic arthritis [88]
	·Anti-IgE: Omalizumab	Binding of IgE to the high-affinity IgE receptor (FcεRI) on the surface of mast cells and basophils.	Unstable angina Myocardial infarction Venous thrombosis Pulmonary embolism [89]	Cytochrome P450 enzymes, efflux pumps and protein-binding mechanisms are not involved in the clearance of omalizumab; thus, there is little potential for drug-drug interactions [90]. None noted [91].
	· Anti IL-4: Dupilumab	Inhibits signaling of IL-4 and IL-13, type 2 cytokines	Cardiovascular deaths, non-fatal myocardial infarctions [92]	Dupilumab is not anticipated to directly interact with cytochrome P450 enzymes, thus no typical drug-drug interactions of dupilumab with other drugs via are expected [93]
	· Anti IL 17-A: Secukinumab Ixekizumab Brodalumab	interleukin-17A inhibitors	too early to conclude if IL-17 targeting will show protective CV effects in patients with chronic inflammatory diseases [94] Ixekizumab-neutral impact [95]	Drug interaction studies have not been conducted for secukinumab. The product labeling cautions that change in the metabolism of CYP-450 substrates, particularly those with a narrow therapeutic index, may be altered during initiation or discontinuation of secukinumab therapy [97].

(continued)

Table 22.1 (continued)

			Brodalumab was link ed to cardiac arrest and cardiomyopathy [96]	
Fusion antibody proteins	Etanercept, Alefacept, Abatacept,	Etanercept: TNF inhibitor Alefacept inhibits the activation of CD4+ and CD8+ T cells . Abatacept prevents antigen-presenting cells from delivering the co - stimulatory signal.	Silent ischemic diastolic dysfunction [98]	Absence of a pharmacokinetic interaction betwe en Etanercept and Warfarin [94] or Digoxin [99] . Alefacept may decrease the blood levels and effects of amiodarone, amlodipine, atorvastatin, felodipine, flecainide, lovastatin, nicardipine, nifedipine, procain amide, quinidine, warfarin [100] . Concurrent therapy with Abatacept and TNF antagonists is not recommended (increased isk of serious infections) [101] . Salicylates may be used during treatment with abatacept [102].
Recombinant human cytokines and growth factors	a) Interferons Interferon α (IFNα) Interferon γ (IFNγ)			
	b) Granulocyte macrophage colony stimulating factor (GM - CSF) c) Platelet derived growth factor (PDGF)	Interferon alpha binds to interferon receptors which, upon dimerization, activate two Jak (Janus kinase) and Tyk2). Acts by stimulating stem cells to produce granulocytes, monocytes and macrophages[103]		

		PDGF is a dimeric glycoprotein which regulates and promotes granulation tissue formation, re-epithelialisation and wound angiogenesis [104]	Atherosclerosis, restenosis, pulmonary hypertension and cardiac fibrosis [107]	
Intravenous immunoglobulin		The mechanism of action of IVIG in most autoimmune diseases remains unclear [111]. IVIGs have an immunomodulatory activity based on biological processes that are implicated in innate or acquired immune response	Arrhythmia (supraventricular tachycardia and bradycardia) occurring during or after immunoglobulin infusion Stroke, myocardial infarction, pulmonary embolism [112]	Ig IV with other drugs and intravenous solutions have not been evaluated. It is recommended to be administered separately from other drugs or medications which the patient may be receiving [113]
Immune checkpoint inhibitors (anti-PD1)	Ipilimumab (cytotoxic T-lymphocyte antigen-4=CTLA-4)	The CTLA-4 is a cell surface molecule that regulates the adaptative immune response. The binding between CTLA-4 and B7 molecules on the antigen presenting cells, interrupts the stimulatory signal which in order blunts T-cell proliferation response [114]. Produce an exacerbated autoimmunity [115].	Myocarditis, myocardial fibrosis [117] Cardiac arrest [118] Congestive heart failure [119] Left ventricular dysfunction, reduction in ejection fraction, paroxysmal atrial fibrillation, ischemia [120] Pericarditis, pericardial effusion [121] Biventricular failure [122]	Clinical pharmacology studies were not performed to evaluate the metabolism and the metabolic pathways of ipilimumab in humans, or to determine the potential for any drug-drug interactions of ipilimumab with other molecules. Ipilimumab is not metabolized by cytochrome P450 enzymes (CYPs) or other drug metabolizing enzymes [123].

(continued)

Table 22.1 (continued)

		Block the acti vity of CTLA -4, thereby sustaining a potent T-cell response against tumor cells [116].		
	Nivolumab (CTLA -4 + Programmed Death-1 (PD-1) Inhibitor)	Nivolumab blocks the immune checkpoint PD-1. This mechanism is related to the reduction of the inhibitory signaling and to restore the patient's natural tumor-specific T-cell immune response [124]	Myocarditis [125] Immune-induced myocarditis and cardiomyopathy [119] Lympho cytic myocarditis [125]	No formal pharmacokinetic drug -drug interaction studies have been conducted with Nivolumab [126]
	Pembrolizumab (Programmed Death-1 (PD-1) Inhibitor)	It binds to the cell surface receptor PD-1 and it antagonizes its interaction with ligands PD-L1 and PD-L2. The binding of Pembrolizumab to PD-1 prevents the inhibitory pathway causing a physiological shift to immune reactivity and enhancing tumor immunosurveillance and anti-tumor immune response [127].	Autoimmune cardiomyopathy (grade 3 CTCAE) and myocarditis [128] Ventricular arrhythmia, left ventricular systolic dysfunction, myocarditis with cardiomyopathy, cardiac atrial flutter, hypertension, sinus tachycardia, stable angina pectoris [129] Congestive cardiac failure [127] Myocar dial infarction [130, 131]	No non-clinical or clinical dedicated pharmacodynamic drug-drug interactions studies with Pembrolizumab have been conducted [132].

References

1. Burgdorf W, Paus R, Sterry W. Thieme clinical companions: dermatology. 1st ed. New York: Thieme; 2006. p. 636.
2. Mladěnka P, Applová L, Patočka J, Costa VM, Remiao F, Pourová J, et al. Comprehensive review of cardiovascular toxicity of drugs and related agents. Med Res Rev. 2018 Jul;38(4):1332–403.
3. O'Brien JJ, Campoli-Richards DM. Acyclovir. Drugs. 1989 Mar 1;37(3):233–309.
4. Chang C, Madkan V, Sra K, Carrasco D, Tyring S. Systemic antiviral agents. In: Wolverton SE, editor. Comprehensive dermatologic drug therapy. 2nd ed. Edinburgh: Elsevier Health Sciences; 2007. p. 101–24.
5. Rabasseda X. Brivudine: a herpes virostatic with rapid antiviral activity and once-daily dosing. Drugs Today. 2003 May 1;39(5):359.
6. Salvaggio MR, Gnann JW Jr. Drugs for herpesvirus infections. Infect Dis Ther. 2017 Jan;1:1309–17.
7. Ashourian N, Cohen P. Systemic antibacterial agents. In: Wolverton SE, editor. Comprehensive dermatologic drug therapy. 2nd ed. Edinburgh: Elsevier Health Sciences; 2007. p. 48–52.
8. Ashourian N, Cohen P. Systemic antibacterial agents. In: Wolverton SE, editor. Comprehensive dermatologic drug therapy. 2nd ed. Edinburgh: Elsevier Health Sciences; 2007. p. 51–5.
9. Ashourian N, Cohen P. Systemic antibacterial agents. In: Wolverton SE, editor. Comprehensive dermatologic drug therapy. 2nd ed. Edinburgh: Elsevier Health Sciences; 2007. p. 54–60.
10. Ashourian N, Cohen P. Systemic antibacterial agents. In: Wolverton SE, editor. Comprehensive dermatologic drug therapy. 2nd ed. Edinburgh: Elsevier Health Sciences; 2007. p. 58–62.
11. Källén BA, Olausson PO, Danielsson BR. Is erythromycin therapy teratogenic in humans? Reprod Toxicol. 2005 Jul 1;20(2):209–14.
12. Romøren M, Lindbæk M, Nordeng H. Pregnancy outcome after gestational exposure to erythromycin–a population-based register study from Norway. Br J Clin Pharmacol. 2012 Dec;74(6):1053–62.
13. Liu X, Ma J, Huang L, Zhu W, Yuan P, Wan R, Hong K. Fluoroquinolones increase the risk of serious arrhythmias: a systematic review and meta-analysis. Medicine. 2017 Nov;96:44.
14. Kagawa N, Senbonmatsu TA, Satoh K, Ichihara K, Yamagata N, Hatano O, Saito T, Nguyen VQ, Waterman MR, Price EJ, Atkinson JB. Tetracycline protects myocardium against ischemic injury. Front Biosci. 2005 Jan 1;10:608–19.
15. Ashourian N, Cohen P. Systemic antibacterial agents. In: Wolverton SE, editor. Comprehensive dermatologic drug therapy. 2nd ed. Edinburgh: Elsevier Health Sciences; 2007. p. 39–43.
16. Ashourian N, Cohen P. Systemic antibacterial agents. In: Wolverton SE, editor. Comprehensive dermatologic drug therapy. 2nd ed. Edinburgh: Elsevier Health Sciences; 2007. p. 43–6.
17. Wozel G, Blasum C. Dapsone in dermatology and beyond. Arch Dermatol Res. 2014 Mar;306(2):103–24.
18. Zhu YI, Stiller MJ. Dapsone and sulfones in dermatology: overview and update. J Am Acad Dermatol. 2001 Sep;45(3):420–34.
19. Kang KS, Kim HI, Kim OH, Cha KC, Kim H, Lee HK, et al. Clinical outcomes of adverse cardiovascular events in patients with acute dapsone poisoning. Clin Exp Emerg Med. 2016;3(1):41–5.
20. Li WH, Liu H-N, Lee D-D. Myocarditis in dapsone-induced drug reaction with eosinophilia and systemic symptoms - a case report and review of the literature. Dermatol Sin. 2011 June;29(2):63–6.
21. Bourgeois GP, Cafardi JA, Groysman V, Hughey LC. A review of DRESS-associated myocarditis. J Am Acad Dermatol. 2012 Jun 1;66(6):e229–36.
22. Gupta A. Systemic antifungal agents. In: Wolverton SE, editor. Comprehensive dermatologic drug therapy. 2nd ed. Edinburgh: Elsevier Health Sciences; 2007. p. 75–99.
23. Odds FC, Brown AJ, Gow NA. Antifungal agents: mechanisms of action. Trends Microbiol. 2003 Jun 1;11(6):272–9.

24. Food and Drug Administration FDA; 2012. Lamisil (Terbinafine Hydrochloride) tablets, 250 mg. [Reviewed: 2012; cited 2020 Mar 7; cited 2020 Mar 7]; [about 22 p]. Highlights of prescribing information [Internet]. Available from: https://www.accessdata.fda.gov/drugsatfda_docs/label/2012/020539s021lbl.pdf
25. Food and Drug Administration FDA; 2013. Lamisil (Terbinafine Hydrochloride) Oral Granules, 125 mg and 187.5 mg: [Reviewed: 2013 June; cited 2020 Mar 7]; [about 7 p]. Highlights Of Prescribing Information [Internet]. Available from: https://www.accessdata.fda.gov/drugsatfda_docs/label/2013/022071s009lbl.pdf
26. Nett JE, Andes DR. Antifungal agents: spectrum of activity, pharmacology, and clinical indications. Infect Dis Clin N Am. 2016 Mar 1;30(1):51–83.
27. Andes D, Pascual A, Marchetti O. Antifungal therapeutic drug monitoring: established and emerging indications. Antimicrob Agents Chemother. 2009 Jan 1;53(1):24–34.
28. Food and Drug Administration FDA (US); 2016. Nizoral (ketoconazole): [about 5 p.]. Drug Safety Communication [Internet] Available from: https://www.fda.gov/Drugs/DrugSafety/ucm500597.html
29. Suspension of marketing authorisations for oral ketoconazole. Benefit of oral ketoconazole does not outweigh risk of liver injury in fungal infections [Internet]. European Medicines Agency's Committee on Medicinal Products for Human Use (CHMP); 2013. Ketoconazole: [Revised: 25 July 2013; Reviewed: 11 October 2013; cited 2020 Mar 7]; [about 6p]. Available from: https://www.ema.europa.eu/en/documents/referral/ketoconazole-article-31-referral-suspension-marketing-authorisations-oral-ketoconazole_en.pdf
30. Nix DE. Cardiotoxicity induced by antifungal drugs. Curr Fungal Infect Rep. 2014 Jun 1;8(2):129–38.
31. Cleary JD, Stover KR, Farley J, Daley W, Kyle PB, Hosler J. Cardiac toxicity of azole antifungals. J Pharm Pharmacol. 2013 May 31;4(03):362.
32. Paul V, Rawal H. Cardiotoxicity with itraconazole. BMJ Case Rep. 2017 Apr 10, 2017; https://doi.org/10.1136/bcr-2017-219376.
33. Page RL, O'Bryant CL, Cheng D, Dow TJ, Ky B, Stein CM, et al. Drugs that may cause or exacerbate heart failure: a scientific statement from the American Heart Association. Circulation. 2016 Aug 9;134(6):e32–69.
34. Olasińska-Wiśniewska A, Olasiński J, Grajek S. Cardiovascular safety of antihistamines. Adv Dermatol Allergol. 2014 Jun;31(3):182.
35. Simons FE, Simons KJ. Histamine and H1-antihistamines: celebrating a century of progress. J Allergy Clin Immunol. 2011 Dec 1;128(6):1139–50.
36. Greaves M. Antihistamins. In: Wolverton SE, editor. Comprehensive dermatologic drug therapy. 2nd ed. Edinburgh: Elsevier Health Sciences; 2007. p. 391–404.
37. Allegra [Internet]. 2005. Food and Drug Administration FDA; Allegra (Fexofenadine Hydrochloride) Tablets: [Reviewed: 2005 September; cited 2020 Mar 7]; [about 13 p]. Available from https://www.accessdata.fda.gov/drugsatfda_docs/label/2005/020872s015lbl.pdf fexofenadine
38. Dávila I, Sastre J, Bartra J, Del Cuvillo A, Jáuregui I, Montoro J, et al. Comparative pharmacology of the H1 antihistamines. J Investig Allergol Clin Immunol. 2006;16(1):13–23.
39. Lee CS, Koo J. Psychotropic Agents. In: Wolverton SE, editor. Comprehensive dermatologic drug therapy. 2nd ed. Edinburgh: Elsevier Health Sciences; 2007. p. 437–58.
40. Rodriguez-Caruncho C, Marsol IB. Antimalarials in dermatology: mechanism of action, indications, and side effects. Actas Dermosifiliogr. 2014 Apr 1;105(3):243–52.
41. Callen JP, Rosenbach M, Camisa C. Antimalarial agents. In: Wolverton SE, Wu JJ, editors. Comprehensive dermatologic drug therapy. 4nd ed. Amsterdam: Elsevier; 2021. p. 234–44.
42. Tselios K, Deeb M, Gladman DD, Harvey P, Urowitz MB. Antimalarial-induced cardiomyopathy: a systematic review of the literature. Lupus. 2018 Apr;27(4):591–9.
43. Patton TJ, Zirwas MJ, Wolverton SE. Systemic Retinoids. In: Wolverton SE, editor. Comprehensive dermatologic drug therapy. 2nd ed. Edinburgh: Elsevier Health Sciences; 2007. p. 275–300.

44. Zouboulis CC. Retinoids–which dermatological indications will benefit in the near future? Skin Pharmacol Physiol. 2001;14(5):303–15.
45. Aryal A, Upreti S. A brief review on systemic retinoids. Int J Pharm Sci Res. 2017 Sep 1;8(9):3630–9.
46. Soriano EA, Azevedo PS, Miot HA, Minicucci MF, Pansani MC, Matsubara LS, et al. Cardiac remodeling induced by 13-cis retinoic acid treatment in acne patients. Int J Cardiol. 2013 Feb 10;163(1):68–71.
47. Güler E, Babur Güler G, Yavuz C, Kizilirmak F. An unknown side effect of isotretinoin pericardial effusion with atrial tachycardia. Anatol J Cardiol. 2015;15:168–9.
48. Alan S, Ünal B, Yildirim A. Premature ventricular contractions associated with isotretinoin use. Bras Dermatol. 2016 Dec;91(6):820–1.
49. Barnetson RS, White AD. The use of corticosteroids in dermatological practice. Med J Aust. 1992 Mar;156(6):428–31.
50. Williams LC, Nesbitt LT Jr. Update on systemic glucocorticosteroids in dermatology. Dermatol Clin. 2001 Jan 1;19(1):63–77.
51. Gollnick H. Systemic therapy. In: WHC B, Braun-Falco O, editors. . 3rd ed. Berlin: Springer; 2009. p. 1573–93.
52. Sholter DE, Armstrong PW. Adverse effects of corticosteroids on the cardiovascular system. Can J Cardiol. 2000 Apr;16(4):505–11.
53. White KP, Driscoll MS, Rothe MJ, Grant-Kels JM. Severe adverse cardiovascular effects of pulse steroid therapy: is continuous cardiac monitoring necessary? J Am Acad Dermatol. 1994 May 1;30(5):768–73.
54. Badalamenti SA, Kerdel FA. Azathioprine. In: Wolverton SE, editor. Comprehensive dermatologic drug therapy. 2nd ed. Edinburgh: Elsevier Health Sciences; 2007. p. 183–95.
55. Gossmann J, Kachel HG, Schoeppe WI, Scheuermann EH. Anemia in renal transplant recipients caused by concomitant therapy with azathioprine and angiotensin-converting enzyme inhibitors. Transplantation. 1993 Sep;56(3):585–9.
56. Product Information [Internet]. May 2011. Imuran (Azathioprine) 50-mg Scored Tablets [about 9 p]. Available from https://www.accessdata.fda.gov/drugsatfda_docs/label/2011/016324s034s035lbl.pdf
57. Kim J, Chan JJ. Cyclophosphamide in dermatology. Australas J Dermatol. 2017 Feb;58(1):5–17.
58. Anber ZNH, Saleh BOM, Al-Rawi SI. The cardiotoxicity effect of different chemotherapeutic regimens in Iraqi patients with breast cancer: a follow up study. Heliyon. 2019;5(8):e02194.
59. Yeh ET, Bickford CL. Cardiovascular complications of cancer therapy: incidence, pathogenesis, diagnosis, and management. J Am Coll Cardiol. 2009 Jun 16;53(24):2231–47.
60. Perlis C, Pan TD, McDonald CJ. Cytotoxic agents. In: Wolverton SE, editor. Comprehensive dermatologic drug therapy. 2nd ed. Edinburgh: Elsevier Health Sciences; 2007. p. 198–205.
61. Miller LW. Cardiovascular toxicities of immunosuppressive agents. Am J Transplant. 2002;2(9):807–18.
62. Lee CS, Koo J. Cyclosporine. In: Wolverton SE, editor. Comprehensive dermatologic drug therapy. 2nd ed. Edinburgh: Elsevier Health Sciences; 2007. p. 219–37.
63. Liu BA, Schwartz R. Potential cardio-protective effects of psoriasis medications. Acta Dermatovener Cr. 2018 Oct 22;26(3):249.
64. Mangoni AA, Zinellu A, Sotgia S, Carru C, Erre GL. Methotrexate and cardiovascular protection: current evidence and future directions. Clin Med Insights Ther. 2017 Nov 9;9:1–12.
65. Mangoni AA, Tommasi S, Zinellu A, Sotgia S, Carru C, Piga M, et al. Repurposing existing drugs for cardiovascular risk management: a focus on methotrexate. Drugs Context. 2018 Nov;14:7.
66. Ridker PM, Everett PM, Pradhan A, MacFadyen JG, Solomon DH, Zaharris E, et al. Low-dose methotrexate for the prevention of atherosclerotic events. N Engl J Med. 2019;380:752–62.
67. Callen J, Klup-Shorten C, Wolverton SE. Methotrexate. In: Wolverton SE, editor. Comprehensive dermatologic drug therapy. 2nd ed. Edinburgh: Elsevier Health Sciences; 2007. p. 163–81.

68. Taylor EB, Ryan MJ. Immunosuppression with mycophenolate mofetil attenuates hypertension in an experimental model of autoimmune disease. J Am Heart Assoc. 2017 Feb 27;6(3):1–11.
69. Herrera J, Ferrebuz A, MacGregor EG, Rodriguez-Iturbe B. Mycophenolate mofetil treatment improves hypertension in patients with psoriasis and rheumatoid arthritis. J Am Soc Nephrol. 2006 Dec 1;17(12 suppl 3):S218–25.
70. De Bastos M, Stegeman BH, Rosendaal FR, Van Hylckama VA, Helmerhorst FM, Stijnen T, et al. Combined oral contraceptives: venous thrombosis. Cochrane Database Syst Rev. 2014 Mar 3;3:1–50.
71. Kromm J, Jeerakathil T. Cyproterone acetate-ethinyl estradiol use in a 23-year-old woman with stroke. CMAJ. 2014 Jun 10;186(9):690–3.
72. Luque-Ramırez M, Lvarez-Blasco, F, Botella-Carretero JI, Martınez-Bermejo E, Escobar-Morreal HF. Comparison of ethinyl-estradiol plus cyproterone acetate versus metformin effects on classic metabolic cardiovascular risk factors in women with the polycystic ovary syndrome. J. Clin. Endocrinol. Metabolism 2007 Jul; 92(7):2453-2461.
73. Sawaya M. Antiandrogens and Androgen Inhibitors. In: Wolverton SE, editor. Comprehensive dermatologic drug therapy. 2nd ed. Edinburgh: Elsevier Health Sciences; 2007. p. 417–35.
74. Product Monograph Mylan-Cyproterone [Internet]. Mylan Pharmaceuticals Ulc. Cyproterone Acetate Tablets 50 mg Antiandrogen: [Reviewed: 2010 Sep 9; cited 2020 Mar 7]; [9 p]. Available from: https://pdf.hres.ca/dpd_pm/00011374.PDF
75. Burgdorf W, Paus R, Sterry W. Miscellaneous agents. Colchicine. In: Burgdorf W, Paus R, Sterry W, editors. Thieme clinical companions: dermatology. 1st ed. New York: Thieme; 2006. p. 634.
76. Hemkens LG, Ewald H, Gloy VL, Arpagaus A, Olu KK, Nidorf M, et al. Cardiovascular effects and safety of long-term colchicine treatment: cochrane review and meta-analysis. Heart. 2016 Apr 15;102(8):590–6.
77. Campbell KB, Cicci TA, Vora AK, Burgess LD. Beyond Gout: Colchicine Use in the Cardiovascular Patient. Hosp Pharm. 2015 Nov 19;50:859–67.
78. Iffat H, Samia A, Gousia S, Parvaiz A. Biologics in dermatology: a brief review. BJMP. 2013;6(4):a629.
79. Cush JJ. Unusual toxicities with TNF inhibition: heart failure and drug-induced lupus. Clin Exp Rheumatol. 2004;22(Suppl. 35):S141–7.
80. Khanna D, Mcmahon M, Furst DL. Anti-tumor necrosis factor alpha therapy and heart failure: what have we learned and where do we go from here? Arthritis Rheum. 2004;50:1040–50.
81. Danila MI, Patkar NM, Curtis JR, Saag KG, Teng GG. Biologics and heart failure in rheumatoid arthritis: are we any wiser? Curr Opin Rheumatol. 2008 May;20(3):327–33.
82. Lis K, Kuzawińska O, Bałkowiec-Iskra E. Tumor necrosis factor inhibitors – state of knowledge. Arch Med Sci. 2014 Dec 22;10(6):1175–85.
83. Foran JM, Rohaitner AZ, Cunningham D, Popescu RA, Solal-Celigny P, Ghielmini M, et al. European Phase II study of rituximab (chimeric anti-CD20 monoclonal antibody) for patients with newly diagnosed mantle cell lymphoma and previously treated mantle cell lymphoma, immunocytoma, and small B lymphocytic lymphoma. J Clin Oncol. 2000;18:317–24.
84. Ng KH, Dearden C, Gruber P. Rituximab-induced Takotsubo syndrome: more cardiotoxic than it appears? BMJ Case Rep. 2015;
85. Litt's Drug Eruptions& Reaction Database [Internet]. Rituximab MabThera (Roche); Rituxan (Genentech): [Revised: 2019 Nov 11, Reviewed: 2019 Nov 11; cited 2020 Mar 7] [1 p]. Available from: https://pdf.hres.ca/dpd_pm/00011374.PDF
86. Reich K, Langley RG, Lebwohl M, Szapary P, Guzzo C, Yeilding N, et al. Cardiovascular safety of ustekinumab in patients with moderate to severe psoriasis: Results of integrated analyses of data from phase II and III clinical studies. Brit J Dermatol. 2011 Apr;164(4):862–72.
87. Menter A, Strober BE, Kaplan DH, Kivelevitch D, Prater EF, Stoff B, Armstrong AW, et al. Joint AAD-NPF guidelines of care for the management and treatment of psoriasis with biologics. J Am Acad Dermatol. 2019 Apr 1;80(4):1029–72.

88. Lee MP, Desai RJ, Jin Y, Brill G, Ogdie A, Kim SC. Association of Ustekinumab vs TNF inhibitor therapy with risk of atrial fibrillation and cardiovascular events in patients with psoriasis or psoriatic arthritis. JAMA Dermatol. 2019 Jun 1;155(6):700–7.
89. Iribarren C, Rahmaoui A, Long AA, Szefler SJ, Bradley MS, Carrigan G, et al. Cardiovascular and cerebrovascular events among patients receiving omalizumab: results from EXCELS, a prospective cohort study in moderate to severe asthma. J Allergy Clin Immunol. 2017 May;139(5):1489–1495.e5.
90. Summary of product characteristics [Internet]. European Medicines Agency. Xolair 75 mg powder and solvent for solution for injection: [Reviewed: 2016; cited 2020 Mar 7] [8 p]. Available from https://www.ema.europa.eu/en/documents/product-information/xolair-epar-product-information_en.pdf
91. Ciccone CD. Davis's drug guide for rehabilitation professionals. 1st ed. Philadelphia: F.A. Davis Company; 2013. 790 p.
92. Food and Drug Administration FDA. 2017. DUPIXENT (dupilumab) injection, for subcutaneous use: [Revised: 2018 Oct, Reviewed: 2018 Oct; cited 2020 Mar 7]; [about 25 p]. Highlights of Prescribing Information [Internet] Available from: https://www.accessdata.fda.gov/drugsatfda_docs/label/2018/761055s007lbl.pdf
93. Summary of opinion (initial authorisation). Assement report [Internet]. London: European Medicines Agency; 2017. Dupixen (Dupilumab); [Revised: 2017 July 20; cited 2020 Mar 7];[about 26 p]. Available from https://www.ema.europa.eu/en/documents/assessment-report/dupixent-epar-public-assessment-report_en.pdf
94. Zhou H, Patat A, Parks V, Buckwalter M, Metzger D, Korth-Bradley J. Absence of a pharmacokinetic interaction between etanercept and Warfarin. J Clin Pharmacol. 2004 May;44(5):543–50.
95. Egeberg A, Wu JJ, Korman N, Solomon JA, Goldblum O, Zhao F, et al. Ixekizumab treatment shows a neutral impact on cardiovascular parameters in patients with moderate-to-severe plaque psoriasis: Results from UNCOVER-1, UNCOVER-2, and UNCOVER-3. J Am Acad Dermatol. 2018 Jul;79(1):104–109.e8.
96. Wasilewska A, Winiarska M, Olszewska M, Rudnicka L. Interleukin-17 inhibitors. A new era in treatment of psoriasis and other skin diseases. Adv Dermatol Allergol. 2016 Aug;33(4):247.
97. Cada DJ, Baker DE, Panther SG, PharmD KI. Secukinumab. Hosp Pharm. 2015 Sep;50(8):714–27.
98. Coondoo A. Biologics in dermatologic therapy–An update. Indian J Dermatol. 2009 Jul;54(3):211.
99. Zhou H, Parks V, Patat A, Le Coz F, Simcoe D, Korth-Bradle J. Absence of a clinically relevant interaction between etanercept and digoxin. J Clin Pharmacol. 2004 Nov;44(11):1244–51.
100. Alefacept Drug Interactions [Internet]. Drugs.com [Revised: 2019 Jun 21; cited 2020 Mar 7]; [about 7 p]. Available from: https://www.drugs.com/cons/alefacept-intramuscular.html
101. Food and Drug Administration FDA; 2005. Orencia (Abatacept) for injection for intravenous use injection, for subcutaneous use: [Revised: 2013 Dec; cited 2020 Mar 7]; [about 16 p]. Highlights Of Prescribing Information [Internet]. Available from: https://www.accessdata.fda.gov/drugsatfda_docs/label/2013/125118s171lbl.pdf
102. Reynolds J, Shojania K, Marra CA. Abatacept: a novel treatment for moderate-to-severe rheumatoid arthritis. Pharmacotherapy. 2007 Dec;27(12):1693–701.
103. Conti L, Gessani S. GM-CSF in the generation of dendritic cells from human blood monocyte precursors: recent advances. Immunobiology. 2008;213(9-10):859–70.
104. Pinkas H, Fisch B, Rozansky G, Felz C, Kessler-Icekson G, Krissi H, et al. Platelet-derived growth factors (PDGF-A and -B) and their receptors in human fetal and adult ovaries. Mol Hum Reprod. 2008;14:199–206.
105. Faisal AWK, Nisar S, Ali SA, Ahmad F. Effects of interferon therapy on heart. J Ayub Med Coll Abbottabad. 2016;28(2):276–80.
106. Kovacic JC, Muller DW, Graham RM. Actions and therapeutic potential of G-CSF and GM-CSF in cardiovascular disease. J Mol Cell Cardiol. 2007 Jan;42(1):19–33.

107. Andrae J, Gallini R, Betsholtz C. Role of platelet-derived growth factors in physiology and medicine. Genes Dev. 2008 May 15;22(10):1276–312.
108. Wong SF, Jakowatz JG, Taheri R. Potential drug-drug interaction between interferon alfa-2b and gemfibrozil in a patient with malignant melanoma. Clin Ther. 2005 Dec;27(12):1942–8.
109. Interferon alfa-2b Drug Interactions [Internet]. Drugs.com: Cerner Multum [Revised: 2018 May 30; cited 2020 Mar 7]; [about 4 p]. Available from: https://www.drugs.com/mtm/interferon-alfa-2b.html
110. Karalliedde LD, Clarke SFJ, Collignon U, Karalliedde J. Adverse drug interactions: a handbook for prescribers. 1st ed. London: Hodder Education; 2010. p. 101.
111. Kazatchkine MD, Kaveri SV. Immunomodulation of autoimmune and inflammatory diseases with intravenous immune globulin. N Engl J Med. 2001 Sep 6;345(10):747–55.
112. Guo Y, Tian X, Wang X, Xiao Z. Adverse Effects of Immunoglobulin Therapy. Front Immunol. 2018;9:1299.
113. Food and Drug Administration FDA; 1994. Gammagard S/D, Immune Globulin Intravenous (Human) IgA less than or equal to 2.2 μg/mL in a 5% Solution. [Revised: 2014; cited 2020 Mar 7] [about 15 p]. Highlights of prescribing information [Internet]. Available from https://www.fda.gov/media/78185/download
114. Trinh VA, Hagen B. Ipilimumab for advanced melanoma: a pharmacologic perspective. J Oncol Pharm Pract. 2013 Sep;19(3):195–201.
115. Thumar JR, Kluger HM. Ipilimumab: a promising immunotherapy for melanoma. Oncology (Williston Park). 2010 Dec;24(14):1280–8.
116. Adis R&D Profile. Ipilimumab. Drugs RD. 2010 Jul;10(2):97–110. https://doi.org/10.2165/11584510-000000000-00000.
117. Voskens CJ, Goldinger SM, Loquai C, Robert C, Kaehler KC, Berking C, et al. The price of tumor control: an analysis of rare side effects of anti-CTLA-4 therapy in metastatic melanoma from the ipilimumab network. PLoS One. 2013 Jan 14;8(1):e53745.
118. Larkin J, Chiarion-Sileni V, Gonzalez R, Grob JJ, Cowey CL, Lao CD, et al. Combined nivolumab and ipilimumab or monotherapy in untreated melanoma. N Engl J Med. 2015 Jul 2;373(1):23–34.
119. Heinzerling L, Ott PA, Hodi FS, Husain AN, Tajmir-Riahi A, Tawbi H, et al. Cardiotoxicity associated with CTLA4 and PD1 blocking immunotherapy. J Immunother Cancer. 2016 Dec 16;4(1):50.
120. Roth ME, Muluneh B, Jensen BC, Madamanchi C, Lee CB. Left ventricular dysfunction after treatment with ipilimumab for metastatic melanoma. Am J Ther. 2016 Nov 1;23(6):e1925–8.
121. Yun S, Vincelette ND, Mansour I, Hariri D, Motamed S. Late onset ipilimumab-induced pericarditis and pericardial effusion: a rare but life threatening complication. Case Rep Oncol Med. 2015; https://doi.org/10.1155/2015/794842. Available from http://downloads.hindawi.com/journals/crionm/2015/794842.pdf
122. Samara Y, Yu CL, Dasanu CA. Acute autoimmune myocarditis and hepatitis due to ipilimumab monotherapy for malignant melanoma. J Oncol Pharm Pract. 2019 Jun;25(4):966–8.
123. Assessment Report For Yervoy (ipilimumab). London: European Medicines Agency 2011. Yervoy (ipilimumab) [about 71 p]. Available from https://www.ema.europa.eu/en/documents/assessment-report/yervoy-epar-public-assessment-report_en.pdf
124. Brahmer JR, Hammers H, Lipson EJ. Nivolumab: targeting PD-1 to bolster antitumor immunity. Future Oncol. 2015 Mar 23;11(9):1307–26.
125. Koelzer VH, Rothschild SI, Zihler D, Wicki A, Willi B, Willi N, et al. Systemic inflammation in a melanoma patient treated with immune checkpoint inhibitors - an autopsy study. J Immunother Cancer. 2016 Dec;4(1):13.
126. Food and Drug Administration FDA; 2014. OPDIVO (nivolumab) injection, for intravenous use: [Revised: 2018 Apr; cited 2020 Mar 7]; [about 47 p]. Highlights of Prescribing Information [Internet]. Available from: https://www.accessdata.fda.gov/drugsatfda_docs/label/2018/125554s058lbl.pdf

127. Seiwert TY, Burtness B, Mehra R, Weiss J, Berger R, Eder JP, et al. Safety and clinical activity of pembrolizumab for treatment of recurrent or metastatic squamous cell carcinoma of the head and neck (KEYNOTE-012): an open-label, multicentre, phase 1b trial. Lancet Oncol. 2016 Jul 1;17(7):956–65.
128. Tajmir-Riahi A, Bergmann T, Schmid M, Agaimy A, Schuler G, Heinzerling L. Life-threatening autoimmune cardiomyopathy reproducibly induced in a patient by checkpoint inhibitor therapy. J Immunother. 2018 Jan 1;41(1):35–8.
129. Zimmer L, Goldinger SM, Hofmann L, Loquai C, Ugurel S, Thomas I, et al. Neurological, respiratory, musculoskeletal, cardiac and ocular side-effects of anti-PD-1 therapy. Eur J Cancer. 2016 Jun 1;60:210–25.
130. Langer CJ, Gadgeel SM, Borghaei H, Papadimitrakopoulou VA, Patnaik A, Powell SF, et al. Carboplatin and pemetrexed with or without pembrolizumab for advanced, non-squamous non-small-cell lung cancer: a randomised, phase 2 cohort of the open-label KEYNOTE-021 study. Lancet Oncol. 2016 Nov 1;17(11):1497–508.
131. Herbst RS, Baas P, Kim DW, Felip E, Pérez-Gracia JL, Han JY, et al. Pembrolizumab versus docetaxel for previously treated, PD-L1-positive, advanced non-small-cell lung cancer (KEYNOTE-010): a randomised controlled trial. Lancet. 2016 Apr 9;387(10027):1540–50.
132. Assessment report Keytruda, International non-proprietary name: pembrolizumab [Internet]. European Medicines Agency; 2015. [Revised: 2015 May 21; cited 2020 Mar 7]; [about 21 p]. Available from https://www.ema.europa.eu/en/documents/assessment-report/keytruda-epar-public-assessment-report_en.pdf
133. Hall RP III, Mickle C. Dapsone. In: Wolverton SE, editor. Comprehensive dermatologic drug therapy. 2nd ed. Edinburgh: Elsevier Health Sciences; 2007. p. 239–57.
134. Sacher F, Fauchier L, Boveda S, de Chillou C, Defaye P, Deharo JC, Gandjbakhch E, Probst V, Cohen A, Leclercq C. Use of drugs with potential cardiac effect in the setting of SARS-CoV-2 infection. Archiv CardiovascDis. 2020; https://doi.org/10.1016/j.acvd.2020.04.003.
135. Van De Kerkhof PC. Update on retinoid therapy of psoriasis in: an update on the use of retinoids in dermatology. Dermatol Ther. 2006 Sep;19(5):252–63.
136. Lammer EJ, Chen DT, Hoar RM, Agnish ND, Benke PJ, Braun JT, Curry CJ, Fernhoff PM, Grix AW Jr, Lott IT, Richard JM. Retinoic acid embryopathy. N Engl J Med. 1985 Oct 3;313(14):837–41.
137. Matsuda S, Koyasu S. Mechanisms of action of cyclosporine. Int Immunopharmacol. 2000 May 1;47(2-3):119–25.
138. Russell G, Graveley R, Seid J, Al-Humidan AK, Skjodt H. Mechanisms of action of cyclosporine and effects on connective tissues. Semin Arthritis Rheum. 1992 Jun 1;21(6):16–22.
139. Dehesa L, Abuchar A, Nuno-Gonzalez A, Vitiello M, Kerdel FA. The use of cyclosporine in dermatology. J Drugs Dermatol. 2012 Aug;11(8):979–87.
140. Amor KT, Ryan C, Menter A. The use of cyclosporine in dermatology: part I. J Am Acad Dermatol. 2010 Dec 1;63(6):925–46.
141. Ryan C, Amor KT, Menter A. The use of cyclosporine in dermatology: part II. J Am Acad Dermatol. 2010 Dec 1;63(6):949–72.
142. Widdifield J, Abrahamowicz M, Paterson JM, Huang A, Thorne JC, Pope JE, et al. Associations between methotrexate use and the risk of cardiovascular events in patients with elderly-onset rheumatoid arthritis. J Rheumatol. 2019 May 1;46(5):467–74.
143. Orvis AK, Wesson SK, Breza TS Jr, Church AA, Mitchell CL, Watkins SW. Mycophenolate mofetil in dermatology. J Am Acad Dermatol. 2009 Feb 1;60(2):183–99.
144. Perlis C, Pan TD, McDonald CJ. Cytotoxic Agents. In: Wolverton SE, editor. Comprehensive dermatologic drug therapy. 2nd ed. Edinburgh: Elsevier Health Sciences; 2007. p. 208–12.
145. Szekanecz Z, Kerekes G, Soltész P. Vascular effects of biologic agents in RA and spondyloarthropathies. Nat Rev Rheumatol. 2009 Dec;5(12):677.
146. Gleghorn K, Wilson J, Wilkerson M. Rituximab: uses in dermatology. Skin Therapy Lett. 2016 Sep 1;21:5–7.
147. Croxtall JD. Ustekinumab. Drugs. 2011 Sep 1;71(13):1733–53.

148. Holm JG, Agner T, Sand C, Thomsen SF. Omalizumab for atopic dermatitis: case series and a systematic review of the literature. Int J Dermatol. 2017 Jan;56(1):18–26.
149. Graves JE, Nunley K, Heffernan MP. Off-label uses of biologics in dermatology: rituximab, omalizumab, infliximab, etanercept, adalimumab, efalizumab, and alefacept (part 2 of 2). J Am Acad Dermatol. 2007 Jan 1;56(1):e55–79.
150. Gooderham MJ, Hong HC, Eshtiaghi P, Papp KA. Dupilumab: A review of its use in the treatment of atopic dermatitis. J Am Acad Dermatol. 2018 Mar 1;78(3):S28–36.
151. Robert M, Miossec P. Effects of Interleukin 17 on the cardiovascular system. Autoimmun Rev. 2017 Sep;16(9):984–91.
152. Tabata MM, Choi S, Hirotsu K, Kwong B, Soleymani T. Cardiotoxicity associated with immune checkpoint inhibitors in cutaneous. J Am Acad Dermatol. 2019 Aug 19;81(2) https://doi.org/10.1016/j.jaad.2019.08.033.
153. Johnson DB, Balko JM, Compton ML, Chalkias S, Gorham J, Xu Y, et al. Fulminant myocarditis with combination immune checkpoint blockade. N Engl J Med. 2016 Nov 3;375(18):1749–55.

The Importance of Cardiac Assessment in the Era of Biologic Therapies for Psoriasis

23

Carmen Salavastru, Dedee F. Murrell, and James Otton

Introduction

Cardiovascular comorbidities are common among patients with psoriasis and cardiovascular risk factor screening of adult patients with psoriasis in primary care has found a high proportion of patients are treated sub-optimally for known cardiovascular risk factors. This can contribute to an increased risk of major cardiovascular events in patients with psoriasis.

Biologic therapies are increasingly used for the treatment of moderate–severe psoriasis, but their cardiovascular safety profile is still unclear [1].

Clinical trials are performed on a specific patient population carefully selected with the help of inclusion criteria and exclusion criteria. These criteria, if too stringent, can dramatically reduce the scope of the trial population and impair the generalizability of the results to the general psoriasis population. Concerning cardiovascular diseases and other organopathies, protocols from the period 2000–2009 excluded patients with symptoms of severe, progressive or uncontrolled disease or history of hospital admission for cardiac disease or stroke within the last year. More restrictive criteria, e.g. systolic blood pressure over 160 mmHg or

C. Salavastru (✉)
Paediatric Dermatology Department, Colentina Clinical Hospital, "Carol Davila" University of Medicine and Pharmacy, Bucharest, Romania
e-mail: carmen.salavastru@umfcd.ro

D. F. Murrell
Head of Department of Dermatology, St George Hospital, University of New South Wales, Sydney, NSW, Australia
e-mail: d.murrell@unsw.edu.au

J. Otton
Department of Cardiology, Liverpool Hospital, University of New South Wales, Sydney, NSW, Australia
e-mail: j.otton@unsw.edu.au

C. Salavastru et al. (eds.), *Skin and the Heart*,
https://doi.org/10.1007/978-3-030-54779-0_23

diastolic over 95 mmHg, were introduced in the 2010–2015 period [2]. Psoriasis patients with abnormal ECGs are now also routinely excluded from clinical trials [3–5].

Evidence-based decision making and management of chronic plaque psoriasis requires both efficacy and safety data. As already recognized, network meta-analysis and similarly randomized clinical trials (included in meta-analyses) have limitations that affect the interpretation of the significance of rare events. These studies are designed to detect differences in the severity of psoriasis in response to therapy over short periods of treatment and are often underpowered and of insufficient duration to detect rare or long-term adverse events [6].

Unlike randomized controlled trials, which enroll patients with less comorbidity as compared to psoriasis patients in real-world settings, the study of Rungapiromnan et al. [1] is more likely to estimate cardiovascular diseases precisely considering of the entire spectrum of patients' comorbidities. The relatively short follow-up used in this study is a disadvantage since cardiovascular diseases may take a long time to manifest. Studies with more extended follow up are required to elucidate if there is a protective effect of biologic therapies in patients with psoriasis. As a conclusion, this large prospective cohort study found no significant differences in the risk of major cardiovascular events between three different biologic therapies and methotrexate. Additional studies with longer term follow-up are needed to investigate the potential effects of biologic therapies on the incidence of major cardiovascular events [1].

Garcia-Doval et al. showed patients ineligible for Randomized Controlled Trials (RCT) are an important proportion (30%) of those receiving systemic therapy for psoriasis [7]. These patients have a higher risk of Severe Adverse Effects (SAE) and should be closely monitored. Patients exposed to biologics (whether these patients are eligible for RCTs or ineligible) are susceptible to the same increase in risk of SAEs, but biologics add a higher baseline risk in patients who are ineligible for RCTs. The risk-benefit ratio in ineligible patients receiving biologics might be different from the ratio in eligible patients [7].

In the era of immunotherapy, monitoring of cardiovascular side effects is essential to optimize patient outcomes [8].

Several clinical studies support the protective effect of treatment with **anti–TNF (tumor necrosis factor)-α** and **anti–IL-6 receptor** monoclonal antibodies on cardiovascular risk in patients with rheumatoid arthritis or psoriasis [8–13].

Anti Tumor Necrosis Factor α

After initial small studies showed promise in treating congestive heart failure (CHF), etanercept was evaluated in two large multicenter trials for treating CHF. Both studies were stopped prematurely due to a failure to show any difference between placebo and treated patients, and one study showed a trend toward increased hospitalization and mortality with etanercept [14]. As with etanercept, infliximab was initially thought to show promise in the treatment of CHF, but at the higher doses of 10 mg/kg, it showed an increase in mortality and morbidity compared with both the placebo group and the 5 mg/kg group. Despite post-marketing case reports of new-onset CHF and worsening of CHF, others have shown conflicting evidence, showing that TNF inhibition does not increase the risk of developing CHF [15]. Patients with known CHF should use these drugs with caution; if used, cardiology co-management is advised [9].

Interleukin 12/23 Inhibitors and Interleukin 17 Inhibitors

Beneficial effects of **antibodies targeting the IL-23/ IL-17 axis** have been reported in patients with psoriasis, but caution about their cardiovascular safety is warranted, especially in patients at high cardiovascular risk [8].

Interleukin 12/23 Inhibitors

Initial analyses of IL-12/23 inhibitors expressed concern regarding an increased risk of Major Adverse Cardiovascular Events (MACE) which led to the discontinuation of briakinumab clinical trials in 2011. Since then, further studies have been performed to assess the risk of MACE with IL-12/23 inhibitors, including ustekinumab [16]. Although there was concern regarding increased risk of MACE with ustekinumab in the phase II trial (five events in the ustekinumab group compared with none in the placebo group), the rate of MACE in phase III trials were shown to be low and not significantly increased [17, 18].

It was also found that a high proportion of patients recruited into the psoriasis clinical trials had cardiovascular risk factors such as obesity, smoking, high blood pressure, and diabetes, which was consistent with previous reports [19]. A recent meta-analysis of randomized clinical trials was conducted to evaluate the risk of MACE in patients with plaque psoriasis that are exposed to biologic therapies including anti-TNF-α agents (adalimumab, etanercept, and infliximab), anti-IL 12/23 agent (ustekinumab), and anti-IL17A agents (secukinumab and ixekizumab) [20].

From a total patient population of 12,596, the rates of MACE were 0.05% for TNF-α inhibitors, 0.09% for anti-IL17A agents, 0.07% for ustekinumab, and 0.04% for placebo. Overall, there was no statistically significant difference in the risk of MACE between patients on biologic therapies and patients on placebo. Also, there was no significant difference in the rate of MACE observed in patients receiving anti-TNF, IL-17A, or IL-12/23 treatments. Furthermore, the use of ustekinumab over 4 years was associated with decreased risk of MACE when compared with the general US population [21]. Thus far, the risk of MACE appears to be primarily caused by the disease status (e.g., severe inflammatory condition) and/or the patient population (e.g., associated comorbidities predisposing to cardiovascular events) [20].

Poizeau et al. found increased MACE in psoriasis patients with high cardiovascular risk treated with IL-12/IL23 inhibitors (n = 9290) in a retrospective study [22].

Interleukin 17 Inhibitors

There is no mention of MACE in the newly published *Comprehensive Dermatologic Drug Therapy* [23].

A review published in 2016 lists case reports relating to Brodalumab including death among patients in brodalumab trials (AMAGINE 2 and AMAGINE 3 [24]) – due to stroke, cardiac arrest, carcinoma of pancreas, cardiomyopathy and hematophagic histiocytosis syndrome [25].

Interleukin 23 Inhibitors [26]

Guselkumab. In Phase III trials in VOYAGE 1 and 2,rates of reported AE and SAE in the Guselkumab group were comparable to those in the Adalimumab group. In each study arm one myocardial infarction was reported. Discontinuation of Guselkimab due to AEs was uncommon [26–28].

With tildrakizumab the frequency of hypertension was noted to appear in a dose related manner; however, the majority of the these patients had hypertension or borderline hypertension at baseline and none discontinued as a result of this AE. Confirmed MACE (e.g., nonfatal myocardial infarction, nonfatal stroke, and cardiovascular deaths that were confirmed as 'cardiovascular' or 'sudden') are reported in the reSURFACE 1 and 2 studies [26, 29].

In the UltMMa-2 trial, risankizumab, randomized to ustekinumab, there was a higher frequency of MACE, malignancy of any kind and death in the risankizumab arm. [26] In the UltIMMa-2 trial, one patient died from sudden cardiac arrest 101 days following the last dose of risankizumab, and another died 161 days after the last dose of risankizumab from an unknown cause (events were not considered to be related to study drug by the investigator) [26, 30].

An additional patient on risankizumab died of an acute myocardial infarction on day 73 of the IMMvent trial, and two MACE occurred in IMMhance in patients receiving risankizumab, one of which resulted in death. [26, 31, 32] All of these patients had a history of cardiovascular risk factors [26].

Further research is needed to determine whether risankizumab can be implicated in the occurrence of MACE [26].

These biologics provide effective options for patients while maintaining a relatively good safety profile.

However, long-term effects will still need to be monitored through further research and postmarketing surveillance.

Treatment with the **anti–IL-1β antibody canakinumab** significantly reduced recurrent cardiovascular events in individuals with stable coronary artery disease well-treated with standard-of-care measures. Other clinical studies support the protective effects of treatment with anti–TNF-α and anti–IL-6 receptor monoclonal antibodies on cardiovascular risk. Blockade of the IL-23/ IL-17 axis, however, warrants caution if the patient has several cardiac risk factors, since targeting this pathway has improved psoriasis but may augment cardiovascular risk in certain patients. Further post-marketing surveillance and registries are therefore important. Thus, careful consideration of the cardiovascular risk profile may influence the choice of the most appropriate treatment for patients with chronic inflammatory diseases [8].

How Important Is to Have a More in Depth Analysis of the Cardiac Function Before Starting a Biologic Treatment in the Psoriasis Patient?

When planning on prescribing a systemic therapy to psoriasis patients, several aspects should be considered:

1. the cardiovascular risk associated with psoriasis
2. the cardiovascular status of the patient: sub-clinical dysfunction or clinically manifest conditions
3. the potential cardiovascular adverse effects of the considered medication

A recent article of Hansen et al. [33] suggests that psoriasis per se is not associated with significant abnormalities of the electrocardiogram.

However, new evidence emerges on various associations between psoriasis and cardiovascular conditions beyond the classical recognition of the cardiovascular comorbidities and cardiovascular risk of these patients.

Cardiac Rate, Rhythms and Conduction Disturbances

Hsien-Yi et al. investigated whether patients with psoriasis have an increased risk of arrhythmia by studying population-based cohort. They identified 40,637 patients with psoriasis and 162,548 subjects without psoriasis matched by age, sex, history of coronary artery disease, hypertension, and diabetes in the Taiwan National Health Insurance Research Database during 2004 through 2006 and the conclusion was that patients with psoriasis were at higher risk of developing arrhythmia, particularly those with psoriatic arthritis, independent of traditional cardiovascular risk factors [34].

Psoriasis vulgaris is a chronic, multisystem disease that results in the development of atrial fibrillation (AF) over time. In one study, the authors' goal was to assess predictors of AF in patients with psoriasis, including total atrial conduction time (TACT) and left atrial global longitudinal strain (LAGLS). A total of 80 individuals, including 40 psoriasis patients and 40 healthy controls, were enrolled in the study. A physical examination was performed, biochemical parameters were studied, and Holter electrocardiography was carried out. Conventional echocardiography, atrial tissue Doppler, and speckle tracking echocardiography were recorded and the authors determined that LAGLS decreased, TACT was prolonged, and PWD increased in patients with psoriasis. There is a relationship between TACT, LAGLS, PWD and the duration and severity of disease. These results demonstrate that LAGLS, TACT, and PWD (P-wave duration difference) are important markers with the ability to predict AF, and are capable of detecting the subclinical electrophysiological changes in psoriasis patients. Since anti-arrhythmic preventive measures may not be effective in this specific patient subset, the authors believe that clinicians should be alert to patients experiencing dyspnoea and palpitations, knowing the increased prevalence of AF [35].

A meta-analysis of prospective studies demonstrated that patients with psoriasis have increased risk of new-onset atrial fibrillation and future interventional studies addressing the impact of psoriasis treatment and prevention of atrial fibrillation should be performed [36].

Increased heart rate and reduced heart-rate variability are associated with subclinical inflammation in healthy middle-aged and elderly subjects. The increased mortality that has been reported in these settings may thus have a common aetiology. An autonomic imbalance in favour of the sympathetic system may interact with inflammatory processes to play a more important role in the process of atherosclerosis than previously thought [37].

Since the Tp-e interval (interval between the peak and the end of the T wave on an ECG) and Tp-e/QT ratio have been accepted as new markers for the assessment of myocardial repolarization and ventricular arrhythmogenesis, Arisoy et al aimed in their study to assess ventricular repolarization in patients with psoriasis using Tp-e interval and Tp-e/QT ratio.

The study population consisted of 74 patients with psoriasis and 74 healthy volunteers. The diagnosis of psoriasis was based on a clinical or histopathological examination of all patients. QT interval, corrected QT (QTc), QT dispersion (QTd), Tp-e interval, corrected Tp-e, and Tp-e/QT ratio were measured from the 12-lead electrocardiogram. These parameters were compared between groups.

According to the electrocardiographic parameters, QT and QTc intervals and QTd were significantly higher in patients with psoriasis than in control subjects. The Tp-e interval, corrected Tp-e, and Tp-e/QT ratio were significantly higher in patients with psoriasis than in control.

Additionally, the CRP value was an independent predictor of an increased Tp-e/QT ratio.

The study revealed that ventricular repolarization features were impaired in patients with psoriasis. Therefore, these patients should be more closely screened for ventricular arrhythmias [38].

P terminal force in lead V1 of a standard 12-lead electrocardiogram (ECG) (PTF) $\geq$ 0.04 mm s is a relatively common finding in a 12-lead ECG of middle-aged subjects. PTF $\geq$ 0.06 mm s is associated with increased risk for atrial fibrillation and death in the general population [39].

Other Sources of Cardiac Dysfunction

Myocardial fibrosis causes the fragmentation of QRS complexes on electrocardiography. It was hypothesized that the frequency of fragmented QRS (fQRS) could be more common in patients with psoriasis vulgaris than in healthy control subjects. In this prospective study, 100 patients with psoriasis vulgaris who did not have any cardiovascular disease were compared with 50 healthy volunteers in control group. The Psoriasis Area Severity Index (PASI) was used for expressing the severity of psoriasis. Patients with psoriasis were categorized according to presence of fQRS in ECG. Patients with psoriasis had higher frequency of fQRS, higher levels of C reactive protein (CRP) and sedimentation rate (ESR) than the control group. Within the patient group there was no statistically significant difference between fQRS (+) and fQRS (−) subgroups with regards to sex, disease duration, CRP, ESR, medications and PASI score. It was suggested that presence of fQRS in ECG may be related with myocardial fibrosis in patients with psoriasis who do not have cardiovascular disease. For this reason, in the authors' opinion, fQRS could be used as a predictive marker for myocardial fibrosis in patients with psoriasis [40].

Although increased CV risks in psoriasis are well established, there are no data about changes of contraction synchrony in psoriasis. Therefore, Bulbul et al. [41] aimed to study the left ventricular (LV) contraction synchrony in patients with psoriasis with narrow QRS and normal ejection fraction.

Fifty patients with psoriasis and 50 age- and sex-matched control subjects were included in the study. LV dyssynchrony was investigated by color-coded tissue Doppler imaging. In the psoriasis group, the mean high-sensitive C-reactive protein values were significantly higher compared with the controls. Peak A velocity, deceleration time, isovolumetric relaxation time, and E/E' values were higher in the psoriasis group; however, E/A ratio and average Em were higher in the control group. LV systolic dyssynchrony parameters [including standard deviation of Ts of the 12 LV segments (Ts-SD-12), maximal difference in Ts between any two of the 12 LV segments, standard deviation of Ts of the six basal LV segments, and maximal difference in Ts between any two of the six basal LV segments] were found to be higher in the psoriasis group. Patients with ventricular dyssynchrony (a Ts-SD-12 > 34.4 ms) were more numerous in the psoriasis group than the control group (34% vs. 6%, $P < 0.01$). Therefore, the authors concluded that in patients with psoriasis with normal ejection fractions and narrow QRS, LV systolic dyssynchrony is an early manifestation of heart involvement and may coexist with diastolic dysfunction [41]

The systemic inflammatory process that characterizes both rheumatoid arthritis and psoriasis may cause adverse structural and functional changes in the walls of the atria, particularly in the left atrium [42].

The resulting inflammation-related atrial myopathy leads to blood stasis, thrombus formation, and thromboembolic stroke.

The concept that many patients with rheumatoid arthritis and psoriasis have a tendency towards undiagnosed atrial myopathy is strongly supported by the available evidence. These patients frequently show abnormalities of electrical activation in the atria, and derangements in atrial geometry and filling, particularly affecting the left atrium.

The magnitude of these abnormalities closely parallels the severity of clinical inflammation. Both rheumatoid arthritis and psoriasis are associated with an expansion of epicardial adipose tissue mass that is proportional to the clinical severity of the disease but independent of body mass. In patients with atrial fibrillation, there is a close association between the thickness and inflammatory state of epicardial fat and the severity of electrical abnormalities in the adjacent myocardium. Accordingly, epicardial fat volume predicts the incidence of atrial fibrillation in the community even in the absence of cardiovascular disease. Epicardial adipose tissue mass increases as atrial fibrillation evolves from a paroxysmal to a persistent arrhythmia. There is a strong association between epicardial adipose tissue mass and derangements in atrial fibrillation geometry and function, potentially explaining why an expansion of epicardial adipose tissue presages an exaggerated risk of thromboembolic events [43].

Clinically Silent Cardiac Malfunction in Psoriasis Patient

Yildiz reported a subclinical impairment of the aortic pulse wave velocity in chronic inflammatory rheumatic disorders, such as SLE, RA, psoriasis and systemic sclerosis, mainly due to the chronic inflammatory status [44].

The analysis of echocardiographic parameters revealed normal dimension, mass and systolic function of the left ventricle. Left ventricular diastolic dysfunction was found in 36.5% patients in the psoriasis group versus 0% in control group, and significant reduction of the E/A ratio was found also for the right ventricle. A significant increase of mitral regurgitation has been found in psoriatic patients. The early recognition of cardiovascular sub-clinical disease in psoriatic patients may guide a strict follow up and an early treatment, potentially improving cardiovascular prognosis [45].

The Need for Cardiology Assessment

As practitioners more readily recognize psoriasis as a systemic disease and place more emphasis on controlling systemic inflammation, treatment goals can be separated into two distinct categories based on the feasibility of achieving desired outcomes. The first and most practically implementable goal is potentially preventing damage associated with systemic inflammation while simultaneously potentially preventing the progression of psoriasis and its comorbidities. The second, perhaps loftier and more forward-thinking goal is potentially reversing existing inflammatory damage and signs and symptoms of comorbidities. Current evidence suggests that preventing damage associated with inflammation, and preventing development of future inflammatory damage and comorbidities, may be a potentially achievable treatment goal for many patients with moderate-to-severe plaque psoriasis when biological therapies are utilized early in the disease [46].

There is mounting evidence that immune diseases, such as ankylosing spondylitis or early severe psoriasis, also increase cardiovascular risk, with risk ratios approaching those in rheumatoid arthritis [47].

The 2019 ACC/AHA Guideline on the Primary Prevention of Cardiovascular Disease lists psoriasis as a Risk-Enhancing Factors for Clinician–Patient Risk Discussion [48].

Psoriasis of any severity was deemed to be associated with an increased risk of myocardial infarction and stroke. Severe psoriasis is also associated with an increased risk of cardiovascular mortality. Future studies should include more complete covariate adjustment and characterization of psoriasis severity [49].

These findings prompt the authors to consider recommending thorough cardiovascular risk factor and symptom review or perhaps initial cardiology consultation, for the psoriasis patients, regardless of the presence of cardiovascular symptoms. This is especially important in patients with severe psoriasis and psoriatic arthritis psoriasis.

The consultation should include:

- Physical examination
- ECG
- Assessment of the cardiovascular risk and assessment of the MACE
- Assessment of the potential adverse effects of the systemic psoriasis medication
- Assessment of the potential benefits of the systemic psoriasis medication
- Consideration of echocardiography in order to detect early, sub-clinical alteration in the cardiac function if any abnormality in the above history, examination or ECG is detected.

Contingent on the initial findings of the cardiovascular assessment, co-management of the patient by the Dermatologist and the Cardiologist can be considered.

The authors consider that assessment of cardiovascular risk factors on a yearly basis may be of benefit to the psoriatic patient.

References

1. Rungapiromnan W, Mason KJ, Lunt M, et al. Risk of major cardiovascular events in patients with psoriasis receiving biologic therapies: a prospective cohort study. J Eur Acad Dermatol Venereol. 2020;34:769–78.
2. Kirsten N, Bulai Livideanu C, Richard MA, Konstantinou MP, Khemis A, Balluteaud C, Goujon C, Beylot-Barry M, Paul C. Inclusion and exclusion criteria in phase III trials with systemic agents in psoriasis: the external validity of drug development. Br J Dermatol. 2016;175:636–8.
3. https://clinicaltrials.gov/ct2/show/NCT01265667; Accessed 16 June 2020
4. https://clinicaltrials.gov/ct2/show/NCT03675542; Accessed 16 June 2020
5. https://clinicaltrials.gov/ct2/show/NCT03478280; Accessed 16 June 2020
6. Sbidian E, Chaimani A, Garcia-Doval I, Do G, Hua C, Mazaud C, Droitcourt C, Hughes C, Ingram JR, Naldi L, Chosidow O, Le Cleach L. Systemic pharmacological treatments for chronic plaque psoriasis: a network meta-analysis. Cochrane Database Syst Rev. 2017;12:CD011535.
7. Garcia-Doval I, Carretero G, Vanaclocha F, et al. Risk of serious adverse events associated with biologic and nonbiologic psoriasis systemic therapy: patients ineligible vs eligible for randomized controlled trials. Arch Dermatol. 2012;148(4):463–70.
8. Ait-Oufella H, Libby P, Tedgui A. Anticytokine immune therapy and atherothrombotic cardiovascular risk. Arterioscler Thromb Vasc Biol. 2019;39:1510–9.
9. Makerowski J, Gordon KB. Tumor necrosis factor inhibitors. In: Wolverton SE, Wu JJ, editors. Comprehensive dermatologic drug therapy. 4th ed. Philadelphia: Elsevier; 2021.

10. Di Minno MN, Iervolino S, Peluso R, Scarpa R, Di Minno G, CaRRDs Study Group. Carotid intima-media thickness in psoriatic arthritis: differences between tumor necrosis factor-α blockers and traditional disease-modifying antirheumatic drugs. Arterioscler Thromb Vasc Biol. 2011;31:705–12. https://doi.org/10.1161/ATVBAHA.110.214585.
11. Jacobsson LT, Turesson C, Gülfe A, Kapetanovic MC, Petersson IF, Saxne T, Geborek P. Treatment with tumor necrosis factor blockers is associated with a lower incidence of first cardiovascular events in patients with rheumatoid arthritis. J Rheumatol. 2005;32:1213–8.
12. Ahlehoff O, Skov L, Gislason G, Gniadecki R, Iversen L, Bryld LE, Lasthein S, Lindhardsen J, Kristensen SL, Torp-Pedersen C, Hansen PR. Cardiovascular outcomes and systemic anti-inflammatory drugs in patients with severe psoriasis: 5-year follow-up of a Danish nationwide cohort. J Eur Acad Dermatol Venereol. 2015;29:1128–34.
13. Ljung L, Rantapää-Dahlqvist S, Jacobsson LT, Askling J. Response to biological treatment and subsequent risk of coronary events in rheumatoid arthritis. Ann Rheum Dis. 2016;75:2087–94.
14. Khanna D, McMahon M, Furst DE. Anti-tumor necrosis factor alpha therapy and heart failure: what have we learned and where do we go from here? Arthritis Rheum. 2004;50(4):1040–50.
15. Listing J, Strangfeld A, Kekow J, et al. Does tumor necrosis factor alpha inhibition promote or prevent heart failure in patients with rheumatoid arthritis? Arthritis Rheum. 2008;58(3):667–77.
16. Kim HJ, Lebwohl M. Interleukin 12/23 Inhibitors. In: Wolverton SE, Wu JJ, editors. Comprehensive dermatologic drug therapy. 4th ed. Philadelphia: Elsevier; 2021.
17. Papp KA, Langley RG, Lebwohl M, et al. Efficacy and safety of ustekinumab, a human interleukin-12/23 monoclonal antibody, in patients with psoriasis: 52-week results from a randomised, double-blind, placebo-controlled trial (PHOENIX 2). Lancet. 2008;371(9625):1675–84.
18. Gordon KB, Papp KA, Langley RG, et al. Long-term safety experience of ustekinumab in patients with moderate to severe psoriasis (Part II of II): results from analyses of infections and malignancy from pooled phase II and III clinical trials. J Am Acad Dermatol. 2012;66(5):742–51.
19. Kimball AB, Wu Y. Cardiovascular disease and classic cardiovascular risk factors in patients with psoriasis. Int J Dermatol. 2009;48(11):1147–56.
20. Rungapiromnan W, Yiu ZZN, Warren RB, Griffiths CEM, Ashcroft DM. Impact of biologic therapies on risk of major adverse cardiovascular events in patients with psoriasis: systematic review and meta-analysis of randomized controlled trials. Br J Dermatol. 2017;176(4):890–901.
21. Hugh J, Van Voorhees AS, Nijhawan RI, et al. From the Medical Board of the National Psoriasis Foundation: the risk of cardiovascular disease in individuals with psoriasis and the potential impact of current therapies. J Am Acad Dermatol. 2014;70(1):168–77.
22. Poizeau F, Nowak E, Kerbrat S, Droitcourt C, Drici M, Sbidian E, Guillot B, Bachelez H, Happe A, Oger E, Dupuy A. Accidents cardiovasculaires précoces sous Ustekinumab. Journes Dermatologiques de Paris: Paris; 2018.
23. Chima MA, Lebwohl M. Interleukin 17 Inhibitors. In: Wolverton SE, Wu JJ, editors. Comprehensive dermatologic drug therapy. 4th ed. Philadelphia: Elsevier; 2021.
24. Lebwohl M, Strober B, Menter A, et al. Phase 3 studies comparing Brodalumab with Ustekinumab in Psoriasis. N Engl J Med. 2015;373(14):1318–28.
25. Wasilewska A, Winiarska M, Olszewska M, Rudnicka L. Interleukin-17 inhibitors. A new era in treatment of psoriasis and other skin diseases. Postepy Dermatol Alergol. 2016 Aug;33(4):247–52.
26. LEE EB, Amin M, Wu JJ. Interleukin23 inhibitors. In: Wolverton SE, Wu JJ, editors. Comprehensive dermatologic drug therapy. 4th ed. Philadelphia: Elsevier; 2021.
27. Blauvelt A, Papp KA, Griffiths CE, et al. Efficacy and safety of guselkumab, an anti-interleukin-23 monoclonal antibody, compared with adalimumab for the continuous treatment of patients with moderate to severe psoriasis: results from the phase III, double-blinded, placebo- and active comparator-controlled VOYAGE 1 trial. J Am Acad Dermatol. 2017;76(3):405–17.
28. Reich K, Armstrong AW, Foley P, et al. Efficacy and safety of guselkumab, an anti-interleukin-23 monoclonal antibody, compared with adalimumab for the treatment of patients with moderate to severe psoriasis with randomized withdrawal and retreatment: Results from

the phase III, double-blind, placebo- and active comparator-controlled VOYAGE 2 trial. J Am Acad Dermatol. 2017;76(3):418–31.
29. Reich K, Papp KA, Blauvelt A, et al. Tildrakizumab versus placebo or etanercept for chronic plaque psoriasis (reSURFACE 1 and reSURFACE 2): results from two randomised controlled, phase 3 trials [published correction appears in Lancet. 2017 Jul 15;390(10091):230]. Lancet. 2017;390(10091):276–88.
30. Gordon KB, Strober B, Lebwohl M, et al. Efficacy and safety of risankizumab in moderate-to-severe plaque psoriasis (UltIMMa-1 and UltIMMa-2): results from two double-blind, randomised, placebo-controlled and ustekinumab-controlled phase 3 trials. Lancet. 2018;392(10148):650–61.
31. Reich K, Gooderham M, Thaçi D, et al. Risankizumab compared with adalimumab in patients with moderate-to-severe plaque psoriasis (IMMvent): a randomised, double-blind, active-comparator-controlled phase 3 trial [published correction appears in Lancet. 2019 Jul 16]. Lancet. 2019;394(10198):576–86.
32. Blauvelt A, Leonardi CL, Gooderham M, et al. Efficacy and safety of continuous Risankizumab therapy vs treatment withdrawal in patients with moderate to severe plaque psoriasis: a phase 3 randomized clinical trial [published online ahead of print, 2020 Apr 8]. JAMA Dermatol. 2020:e200723.
33. Hansen RP, Juhl CR, Idaksen JL, Jemec GB, Ellervik Kanters JKC. Am J Cardiol. 2018;121:1004–7.
34. Hsien-Yi C, Chang WL, Huang WF, Wen YW, Tsai YW, Tsai TF. Increased risk of arrhythmia in patients with psoriatic disease: a nationwide population-based matched cohort study. J Am Acad Dermatol. 2015;73(3):429–38.
35. Duman H, Dilek N, Demirelli S, Inci S, Duman H, Çetin M, Durakoğlugil ME. The relationship between total atrial conduction time and left atrial global strain in patients with psoriasis vulgaris. Arch Med Sci. 2019;15(4):865–71.
36. Upala S, Shahnawaz A, Sanguankeo A. Psoriasis increases risk of new-onset atrial fibrillation: a systematic review and meta-analysis of prospective observational studies. J Dermatol Treat. 2017;28(5):406–10.
37. Sajadieh A, Nielsen OW, Rasmussen V, Hein HO, Abedini S, Hansen JF. Increased heart rate and reduced heart-rate variability are associated with subclinical inflammation in middle-aged and elderly subjects with no apparent heart disease. Eur Heart J. 2004;25(5):363–70.
38. Arısoy A, Karaman K, Karayakalı M, Demirelli S, Seçkin HY, Çelik A, Ceyhan K. Evaluation of ventricular repolarization features with novel electrocardiographic parameters (Tp-e, Tp-e/QT) in patients with psoriasis. Anatol J Cardiol. 2017;18:397–401.
39. Eranti A, Aro AL, Kerola T, Anttonen O, Rissanen HA, Tikkanen JT, Junttila MJ, Kenttä TV, Knekt P, Huikuri HV. Prevalence and prognostic significance of abnormal P terminal force in lead V1 of the ECG in the general population. Circ Arrhythm Electrophysiol. 2014;7:1116–21.
40. Baş Y, Altunkaş F, Seçkin HY, et al. Frequency of fragmented QRS in patient with psoriasis vulgaris without cardiovascular disease. Arch Dermatol Res. 2016;308:367–71.
41. Bulbul Sen B, Rifaioglu EN, Ekiz O, Buyukkaya E, Kurt M, Karakas MF, Buyukkaya S, Bilen P, Akcay AB, Sen N. Assessment of left ventricular dyssynchrony in patients with psoriasis. Int J Dermatol. 2014;53(10):1221–7.
42. Dai H, Wang X, Yin S, Zhang Y, Han Y, Yang N, Xu J, Sun L, Yuan Y, Sheng L, Gong Y, Li Y. Atrial fibrillation promotion in a rat model of rheumatoid arthritis. J Am Heart Assoc. 2017;6:e007320.
43. Parker M. Potential role of atrial myopathy in the pathogenesis of stroke in rheumatoid arthritis and psoriasis: a conceptual framework and implications for prophylaxis. J Am Heart Assoc. 2020;9:e014764.
44. Yildiz M. Arterial distensibility in chronic inflammatory rheumatic disorders. Open Cardiovasc Med J. 2010;4:83–8.
45. Gorga E, Scodro M, Valentini F, D'Ortona R, Arisi M, Sciatti E, Bonadei I, Regazzoni V, Vizzardi E, Metra M, Calzavara Pinton P. Echocardiographic evaluation of diastolic dysfunction

in young and healthy patients with psoriasis: a case-control study. Monaldi Arch Chest Dis. 2018;88(3):934.

46. Korman NJ. Management of psoriasis as a systemic disease: what is the evidence? Br. J Dermatol. 2020;182:840–8.
47. Piepoli MF, Hoes AW, Agewall S, et al. 2016 European Guidelines on cardiovascular disease prevention in clinical practice: The Sixth Joint Task Force of the European Society of Cardiology and Other Societies on Cardiovascular Disease Prevention in Clinical Practice (constituted by representatives of 10 societies and by invited experts)Developed with the special contribution of the European Association for Cardiovascular Prevention & Rehabilitation (EACPR). Eur Heart J. 2016;37(29):2315–81.
48. Arnett DK, Blumenthal RS, Albert MA, Buroker AB, Goldberger ZD, Hahn EJ, Himmelfarb CD, Khera A, Lloyd-Jones D, McEvoy JW, Michos ED, Miedema MD, Muoz D, Smith SC Jr, Virani SS, Williams KA Sr, Yeboah J, Ziaeian B. 2019 ACC/AHA guideline on the primary prevention of cardiovascular disease: a report of the American College of Cardiology/American Heart Association Task Force on Clinical Practice Guidelines. Circulation. 2019;140:e596–646.
49. Armstrong EJ, Harskamp CT, Armstrong AW. Psoriasis and major adverse cardiovascular events: a systematic review and meta-analysis of observational studies. J Am Heart Assoc. 2013;2:e000062.

Part VII

Erythroderma and High Output Cardiac Failure

Erythroderma and Cardiac Function

24

Carmen Salavastru, Stefana Cretu,
and George Sorin Tiplica

Introduction

Erythroderma is a clinical syndrome characterized by cutaneous inflammation, manifested as erythema and scaling involving 90% or more of the body surface area [1–4]. Also referred to as exfoliative dermatitis, erythroderma is not a common occurrence and its true incidence is not known [1, 5]. It may affect both adults and children. Sometimes it can be part of genetic conditions, such as ichtyosis [6]. The cutaneous inflammation underlying erythroderma is accompanied by vasodilatation, increased capillary permeability, edema, loss of fluids, proteins and electrolytes [3]. All of these events can have a significant impact on all organ systems, particularly on the cardiovascular function, threatening survival [1].

Etiology and Population Affected

Erythroderma is a severe clinical endpoint of several conditions. It may develop slowly, over time or abruptly. Most studies report that the majority of cases are exacerbations of a previous dermatological disease. Psoriasis (Fig. 24.1) or eczema

C. Salavastru (✉)
Paediatric Dermatology Department, Carol Davila University of Medicine and Pharmacy, Bucharest, Romania

S. Cretu
Dermatology Department, Carol Davila University of Medicine and Pharmacy, Bucharest, Romania

G. S. Tiplica
"Carol Davila" University of Medicine and Pharmacy, Dermatology II, Colentina Clinical Hospital, Bucharest, Romania
e-mail: george.tiplica@umfcd.ro

C. Salavastru et al. (eds.), *Skin and the Heart*,
https://doi.org/10.1007/978-3-030-54779-0_24

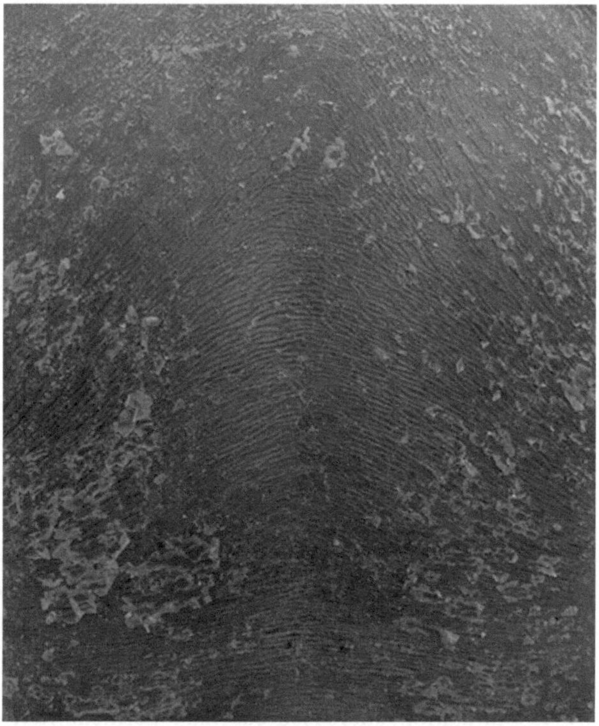

Fig. 24.1 Erythrodermic psoriasis

are the most frequent causes, although pityriazis rubra pilaris or genetic diseases, such as congenital ichtyosiforme erythroderma (Fig. 24.2), lamellar ichtyosis or Darier's disease might also be involved. Other etiologies are cutaneous T cell lymphoma (CTLC) and drug reactions. However, in a small number of cases, etiology remains unknown [4, 6–8]. Incidence of erythroderma and distribution of etiology are difficult to assess. One reason is that most of the available literature consists of retrospective studies. Another reason is the variation amongst study populations, different genetic backgrounds and patient related features, diverse environments, both from the geographical and social perspective [7]. Reported incidence of erythroderma in one Portuguese study was 9.4 cases/year. Other several studies found that between 13–35 in 100.000 dermatologic patients present with erythroderma [1, 7, 8]. Elderly patients and those with large body surface areas involvement are most at risk for developing life-threatening complications [3, 9]. Patients already suffering from heart failure or with low cardiac reserve are particularly at risk for the development pulmonary edema [10].

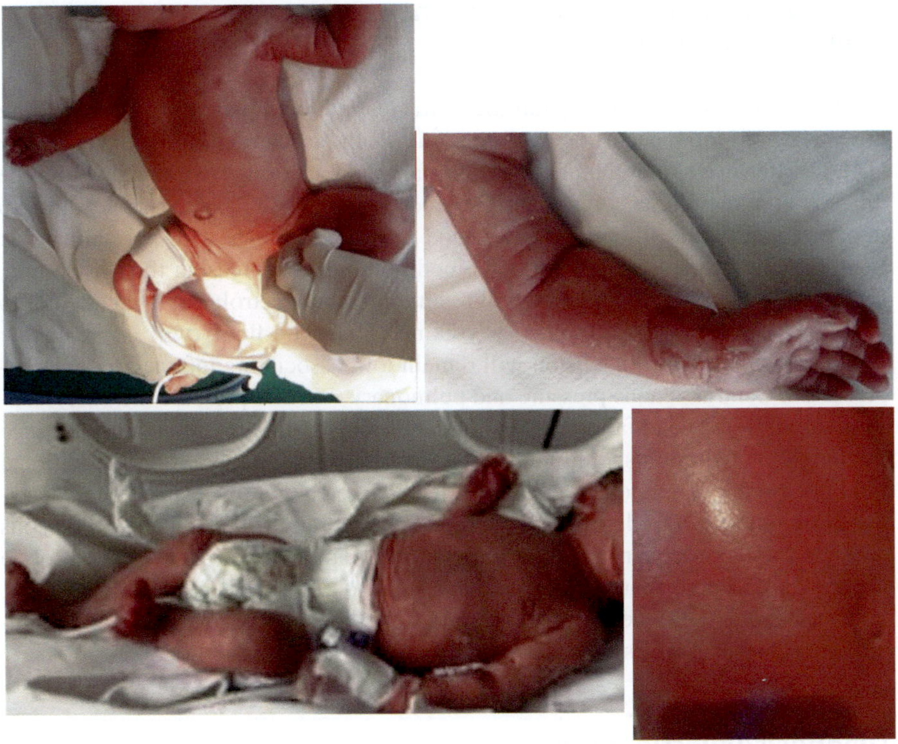

Fig. 24.2 Congenital ichtyosiform erythroderma in an infant with Netherton syndrome

Pathogenesis of Erythrodema

The mechanisms underlying erythroderma are not fully understood. Some studies have suggested that mechanisms may not be the same in all etiologies [1, 11]. Interplay between cytokines IL-1, IL-2, IL-8, tumor necrosis factor, interferon gamma and cellular adhesion molecules, particularly ICAM-1 results in increased leukocyte trafficking within the dermis, which then leads to increased proliferation of basal epidermal cells, with accelerated turnover and sheading at the skin surface. Increased endothelial-leukocyte interaction, mediated by adhesion molecules, stimulates inflammation of the dermis, an event clinically perceived as erythema. Scaling is the clinical image of the accelerated sheading of keratinocytes. Protein loss as a result of scaling is high in erythrodermic patients. The highest increase in protein loss, compared to normal levels is found in psoriasic erythroderma, 25–30%. In other etiologies, protein loss increases by 10–15% [1, 6, 11].

Pathogenesis of Cardiovascular Changes in Erythrodermic Patients

Cardiac failure is a complex syndrome characterized by impaired ventricular filling or ejection of blood, occurring as a consequence of structural or functional damage [12]. In extensive skin inflammation important fluid amounts are trapped within the dilated skin capillaries. Circulating blood volume, thus decreases leading to impaired ventricular filling and low blood pressure. Patients with normal cardiac function can compensate for the low blood volume by increasing their heart rate. However, without treatment, they will retain fluid and electrolytes, in an attempt to compensate for the low circulatory volume. The extra-fluids will arrive in the peripheral capillaries and tension will remain low, associating internal organ hypoperfusion. Central venous pressure and pulmonary vascular pressure increase, leading to high-output heart failure and pulmonary edema [10].Correcting this imbalance by fluid administration should not be attempted because it may produce additional fluid retention and pulmonary edema. Instead, targeted therapy against the underlying cause of the erythroderma and glucocorticoid therapy will resolve the cutaneous inflammation, consequently returning the blood volume to normal [10]. Electrolyte imbalance can contribute to the cardiovascular strain in erythrodermic patients. Hypocalcaemia is frequently observed and sometimes hypophosphatemia, particularly in erythrodermic psoriasis [13].

Diagnosis/Investigations

Erythrodermic patients should undergo a full clinical examination, with particular focus on the cardiovascular system, pulmonary and kidney functions. Urine levels should be monitored. A complete blood count, serum protein electrophoresis, erythrocyte sedimentation rate, electrolytes levels are all necessary. Cardiovascular ultrasound is also very important [10, 13, 14]. Skin biopsy in erythrodermic patients may reveal the etiology in some cases (Fig. 24.2), although in others, findings might prove non-specific [1, 3, 4, 6, 7].

Treatment

Patients already suffering from heart failure or with low cardiac reserve will not be able to compensate for the blood shunting at the dermal level by pumping more blood volume and are more at risk for pulmonary edema [10]. Additional fluid administration should be avoided. In these patients, systemic glucocorticoids must be started with caution, at low doses, as they can precipitate cardiogenic pulmonary edema. If the patient is already intubated and artificially ventilated, therapy can be started at the usual recommended doses [10]. Treatment of erythroderma should be direct towards the underlying cause, in addition to supportive measure [3, 4]. Good hygiene measures amongst the personnel caring for the patient and the patient's own personal hygiene are important in order to prevent infections. Topical therapy includes antiseptics, low to medium-potency corticosteroids and emollients. The latter are very important for restoring the barrier function of the skin [3].

Prognosis/Complications

Patients suffering from erythroderma have a higher death rate compared to age and gender matched controls, even if properly managed [1, 3, 5, 15]. These patients need to be hospitalized, etiology must be uncovered, anti-inflammatory medication and topical therapy should be started as soon as possible. Supportive care measures must be implemented [3]. Relapse rates vary between 26.2%-31.2% depending on study, etiology and follow-up period. Some authors have observed relapse rates as high as 100% in patients suffering from psoriasis or CTCL. In cases of drug induced erythroderma, identification and avoidance of the culprit drug are of paramount importance [5, 6, 8]. In a study conducted by Akhyani, drug induced erythroderma had the best prognosis [9].

References

1. Okoduwa C, Lambert WC, Schwartz RA, Kubeyinje E, Eitokpah A, Sinha S, Chen W. Erythroderma: review of a potentially life-threatening dermatosis. Indian J Dermatol. 2009 Jan;54(1):1.
2. Dobson JS, Levell NJ. Erythroderma. Medicine. 2017 Jul 1;45(7):417–21.
3. Inamadar AC, Palit A. Acute skin failure: concept, causes, consequences and care. Indian J Dermatol Venereol Leprol. 2005 Nov 1;71(6):379.
4. Vasconcellos C, Domingues PP, Aoki V, Miyake RK, Sauaia N, Martins JE. Erythroderma: analysis of 247 cases. Rev Saude Publica. 1995;29:177–82.
5. Rym BM, Mourad M, Bechir Z, Dalenda E, Faika C, Iadh AM, Amel BO. Erythroderma in adults: a report of 80 cases. Int J Dermatol. 2005 Sep;44(9):731–5
6. Cuellar-Barboza A, Ocampo-Candiani J, Herz-Ruelas ME. A practical approach to the diagnosis and treatment of adult erythroderma. Actas Dermo-Sifiliográficas (English Edition). 2018 Nov 1;109(9):777–90.
7. César A, Cruz M, Mota A, Azevedo F. Erythroderma. A clinical and etiological study of 103 patients. J Dermatol Case Rep. 2016 Mar 31;10(1):1.
8. Li J, Zheng HY. Erythroderma: a clinical and prognostic study. Dermatology. 2012;225(2):154–62.
9. Akhyani M, Ghodsi ZS, Toosi S, Dabbaghian H. Erythroderma: a clinical study of 97 cases. BMC Dermatol. 2005 Dec;5(1):5.
10. Taheri A, Mansouri AD, Mansoori P, Asad RI. Management of fluid status and cardiovascular function in patients with diffuse skin inflammation. J Dermatol Treat. 2019 Jul 4;30(5):506–10.
11. Sehgal VN, Srivastava G, Sardana K. Erythroderma/exfoliative dermatitis: a synopsis. Int J Dermatol. 2004 Jan;43(1):39–47.
12. Januzzi JLJR, Mann DL. Chapter 21: Approach to the patient with heart failure. In: Zipes DP, Libby P, Bonow RO, Mann DL, Tomaselli GF, editors. Braunwald's heart disease: a textbook of cardiovascular medicine, vol. 1. 7th ed. Philadelphia, PA: Elsevier Health Sciences; 2018.

13. McElhenny BE, Todd DJ, McCance D, Young I, Burrows D. Erythrodermic psoriasis. Report of a case associated with symptomatic hypophosphataemia. Clin Exp Dermatol. 1993 Mar;18(2):167–8.
14. Tan GF, Kong YL, Tan AS, Tey HL. Causes and features of erythroderma. Ann Acad Med Singapore. 2014 Aug 1;43(8):391–4.
15. Voigt GC, Kronthal HL, Crounse RG. Cardiac output in erythrodermic skin disease. Am Heart J. 1966 Nov 1;72(5):615–20.

Part VIII

Miscellaneous

Disorders of Fluid Regulation

25

Shruti Rateesh, Patrick Pender, and James Otton

From an evolutionary standpoint, the human body is designed to preserve circulating volumes in times of hypovolemia (or perceived hypovolemia). Low and high-pressure baroreceptors in various circulatory beds (most notably the carotid sinuses and the afferent glomerular arterioles), as well as ion channels in the distal tubule of the kidney, infer the body's volume. Ion channels in the hypothalamus sense the sodium concentration and extracellular fluid osmolality. Glomerular filtration rate, physical forces along the nephron, the sympathetic nervous system, and the renin-angiotensin-aldosterone system (RAAS) are the mechanisms by which volume balance is restored. Osmolality effectors include the stimulation of thirst, which results in the release of the antidiuretic hormone vasopressin, and the placement of aquaporin water channels in the renal collecting ducts so that concentrated urine can be made.

Survival depends on adequate blood perfusion of organ systems. The part of the intravascular, extracellular, volume within the arterial system effectively perfusing tissues is conceptualized as the effective arterial blood volume (EABV) [1]. Normal cell function and survival requires an uninterrupted supply of oxygen and nutrients, and elimination of carbon dioxide and metabolic by-products. Effective arterial blood volume is affected by red blood cell mass, plasma volume (which is a direct reflection of extracellular fluid volume), cardiac output, vascular capacity (total and regional arterial resistance), venous capacity, Starling forces at a capillary level, endothelial barrier integrity, and gravity.

S. Rateesh · P. Pender
Department of Cardiology, Liverpool Hospital, Sydney, NSW, Australia

J. Otton (✉)
Department of Cardiology, Liverpool Hospital, University of New South Wales, Sydney, NSW, Australia
e-mail: j.otton@unsw.edu.au

C. Salavastru et al. (eds.), *Skin and the Heart*,
https://doi.org/10.1007/978-3-030-54779-0_25

Plasma Osmolality, Glycosaminoglycans, Sodium and Their Effects on Fluid Balance

Recent evidence has demonstrated that a large part of total body sodium is bound to glycosaminoglycan (GAG) networks within the interstitium. These GAG networks function as sodium buffers and play an important role in fluid homeostasis and endothelial function. Sodium cations are predominantly extracellular and largely bound to the negative glycosaminoglycans. Multiple GAG chains anchor to a linear linking protein, forming a large, brush-shaped proteoglycan that contains numerous anionic charges. These are connected, via intramolecular hydrogen bonds, to form a compact macromolecule. The extremely polyanionic nature of these macromolecules leads to electrostatic interactions between negatively charged surfaces, such as collagen fibrils, proteins, and positive electrolytes, thus creating a network of high oncotic pressure [2].

The interstitium connects and supports tissues while serving as a transition medium for nutrients, water products, and signaling molecules. GAGs are the main constituents of the interstitium. Together with collagen and/or elastin fibres, they comprise the solid phase and determine the structure and compliance of the interstitium. One GAG molecule can bind a large quantity of sodium cations; therefore, the interstitium can accumulate or buffer a high amount of sodium. In vitro studies have demonstrated that the interstitial GAG network can adapt to short periods of higher salt intake, because a high concentration of sodium cations alters the sulfation pattern, thereby increasing GAG charge density. High sodium concentrations also promote gene expression of GAG polymerization enzymes, which further increases GAG content, thus activating a positive feedback pathway to expand sodium storage capacity. In the reverse scenario of salt scarcity, GAG polymerization and sulfation are reduced, and a subsequent reduction in the matrix is associated with gradual mobilization of sodium from tissue reservoirs [2].

Glycosaminoglycans create a high osmotic pressure microenvironment. As described by the Starling equation, high interstitial oncotic (π_I) pressures and low interstitial hydrostatic pressures promote transudation of plasma fluid into the interstitium, whereas low interstitial compliance opposes fluid accumulation. Subjects with a more dense interstitial GAG network—and consequently a higher interstitial oncotic pressure (π_i)—will have more filtration over the capillary membrane into the interstitium. However, the limited elastic properties (and thus, low compliance) of the interstitial GAG network prevent fluid accumulation. Small increases in interstitial fluid content lead to appreciable increases in interstitial tensile stress. This forces interstitial fluid into lymphatic vessels. As fluid quickly drains into the systemic circulation, interstitial hydrostatic pressure remains low, and protein osmotic pressure remains high (compensated state) [3, 4].

Interstitial fluid accumulates when the rate of transudation from capillaries into the interstitium exceeds the rate at which the lymphatic system can efficiently drain the fluid. Venous pressure, more than arterial pressure, increases capillary hydrostatic pressure. Therefore, increased central venous pressure and pulmonary capillary wedge pressure in heart failure promote interstitial fluid accumulation. In response, lymphatic capacity gradually increases, parallel to a rise in venous pressure, and only in high ranges of venous pressure is the return of lymph to the great veins impeded. Elevated filling pressures are a hallmark of decompensated heart failure; however, the occurrence of pulmonary and/or peripheral edema correlates poorly with pulmonary capillary wedge pressure and central venous pressure. Therefore, factors additional to increased capillary pressure must play a role in determining the occurrence of edema.

A prolonged, excessively high sodium concentration leads to a dense interstitial GAG network with the accumulation of sodium cations and an altered conformation of the GAG macromolecules, creating a dysfunctional GAG network with altered sodium buffering capacity. This may result in decreased tensile stress, and thus, a high compliance state of the interstitial matrix. The combination of high interstitial oncotic pressure and high compliance facilitates fluid transudation. This results in a reduction of effective arterial blood volume, with subsequent unrestrained neurohumoral stimulation in heart failure, which further contributes to the dysfunction of the GAG network. Lymphatic vessel integrity is altered as lymph vessels start to widen, leading to leakage of lymph into the interstitium. Thus, when interstitial GAG networks become dysfunctional, even mildly elevated venous pressures in heart failure might lead to pulmonary congestion and peripheral edema [2].

Renin-Angiotensin-Aldosterone System

As alluded to previously, fluid balance hinges on several evolutionary mechanisms and it is the maladaptation of these which result in net fluid accumulation. Angiotensinogen, a precursor to angiotensin I, is produced primarily in the liver. Renin is produced by the juxtaglomerular apparatus (JGA) in the kidney, the release of which is stimulated by baroreflex mechanisms in the JGA, by beta-adrenergic sympathetic innervation of these cells, and by solute delivery, notably chloride in the tubular fluid at the macula densa segment of the distal tubule. Renin cleaves angiotensinogen into the decapeptide, angiotensin I. Angiotensin I is then converted into the octapeptide angiotensin II, by angiotensin converting enzyme (ACE), located predominantly in endothelial cells of capillaries, within the lungs, and within the epithelial cells of the kidneys. Angiotensin II acts on the collecting duct cells, causing reabsorption of sodium (and chloride). Angiotensin II also exhibits its own independent sodium reabsorptive effects in the kidney, acts in the brain to stimulate thirst and salt appetite, as well as to increase sympathetic tone, and acts directly on the vascular wall (primarily arterioles) to promote vasoconstriction and thus increase blood pressure. In the adrenal cortex, angiotensin II stimulates the release of the mineralocorticoid, aldosterone, which acts on the distal convoluted tubules and cortical collecting ducts of the kidneys, resulting in sodium and water reabsorption from the urine. Finally, angiotensin II causes release of vasopressin (antidiuretic hormone) from the posterior pituitary gland. A potent vasoconstrictor, vasopressin also stimulates reabsorption of water by promoting the expression of aquaporin channels in the kidneys. Additionally, vasopressin stimulates an individual's appetite for salt and the sensation of thirst. These effects directly act to increase blood pressure [5–7].

Congestive Cardiac Failure and Fluid Retention

Cardiac output is a product of heart rate and stroke volume. A decrease in cardiac output is the primary cause of fluid retention in congestive cardiac failure (CCF) secondary to left ventricular failure. The Frank-Starling law of the heart states that the stroke volume increases as end-diastolic volume increases when all other factors affecting myocardial performance are unchanged. In early-compensated stages of CCF, elevated left ventricular end diastolic volume secondary to both decreased cardiac performance and expansion of the ECFV leads to an increase in stroke volume and restoration of cardiac output. As CCF progresses, through the mechanisms explained above, low EABV leads to progressive renal retention of salt and water, potentiating ECFV expansion and progressive distention of the myocardium, with deleterious effects on cardiac performance.

The term cardio-renal syndrome (CRS) defines disorders of the heart and kidneys whereby "acute or chronic dysfunction in one organ may induce acute or chronic dysfunction of the other". CRS requires a tailored approach to manage a patient's clinical picture and thus provide better outcomes. Precise prescription of fluid removal by diuretics or extracorporeal therapies is a key element of this approach. Adequate monitoring of fluid balance is essential to prevent worsening of renal function or other complications while delivering these therapies. The range of optimal ECFV values appears to be very narrow in patients with CCF. Hypervolemia results in myocardial stretching and decompensation, whereas hypovolemia leads to low EABV that can result in end-organ malperfusion [1, 8].

Increased Capillary Permeability

Capillary permeability characterizes the capacity of a blood vessel wall to allow for the flow of small molecules/cells into and of out the vessel. Vascular walls are lined by a single layer of endothelial cells. The spaces between these cells (cellular junctions) are tightly regulated.

Cytokines (such as interleukin-1 and tumor necrosis factor- alpha) and other inflammatory mediators induce gaps between endothelial cells by disassembly of intercellular junctions. This creation of gaps can result in microvascular leak, allowing for the movement of fluid into the interstitial space. Increased capillary permeability is one of the major contributors to edema in sepsis, trauma, burns, and anaphylaxis, amongst others [1, 9].

Idiopathic systemic capillary leak syndrome (ISCLS) is a rare disorder resembling anaphylaxis in its clinical presentation. Typically starting in midlife, it is characterized by episodes of severe hypotension, hypoalbinunemia, and hemoconcentration related to fluid extravasation through the capillary membrane. Its underlying pathogenesis remains unclear although some studies allude to abnormalities in vascular endothelial growth factor (VEGF), and angiopoetin 2 [10]. Tumor necrosis factor-alpha, leukotrienes, and interleukin 2 also play a role. Tissue biopsies obtained during acute attacks demonstrate endothelial cell apoptosis [11].

Some studies have found an association with monoclonal gammopathies [12]; it is unclear at this stage whether the elevated serum paraproteins detected during the acute phase of ISCLS represents pathogenesis versus epiphenomenon. ISCLS has three phases: a prodromal phase (during which there are non-specific symptoms of fatigue, irritability, nausea, abdominal discomfort, myalgias, polydipsia, and an unheralded increase in body weight), a fluid extravasation phase (during which endothelial permeability results in hypoalbuminema, hypotension, and hemoconcentration), and a fluid recovery phase (during which capillary permeability is restored, with a shift towards fluid recruitment back into the intravascular space). Severe extravasation may result in distributive shock [13], which has been fatal in some cases [14]. Cutaneous changes include sclerosis, livedo, purpura, and photodistributed maculopapular rash; dermal mucinosis has been confirmed on biopsy of one patient [15]. Several disorders may mimic ISCLS, including sepsis, toxic shock syndrome (TSS), anaphylaxis, drug reactions and hereditary angioedema, thus rendering ISCLS a diagnosis of exclusion. Treatment is supportive, with initial fluid resuscitation balanced with avoidance of intravascular volume overload, the latter of which may require diuretics and or renal replacement therapy/ultrafiltration. Some case reports describe the use of intravenous immunoglobulin, theophylline, terbutaline [16], infliximab, glucocorticoids, spironolactone, indomethacin, leukotriene-modifying agents, cyclosporine, thalidomide, and Ginkgo biloba, in the treatment of ISCLS [13, 17]. None of these have been established to routinely treat/prevent ISCLS.

Albumin and its Role in Fluid Homeostasis

Serum albumin is the main protein of human blood plasma. Its main function is to regulate the oncotic pressure of intravascular blood. It binds water, cations (such a calcium, sodium, and potassium), fatty acids, hormones, bilirubin, ii, and drugs (e.g., barbiturates). It is produced in the liver.

Conditions predisposing to hypoalbuminemia (reduced synthesis from liver cirrhosis, or losses due to protein losing enteropathy, nephrotic syndrome, malabsorption, malnutrition, late pregnancy, burns) will result in a decrease in the capillary oncotic pressure with the net result favoring movement of fluid into the interstitial space. Increased capillary permeability due to reasons listed above will result in leakage of albumin through the leaky intercellular junctions, increasing the interstitial oncotic pressure, once again promoting the movement of fluid into the interstitium.

Edema

Edema is the palpable swelling produced by expansion of the interstitial fluid volume through the mechanisms described above (alone or in combination). In its most extreme form, it is generalized, occupying all third spaces, and is referred to as anasarca [18] (Table 25.1).

Table 25.1 Pathophysiologic categories of edema (adapted from Robbins and Cotran: Ref. [19])

Increased hydrostatic pressure

Impaired venous return
  Congestive cardiac failure
  Constrictive pericarditis
  Tricuspid regurgitation
  Ascites (liver cirrhosis)
  Venous obstruction or compression
    Thrombosis/stenosis
    External pressure (e.g., mass)
    Lower extremity inactivity with prolonged dependency
  Chronic venous insufficiency

Arteriolar dilatation/increased capillary permeability
  Heat
  Neurohumoral dysregulation
  Idiopathic edema
  Burns
  Trauma
  Sepsis/inflammation
  Allergic reactions/angioedema
  Acute respiratory distress syndrome
  Diabetes mellitus
  Interleukin-2 therapy
  Malignant ascites
  Idiopathic systemic capillary leak syndrome

Reduced plasma osmotic pressure (hypoproteinemia)
  Protein-losing glomerulopathies
  Protein-losing gastroenteropathy
  Ascites (liver cirrhosis)
  Malnutrition

Lymphatic obstruction
  Inflammatory
  Infective (e.g., filariasis)
  Neoplastic
  Postsurgical (e.g., post lymph node dissection)
  Postirradiation

Sodium retention
  Excessive salt intake with renal insufficiency
  Increased tubular reabsorption of sodium
    Renal hypoperfusion
    Increased renin-angiotensin-aldosterone secretion

Inflammation
  Acute inflammation
  Chronic inflammation
  Angiogenesis

Drugs
  Nonsteroidal anti-inflammatory drugs
  Glucocorticoids
  Fludrocortisone
  Thiazolidinediones
  Insulins
  Estrogens/progestins/androgens/testosterone
  Aromatase inhibitors
  Tamoxifen
  Vasodilator drugs: Hydralazine, minoxidil, diazoxide, calcium channel blockers (particularly dihydropyridines)

Cardiological manifestations of elevated venous pressures are those of congestive cardiac failure: increase in dry weight, pulmonary congestion, peripheral edema and general fluid overload (including intraabdominal third space edema, gastrointestinal wall edema). Chronic lower limb edema is subsequently compounded by venous stasis, resulting in soft tissue tenderness, even of normal appearing skin, discovered when examining for the presence of edema by palpation (Fig. 25.1). Its association with other cutaneous signs of chronic venous disease (in particular, chronic venous insufficiency), is common.

The soft tissue injury begins in the subcutis, and visible changes may not appear for some time. Frequently, non-specific petechial lesions are present. As the hemoglobin in the petechial lesions breaks down, the iron remains in the skin as hemosiderin and may cause impressive brown pigmentation (Fig. 25.2). Stasis dermatitis arises from chronic fibrin and hemosiderin deposition, and is characterized by erythema, scaling, pruritus, erosions, oozing, crusting, and occasional vesicles may occur during any stage of chronic venous insufficiency [20].

Untreated venous insufficiency can result in tortuous dilated veins, telangiectasias, and reticular veins [21]. Telangiectasias can be stellate, sunburst and arborizing patterns and may gradually spread over the entire lower limbs, giving them a blue-purplish discoloration (Fig. 25.3).

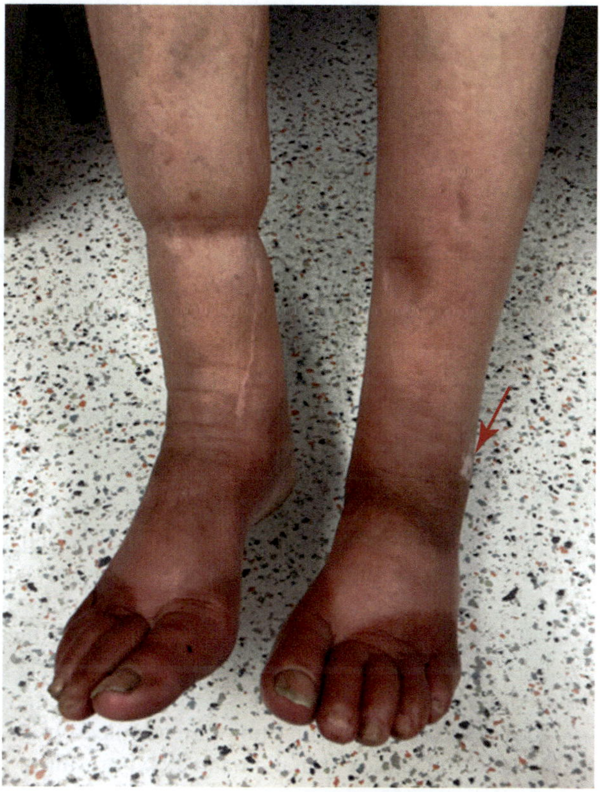

Fig. 25.1 Bilateral pitting edema. Right leg depicts healed scar from harvesting of the great saphenous vein for coronary artery bypass grafting. Atrophie blanche lesion demonstrated on left lateral malleolus (arrow)

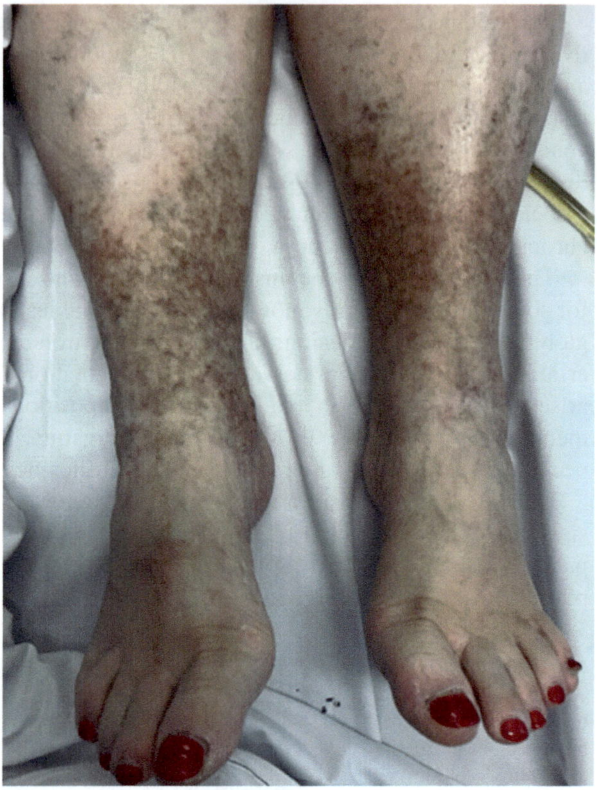

Fig. 25.2 Thickened skin and hyperpigmentation due to hemosiderin deposition in chronic venous insufficiency. Indwelling urinary catheter seen in background

Chronic venous hypertension induces progressive fibrosis of the skin and subcutaneous tissues, a condition referred to as lipodermatosclerosis. In its acute phase, it is painful and disabling and typically appears as a thickened raised red-brown area in the skin of the lower limb [22]. There is a constant perceived sensation of heat. The acute form eventually progresses to become chronic; however, the chronic variety can develop spontaneously. Chronic lipodermatosclerosis is stiff and shiny skin that is fixed, hard, indurated, and contracting the subcutaneous tissues. Progressive contraction of the skin and subcutaneous tissues results in shrinking of the gaiter area which, in conjunction with edema in the calf, gives the leg a stick-like or inverted bottle shape (Fig. 25.3).

Skin necrosis with replacement by scar tissue without ulceration or sloughing results in small areas or patches of skin that are usually gray-white in color and only a few millimeters in size. These lesions, known as atrophie blanche, are small depressions in the skin surface, covered with thin, transparent epithelium, and a sometimes surrounded by a halo of fine, dilated venules. Multiple areas may coalesce to form a large scar which, due to its delicate structure, may spontaneously break down or form ulcers.

The above cutaneous conditions are pre-ulcerous. Left untreated, they can impair tissue nutrition and oxygenation and slowly result in tissue death. Any injury may

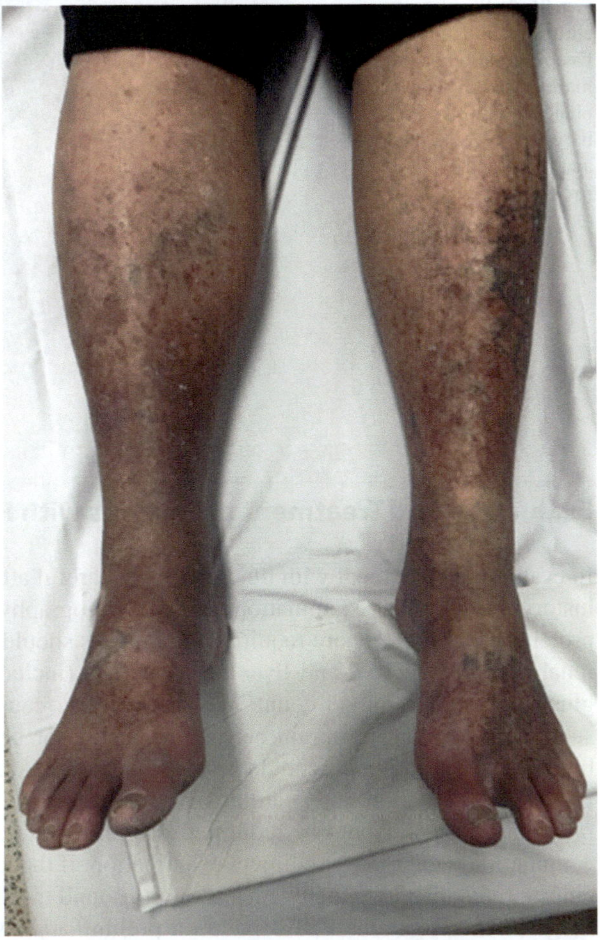

Fig. 25.3 Venous stasis dermatitis. Bilateral hyperpigmentation from hemosiderin. Note the 'inverted champagne bottle' appearance of the lower limb, characteristic of lipodermatosclerosis

rapidly progress to ulceration. Ulcerations begins in an already abnormal area. There is partial skin loss which due to poor tissue nutrition, poor oxygen delivery and poor removal of metabolic byproducts, causes necrosis to the extent of full-thickness skin loss. Necrosis can extend into the subcutaneous fat, superficial fascia, deep fascia, muscles, and even the periosteum. Although peripheral nerve endings are directly involved in the inflammatory process and may give rise to local pain, in large, infected ulcers pain may be a minor feature.

Ulcers that are not aggressively treated may become secondarily infected (especially in individuals with diabetes mellitus). If infection extends into tendons and periosteum, amputation may be required.

In their extreme form, ulcers cause much morbidity from pain, discomfort, and fluid discharge (Fig. 25.4). They can give rise to anemia and hypoproteinemia (which exacerbates edema). On rare occasions they can become malignant (Marjolin's ulcer) [23].

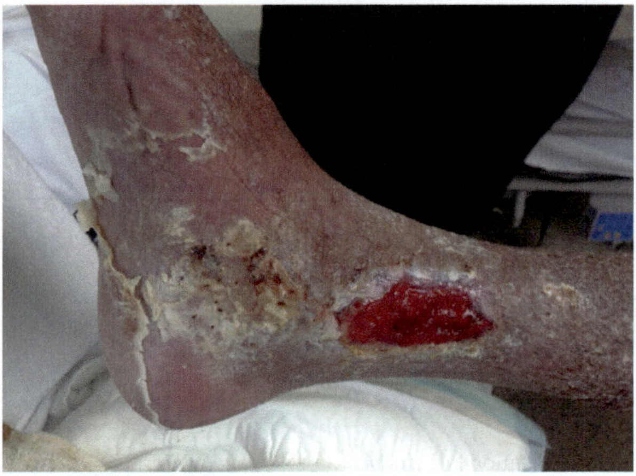

Fig. 25.4 Seqelae of chronic venous stasis. Deep ulceration on medial malleolus with atrophie blanche, with sloughy base. The ulcer is shallow and red-based, with irregular borders

Evaluation and Treatment of Patients with Fluid Overload

In evaluating the patient with fluid overload, careful attention should be paid to the history and physical examination. Electrocardiography, urine dipstick looking for proteinuria, chest-xray are required. Blood tests should include serum electrolytes, renal function, thyroid and liver function tests (including albumin), lipid profile, glucose, complete blood count. Where a cardiac cause is suspected, biomarkers such as N-terminal pro-brain natriuretic peptide or brain natriuretic peptide, and high sensitivity troponins should be considered. Transthoracic echocardiogram will provide information on cardiac function. 24 h urine collection, urinary protein:creatinine should be requested where nephrotic syndrome is suspected, in conjunction with urinary sediment examination. If the kidneys are deemed to be the culprit, renal tract imaging by means of ultrasound in the first instance should occur. Targeted investigations will depend on preliminary results and are not limited to further cardiac investigations, liver imaging, vasculitis screening, and exclusion of infective causes. Doppler ultrasound of the lower limbs is helpful in excluding venoocclusive disease. Wound swabs from ulcers may be helpful in targeting anti-microbial therapy.

Treatment of fluid overload is once again targeted at the cause; the mainstays include diuretic agents, and extracorporeal removal by dialysis [1, 8, 24].

References

1. Roumelioti M, Glew R, Khitan Z, Rondon-Berrios H, Argyropoulos CP, Malhotra D, Raj DS, Agaba EI, Rohrscheib M, Murata GH, Shapiro JI, Tzamaloukas AH. Fluid balance concepts in medicine: principles and practice. World J Nephrol. 2018;7:1–28. https://doi.org/10.5527/wjn.v7.i1.1.

2. Nijst P, Verbrugge FH, Grieten L, Dupont M, Steels P, Tang WHW, Mullens W. The pathophysiological role of interstitial sodium in heart failure. J Am Coll Cardiol. 2015;65:378–88. https://doi.org/10.1016/j.jacc.2014.11.025.
3. Levick JR, Michel CC. Microvascular fluid exchange and the revised Starling principle. Cardiovasc Res. 2010;87:198–210. https://doi.org/10.1093/cvr/cvq062.
4. Starling EH. On the absorption of fluids from the connective tissue spaces. J Physiol. 1896;19:312–26.
5. Paul M, Mehr AP, Kreutz R. Physiology of local renin-angiotensin systems. Physiol Rev. 2006;86:747–803. https://doi.org/10.1152/physrev.00036.2005.
6. Knepper MA, Kwon TH, Nielsen S. Molecular physiology of water balance. N Engl J Med. 2015;372:1349–58. https://doi.org/10.1056/NEJMra1404726.
7. Fournier D, Luft FC, Bader M, Ganten D, Andrade-Navarro MA. Emergence and evolution of the renin-angiotensin-aldosterone system. J Mol Med. 2012;90:495–508. https://doi.org/10.1007/s00109-012-0894-z.
8. Irfan M. The hands-on guide to clinical reasoning in medicine. Oedema. 2018; https://doi.org/10.1002/9781119578055.
9. Angus DC, Van Der Poll T. Severe sepsis and septic shock. N Engl J Med. 2013;369:840–51. https://doi.org/10.1056/NEJMra1208623.
10. Lesterhuis WJ, Rennings AJ, Leenders WP, et al. Vascular endothelial growth factor in systemic capillary leak syndrome. Am J Med. 2009;122(6):e5–7.
11. Johansson BR, Löfdahl CG. Ultrastructure of the microvessels in skeletal muscle in a case of systemic capillary leak syndrome. Acta Med Scand. 1979;206:413.
12. Ewan PW, Lachmann PJ, Morice AH, Forster PJG, Doorenbos CJ. Treatment of systemic capillary leak syndrome. Lancet. 1988;332:1496.
13. Dhir V, Arya V, Malav IC, et al. Idiopathic systemic capillary leak syndrome (SCLS): case report and systematic review of cases reported in the last 16 years. Intern Med. 2007;46:899.
14. Clarkson B, Thompson D, Horwith M, Luckey EH. Cyclical edema and shock due to increased capillary permeability. Am J Med. 1960;29:193–216.
15. Fardet L, Kerob D, Rybojad M, Vignon-Pennamen MD, Schlemmer B, Guermazi A, Morel P, Lebbé C. Idiopathic systemic capillary leak syndrome: cutaneous involvement can be misleading. Dermatology. 2004;209:291–5. https://doi.org/10.1159/000080851.
16. Tahirkheli NK, Greipp PR. Treatment of the systemic capillary leak syndrome with terbutaline and theophylline: a case series. Ann Intern Med. 1999;130:905.
17. Kapoor P, Greipp PT, Schaefer EW, et al. Idiopathic systemic capillary leak syndrome (Clarkson's disease): the Mayo Clinic experience. Mayo Clin Proc. 2010;85:905.
18. Newman SA. Cutaneous changes in arterial, venous, and lymphatic dysfunction. In: Kang S, et al., editors. Fitzpatrick's dermatology. 9th ed. New York: McGraw-Hill.
19. Mitchell RN. Hemodynamic disorders, thromboembolic disease, and shock. In: Kumar V, Abbas AK, Aster JC, editors. Robbins and cotran pathologic basis of disease. 9th ed. Amsterdam: Elsevier; 2020.
20. Nicholls SC. Sequelae of untreated venous insufficiency. Semin Interv Radiol. 2005;22(3):162–8. https://doi.org/10.1055/s-2005-921960.
21. Sadick NS. Predisposing factors of varicose and telangiectatic leg veins. J Dermatol Surg Oncol. 1992;18:883.
22. Chiesa R, Marone EM, Limoni C, et al. Chronic venous disorders: correlation between visible signs, symptoms, and presence of functional disease. J Vasc Surg. 2007;46:322.
23. Tanai E, Frantz S. Pathophysiology of heart failure. Compr Physiol. 2016;6:187–214. https://doi.org/10.1002/cphy.c140055.
24. Patarroyo-Aponte M, Colvin-Adams M. Evaluation of patients with heart failure. Cardiol Clin. 2014;32:47–62. https://doi.org/10.1016/j.ccl.2013.09.014.

Infantile Hemangiomas and the Heart

26

Kristina Semkova, Sonya Marina, and Jana Kazandjieva

Introduction and Pathophysiology

Infantile hemangiomas (IHs) are the most common benign vascular tumors of infancy with a well-established natural evolution consisting of an initial phase of proliferation followed by spontaneous involution over months to years. The programmed life cycle of IHs has given many clues to the pathogenesis but the exact triggering mechanisms at each phase are still unknown and the etiology is poorly understood. Despite the consistent course of progression and regression, there is a significant variation in clinical presentation, localization, life-cycle and associations, hence it is highly likely that several different endogenous and exogenous factors determine the occurrence, development and outcome of IHs [1] (Table 26.1).

Table 26.1 Association between infantile hemangiomas and the heart

Infantile hemangiomas	Heart
Organ involvement • *Liver hemangiomas*	High-output congestive cardiac failure
Treatment for IH • *Beta blockers (propranolol, acebutalol, nadolol)* • *Systemic corticosteroidss*	Hypotension and bradycardia (beta blockers) Hypertension (systemic steroids)
Syndromic associations • *PHACES*	Aortic arch anomalies Ventricular septal defect, vascular ring and systemic venous anomalies

K. Semkova (✉)
St John's Institute of Dermatology, St Thomas' Hospital, London, UK

S. Marina
Department of Dermatology, Medical University, Varna, Bulgaria

J. Kazandjieva
Department of Dermatology, Medical University, Sofia, Bulgaria

C. Salavastru et al. (eds.), *Skin and the Heart*,
https://doi.org/10.1007/978-3-030-54779-0_26

Multiple gestations, female sex, maternal age, in vitro fertilization, low birth weight, prematurity, gestational hypertension, pre-eclampsia, gestational diabetes mellitus, use of progesterone during pregnancy, invasive antepartum procedures and placental ischemic abnormalities increase the risk for IHs [2]. Many of these etiological factors induce hypoxic stress for the fetus and the difference in the type and timing of hypoxic stimuli likely affects precursor cells and results in the characteristic clinical pattern [3, 4]. Generalized pre-delivery hypoxia in placental insufficiency or pre-eclamsia is associated with small, localized hemangiomas, whilst regional hypoxia secondary to abnormal vasculature carries a risk for segmental hemangiomas. The different timing and type of hypoxic stimuli most probably accounts for a different timing of deposition of precursor cells and hence a different characteristic pattern of tissue involvement.

Low levels of oxygen (tissue hypoxia) prompt cells to modify gene expression stimulating angiogenesis as a survival mechanism. The major regulator of this cellular response is the hypoxia-inducible factor 1α (HIF-1α) which up-regulates VEGF, GLUT-1 and insulin growth factor-2 (IGF-2) [5, 6]. GLUT-1 is a specific marker of IHs expressed by micro-vascular endothelial cells at sites of blood-tissue barriers, such as the placenta and in the brain [7].

De novo formation of vessels (vasculogenesis) followed by angiogenesis is the current concept for IHs development. Hemangioma endothelial progenitor cells (HemEPCs) are isolated from proliferating hemangiomas and defined as potential precursors of hemangioma endothelial cells (HemECs) by co-expression of the human stem cell marker CD133 and the endothelial marker CD34 [8]. Cells with the CD133+/CD34+ phenotype decrease in number during the involution phase thus confirming their role in angiogenesis [8, 9]. As hemangioma endothelial cells co-express primitive mesodermal, mesenchymal and neural crest markers, there may be a shift to differentiation into mesenchymal cells to form the fibro-fatty tissue [10, 11]. Terminal mesenchymal differentiation is likely inhibited during the proliferating phase by Pref-1 and angiotensin II and down-regulation of these cytokines at a later stage might account for a default adipogenesis during involution, as shown in cultures of hemangioma endothelial cells recovered from IHs explants [11].

Placental origin of IHs due to embolization of placental stem cells to receptive fetal tissues during gestation is another hypothesis which is supported by the unique immunohistochemical similarities between the placenta and the IHs endothelium which co-expresses surface markers such as glucose-transporter protein 1 (GLUT-1), Lewis Y antigen (CD14), CD32, CD15, merosin and indoleamine 2,3-deoxygenase (IDO) [12, 13]. These proteins are not found in other vascular tumors/malformations and non-hemangioma tumor vasculature. A placental origin could well explain the programmed life-cycle of IHs that resembles the development of the placenta with an initial proliferation phase followed by a subsequent phase of stabilisation.

Prevalence/Population Affected

Infantile hemangiomas affect between 3% and 10% of infants. The incidence increases with decreasing of gestational age and is about 23% for those born at <1000 g compared to 1–4% for term infants. There is clear female predominance (3:1 ratio) and a predilection for Caucasian infants as compared with other ethnicities [14, 15].

In pre-term infants the incidence of multiple hemangiomas is higher, about 40%, compared to about 25% for infants born at term. Lower birth weight also correlates with increased numbers of IHs. Segmental hemangiomas occur with similar incidence but facial involvement is more common in term infants [16].

Dermatological Manifestations

Most IHs present as sporadic single cutaneous lesions. They are subclassified into superficial, subcutaneous (deep) or combined (mixed) based on the depth of the vascular proliferation. The superficial hemangiomas are bright erythematous plaques with irregular surface or nodules, whilst the deep lesions present as areas of swelling underlying normal skin or skin with bluish tinge without surface change (Fig. 26.1).

Sixty per cent of IHs develop on the head/neck area, 25% are seen on the trunk and 15% on the extremities [15, 17]. Facial distribution is non-random as nodular IHs are localized along the lines of embryological fusion (mainly on the cheek, upper lip and upper eyelid) and diffuse IHs follow a segmental distribution pattern [4]. Multiple hemangiomas are present in approximately 20% of all affected children.

IHs follow a characteristic natural course of spontaneous involution over months to years after a rapid initial phase of proliferation. Most lesions appear de novo at around 3 weeks of age, although a precursor lesion (erythematous or telangiectatic macule, or bruise) may be seen at birth in about 50% of children. The growth phase is usually completed within the first 6 to 10 months of life with complete regression in as much as 90% by the age of 9 [18, 19]. Some hemangiomas may have minimal or arrested growth [20], whilst deep and segmental lesions show a tendency for a prolonged growth phase [21].

Diagnosis/Investigations

The diagnosis is clinical for most cases and laboratory investigations and imaging are only rarely required.

Histological examination reveals a dermal and/or subcutaneous multilobular proliferation of vascular spaces lined by plump endothelial cells. A feeding arteriole is commonly seen at the base. With involution, in older lesions the vessels are gradually replaced by fibrosis. By immunohistochemistry, the proliferation is invariably positive for the marker GLUT-1.

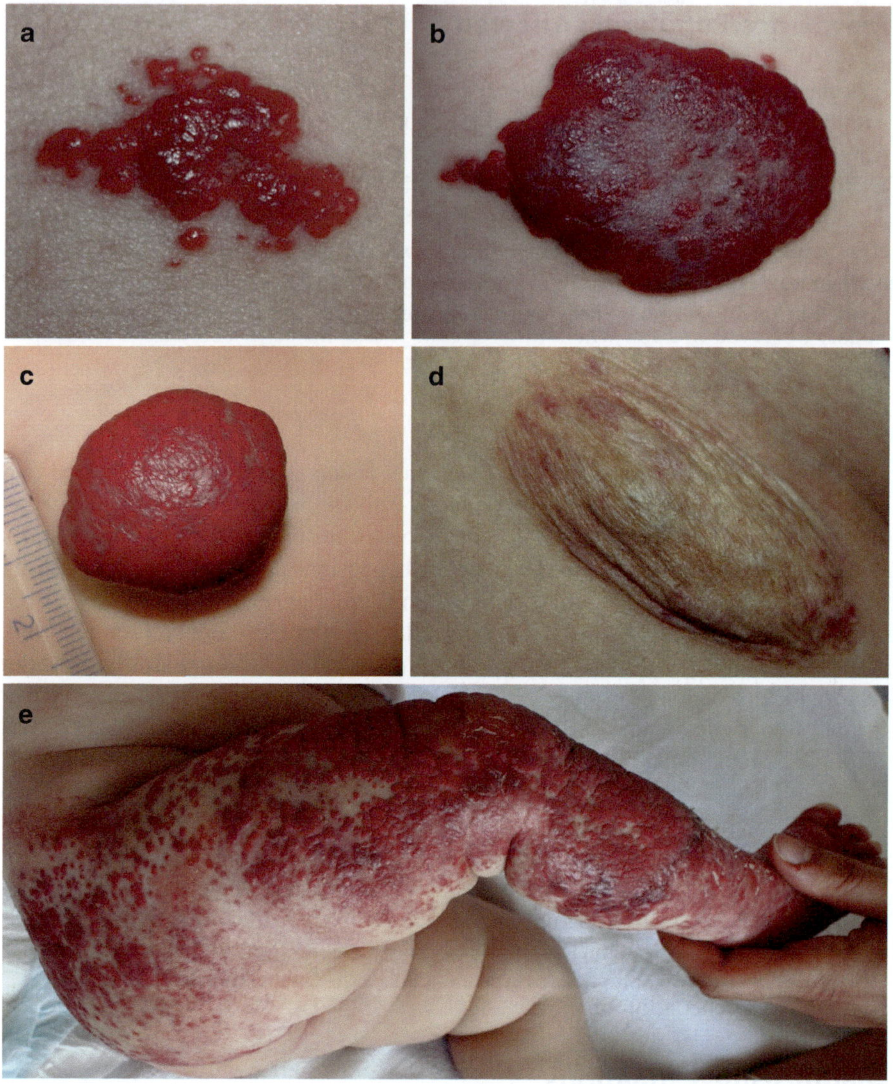

Fig. 26.1 (**a**) Superficial IH; (**b**) combined superficial and deep IH; (**c**) nodular IH; (**d**) residual fibro-fatty tissue after resolution of IH; (**e**) segmental IH

Imaging investigations such as MRI and ultrasonography should be performed only in patients with suspected deep involvement or associated abnormalities.

Treatment

Most IHs can be left without active treatment until spontaneous involution, an approach known as active non-intervention. Treatment is warranted for very large hemangiomas or hemangiomas in specific anatomic areas to prevent or improve scarring, disfigurement or functional and life-threatening complications [22]. Propranolol is the first-line systemic agent in the latter cases. Other options include corticosteroids, interferon, chemotherapeutics and surgical/laser treatments, but the relatively high morbidity of these interventions limits their use to the exceptional cases of propranolol contraindications. Small lesions without risk of significant cosmetic or function threatening sequelae may be monitored without treatment until spontaneous resolution or treated with topical agents such as timolol maleate.

Propranolol, a non-selective β-adrenergic antagonist competitively inhibiting the β_1 and β_2-adrenoreceptors expressed on endothelial cells, has been used in pediatric cardiology for over 50 years. Its anti-proliferative effect in IHs has been serendipitously observed in 2008 when used to manage a child with secondary hypertrophic obstructive cardiomyopathy induced by systemic corticosteroid treatment for a nasal capillary IH [23]. Rapid regression with propranolol can be achieved in segmental and complicated cutaneous hemangiomas [24], airway hemangiomas [25], vision affecting peri-orbital and orbital hemangiomas [26, 27], PHACES [28, 29], liver hemangiomas [30–33] and hemangiomatosis [34]. Propranolol is similarly effective in involuting hemangiomas and could be used in patients who failed to respond to other active interventions during the proliferative phase or have not sought adequate early therapy [35].

The safety profile of propranolol is relatively good and well-known due to its long-term use as a chronic therapy for children with hypertension and cardiovascular disease [36, 37]. Most adverse events develop as a result of the receptor blockade, but the risk of toxicity cannot be predicted because bioavailability of propranolol in children is inconsistent and not dose related [38]. The most common side effects are hypotension, sinus bradycardia, hypoglycemia and bronchospasm/bronchiolitis that are not life-threatening, but require patient monitoring at baseline and during treatment [39]. Other minor side effects include restless sleep, nightmares, agitation, diarrhoea and peripheral coldness [40, 41]. Special attention is required in patients at risk of cardiac compromise, including patients with very large hemangiomas, PHACES syndrome, PELVIS syndrome and miliary hemangiomatosis [39]. Although propranolol is lipophilic and crosses the blood-brain barrier, there are no long-term effects on intelligence and memory development in children treated with propranolol for IHs during infancy [42].

Propranolol is usually started at a dose of 1 mg/kg/day which is up-titrated to a dose of 2–3 mg/kg/day in two or three divided doses. Treatment is continued for 6 months or longer and should be discontinued after the end of the proliferation phase to prevent rebound growth.

Timolol maleate is a topical non-selective beta-adrenergic antagonist which is a highly effective and relatively safe treatment option for superficial IHs, primarily for small, localised lesions, to ensure a predictable cosmetic outcome [15, 43]. Timolol is available in different formulations, including 0.5% drops and 0.1% gel-forming solution, and can be applied two to three times daily. It may be systemically absorbed, yet the risk of beta-blocker side effects is low [44]. Bronchospasm and sleep disturbances are exceedingly rare. Even though treatment is by default not warranted for small and superficial IHs, since the overall outcome might be comparable to that of spontaneous involution in the long term, early non-aggressive therapeutic intervention with a safe and effective topical modality has its advantages over ‘active non-intervention’. These include prophylaxis for a better cosmetic outcome by prevention of fibro-fatty tissue deposition and alleviation of parents’ and patient’s psychological distress.

Prognosis/Complications

Most small infantile hemangiomas resolve spontaneously without any or with minimal scarring. Large lesions usually leave behind residual life-long lesions, including telangiectasia, fibro-fatty deposits, depigmentation and scars following ulceration. Residual changes are seen in 25 to 69% of untreated hemangiomas, depending on the studied population [15, 18].

Ulceration, seen predominantly in the proliferative phase [42], is the most common complication of IHs and occurs in up to about 16% of all patients [43]. Treatment of ulcerated lesions is important because tissue destruction leads to an increased risk of local and systemic infections, bleeding, pain and scarring [42, 43]. The first line treatment for ulcerated IHs is propranolol but other conventional therapeutic options include wound care, topical antiseptics and antibiotics, systemic and intralesional corticosteroids and lasers. The mean time of healing with propranolol is about 4 weeks and depends on the size and location [44, 45].

Cardiological Manifestations

Infantile hemangiomas can develop in various extracutaneous sites but not the heart. The heart can be, however, indirectly involved as cardiac failure may develop with multiple liver hemangiomas, in diffuse neonatal hemangiomatosis and as a side effect from some of the systemic treatments for IHs. Cardio-vascular anomalies are part of the PHACE syndrome.

Liver Hemangiomas and the Heart

Hepatic infantile hemangiomas (HIH) have been described in association with IHs. Infants with multiple cutaneous lesions and under the age of 6 months should be screened for liver hemangiomas. They are usually multifocal or diffuse and present with similar course of initial sudden and rapid growth after birth followed by slow spontaneous involution. Although many HIH have no clinical symptoms, complications including high-output congestive cardiac failure, consumptive coagulopathy, liver failure, consumptive hypothyroidism and abdominal compartment syndrome are well documented [46, 47]. Cardiac failure develops as a result of the high flow within the vascular lesions and is usually seen during the proliferation phase with increase in shunting. Consumptive hypothyroidism is specific to HIH as they express type 3 iodothyronine deiodinase that inactivates the thyroid hormone. This complication also develops as the lesions proliferate [46]. Diffuse HIH are associated with a higher risk of complications and mortality as compared to multifocal lesions and should be monitored more closely and for longer period. Mortality in diffuse and multifocal HIH is about 16% [48]. Consumptive coagulopathy with low thrombocyte count and high prothrombin time not responding to therapy is a predictor for poor outcome [49].

HIH should be differentiated from congenital hemangiomas which proliferate in utero and reach their maximum size prior to or before birth. In these patients, complications such as high-output cardiac failure, usually develop at birth or shortly thereafter.

Investigations and Management

Doppler ultrasound is the preferred screening and monitoring diagnostic imaging as the specific radiologic features are well-defined. On ultrasound, hemangiomas appear as solitary or multifocal, uniformly hypo- or hyperechoic mass. Large hemangiomas may have a more complex heterogenous appearance as they may contain calcifications, cystic spaces, and areas of fibrosis that give them a heterogeneous aspect. MRI of the liver with dynamic acquisition pattern and consideration for a biopsy are recommended when the ultrasound findings are not classic, the clinical history is discrepant or the hemangioma is detected after infancy. MRI of congenital and infantile hemangiomas usually shows hyperintensity on standard T2-weighted sequences and hypointensity relative to the normal liver parenchyma on the T1-weighted images [46]. It is recommended that liver ultrasound be performed at progressively longer intervals, with an initial 2-week interval and decreasing the frequency with 2 weeks after each stable evaluation. Regular monitoring is required until complete involution.

Current recommendations [46] for investigating HIH include full blood count at diagnosis and then as needed, alpha-fetoprotein at diagnosis and until normalized, serial liver ultrasounds, thyroid function tests (TSH and free T4) at diagnosis and then monthly until at least 6 months of age for diffuse hemangiomas or at diagnosis and then as needed if symptomatic for multifocal hemangiomas. Echocardiogram should be considered in clinical signs of cardiac failure or if the ultrasound examination shows evidence of shunting or massive flow. In case of normal findings on the echocardiogram, repeat testing should be performed only if/when the patient develops new clinical symptoms, increasing liver shunting or hypothyroidism [46].

Treatment decision should be based on the type of HIH, the symptoms and signs and the ultrasound findings. Asymptomatic patients with multifocal HIH but no evidence of cardiac failure or hemodynamically significant shunting, should be followed up with ultrasonography until complete regression. Patients with hemodynamically significant shunting benefit from propranolol or corticosteroid therapy and should be monitored closely by a specialist [32, 33, 50]. Propranolol has been used at doses of 2.5 to 5 mg/kg and was suggested as the first line pharmacological treatment in view of the minimal side effects and marked efficacy [32]. In about one third of patients the pharmacologic therapy fails and for them embolization should be considered as the next step. Early embolization is necessary in infants with large shunts presenting with cardiac failure. Resection can be considered in recalcitrant cases. Diffuse HIH require a more aggressive approach as the risk of death is higher, including with high doses of pharmacotherapy and thyroid hormone monitoring and replacement. Embolization does not normally work for these patients as there are no high-flow shunts. Sirolimus has also been used with success to treat HIH that fail conventional therapies [51]. Hepatic transplantation should be considered in case of poor response to medical therapies [50].

Treatment for IH and the Heart

Propranolol

In the pediatric population, propranolol is indicated for the treatment of various cardiological and other conditions, including arrythmias, hypertension, tetralogy of Fallot, hyperthyroidism and migraines. Its mechanism of action via a non-selective beta-blockade can, however, result in potential cardio-vascular side effects.

Cardiovascular Side Effects

Hypotension and bradycardia are expected adverse events and have been reported rarely in children on propranolol. Hypotension may be seen within the first 12 weeks after treatment initiation in about 5% of infants and is usually transient and asymptomatic warranting no treatment change. Bradycardia commonly develops within the first week of treatment and is also transient and asymptomatic in the majority of cases usually resolving with treatment adjustments or upon discontinuation of propranolol [36, 52]. Drop in the heart rate with more than 20% may be an early indication for treatment response [53].

Conduction disturbances, such as syncope and atrioventricular block, may also occur, in particular in infants with underlying cardiovascular conditions [15, 36, 52]. Exceedingly rare nearly fatal or fatal cardiac outcomes have been reported in the literature in the setting of other medical issues and propranolol treatment. These include a cardiac arrest, possibly following a neurally-mediated syncope in a dehydrated toddler with a viral infection, a third degree atrioventricular block [54] and fatal acute cardiac failure during sclerotherapy of esophageal varices secondary to biliary atresia [36].

Pre-treatment Cardiovascular Assessment

Prior to treatment initiation, infants should be assessed with thorough cardiovascular and respiratory history and history about previous hypoglycemic episodes and feeding concerns, as well as a comprehensive physical examination, including heart auscultation, palpation of peripheral pulses, abdominal examination for liver enlargement, and measurement of heart rate and blood pressure. Further investigations are warranted only in special circumstances. Pre-treatment ECG is required in patients with a heart rate abnormal for age, a strong family history of sudden death/arrhythmia, episodes of loss of consciousness and maternal history of connective tissue disease. Pre-treatment ECHO is required in patients with heart rate abnormal for age, heart murmurs, and in patients with segmental IH. Cardiology assessment is warranted only for patients with positive examination findings or with segmental IHs. Routine screening blood tests are not recommended and blood glucose screening should be considered only for infants who are pre-term, small for age, feeding poorly or with a history of hypoglycaemic episodes [55].

Systemic Corticosteroids

Systemic corticosteroids were the mainstay of treatment for infantile hemangiomas prior to the introduction of propranolol therapy. They are fairly safe when used at the recommended dose of 2–4 mg/kg/day with gradual weaning [56]. Cardiovascular adverse events are rare at this dose. Hypertension may develop after a mean of 25 days of treatment and is usually asymptomatic and of unknown clinical significance [57, 58]. Treatment with a single or multiple antihypertensive agents is sometimes necessary to achieve control of the blood pressure [57].

Other Treatments

Different other agents may be used for treatment of IH but the literature data as to efficacy and adverse effects is scarce. Captopril has been used and associated with hypotension [59]. Other beta-blockers, such as atenolol [60] and nadolol [61], have been associated with lower incidence of cardiovascular side effects. Temporary reduction of the dose or discontinuation of therapy may be considered.

PHACE Syndrome

Clinical Presentation

PHACE syndrome (posterior fossa anomalies, hemangioma, arterial lesions, cardiac abnormalities/coarctation of the aorta, eye anomalies) presents with large IHs in the head and neck area and developmental abnormalities. Screening for PHACE syndrome is currently recommended for patients with segmental IH on the head, infants with IH (smaller or lacking typical morphology or distribution) and characteristic/major anomalies found in PHACE, infants without cutaneous IHs but with other characteristic anomalies found in PHACE [62].

Congenital heart disease in patients with PHACE is significantly higher than the general population and ranges from 41% to 67% with coarctation of the aorta in 19%–30% [62, 63]. Aortic arch anomalies in PHACE involve the transverse and descending aorta arch with segments of narrowing and obstruction adjacent to segments with aneurysmal dilatation. This is often associated with aberrant subclavian origin which may be seen in as many as 50% of patients with PHACE and in which both subclavian arteries are distal to the obstruction [63]. In such cases the four-extremity blood pressure assessment of gradient between upper and lower extremities is inaccurate for arch obstruction identification and repeat annual echocardiogram is warranted even in asymptomatic children [62].

Additional cardiovascular abnormalities described in the literature with PHACE syndrome include a right or double aortic arch, a ventricular septal defect, vascular ring and systemic venous anomalies [63]. Individual reports of tetralogy of Fallot, ectopia cordis, pulmonary stenosis and atrial septal defects can also be found in the literature [62].

Aplasia, hypoplasia, or occlusion of a major cerebral artery is a significant risk factor for acute ischemic stroke in children with PHACE, in particular when more than one vessel is involved or when there is coarctation of the aorta [64]. Based on the risk of acute ischaemic stroke, patients are stratified into low, intermediate and high risk [62].

Low risk patients present with arterial anomalies frequently seen in the general population or anomalies that have no or have very minimal clinical significance such as persistent embryonic arteries, anomalous arterial origin or course, circle of Willis variants. Intermediate risk patients have non-stenotic dysgenesis, narrowing or occlusion of arteries proximal to the circle of Willis without hemodynamic risk. High risk patients have at least one of three criteria: 1) narrowing of >25% or occlusion of principal cerebral vessels within or above the circle of Willis that results in an "isolated" circulation; 2) tandem or multiple arterial stenoses with complex blood flow or cerebrovascular stenosis in the setting of coarctation of the aorta that may result in diminished cerebral perfusion; 3) imaging findings suggestive of chronic/silent ischemia or progressive steno-occlusive disease, such as existing infarction, chronic or border zone ischemic changes, lenticulostriate collateral dilation or pial collaterals [62].

Investigations and Management

Screening investigations and monitoring depend on the clinical presentation and the assigned risk. Physical examination with focus on midline fusion defects, screening echocardiogram, ophthalmology assessment and MRI brain/neck/arch are the currently recommended initial screening evaluations in all children at risk [62].

When intracardiac and aortic arch anomalies are identified on the echocardiogram, the child should be referred to a paediatric cardiologist for urgent assessment and, in case of arch abnormalities, for cardiac MRI/MRA as this will delineate better the arch and brachiocephalic anatomy. About 15% of children require surgical intervention for correction of aortic abnormalities and complex reconstruction techniques are usually required, including interposition grafts, bypass grafts, patch aortoplasty and subclavian flap angioplasty [65]. End-to-end repair, which is the preferred procedure for coarctation in patients without PHACE, is usually not feasible due to the long segmental involvement [65]. The use of non-native tissue techniques results in high rate of recurrent obstruction.

If there is no obstruction of the aortic arch, yearly echocardiograms and pediatric cardiology follow up are recommended as progressive narrowing of coarctation and/or progressive aneurysmal dilation are known, albeit rare, potential complications in children with PHACE with congenital abnormalities of the aortic arch [63, 65].

MRA is used to screen for the common cerebral vascular anomalies of PHACE and, if required, other modalities can also be used.

Low risk patients do not need further imaging unless new neurological symptoms develop. Intermediate risk patients should be followed up by pediatric neurologist. Elective imaging should be best postponed until no anaesthesia is required. These patients should avoid contact sports and sports that involve extreme neck positions (wrestling for example). The risk of aneurysm and thrombus formation is increased in adulthood for patients with significant vessel tortuosity and turbulent flow [62]. Patients with high risk should be assessed regularly by a paediatric neurologist with repeat imaging at 6 and 12 months. Although anesthetics pose potential risk for this group, the risk of progressive vascular changes and stroke is deemed much higher [62]. High-risk patients should also avoid contact sports and prophylactic aspirin at a dose of 4–5 mg/kg/d up to 81 mg could be considered for this group [62]. Pediatric neurologists and neurosurgeons with expertise in vascular pathology should be consulted in case of progressive vascular changes, such as moyamoya vasculopathy.

Surgical intervention, including extensive arch reconstruction, is required in about 37% of patients with arch anomalies [63]. Preoperative assessment should include full assessment not only of the aortic but also of the cerebrovascular abnormalities in view of the higher risk of ischemic brain injury.

Treatment of hemagiomas in PHACE is challenging and often a systemic medication is required as the lesions are usually extensive, may involve functional areas such as the airways and carry a high risk of scarring and disfigurement. Propranolol should be used with caution in patients with PHACES and cervical or cerebral arteriopathy as systemic hypotension may reduce the blood flow through the stenotic/occluded vessels supplying the brain and increase the risk of acute ischemic stroke. The risk is particularly high in infants with severe narrowing/stenosis or nonvisualization of major vessels without adequate anatomic evidence of collateral circulation [66]. The recommended approach in patients with PHACE who are initiated on propranolol is multidisciplinary consultation with neurology and/or cardiology prior to the start of treatment, use of the lowest possible dose with slow upward dosage titration, and three times daily dosing in order to minimize abrupt changes in systolic blood pressure [66]. Systemic steroids, alone or in combination with betablockers, is an alternative for patients at risk.

References

1. Semkova K, Kazandjieva J, Tsankov N. What's new in infantile hemangiomas. Current insights and future perspectives. SKINMed. 2013;11:341–9.
2. Hunjan MK, Schoch JJ, Anderson KR, Lohse CM, Marnach ML, Hand JL, Davis DMR, Tollefson MM. Prenatal risk factors for infantile hemangioma development. J Invest Dermatol. 2017;137(4):954–7.
3. Drolet BA, Frieden IJ. Characteristics of infantile hemangiomas as clues to pathogenesis: does hypoxia connect the dots? Arch Dermatol. 2010;146:1295–9.
4. Waner M, North PE, Scherer KA, et al. The nonrandom distribution of facial hemangiomas. Arch Dermatol. 2003;139:869–75.

5. Ritter MR, Butschek RA, Friedlander M, Friedlander SF. Pathogenesis of infantile haemangioma: new molecular and cellular insights. Expert Rev Mol Med. 2007;9:1–19.
6. Storch CH, Hoeger PH. Propranolol for infantile haemangiomas: insights into the molecular mechanisms of action. Br J Dermatol. 2010;163:269–74.
7. North PE, Waner M, Mizeracki A, Mihm MC Jr. GLUT1: a newly discovered immunohistochemical marker for juvenile hemangiomas. Hum Pathol. 2000;31:11–22.
8. Yu Y, Flint AF, Mulliken JB, et al. Endothelial progenitor cells in infantile hemangioma. Blood. 2004;103:1373–5.
9. Kleinman ME, Greives MR, Churgin SS, et al. Hypoxia-induced mediators of stem/progenitor cell trafficking are increased in children with hemangioma. Arterioscler Thromb Vasc Biol. 2007;27:2664–70.
10. Itinteang T, Tan ST, Brasch H, Day DJ. Primitive mesodermal cells with a neural crest stem cell phenotype predominate proliferating infantile haemangioma. J Clin Pathol. 2010;63:771–6.
11. Itinteang T, Vishvanath A, Day DJ, Tan ST. Mesenchymal stem cells in infantile haemangioma. J Clin Pathol. 2011;64:232–6.
12. North PE, Waner M, Mizeracki A, et al. A unique microvascular phenotype shared by juvenile hemangiomas and human placenta. Arch Dermatol. 2001;137:559–70.
13. Barnés CM, Huang S, Kaipainen A, et al. Evidence by molecular profiling for a placental origin of infantile hemangioma. Proc Natl Acad Sci U S A. 2005;102:19097–102.
14. Goelz R, Poets CF. Incidence and treatment of infantile haemangioma in preterm infantsArchives of Disease in Childhood. Fetal and Neonatal Edition. 2015;100:F85–91.
15. Novoa M, Baselga E, Beltran S, Giraldo L, Shahbaz A, Pardo-Hernandez H, Arevalo-Rodriguez I. Interventions for infantile haemangiomas of the skin. Cochrane Database Syst Rev. 2018;18(4):CD006545.
16. Garzon MC, Drolet BA, Baselga E, et al. Comparison of infantile hemangiomas in preterm and term infants: a prospective study. Arch Dermatol. 2008;144:1231–2.
17. Hochman M, Adams DM, Reeves TD. Current knowledge and management of vascular anomalies: I. Hemangiomas. Arch Facial Plast Surg. 2011;13:145–51.
18. Bauland CG, Lüning TH, Smit JM, et al. Untreated hemangiomas: growth pattern and residual lesions. Plast Reconstr Surg. 2011;127:1643–8.
19. Chang LC, Haggstrom AN, Drolet BA, et al. Growth characteristics of infantile hemangiomas: implications for management. Pediatrics. 2008;122:360–7.
20. Suh K-Y, Frieden IJ. Infantile hemangiomas with minimal or arrested growth: a retrospective case series. Arch Dermatol. 2010;146:971–6.
21. Brandling-Bennett HA, Metry DW, Baselga E, et al. Infantile hemangiomas with unusually prolonged growth phase: a case series. Arch Dermatol. 2008;144:1632–7.
22. Maguiness SM, Frieden IJ. Current management of infantile hemangiomas. Semin Cutan Med Surg. 2010;29:106–14.
23. Léauté-Labrèze C, Dumas, de la Roque E, Hubiche T, et al. Propranolol for severe hemangiomas of infancy. N Engl J Med. 2008;358:2649–51.
24. Manunza F, Syed S, Laguda B, et al. Propranolol for complicated infantile haemangiomas: a case series of 30 infants. Br J Dermatol. 2010;162:466–8.
25. Peridis S, Pilgrim G, Athanasopoulos I, Parpounas K. A meta-analysis on the effectiveness of propranolol for the treatment of infantile airway haemangiomas. Int J Pediatr Otorhinolaryngol. 2011;75:455–60.
26. Claerhout I, Buijsrogge M, Delbeke P, et al. The use of propranolol in the treatment of periocular infantile haemangiomas: a review. Br J Ophthalmol. 2010;95(9) https://doi.org/10.1136/bjo.2010.192245.
27. Fay A, Nguyen J, Jakobiec FA, et al. Propranolol for isolated orbital infantile hemangioma. Arch Ophthalmol. 2010;128:256–8.
28. Denoyelle F, Leboulanger N, Enjolras O, et al. Role of propranolol in the therapeutic strategy of infantile laryngotracheal hemangioma. Int J Pediatr Otorhinolaryngol. 2009;73:1168–72.
29. Theletsane T, Redfern A, Raynham O, et al. Life-threatening infantile haemangioma: a dramatic response to propranolol. J Eur Acad Dermatol Venereol. 2009;23:1465–6.

30. Muthamilselvan S, Vinoth PN, Vilvanathan V, et al. Hepatic haemangioma of infancy: role of propranolol. Ann Trop Paediatr. 2010;30:335–8.
31. Sarialioglu F, Erbay A, Demir S. Response of infantile hepatic hemangioma to propranolol resistant to high-dose methylprednisolone and interferon-α therapy. Pediatr Blood Cancer. 2010;15:1433–4.
32. Mazereeuw-Hautier J, Hoeger PH, Benlahrech S, Ammour A, Broue P, Vial J, Ohanessian G, Léauté-Labrèze C, Labenne M, Vabres P, Rössler J, Bodemer C. Efficacy of propranolol in hepatic infantile hemangiomas with diffuse neonatal hemangiomatosis. J Pediatr. 2010 Aug;157(2):340–2.
33. Yang K, Peng S, Chen L, Chen S, Ji Y. Efficacy of propranolol treatment in infantile hepatic haemangioma. J Paediatr Child Health. 2019 Jan 9;55:1194–200. https://doi.org/10.1111/jpc.14375.
34. Mazereeuw-Hautier J, Hoeger PH, Benlahrech S, et al. Efficacy of propranolol in hepatic infantile hemangiomas with diffuse neonatal hemangiomatosis. J Pediatr. 2010;157:340–2.
35. O'Loughlin A, O'Donnell B, Watson R. Mature infantile haemangiomas role for propranolol. J Eur Acad Dermatol Venereol. 2010;25(11):1363–4. [Epub ahead of print]
36. Léaute-Labrèze C, Boccara O, Degrugillier-Chopinet C, Mazereeuw-Hautier J, Prey S, Lebbé G, Gautier S, Ortis V, Lafon M, Montagne A, Delarue A, Voisard JJ. Safety of Oral Propranolol for the Treatment of Infantile Hemangioma: A Systematic Review. Pediatrics. 2016 Oct;138(4):e20160353.
37. Love JN, Sikka N. Are 1-2 tablets dangerous? Beta-blocker exposure in toddlers. J Emerg Med. 2004;26:309–14.
38. Blatt J, Morrell DS, Buck S, et al. {beta}-blockers for infantile hemangiomas: a single-institution experience. Clin Pediatr (Phila). 2011;50(8):757–63. [Epub ahead of print]
39. Lawley LP, Siegfried E, Todd JL. Propranolol treatment for hemangioma of infancy: risks and recommendations. Pediatr Dermatol. 2009;26:610–4.
40. de Graaf M, Breur MPJ, Raphaël MF, et al. Adverse effects of propranolol when used in the treatment of hemangiomas: a case series of 28 infants. J Am Acad Dermatol. 2011;65(2):320–7. [Epub ahead of print]
41. Sans V, de la Roque ED, Berge J, et al. Propranolol for severe infantile hemangiomas: follow-up report. Pediatrics. 2009;124:e423–31.
42. Hermans DJ, Boezeman JB, Van de Kerkhof PC, et al. Differences between ulcerated and non ulcerated hemangiomas, a retrospective study of 465 cases. Eur J Dermatol. 2009;19:152–6.
43. Chamlin SL, Haggstrom AN, Drolet BA, et al. Multicenter prospective study of ulcerated hemangiomas. J Pediatr. 2007;151:684–9.
44. Hermans DJ, van Beynum IM, Schultze Kool LJ, et al. Propranolol, a very promising treatment for ulceration in infantile hemangiomas: a study of 20 cases with matched historical controls. J Am Acad Dermatol. 2011;64:833–8.
45. Naouri M, Schill T, Maruani A, et al. Successful treatment of ulcerated haemangioma with propranolol. J Eur Acad Dermatol Venereol. 2010;24:1109–12.
46. Iacobas I, Phung TL, Adams DM, Trenor CC 3rd, Blei F, Fishman DS, Hammill A, Masand PM, Fishman SJ. Guidance document for hepatic hemangioma (infantile and congenital) evaluation and monitoring. J Pediatr. 2018;203:294–300.
47. Rialon KL, Murillo R, Fevurly RD, Kulungowski AM, Zurakowski D, Liang M, Kozakewich HP, Alomari AI, Fishman SJ. Impact of screening for hepatic hemangiomas in patients with multiple cutaneous infantile hemangiomas. Pediatr Dermatol. 2015;32(6):808–12.
48. Rialon KL, Murillo R, Fevurly RD, Kulungowski AM, Christison-Lagay ER, Zurakowski D, Kozakewich HP, Alomari AI, Fishman SJ. Risk factors for mortality in patients with multifocal and diffuse hepatic hemangiomas. J Pediatr Surg. 2015;50(5):837–41.
49. Kuroda T, Hoshino K, Nosaka S, Shiota Y, Nakazawa A, Takimoto T. Critical hepatic hemangioma in infants: recent nationwide survey in Japan. Pediatr Int. 2014 Jun;56(3):304–8.
50. Christison-Lagay ER, Burrows PE, Alomari A, et al. Hepatic hemangiomas: subtype classification and development of a clinical practice algorithm and registry. J Pediatr Surg. 2007;42:62–7. 67–68, Discussion

51. Hutchins KK, Ross RD, Kobayashi D, Martin A, Rajpurkar M. Treatment of refractory infantile hemangiomas and pulmonary hypertension with Sirolimus in a pediatric patient. J Pediatr Hematol Oncol. 2017;39(7):e391–3.
52. Droitcourt C, Kerbrat S, Rault C, Botrel MA, Happe A, Garlantezec R, Guillot B, Schleich JM, Oger E, Dupuy A. Safety of oral propranolol for infantile hemangioma. Pediatrics. 2018 Jun;141(6):e20173783.
53. Sondhi V, Patnaik SK. Propranolol for infantile hemangioma (PINCH): an open-label trial to assess the efficacy of propranolol for treating infantile hemangiomas and for determining the decline in heart rate to predict response to propranolol. J Pediatr Hematol Oncol. 2013 Oct;35(7):493–9.
54. Tosoni A, Cutrone M, Dalle Carbonare M, Pettenazzo A, Perilongo G, Sartori S. Cardiac arrest in a toddler treated with propranolol for infantile hemangioma: a case report. Ital J Pediatr. 2017 Nov 17;43(1):103.
55. Solman L, Glover M, Beattie PE, Buckley H, Clark S, Gach JE, Giardini A, Helbling I, Hewitt RJ, Laguda B, Langan SM, Martinez AE, Murphy R, Proudfoot L, Ravenscroft J, Shahidullah H, Shaw L, Syed SB, Wells L, Flohr C. Oral propranolol in the treatment of proliferating infantile haemangiomas: British Society for Paediatric Dermatology consensus guidelines. Br J Dermatol. 2018 Sep;179(3):582–9.
56. Greene AK. Systemic corticosteroid is effective and safe treatment for problematic infantile hemangioma. Pediatr Dermatol. 2010 May-Jun;27(3):322–3.
57. Christou EM, Wargon O. Effect of captopril on infantile haemangiomas: a retrospective case series. Australas J Dermatol. 2012 Aug;53(3):216–8.
58. Kim KH, Choi TH, Choi Y, Park YW, Hong KY, Kim DY, Choe YS, Lee H, Cheon JE, Park J, Park KD, Kang HJ, Shin HY, Jeong JH. Comparison of efficacy and safety between propranolol and steroid for infantile hemangioma: a randomized clinical trial. JAMA Dermatol. 2017 Jun 1;153(6):529–36.
59. Zaher H, Rasheed H, El-Komy MM, Hegazy RA, Gawdat HI, Abdel Halim DM, Abdel Hay RM, Hegazy RA, Mohy AM. Propranolol versus captopril in the treatment of infantile hemangioma (IH): a randomized controlled trial. J Am Acad Dermatol. 2016 Mar;74(3):499–505.
60. Wang Q, Xiang B, Chen S, Ji Y. Efficacy and safety of oral atenolol for the treatment of infantile haemangioma: a systematic review. Australas J Dermatol. 2018 Dec 4;60:181–5. https://doi.org/10.1111/ajd.12966.
61. Bernabeu-Wittel J, Narváez-Moreno B, de la Torre-García JM, Fernández-Pineda I, Domínguez-Cruz JJ, Coserría-Sánchez F, Álvarez-del-Vayo C, Conejo-Mir J. Oral Nadolol for the treatment of infantile hemangiomas: a single-institution retrospective cohort study. Pediatr Dermatol. 2015 Nov-Dec;32(6):853–7.
62. Garzon MC, Epstein LG, Heyer GL, Frommelt PC, Orbach DB, Baylis AL, et al. PHACE syndrome: consensus-derived diagnosis and care recommendations. J Pediatr. 2016;178:24–33.e2.
63. Bayer ML, Frommelt PC, Blei F, et al. Congenital cardiac, aortic arch, and vascular bed anomalies in PHACE syndrome (from the International PHACE Syndrome Registry). Am J Cardiol. 2013;112(12):1948–52.
64. Siegel DH, Tefft KA, Kelly T, Johnson C, Metry D, Burrows P, Pope E, Cordisco M, Holland KE, Maheshwari M, Keith P, Garzon M, Hess C, Frieden IJ, Fullerton HJ, Drolet BA. Stroke in children with posterior fossa brain malformations, hemangiomas, arterial anomalies, coarctation of the aorta and cardiac defects, and eye abnormalities (PHACE) syndrome: a systematic review of the literature. Stroke. 2012;43:1672–4.
65. Caragher SP, Scott JP, Siegel DH, Mitchell ME, Frommelt PC, Drolet BA. Aortic arch repair in children with PHACE syndrome. J Thorac Cardiovasc Surg. 2016;152(3):709–17.
66. Metry D, Frieden IJ, Hess C, Siegel D, Maheshwari M, Baselga E, Chamlin S, Garzon M, Mancini AJ, Powell J, Drolet BA. Propranolol use in PHACE syndrome with cervical and intracranial arterial anomalies: collective experience in 32 infants. Pediatr Dermatol. 2013 Jan-Feb;30(1):71–89.

Erdheim-Chester Disease

27

Can Baykal and Muhammed Burak Günay

Introduction

Erdheim-Chester disease (ECD) is a rare chronic systemic disorder with non-specific skin involvement, formerly included in the non-Langerhans cell histiocytosis group [1]. However, in the recent revised classification of histiocytoses and neoplasms of the macrophage-dendritic cell lineages, ECD is classified in the "Langerhans-related group" [2] due to its clonal mutations involving genes of RAS-RAF-MEK-ERK protein kinase pathways in more than 80% of the patients similar to Langerhans cell histiocytosis. The heterogenous manifestations of ECD caused by infiltration of histiocytes on many organs may vary from an indolent focal disease to a life-threatening multisystemic disease [3]. The skeleton, central nervous system (CNS), cardiovascular system (CVS), lungs, orbits, kidneys, pituitary gland and skin are cited among the more common sites of involvement. However, testes, thyroid and lymph node involvement have also been reported [4]. Hence, ECD may await interest of different specialities including cardiologists and dermatologists.

Etiology and Pathogenesis

ECD occurs sporadically and its etiology is still unknown. There are no documented infectious or genetic mechanism to explain the whole pathogenesis of ECD [5]. However, encouraging progress about pathogenesis of ECD has been observed in the last years. Some local and systemic chemokines/cytokines seem to be responsible for the recruitment and activations of histiocytes into ECD lesions [5]. Elevated levels of interferon (IFN)-α, interleukin (IL)-12, monocyte chemotactic protein-1 and decreased levels of IL-4 and IL-7 have been shown in some cases [5].

C. Baykal · M. B. Günay (✉)
Dermatology and Venereology, Istanbul Faculty of Medicine, Istanbul, Turkey
e-mail: baykalc@istanbul.edu.tr; muhammed.gunay@istanbul.edu.tr

C. Salavastru et al. (eds.), *Skin and the Heart*,
https://doi.org/10.1007/978-3-030-54779-0_27

Furthermore, IL-6 may have a crucial role in the pathogenesis of ECD, because this cytokine is involved in osteoclast differentiation that can eventually lead to osteosclerosis, one of the major features of the disease.

Recent genetic studies of ECD revealed BRAF mutations in pathologic histiocytes [3]. BRAF is a serine/threonine protein kinase, with a crucial role in the regulation of cell proliferation and survival, as it contributes to the RAS-RAF-MEK-ERK protein kinase pathway. In many other malignancies such as melanoma, papillary thyroid carcinoma, colorectal cancer and non-small-cell lung cancer, BRAF mutations have been shown with different rates. More than 30 BRAF gene mutations associated with human cancers have been identified, but the most prevalent one is the mutation of V600E which causes the amino acid substitution of glutamic acid for valine at position 600 of the BRAF protein. Nearly half of the ECD patients showed this BRAF V600E mutation [6]. This pathway also plays a role as a therapeutic target in some patients with ECD [6].

Epidemiology

The incidence of ECD is unknown [3]. Since its first description by Jakop Erdheim and William Chester in 1930 [7], approximately 600 cases have been reported only in the relevant medical literature. Although it has been diagnosed in all age groups, most of the patients are adults and the mean age at diagnosis is 53 years [3]. There is no gender predilection.

Clinical Manifestations

As there are no specific symptoms of ECD, awareness of its multisystemic involvement and multidisciplinary approaches are very important in diagnosis. Some clinical features such as bone pain, diabetes insipidus and skin findings may have a particular diagnostic value. However, CVS, pulmonary and CNS involvements cause the most valuable prognostic manifestations [8]. Especially, cardiovascular manifestations are the major cause of mortality in ECD patients and about 60% of patients perish due to a cardiac complication [9].

Cutaneous Findings

Cutaneous involvement is found in about 25–30% of ECD patients [10] and may be the first symptom of the disorder. It most commonly presents as xanthelasma-like eyelid lesions and/or xanthomatous papulonodular lesions on other sites of the body or rarely as not well described lesions such as erythematous patches. Eyelid involvement is the most charachteristic cutaneous manifestations of ECD occuring more commonly on the inner canthus of the upper eyelids as flat yellowish to brown-gray asymptomatic plaques [10]. Unlike xanthelasma palpebrarum usually associated with dislipidemias, the flat eyelid plaques of ECD tend to be more diffuse (Fig. 27.1) extending into the neighbouring skin of temporal region and cheeks and can also affect bulbar conjunctiva and sclera (Fig. 27.2) [11, 12]. The eyelid lesions in ECD could also be differentiated histopathologically from xanthelasma palpebrarum [10]. Moreover xanthelasma-like lesions of eyelids can also be seen in late stage of Langerhans cell histiocytosis and some other subtypes of non-Langerhans cell histiocytoses [11]. Diffuse plane normolipemic xanthomatosis may locate as diffuse flat xanthomatous plaques on the eyelids also extending to neighbouring areas but similar yellow plaques may be seen on other body sites and association of monoclonal gammopathies is common in these patients. Xanthomatous lesions on the eyelids seen in necrobiotic xanthogranuloma are typically indurated and sometimes ulcerated [11].

Papulonodular lesions on the other sites of body have also been reported in ECD patients [10]. They may begin as irregularly distributed reddish-brown, non-painful papules (Fig. 27.3) or nodules located on trunk and extremities [10, 12, 13]. These lesions could be clinically indistinguishable from those found in juvenile xanthogranuloma, generalized eruptive histiocytosis and xanthoma disseminatum patients [3]. Juvenile xanthogranuloma, the commonest variant of non-Langerhans cell histiocytosis, is most frequently seen in early childhood locating anywhere on the body and may sometimes present with disseminated papular lesions. However, it very rarely shows systemic manifestations including focal lytic bone lesions (femur, proximal tibia, fibula) in contrast to severe multi-systemic manifestations seen in ECD including osteosclerosis. Generalized eruptive histiocytosis, an indolent disease of adults, is restricted to the skin as brown, irregularly distributed papular lesions. In xanthoma disseminatum, a progressive variant of non-Langerhans histiocytoses, xanthoma-like papulonodular lesions of variable size tend to locate remarkably on intertriginous areas showing tendency to confluence and sometimes may involve the eyelids [11]. Diabetes insipidus is a common systemic manifestation of xanthoma disseminatum and ECD.

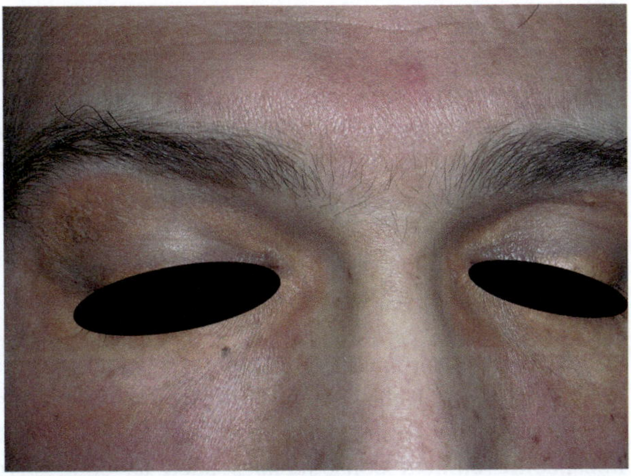

Fig. 27.1 Symmetrically located flat yellow plaques involving both eyelids in a diffuse pattern and extending to the neighbouring area

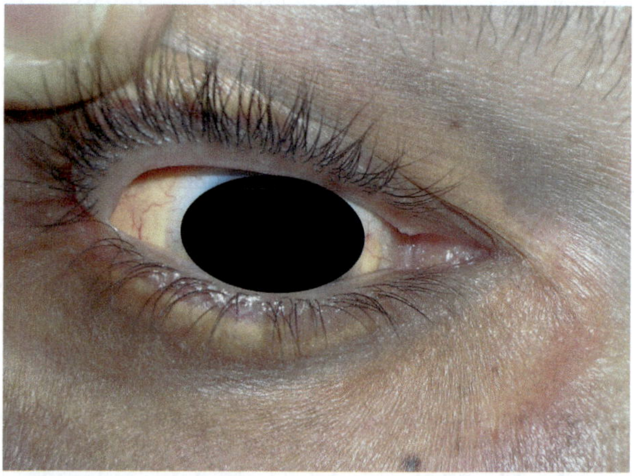

Fig. 27.2 Yellow plaque on the bulbar conjunctiva and sclera accompanying to the eyelid involvement

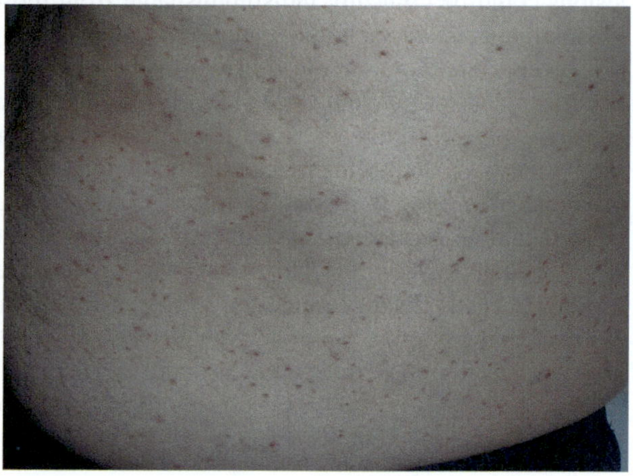

Fig. 27.3 Disseminated yellowish brown small papules on the trunk

Erythematous or brown patches located on extremities and trunk varying from 5 to 15 cm in size have also been reported in ECD patients [10]. Crusty papules [10], verruca plana-like papules [14] and hyperpigmentation of oral mucosa are occasionally reported findings of ECD [14]. None of the mucocutaneous manifestations of ECD has a known risk of morbidity but they may play an important role in the diagnosis of the disorder.

Cardiovascular Involvement

Involvement patterns of CVS evident in the disease may vary depending on the location and size of the lesions. Pericardium and perivascular area of the big vessels are the most frequently affected parts of CVS [8]. These lesions account for various nonspecific clinical consequences such as congestive heart failure, myocardial infarction, valvular dysfunction, pericardial tamponade, thromboembolism, ischemia and peripheral edema [9]. Pericardial infiltration, the most frequent form of cardiac involvement, may lead to thickened pericardium, pericardial effusion or pericardial tamponade which can be detected by echocardiography and computed tomography [9]. In notable pericardial effusions, pericardiocentesis can be a rational method both for diagnostic and therapeutic purposes. Myocardium is another common site of cardiac involvement, mainly presenting with myocardial hypertrophy and thickening. Ventricular walls, atrial walls, interatrial septum and coronary sulcus can be infiltrated by histiocytes and pseudo-tumoral infiltration of right atrium has also been frequently reported [4]. If ECD presents with an atrial mass, it should be differentiated from solid cardiac tumours especially cardiac myxomas. In ECD patients many electrocardiographic abnormalities such as short PR segments, sinoatrial blocks, sinus bradycardia, myocardial infarction compatible with Q wave abnormalities without a history of myocardial infarction, ST-T wave abnormalities and a slight ST elevation have been described, but all of these findings can also be seen in many different diseases [8].

Perivascular histiocytic infiltration of ECD affects especially large arteries such as aorta and renal arteries. Infiltration of small vessels like coronary arteries and venous involvement have also been reported rarely [8]. Perivascular infiltration and fibrosis of the thoracic or abdominal aorta are among the frequently reported vascular involvement patterns of ECD. Periaortic fibrosis can be limited only to a segment of aorta or may affect the entire vessel and appears as a "coated aorta" on CT scans [15]. The differential diagnosis of this "coated aorta" appearance includes retroperitoneal fibrosis and Takayasu arteritis. As most of the CVS findings of ECD are nonspecific, other findings such as associated skeletal involvement might be helpful in substantiating a diagnosis of ECD. Vascular involvement of ECD can also cause arterial stenosis which may lead to cerebral ischemia with carotid involvement, myocardial infarction due to coronary involvement and mesenteric ischemia with superior mesenteric artery involvement. Renovascular hypertension may occur due to ostial stenosis of renal arteries. This long list of life-threatening complications clearly shows that CVS involvement is a poor prognostic sign and it also confers a lower response rate to treatment. In essence, there are no specific CVS findings of ECD and the symptoms may mimic many other CVS disorders of different origins such as atherosclerotic or inflammatory diseases and even neoplasms. So high suspicion and multidisciplinary approach are essential for diagnosis of cardiovascular involvement of ECD.

Other Clinical Manifestations

Skeletal Involvement

The most common clinical feature of ECD is mild but persistent pain of long bones [3]. Distal ends of the femurs, proximal and distal tibia are the most typical sites of involvement which may be a useful indicator to differentiate ECD from Langerhans cell histiocytosis; the latter tending to affect axial skeleton primarily. Axial skeleton and epiphyseal regions are classically spared in ECD. In about 50% of cases skeletal involvement is subclinical and only radiological screening including plain radiographs and Tc99m-bone scintigraphy can be diagnostic [16]. Plain radiographs of lower or sometimes upper extremity bones usually show bilateral, symmetrical cortical osteosclerosis of the diaphyseal and/or metaphyseal regions of the distal ends [17].

Neurological and Orbital Involvement

CNS involvement appears in approximately 51% of ECD patients and accounts for 29% of all deaths, remarkably [3]. Invasion of ECD to the CNS and adjacent structures, such as meninges, facial bones, orbits and intracranial vasculature may manifest with a wide range of symptoms. The location and size of the lesions determine whether the patient will be completely asymptomatic, or suffer from various neurological deficits, including severe disability. Most common related manifestations are diabetes insipidus, exophthalmos and loss of vision due to retrobulbar infiltration, cerebellar ataxia, panhypopituitarism and papilledema [18].

Pulmonary Involvement

ECD is known among rare causes of interstitial lung disease and pleural thickening [19]. Pulmonary involvement presents with nonspecific symptoms such as dry cough, progressive dyspnea and less commonly with cyanosis. Pulmonary function tests reveal typically restrictive ventilation pattern with normal or reduced carbon monoxide diffusion capacity. High resolution computed tomography scans may show parenchymal and/or pleural changes including interlobular septal thickening, centrilobular micronodular opacities, thickening of the interlobar fissures, parenchymal consolidations, microcystic lesions, pleural effusions and pleural thickening [20]. However, definite diagnosis of pulmonary involvement of ECD relies on the detection of typical histiocytic infiltrates in the lung biopsy. Respiratory failure resulting from lung involvement is among causes of death in ECD [20].

Endocrine System Involvement

Pathologic histiocytes may infiltrate the pituitary gland, leading to endocrine manifestations of ECD, such as hyperprolactinemia, gonadotropin insufficiency or deficiency of insulin-like growth factor. The most common endocrinopathy is diabetes insipidus occurring in about 25% of ECD patients [21]. Symptoms of diabetes insipidus usually appear at the disease onset, but it is still most overlooked presentation of ECD, with a median diagnostic delay of 5 years [3]. This endocrinopathy may also be seen in Langerhans cell histiocytosis and in some variants of non-Langerhans cell histiocytoses such as xanthoma disseminatum.

Retroperitoneal and Renal Involvement

Retroperitoneal involvement of ECD may manifest as a mass-like infiltrative lesion surrounding the kidneys. These infiltration can be detected by abdominal computed tomography scan and is named as "hairy kidney" representing a typical sign of ECD [22]. Retroperitoneal fibrosis may remain silent, but it may also lead to hydroureteronephrosis and eventually renal failure by causing ureteral compression.

Diagnosis

As ECD is a very rare disease with protean, nonspecific manifestations of many organ systems, its diagnosis is usually delayed. In case of suspicion of ECD by clinical findings multidisciplinary consultations, radiological imaging, and biopsy of involved organs are indicated [22]. Radiological imaging studies should be done to detect the typical findings such as symmetrical diaphyseal and metaphyseal osteosclerosis of the long bones, infiltration of perinephric fat (hairy kidney) and infiltration of perivascular tissue (coated aorta) [3, 15]. If cutaneous findings are prominent skin biopsy may be preferred rather than visceral organs. Histopathological examination of skin lesions shows diffuse dermal infiltration of variably lipidized histiocytes and multinucleated Touton type giant cells with intervening fibrosis but similar findings can also be seen in other histiocytoses such as juvenile xanthogranuloma [10, 11]. Immunohistochemical profile of ECD is CD68+, CD163+, FXIIIa+, CD1a- and langerin (CD207)-. The pattern of S-100 positivity is variable [12]. In relation with site of involvement perirenal fat, cerebral tissue, lungs, bones and other organs can also be targeted for biopsy and they yield similar histologic findings [10].

As clinical, radiological and even histopathological findings are not pathognomonic, correlation of all these findings is crucial in accurate diagnosis of ECD.

Therapy and Prognosis

As the severity of organ involvement in ECD is variable, not all patients require treatment at the time of diagnosis [22]. Furthermore some patients of ECD follow an indolent clinical course [22]. Active treatment is necessary for symptomatic disease, CNS involvement or evidence of organ dysfunction. There is not a confirmed therapy against skin involvement. As first-line therapeutic option is IFN-α/pegIFN-α2a, various drugs have been used [22, 23]. IFN-α is administered at dosages ranging from 3 to nine million units three times per week [24]. Optimal duration of IFN-α is unclear, but in the literature there are cases which used IFN-α almost four years long. PegIFN-α2a administered at dosages ranging from 135–200 μg per week have less side-effects than IFN-α [22]. In a case series patients treated with IFN-α showed five-year overall survival rate of approximately 70% [3].

BRAF inhibition is also a promising therapeutic target in ECD similar to melanoma. Xanthelasma-like skin lesions can be chosen for biopsy to determine BRAF mutation status [10]. In ECD patients harboring the BRAF V600E mutation vemurafenib, a potent inhibitor of the kinase domain in mutant BRAF, is an effective agent [25]. Vemurafenib, also one of the main therapeutic alternatives in melanoma, has a rich spectrum of adverse effects such as arthralgia, alopecia, fatigue, rash, hyperkeratotic lesions, squamous cell carcinoma and QT interval prolongation on the electrocardiogram. Suggested dosage of vemurafenib in ECD is 960 mg twice daily, but the optimal duration of therapy is unclear [22]. The efficacy of the combination therapy of BRAF and MEK inhibitors such as cobimetinib in ECD is still under investigation [26]. Other treatment alternatives are cladribine, anakinra, glucocorticoids, cyclophosphamide and infliximab [6]. However all of these treatment options except for IFN-α have low level of evidence for survival benefit and there is still no known cure for ECD.

References

1. The Writing Group of the Histiocyte S. Histiocytosis syndromes in children. Lancet. 1987;329:208–9.
2. Emile JF, Abla O, Fraitag S, Horne A, Haroche J, Donadieu J, Requena-Caballero L, Jordan MB, Abdel-Wahab O, Allen CE, Charlotte F, Diamond EL, Egeler RM, Fischer A, Herrera JG, Henter JI, Janku F, Merad M, Picarsic J, Rodriguez-Galindo C, Rollins BJ, Tazi A, Vassallo R, Weiss LM, Histiocyte S. Revised classification of histiocytoses and neoplasms of the macrophage-dendritic cell lineages. Blood. 2016;127:2672–81.
3. Campochiaro C, Tomelleri A, Cavalli G, Berti A, Dagna L. Erdheim-Chester disease. Eur J Intern Med. 2015;26:223–9.
4. Sheu SY, Wenzel RR, Kersting C, Merten R, Otterbach F, Schmid KW. Erdheim-Chester disease: case report with multisystemic manifestations including testes, thyroid, and lymph nodes, and a review of literature. J Clin Pathol. 2004;57:1225–8.
5. Arnaud L, Gorochov G, Charlotte F, Lvovschi V, Parizot C, Larsen M, Ghillani-Dalbin P, Hervier B, Kahn JE, Deback C, Musset L, Amoura Z, Haroche J. Systemic perturbation of cytokine and chemokine networks in Erdheim-Chester disease: a single-center series of 37 patients. Blood. 2011;117:2783–90.
6. Munoz J, Janku F, Cohen PR, Kurzrock R. Erdheim-Chester disease: characteristics and management. Mayo Clin Proc. 2014;89:985–96.
7. Chester W. Über Lipoidgranulomatose. Virchows Arch Pathol Anat Physiol Klin Med. 1930;279:561–602.
8. Nicolazzi MA, Carnicelli A, Fuorlo M, Favuzzi AM, Landolfi R. Cardiovascular involvement in Erdheim-Chester disease: a case report and review of the literature. Medicine (Baltimore). 2015;94:1365.
9. Haroche J, Cluzel P, Toledano D, Montalescot G, Touitou D, Grenier PA, Piette JC, Amoura Z. Cardiac involvement in Erdheim-Chester disease: magnetic resonance and computed tomographic scan imaging in a monocentric series of 37 patients. Circulation. 2009;119:597–8.
10. Chasset F, Barete S, Charlotte F, Cohen-Aubart F, Arnaud L, Le Pelletier F, Emile JF, Frances C, Amoura Z, Haroche J. Cutaneous manifestations of Erdheim-Chester disease (ECD): clinical, pathological, and molecular features in a monocentric series of 40 patients. J Am Acad Dermatol. 2016;74:513–20.
11. Baykal C, Polat Ekinci A, Yazganoglu KD, Buyukbabani N. The clinical spectrum of xanthomatous lesions of the eyelids. Int J Dermatol. 2017;56:981–92.
12. Volpicelli ER, Doyle L, Annes JP, Murray MF, Jacobsen E, Murphy GF, Saavedra AP. Erdheim-Chester disease presenting with cutaneous involvement: a case report and literature review. J Cutan Pathol. 2011;38:280–5.
13. Di Lernia V, Ricci C. Papulonodular lesions, gynaecomastia and retroperitoneal fibrosis. Clin Exp Dermatol. 2010;35:187–9.
14. Yanagi T, Kato N, Yamane N, Osawa R, Hiraga H. Verruca plana-like papules as a new manifestation of Erdheim-Chester disease. Arch Dermatol. 2007;143:945–55.
15. Serratrice J, Granel B, De Roux C, Pellissier JF, Swiader L, Bartoli JM, Disdier P, Weiller PJ. Coated aorta: a new sign of Erdheim-Chester disease. J Rheumatol. 2000;27:1550–3.
16. Wilejto M, Abla O. Langerhans cell histiocytosis and Erdheim-Chester disease. Curr Opin Rheumatol. 2012;24:90–6.

17. Dion E, Graef C, Miquel A, Haroche J, Wechsler B, Amoura Z, Zeitoun D, Grenier PA, Piette JC, Laredo JD. Bone involvement in Erdheim-Chester disease: imaging findings including periostitis and partial epiphyseal involvement. Radiology. 2006;238:632–9.
18. Cavalli G, Guglielmi B, Berti A, Campochiaro C, Sabbadini MG, Dagna L. The multifaceted clinical presentations and manifestations of Erdheim-Chester disease: comprehensive review of the literature and of 10 new cases. Ann Rheum Dis. 2013;72:1691–5.
19. Park JW, Chung CU, Shin JY, Jung SY, Yoo SJ, Lee JE, Jung SS, Kim JO, Kim SY, Park HS. Erdheim-Chester disease with hepatitis, glomerulonephritis, aplastic anemia and lung involvement. Tuberc Respir Dis. 2009;67:345–50.
20. Wittenberg KH, Swensen SJ, Myers JL. Pulmonary involvement with Erdheim-Chester disease: radiographic and CT findings. Am J Roentgenol. 2000;174:1327–31.
21. Haroche J, Arnaud L, Amoura Z. Erdheim-Chester disease. Curr Opin Rheumatol. 2012;24:53–9.
22. Diamond EL, Dagna L, Hyman DM, Cavalli G, Janku F, Estrada-Veras J, Ferrarini M, Abdel-Wahab O, Heaney ML, Scheel PJ, Feeley NK, Ferrero E, McClain KL, Vaglio A, Colby T, Arnaud L, Haroche J. Consensus guidelines for the diagnosis and clinical management of Erdheim-Chester disease. Blood. 2014;124:483–92.
23. Braiteh F, Boxrud C, Esmaeli B, Kurzrock R. Successful treatment of Erdheim-Chester disease, a non-Langerhans-cell histiocytosis, with interferon-alpha. Blood. 2005;106:2992–4.
24. Esmaeli B, Ahmadi A, Tang R, Schiffman J, Kurzrock R. Interferon therapy for orbital infiltration secondary to Erdheim-Chester disease. Am J Ophthalmol. 2001;132:945–7.
25. Haroche J, Cohen-Aubart F, Emile JF, Arnaud L, Maksud P, Charlotte F, Cluzel P, Drier A, Hervier B, Benameur N, Besnard S, Donadieu J, Amoura Z. Dramatic efficacy of vemurafenib in both multisystemic and refractory Erdheim-Chester disease and Langerhans cell histiocytosis harboring the BRAF V600E mutation. Blood. 2013;121:1495–500.
26. Cohen Aubart F, Emile JF, Maksud P, Galanaud D, Cluzel P, Benameur N, Aumaitre O, Amoura Z, Haroche J. Efficacy of the MEK inhibitor cobimetinib for wild-type BRAF Erdheim-Chester disease. Br J Haematol. 2018;180:150–3.

[illegible]

Cardiac Implantable Device Related Complications

28

Justin Phan and Rajesh Subbiah

Introduction

Since the insertion of the first implantable pacemaker in 1958 and the first implantable cardioverter-defibrillator (ICD) in 1980, there has been a rapid uptake and evolution in cardiac implantable device therapies. These cardiac devices have dramatically improved the survival and provided symptomatic relief for a broad range of cardiac conditions., and rates of device implantation have increased rapidly. As a result, both cardiologists and non-cardiologists will need to be familiar with complications associated with device therapy.

Types of Devices

Cardiac implantable electronic devices (CIEDs) may be broadly divided into having four functions: pacing therapies for symptomatic bradyarrhythmias, device therapies for the management of tachyarrhythmias, cardiac resynchronisation therapy (CRT) for the management of left ventricular systolic dysfunction [1] and cardiac monitoring with implantable loop recorders. There may be overlap, as ICDs are able to provide pacing therapy for bradyarrhythmias or may be combined with a

J. Phan (✉)
Department of Cardiology, St Vincent's Hospital, Darlinghurst, NSW, Australia

University of New South Wales, Kensington, NSW, Australia
e-mail: justin.phan@svha.org.au

R. Subbiah
Department of Cardiology, St Vincent's Hospital, Darlinghurst, NSW, Australia

University of New South Wales, Kensington, NSW, Australia

Victor Chang Cardiac Research Institute, Darlinghurst, NSW, Australia
e-mail: rajesh.subbiah@svha.org.au

C. Salavastru et al. (eds.), *Skin and the Heart*,
https://doi.org/10.1007/978-3-030-54779-0_28

biventricular pacing system to provide both resynchronisation and tachyarrhythmia therapies.

A typical cardiac device includes a pulse generator, which generates electrical impulses, and one or more electrodes transmitting and receiving electrical impulses to and from the heart. The pulse generator is typically inserted in a pre-pectoral pocket inferior to the clavicle. Older devices, or devices inserted into infants, may be placed surgically into the abdomen. The cardiac leads are typically inserted by transvenous access through the axillary or subclavian vein, and are usually fixated in the right atrium, right ventricle or the coronary sinus in the case of CRT. In circumstances where transvenous lead placement is unsuccessful or not possible, leads may need to be surgically placed on the epicardial surface of the heart.

A more recently developed defibrillator device is the subcutaneous ICD (S-ICD), where the pulse generator and electrodes are entirely subcutaneous without the need for an endovascular approach. Although there are ongoing trials comparing this device with transvenous ICDs, there is registry data to suggest good mid-term safety and efficacy of these devices [2]. This device may be an attractive option for patients in whom only defibrillator, but not pacing therapy, is required as there are fewer lead-related complications [3].

Complications of Cardiac Devices

Complications arising from CIEDs may be divided into acute and long-term complications as summarised in Table 28.1. The incidence of complications is variable due to differences in definitions, however, one recent study found that complications may occur acutely in up to 9% of patients and in the long term in up to 6% of patients [4]. Complications may also occur during generator replacement and lead revision procedures [5]. These complications are important source of morbidity associated with CIEDs and are associated with significant healthcare utilisation.

Table 28.1 Acute and long-term complications of patients with transvenous pacemakers

	Acute (0–1 months)	Long-term (1–36 months)
All	8.94	5.94
Infection	1.15	2.42
Thoracic trauma	3.71	–
Pocket complication (Haematoma/pocket revision	0.26	0.96
Generator complication	0.06	0.06
Lead complication requiring revision	3.51	2.84
Venous embolism/thrombosis	0.49	–
Cardiac perforation	0.56	–

Adapted from Cantillon et al. [4] with permission from the publisher. Numbers are displayed as frequency (%)

Cutaneous Complications

Pocket Haematoma

Pocket haematomas are an important complication as it is associated with patient discomfort and an increased risk of subsequent device infection [6]. Pocket haematomas typically occur early following device implant and present as localised swelling, bruising and pain overlying the pulse generator pocket. The reported incidence of pocket haematoma varies from 1–5% [4, 7] and may be higher in patients undergoing implantation of an ICD compared to a pacemaker [8].

Pocket haematomas occur more frequently in patients on antithrombotic treatment [9]. Given the expanding indications for antiplatelet and anticoagulant therapy, balancing the thromboembolic and bleeding risks will become increasingly important in patients undergoing CIED implantation. Clopidogrel cessation, where possible, at least 4 days prior to CIED implantation is associated with a lower risk of pocket haematoma [8]. For patients in whom anticoagulant therapy cannot be interrupted due to unacceptably high thromboembolic risk, warfarin is associated with a five-fold reduction in pocket haematoma compared to heparin bridging [10]. The safety of uninterrupted direct-acting oral anticoagulant therapy during CIED implantation is the subject of ongoing clinical trials, however, there are small trials suggesting that this approach is safe [11].

Pocket haematomas typically resolve with local compression. In some instances, pocket exploration is necessary to prevent haematoma expansion, which may compromise skin perfusion and lead to skin necrosis and wound dehiscence (see Figs. 28.1 and 28.2). There are few data on methods for preventing pocket haematoma with

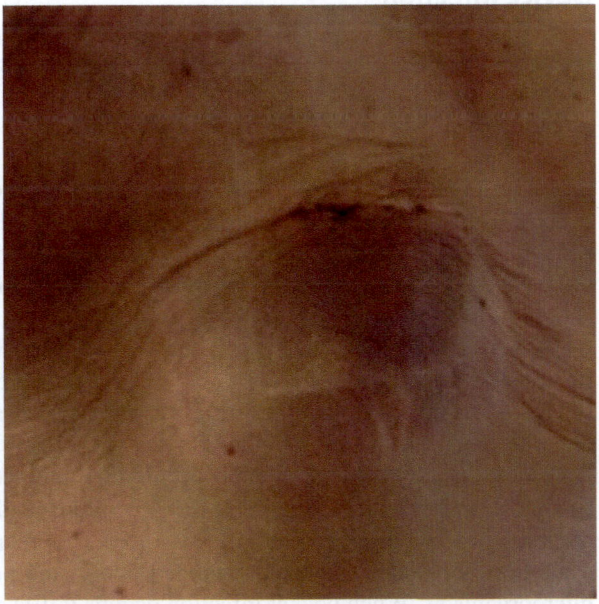

Fig. 28.1 Small pocket haematoma that did not require further intervention. Reproduced from [12] with permission from the publisher

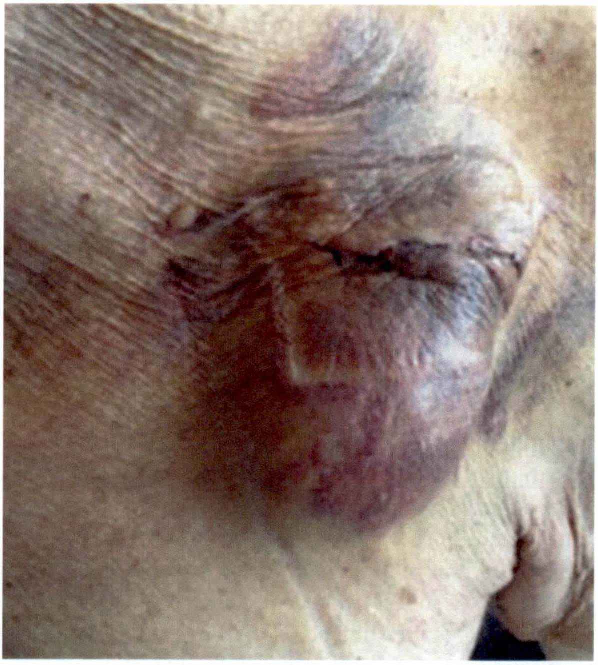

Fig. 28.2 Large pocket haematoma that required evacuation. Reproduced from [12] with permission from the publisher

some small studies examining the use of a fibrin sealant [13] and pocket compression devices [14], however, there are conflicting results on their efficacy.

Device Infection

Device infection is a serious complication of CIED implantation and is associated with increased short and long term mortality [15]. CIED pocket infection refers to infection involving the pulse generator pocket and the subcutaneous segment of the leads. Pocket infection may extend and involve the intravascular components, leading to systemic infection. *Staphylococcus aureus* and coagulase-negative staphylococci are the predominant causative organisms in CIED infection, and may be responsible for up to 89% of cases of device-associated endocarditis [16]. Empiric intravenous antibiotic therapy typically includes anti-staphylococcal cover and should follow local surgical antibiotic guidelines.

Pocket infection is typically a result of perioperative contamination with skin flora, as demonstrated in a study of 103 patients whereby three out of four device infections involved a coagulase-negative staphylococcal species that was isolated on swab specimens taken from the skin and pocket before and after device insertion [17]. When there is inflammation overlying the implanted device, pocket infection should be suspected (see Fig. 28.3). Blood cultures and transoesophageal echocardiography should be performed to assess for CIED related infection. Percutaneous aspiration is typically not recommended due to the potential risk of introducing microorganisms. When pocket infection occurs, CIED removal is usually required.

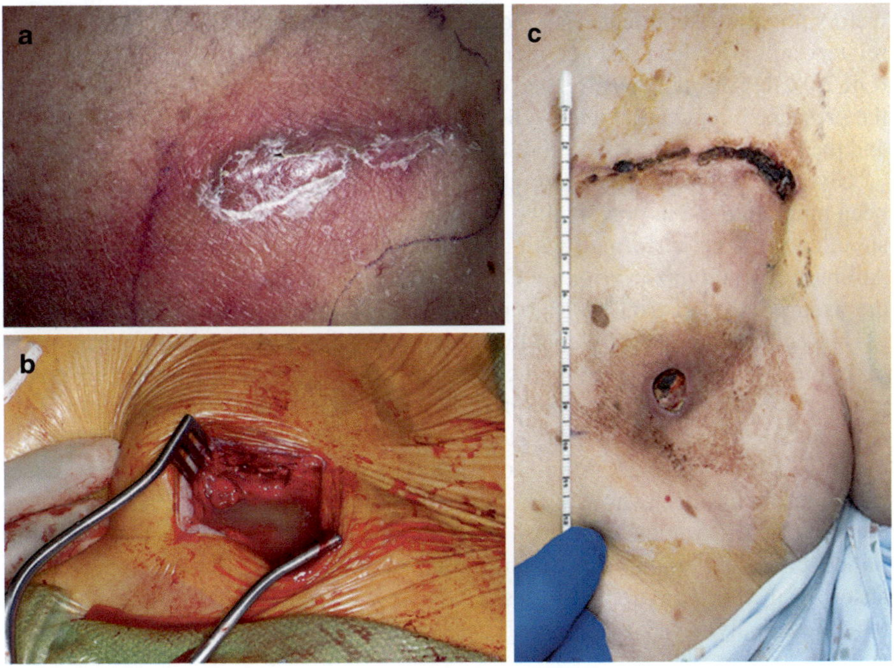

Fig. 28.3 Signs of Pocket Infection. (**a**) Redness and skin changes in a patient 2 weeks after device surgery. (**b**) Purulence within the pocket. (**c**) Erosion in a patient who subsequently developed systemic signs of infection. Reproduced from [18] with permission from the publisher

Pocket infection must be distinguished from post-implantation inflammation/haematoma and superficial site infection, as these may produce similar cutaneous findings. In uncertain cases, fluorine-18 fluorodeoxyglucose positron emission tomography /computed tomography may be useful, with a reported 96% sensitivity and 97% specificity for diagnosing pocket infections [19].

Systemic CIED infection refers to infection involving the transvenous portion of the device leads (lead endocarditis) or the tricuspid valve. Epicardial leads may also be affected. The clinical findings are similar to those of right-sided endocarditis, including fever, bacteraemia, pulmonary abnormalities and metastatic seeding. Patients with suspected systemic CIED infection should receive empiric therapy whilst awaiting a microbiological diagnosis. In most cases, patients will require lead and device extraction as device retention with antibiotic therapy is associated with increased risk of mortality [20]. The optimal timing for a new replacement CIED implantation is variable, with clinical resolution of infection and negative surveillance blood cultures typically required to reduce the risk of reinfection.

Risk factors for CIED infection have been studied in one large systematic review and meta-analysis, and were divided into host-related, procedure-related and device-related factors [6]. Regarding host-related factors, the most significant risk factors were end-stage renal disease [odds ratio (OR) 8.7], history of previous device infection (OR 7.8), and corticosteroid usage (OR 3.4). Regarding procedure-related factors, the most significant risk factors were post-operative haematoma (OR 8.5), reintervention for lead dislodgement (OR 6.4) and device replacement or revision (OR 2.0). Regarding device-related characteristics, the most significant factors were the presence of epicardial leads (OR 8.1), an abdominal generator pocket (OR 4.0) and the positioning of two or more leads (OR 2.0).

Given the morbidity and mortality associated with CIED infection, there has been much interest in preventative measures. Device implantation or replacement should always be performed with aseptic technique in a controlled environment. Antibiotic prophylaxis prior to CIED implantation has been shown in a randomised controlled trial of 1000 patients to reduce the risk of CIED infection [21]. Regimens for prophylaxis may vary according to local antibiotic prophylaxis guidelines, but typically include anti-staphylococcal cover, such as with intravenous cephazolin, or vancomycin in patients at high risk for methicillin-resistant staphylococcal aureus. More recently, an absorbable antibacterial envelope (TYRX, Medtronic, Minnesota) designed to hold a CIED at the time of implantation has been shown in a randomised controlled trial of 6983 patients to the rate of CIED infection by 40% at 12 months [22]. The TYRX envelope elutes minocycline and rifampin for a minimum of 7 days, and the envelope is fully absorbed in approximately 9 weeks. There were no reported allergies to the envelope mesh, polymer or antibiotics reported in the study.

Scarring

Scarring following CIED implantation may result in an undesirable cosmetic outcome and may cause discomfort. Hypertrophic scar and keloid formation (see Fig. 28.4) are a result of excess tissue formation. The risk may be reduced by good suture technique and avoiding excess skin tension. Keloids may be treated by intralesional steroid injection and laser phototherapy [18].

Pacemaker Allergy

Allergic reactions to pacemakers are rare, and clinical manifestations range from localised skin irritation overlying the pulse generator to generalised dermatitis and pruritis [23, 24]. Hypersensitivity reactions to various components in the pulse generator and pacing leads have been reported. Titanium is typically used to encase the pulse generator and circuitry, and reduces electromagnetic interference [25]. Several case reports have documented hypersensitivity reactions to the titanium casing by patch testing, with improvement by various methods, including wrapping the device in a polytetrafluoroethylene sheet [26] and replacing the pulse generator with a gold-coated generator [27], with subsequent resolution of localised erythema.

Other reported hypersensitivity reactions that were confirmed by patch testing include nickel, cobalt and chromium, which are found in the pacing leads.

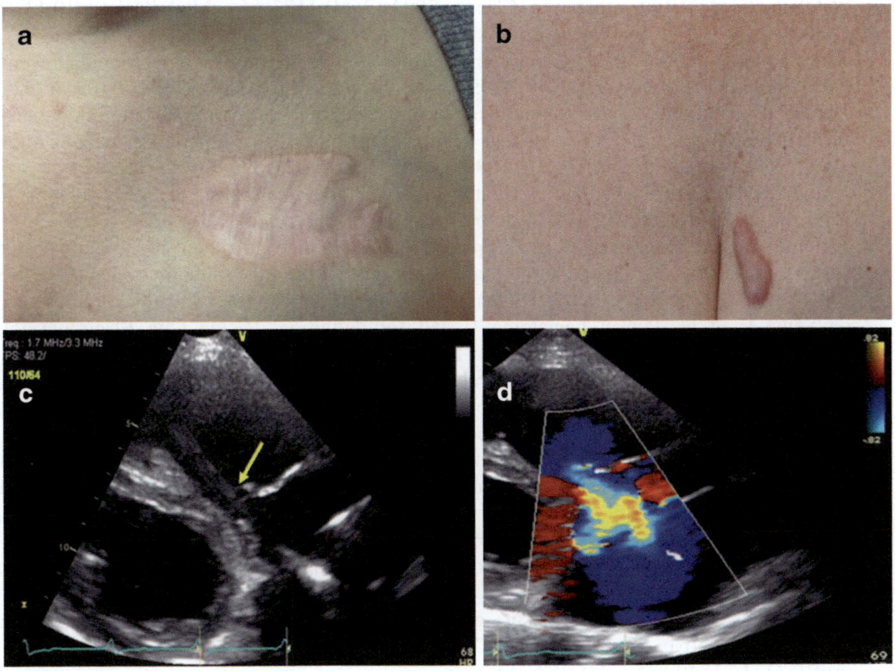

Fig. 28.4 (**a**) Hypertrophic scar after pacemaker implantation (**b**) Keloid formation at the site of device surgery. Adapted from [18] with permission from the publisher

References

1. Epstein AE, et al. ACC/AHA/HRS 2008 guidelines for device-based therapy of cardiac rhythm abnormalities: executive summary. Circulation. 2008;117(21):2820–40. https://doi.org/10.1161/CIRCUALTIONAHA.108.189741.
2. Boersma L, et al. Implant and midterm outcomes of the subcutaneous implantable cardioverter-defibrillator registry: the EFFORTLESS Study. J Am Coll Cardiol. 2017;70(7):830–41. https://doi.org/10.1016/j.jacc.2017.06.040.
3. Basu-Ray I, et al. Subcutaneous versus Transvenous implantable defibrillator therapy: a meta-analysis of case-control studies. JACC Clin Electrophysiol. 2017;3(13):1475–83. https://doi.org/10.1016/j.jacep.2017.07.017.
4. Cantillon DJ, et al. Complications and health care costs associated with transvenous cardiac pacemakers in a nationwide assessment. JACC Clin Electrophysiol. 2017;3(11):1296–305. https://doi.org/10.1016/j.jacep.2017.05.007.
5. Poole JE, et al. Complication rates associated with pacemaker or implantable cardioverter-defibrillator generator replacements and upgrade procedures: results from the REPLACE registry. Circulation. 2010;122(16):1553–61. https://doi.org/10.1161/CIRCULATIONAHA.110.976076.
6. Polyzos KA, Konstantelias AA, Falagas ME. Risk factors for cardiac implantable electronic device infection: a systematic review and meta-analysis. Europace. 2015;17(5):767–77. https://doi.org/10.1093/europace/euv053.
7. Wiegand UKH, et al. Pocket hematoma after pacemaker or implantable cardioverter defibrillator surgery: influence of patient morbidity, operation strategy, and perioperative anti-

platelet/anticoagulation therapy. Chest. 2004;126(4):1177–86. https://doi.org/10.1378/chest.126.4.1177.
8. Kutinsky IB, et al. Risk of hematoma complications after device implant in the clopidogrel era. Circ Arrhythm Electrophysiol. 2010;3(4):312–8. https://doi.org/10.1161/CIRCEP.109.917625.
9. Demir GG, et al. Pocket haematoma after cardiac electronic device implantation in patients receiving antiplatelet and anticoagulant treatment: a single-centre experience. Acta Cardiol. 2017;72(1):47–52. https://doi.org/10.1080/00015385.2017.1281539.
10. Birnie DH, et al. Pacemaker or defibrillator surgery without interruption of anticoagulation. N Engl J Med. 2013;368(22):2084–93. https://doi.org/10.1056/nejmoa1302946.
11. Birnie DH, et al. Continued vs. interrupted direct oral anticoagulants at the time of device surgery, in patients with moderate to high risk of arterial thrombo-embolic events (BRUISE CONTROL-2). Eur Heart J. 2018;39(44):3973–9. https://doi.org/10.1093/eurheartj/ehy413.
12. de Sensi F, et al. Pocket hematoma: a call for definition. Pacing Clin Electrophysiol. 2015;38(8):909–13. https://doi.org/10.1111/pace.12665.
13. Milic DJ, et al. Prevention of pocket related complications with fibrin sealant in patients undergoing pacemaker implantation who are receiving anticoagulant treatment. EP Europace. 2005;7(4):374–9. https://doi.org/10.1016/j.eupc.2005.03.007.
14. Turagam MK, et al. Use of a pocket compression device for the prevention and treatment of pocket hematoma after pacemaker and defibrillator implantation (STOP-HEMATOMA-I). J Interv Card Electrophysiol. 2017;49(2):197–204. https://doi.org/10.1007/s10840-017-0235-9.
15. Le KY, et al. Impact of timing of device removal on mortality in patients with cardiovascular implantable electronic device infections. Heart Rhythm. 2011;8(11):1678–85. https://doi.org/10.1016/j.hrthm.2011.05.015.
16. Massoure P-L, et al. Pacemaker endocarditis: clinical features and management of 60 consecutive cases. Pacing Clin Electrophysiol. 2007;30(1):12–9. https://doi.org/10.1111/j.1540-8159.2007.00574.x.
17. Da Costa A, et al. Role of the preaxillary flora in pacemaker infections: a prospective study. Circulation. 1998;97(18):1791–5.
18. Mulpuru SK, et al. Cardiac pacemakers: function, troubleshooting, and management. J Am Coll Cardiol. 2017;69(2):189–210. https://doi.org/10.1016/j.jacc.2016.10.061.
19. Mahmood M, et al. Role of (18)F-FDG PET/CT in the diagnosis of cardiovascular implantable electronic device infections: a meta-analysis. J Nucl Cardiol. 2017;26:958–70. https://doi.org/10.1007/s12350-017-1063-0.
20. Sohail MR, et al. Infective endocarditis complicating permanent pacemaker and implantable cardioverter-defibrillator infection. Mayo Clin Proc. 2008;83(1):46–53. https://doi.org/10.4065/83.1.46.
21. de Cesar OJ, et al. Efficacy of antibiotic prophylaxis before the implantation of pacemakers and cardioverter-defibrillators. Circ Arrhythm Electrophysiol. 2009;2(1):29–34. https://doi.org/10.1161/CIRCEP.108.795906.
22. Tarakji KG, et al. Antibacterial envelope to prevent cardiac implantable device infection. N Engl J Med. 2019;380(20):1895–905. https://doi.org/10.1056/NEJMoa1901111.
23. Buchet S, et al. Pacemaker dermatitis. Contact Dermatitis. 1992;26(1):46–7. https://doi.org/10.1111/j.1600-0536.1992.tb00867.x.
24. Weiss R. Pacemaker dermatitis. Contact Dermatitis. 1989;21(5):343–4. https://doi.org/10.1111/j.1600-0536.1989.tb04759.x.
25. Onari GOH, et al. Hypersensitivity reactions associated with endovascular devices. Contact Dermatitis. 2008;2:7–22.
26. Ishii K, et al. Pacemaker contact dermatitis: The effective use of a polytetrafluoroethylene sheet. Pacing Clin Electrophysiol. 2006;29(11):1299–302. https://doi.org/10.1111/j.1540-8159.2006.00535.x.
27. Goli A, Shroff S, Osman MN. A case of gold-coated pacemaker for pacemaker allergy. J Innov Cardiac Rhythm Manag. 2012;3:944–7. https://doi.org/10.19102/icrm.2012.0309.

Correction to: The Skin and Diabetes

J. W. J. Lasschuit, J. R. Snaith, and J. W. Frew

Correction to: C. Salavastru et al. (eds.), *Skin and the Heart*, https://doi.org/10.1007/978-3-030-54779-0_18

This book was inadvertently published with incorrect captions to the figures 2 and 3 in chapter 18. This has now been corrected in the book.

The updated online version of this chapter can be found at https://doi.org/10.1007/978-3-030-54779-0_18

C. Salavastru et al. (eds.), *Skin and the Heart*,
https://doi.org/10.1007/978-3-030-54779-0_29

Index

C. Salavastru et al. (eds.), *Skin and the Heart*,
https://doi.org/10.1007/978-3-030-54779-0

GPSR Compliance

The European Union's (EU) General Product Safety Regulation (GPSR) is a set of rules that requires consumer products to be safe and our obligations to ensure this.

If you have any concerns about our products, you can contact us on ProductSafety@springernature.com

In case Publisher is established outside the EU, the EU authorized representative is:

Springer Nature Customer Service Center GmbH
Europaplatz 3
69115 Heidelberg, Germany

Batch number: 10732076

Printed by Printforce, the Netherlands